# Nerve Injuries

Operative Results for Major Nerve
Injuries, Entrapments, and Tumors

**DAVID G. KLINE, A.B., M.D.**
Professor and Chairman
Department of Neurosurgery
School of Medicine in New Orleans
Louisiana State University
    Medical Center
Attending Charity, Ochsner, and
    University Hospitals
New Orleans, Louisiana


**ALAN R. HUDSON, MB, ChB, FRCS(C),
FRCS(Ed), FCS(SA)(Hon)**
President, The Toronto Hospital
Professor, Neurosurgery, University of Toronto
Toronto, Ontario
Canada

MEDICAL ILLUSTRATOR
**Eugene New**

# Nerve Injuries

## Operative Results for Major Nerve Injuries, Entrapments, and Tumors

**W.B. SAUNDERS COMPANY**
*A Division of Harcourt Brace & Company*
Philadelphia   London   Toronto   Montreal   Sydney   Tokyo

**W.B. SAUNDERS COMPANY**
*A Division of Harcourt Brace & Company*

The Curtis Center
Independence Square West
Philadelphia, Pennsylvania 19106

**Library of Congress Cataloging-in-Publication Data**

Kline, David G.
    Nerve injuries / David G. Kline, Alan R. Hudson; medical
illustrator, Eugene New — 1st ed.

        p.   cm.

    Includes bibliographical references and index.
    ISBN 0-7216-3264-5

    1. Nervous system—wounds and injuries.   I. Kline, David
G., Hudson, Alan R.   II. Title.
        [DNLM:   1. Nervous System—injuries.     WL 100 K65n 1995]

    RD595.K57   1995        617.4'83044—dc20

    DNLM/DLC                                      94-12233

Nerve Injuries: Operative Results for Major Nerve Injuries, Entrapments, and Tumors          ISBN 0-7216-3264-5

Copyright © 1995 W.B. Saunders Company

All rights reserved. No part of this publication may be reproduced or transmitted in any form or by any means, electronic or mechanical, including photocopy, recording, or any information storage and retrieval system, without permission in writing from the publisher.

Printed in the United States of America.

Last digit is the print number:     9     8     7     6     5     4     3     2     1

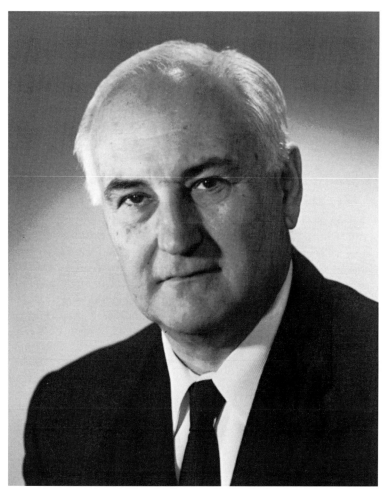

SIR SYDNEY SUNDERLAND
December 31, 1910–August 27, 1993

## DEDICATION TO SYDNEY SUNDERLAND

Sir Sydney Sunderland was born in 1910 in Brisbane, Australia, and received his M.B., D.Sc., M.D., and LL.D. (honorary) degrees from the University of Melbourne, where he began his career as a Lecturer in Anatomy and Neurology in 1937. He was influenced greatly by work with Frederick Wood Jones, Professor of Anatomy; with Dr. Leonard Cox, who established a neurologic clinic in Australia; and subsequently with Hugh Cairns, a neurosurgeon in Oxford, England. Sydney Sunderland was appointed to the Chair of Anatomy when he was only 27 years of age. He became Professor of Anatomy and then of Experimental Neurology at the same institution, publishing a remarkably large

volume of original experimental work concerning the anatomy and regeneration of the peripheral nervous system. He was a Visiting Specialist in Peripheral Nerve Injuries at the 115th Australian Hospital Unit from 1941 to 1945, working with Mr. Hugh Trumble, a neurosurgeon. He served as Dean of the University of Melbourne from 1953 to 1971, worked as a member and eventually Chairman of the Royal Australasian College of Surgeons Certification Committee between 1945 and 1969, and served on many governmental and academic councils in Australia and New Zealand.

In addition to being knighted by the Queen of England in 1971, Sir Sydney worked as a Demonstrator in Anatomy at Oxford, as a Visiting Professor in Anatomy at Johns Hopkins, and as a Fogarty Scholar at the National Institutes of Health in Washington, D.C., gave a number of honorary lectures, and had an international peripheral nerve society named after him. His professional life's work was with peripheral nerve, and this was highlighted by publication of a reference text of encyclopedic proportions, *Nerves and Nerve Injuries*, in 1968. He extensively revised, updated, and republished this large reference work in 1978.

In 1991, Sir Sydney published a book entitled *Nerve Injuries and Their Repair: A Critical Appraisal*. This work is based on his lifetime study of nerves and reflects on selected and, at times, controversial topics concerning nerve injury and repair. He is best known for his work with fascicular anatomy and the changing topography of these intraneural structures. He also made singular contributions to our understanding of oculomotor function and its involvement by uncal herniation and of the mechanisms involved in nerve root or spinal nerve stretch and avulsion. He was married for 53 years to Nina Gwendoline, or "Lady Gwen." This wonderful woman was educated as a lawyer and yet helped Sir Sydney type and edit his many manuscripts. They had one son, who has served as Deputy Medical Director at the Alfred Hospital in Melbourne, the same hospital at which his father had his medical roots. Sir Sydney died in Melbourne on August 27, 1993, at the age of 82, having had a very full life.

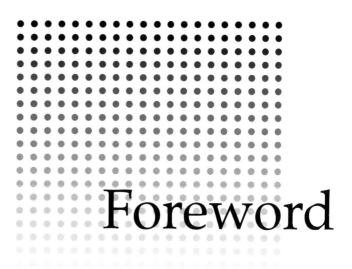

# Foreword

Although peripheral nerve surgery has been done since the 19th century, significant progress was not demonstrated until the use of the operating microscope in the mid-1960s, accompanied by appropriate suture materials and instruments. A second major advance has been the utilization of electrophysiologic testing for the evaluation of peripheral nerve injury and repair.

The senior author of this text has been in the vanguard of these technical advances as well as of many other aspects of patient care. I have enjoyed a professional relationship with David G. Kline since we met at the Walter Reed Army Medical Center more than 30 years ago. During that two-year period, he published eight research papers and participated in routine patient care activities. Subsequently, David Kline developed productive research facilities and a neurosurgical postgraduate education program at the Louisiana State University in New Orleans. He has achieved worldwide recognition for his research in peripheral nerve injuries, neurophysiology of nerve regeneration, and nerve tumors. In these efforts, he has published more than 165 medical articles and has served on the editorial boards of 11 medical journals. David Kline is Professor of Neurosurgery and Head of the Department of Neurosurgery at the Louisiana State University. His many administrative activities in education have included appointments as chairman of the American Board of Neurologic Surgeons and as president of the Sunderland Society for international peripheral nerve study.

Alan R. Hudson completed his neurosurgical postgraduate training program at the University of Toronto in Ontario, where he is Professor of Neurosurgery and was Chairman of the Division of Neurosurgery. His research activities have produced more than 120 medical articles. During his tenure at the University of Toronto, he has received international recognition for his professional and research activities, including the presidency of the Canadian Neurosurgical Society. Professor Hudson has held the McCutcheon Chair as Surgeon-in-Chief of the Toronto Hospital from 1989 to 1991; in 1991 he was made president and chief executive officer of that hospital, Canada's largest for acute care.

In 1970, Alan Hudson established a peripheral nerve research laboratory and received a Clinical Traineeship Award from the Royal College of Surgeons. He chose to spend the Award with David Kline in New Orleans. From that experience grew a very productive relationship for on-going research, and these two physicians have collaborated on more than 30 published medical articles. This text is the result of their agreed-upon approach to major problems and brings together two experts with international reputations in the field of peripheral nerve surgery.

This book discusses in detail the varied etiologic mechanisms, the appropriate clinical and laboratory evaluation, and the operative techniques, including intraoperative electrophysiologic studies and their potential complications, that are involved in the treatment of major peripheral nerve injuries, entrapments, and tumors of both the upper and lower extremities.

The text of this book is unique in that it presents not only a comprehensive review but also attempts to portray in some detail results of treatment. It has been written by only two authors, in contrast to the usual text by multiple authors. The result is a presentation of personal experiences with proven approaches to very complex problems. Further, the statistical conclusions are based on a single database from the Louisiana State University Medical Center, which documents actual experience in a single-practice location.

This book will be of great assistance to all medical personnel who have taken up the challenge of managing major problems of the peripheral nervous system.

GEORGE E. OMER, JR., M.D., M.S., F.A.C.S.
Professor and Chairman Emeritus
Department of Orthopaedics and Rehabilitation
The University of New Mexico

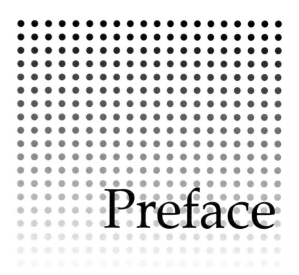

# Preface

When we began work on this book more than 9 years ago, there were already several excellent texts available on nerve injuries and entrapments. In the interim, several more books have been published. We set to work on a relatively comprehensive manuscript because we wished to present results from a large personal series of major injuries and other nerve lesions. We believe that outcome analysis will be demanded by society in general and by third-party payers in particular in this last decade of the twentieth century or in the early years of the twenty-first century. Analysis of such results was thought to be necessary to provide future directions for patient care and for research and development concerning nerve lesions. A comprehensive and yet readable analysis of results in this field appeared to be indicated and had not been done since publication of the VA Monograph, *Peripheral Nerve Injury*, in 1957. Although correcting loss caused by nerve injury is very demanding, analysis of outcomes in a usable fashion proved to be even more difficult.

The series of cases presented here come primarily from one institution (Louisiana State University Medical Center and related hospitals such as Charity, Ochsner, and University), but we have tried to reflect on and extrapolate from the data. We have similar philosophies concerning clinical investigation, timing for operations, and techniques used. The information presented represents our joint and current recommendations for care of these difficult lesions.

We are presenting these data in the hope that they will be improved on in future years. We expect that others who follow us will contribute in a fashion that will lead to better results than ours. Rather than editing a multi-authored book, we have tried to consolidate the personal experiences of two clinicians who have been involved in the surgery of nerve injuries and repairs for the past 30 years, including major nerve injuries, entrapments, and tumors. Not included in this text are injuries to the cranial nerves. The only exception is the eleventh cranial or accessory nerve, because this is an important part of shoulder and upper limb function. Several excellent texts already exist on the facial nerve and some of the other cranial nerves less frequently involved in injury.

We both feel strongly that workers in this field need to have a thorough background in the gross anatomy and microanatomy of the limbs; therefore each chapter has this background as a core. We also believe that there is a great need for clinicians to have a good grasp of the basic physiologic principles involved in both the intact and injured or regenerating nerve. There are advantages as well as drawbacks to the various electrophysiologic tests used to help guide the care of a patient with a peripheral nerve problem, and these are commented on throughout the text. Neither of us are electromyographers but we have tried to weight such information and to provide some detail especially about intraoperative electrical studies. There is also great value to laboratory research, but this is primarily a clinical book, so only selected basic science findings related to nerve repair are presented.

The outline for each chapter in this book, even those on individual nerves, is not the same. We tried to mold each section along selected and important areas to be addressed for each nerve or region of anatomy. The book is not intended to provide answers for the many variations in anatomy and function of each nerve and the many things that can occur connected with it but rather to emphasize major injury, an area with which we do have experience. Our efforts for this text have focused on providing detail about major nerve injury management and especially about degree of recovery. The tables presenting the data analyzed and their outcomes in terms of results are central to the book and require close and repetitive study. In this regard, an initial survey of the chapters on mechanisms of injury, clinical evaluation, and grading of loss and subsequent recovery is very important, especially if the tables are to be used to apply the lessons gained from these outcomes to future problems.

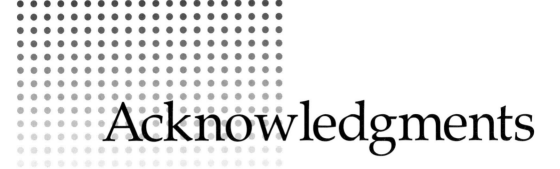

# Acknowledgments

We shall always be in debt to those who have taught us, and they are many. These people include George Hayes of Washington, DC, Frank Nulsen of Cleveland, Eddie Kahn and Dick Schneider of Ann Arbor, Graham Weddell of Oxford, Bill Horsey of Toronto, and Jannie Louw of Capetown. We have also been fortunate to work with excellent electrophysiologists, including Henry Berry, George Koepke, Earl Hackett, Leo Happel, and Austin Sumner. Input from other specialists, such as Robin Richards, Susan Mackinnon, Juan Bilbao, Rand Voorhies, Mike Carey, Hector LeBlanc, Carlos Garcia, Roger Smith, and Dick Coulon, is also appreciated. Many others in our university units have been of great help to us. They have tolerated our passion for this area, supported us, assisted us, and at times covered for us while we worked on this manuscript. Of especial note is the input from our residents and fellows without which neither the extensive clinical work nor text would have been possible. We are particularly indebted to our families and our loved ones, our wives and children, who permitted us the time and especially the equanimity to complete this task.

We certainly thank the many physicians in North America and abroad who have referred cases to us and who for the most part have been willing to provide follow-up care and in many instances even follow-up evaluation. Finally, we are indebted to WB Saunders Company and their editors, especially Richard Zorab, who have been extremely patient throughout the period during which this book was written and then edited.

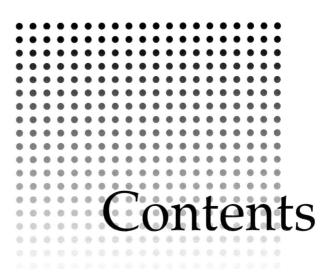

# Contents

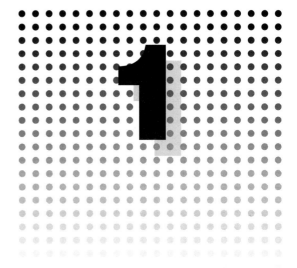

# Basic
# Considerations

# SUMMARY

The majority of nerve volume is composed of connective tissue and not axons and their coverings with myelin. These connective tissue layers, including the endoneurium, perineurium, interfascicular epineurium, and epineurium, along with their accompanying fibroblasts, respond to serious injury with a proliferative and disorganized pattern of regeneration. Despite a rich and forgiving blood supply and a substantial neuronal ability to reform axons, serious injury to nerve results in poor spontaneous recovery. A firm understanding of both the Wallerian process of degeneration and the human nerve's ability to recover from a given injury is extremely important, as is some method to gradate damage. Appreciation of some of the recent information developed concerning neuronal response to injury, neurotropism, and axonal metabolism is necessary, but not without a firm understanding of the more basic elements of a nerve's response to serious injury.

It is not our intent to review the large literature available in this area but rather to present the more important basic information needed by the clinician caring for patients with nerve lesions. In many cases, other publications provide more basic detail.

# CONNECTIVE TISSUE LAYERS

The major tissue component of peripheral nerve is connective tissue[111-119] (Figure 1–1). This provides the skeleton or framework for the conductive elements, the axons, and their Schwann cells. The connective tissue layers help to protect and to provide nutrition for their enclosed nerve fibers. Estimates as to the amount of connective tissue in nerve vary, but its volume is greater than that of axons and their coverings.[50] The area occupied by fascicles, compared with that containing epineurium and interfascicular epineurium, varies from nerve to nerve and also at given levels or cross-sectional areas in the same nerve[115] (Figure 1–2). For example, almost 85% of the cross-sectional area of the sciatic nerve at the level of the hip is connective tissue.

The outer covering of nerve is provided by epineurium, which is connective tissue containing both collagen and elastic fibers. This layer serves to invest the fascicles and also provides a slight undulation to nerve. This undulation provides some longitudinal mobility, relative fixation being provided by neural branches entering musculature and the subcutaneous spaces.[111] Some investigators identify a mesoneurium external to the epineurium.[57,112] In health, this connective tissue layer or mesoneurium is filmy and transparent and helps to tether or secure nerve to adjacent structures such as tendons, vessels, muscles, and fascial planes.

Epineurial connective tissue is continuous with that between and surrounding the fascicles, which is termed the interfascicular epineurium. The latter is not as compact as the epineurium itself, and its volume varies from nerve to nerve and from level to level in the same nerve.

Fascicles vary in number as well as in size, depending on the nerve and level of nerve examined. Each fascicle is encircled by perineurium, which consists of oblique, circular, and longitudinal collagen fibrils dispersed among perineurial cells.[86] The latter have some morphologic features in common with Schwann cells, including the presence of a basement lamella.[67,119] Because the perineurial cells have tight junctions, the perineurium is a major site for a blood-nerve barrier.[71,85] Interruption of the perineurium can affect the function of the axons that it encloses[103,107] (Figure 1–3). Injury to the perineurium alone, such as resecting a portion of it, has an adverse effect on nerve function.[61] Such damage can be prolonged, because the perineurium does not reconstitute itself well.[10,117] The conductive properties of axons are dampened (Figure 1–4), and, in some cases, the fibers undergo partial demyelination as well as loss of axonal diameter.[52,61]

Perineurium is traversed by vessels which carry a perineurial sleeve of connective tissue with them to mingle somewhat with the endoneurium.[70,104] The perineurial sleeves have

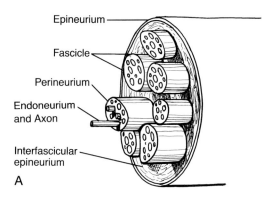

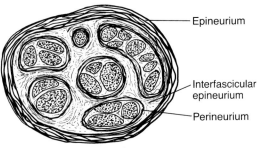

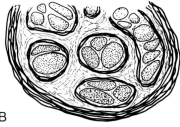

**Figure 1–1.** (*A*) This drawing shows the connective tissue layers of nerve. The epineurium is more compact than the interfascicular epineurium but not as compact as the more tightly woven three layers of the perineurium. Endoneurium surrounds each myelinated fiber and groups of unmyelinated or poorly myelinated fibers. (*B*) This drawing of a cross section of nerve shows the disposition of the connective tissue layers from another perspective (*top*) and with a portion of epineurium and perineurium resected with resultant changes in fascicular structure (*bottom*).

close approximation to vessel walls. This anatomic feature may provide a potential vascular communication between the connective tissues of the epineurium and those of the endoneurium. Endoneurium encircles each myelinated axon and groups of unmyelinated or poorly myelinated axons. Microvessels with tight junctions are found at this level, and the endothe-

lium of these capillaries serves as a second blood-nerve barrier, along with the endoneurial tissue itself[69,84] (Figure 1–5). These endoneurial microvessels are morphologically similar to the capillaries and their related astrocytic connections seen in the central nervous system (CNS). Changes in the permeability of these vessels occur frequently, even after relatively mild nerve trauma.[95] Endoneurial fibroblasts occasionally can be seen in the connective tissues between the nerve fibers. Endoneurium is the final protective investiture for the axon and protects it if the nerve is mildly elongated or stretched.[66,111] Endoneurium also provides a constraint for the intracellular pressure provided by the axon and its myelin sheath.[112]

## NERVE FIBERS AND SCHWANN CELLS

The neural structure is comprised of axons and their accompanying Schwann cells. In a healthy nerve, the nerve fibers, or axons, reside within the fascicular structure. Even the neural fibers and their Schwann cells are surrounded not only by ground substance but by collagen fibrils, which have some degree of condensation immediately superficial to the basement lamellae of the Schwann cells (Figure 1–6). Thus, the connective tissue component of nerve exists even at this central microscopic level.

Axons originate from their cell bodies, which are in the spinal cord, dorsal root ganglia, and autonomic ganglia. On the other hand, most of the neuron's cytoplasm is included in the volume of the axon because it is very long compared with the size of the neuron.[32,126] In healthy nerve, there tend to be two sizes of fibers, large and small. The larger fibers are better myelinated than the smaller fibers and are concerned with conduction of afferent and efferent messages connected with muscles as well as afferent messages connected with touch, pressure, and some painful sensations. Smaller fibers conduct efferent messages concerned with autonomic function and afferent messages for most painful sensations.

Schwann cells are placed along the longitudinal extent of the axon.[99] In the case of larger fibers, the membrane of each Schwann cell

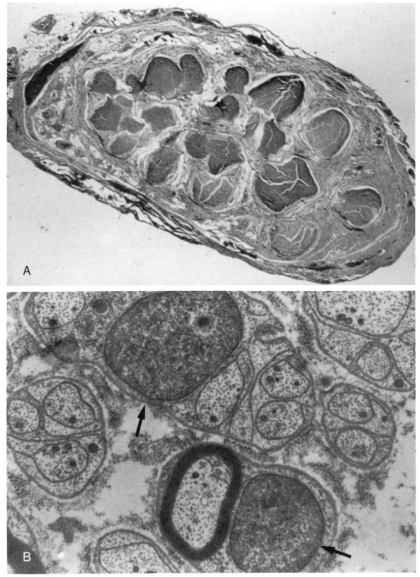

**Figure 1–2.** (*A*) Cross section of a large nerve to show its fascicular disposition. This is a healthy primate nerve, and yet one can see the extensive connective tissue components at an epineurial and interfascicular level. Masson stain × 12. (*B*) Electron micrograph of normal nerve showing a myelinated nerve with attendant Schwann cell (*lower arrow*) and surrounding endoneurium at the lower right. In the upper portion of the picture is a group of unmyelinated fibers and a Schwann cell (*upper arrow*) surrounded by an endoneurial envelope. A similar grouping of three small fibers is seen to the left.

wraps serially around a segment of axon, providing a lipoprotein coating or covering of myelin.[14] There is less envelopment of the axon as the edge of one Schwann cell approaches that of another[91]; this is known as the node of Ranvier. Processes from adjacent Schwann cells interdigitate with each other at these nodal areas. The node of Ranvier permits ionic exchanges between the axoplasm of a nerve fiber and the

extracellular space. This exchange, in turn, permits saltatory conduction of an impulse, which travels from one node to the next.

Small and less myelinated fibers are enveloped by the membrane of a Schwann cell but by no lipoprotein sheath, or less than in the larger and better myelinated fibers.[18,19,79] Nonmyelinated fibers do not have the structural capacity for saltatory conduction, and impulses transmit

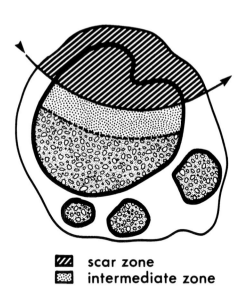

☑ scar zone
▨ intermediate zone

A

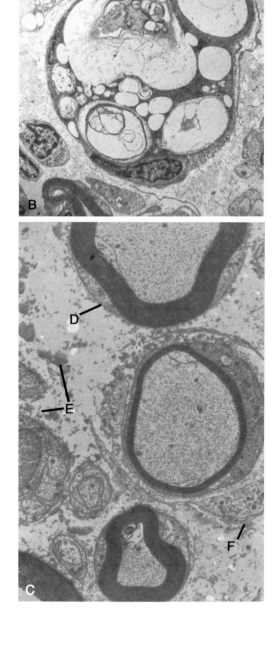

**Figure 1-3.** (*A*) The effect on a nerve of a partial injury in which the perineurium has been interrupted. Initial physical injury in this case leads to an area of complete axonal destruction and subsequent scar formation. (*B*) In the intermediate zone, some axons undergo degeneration amid ones that are maintained. (*C*) In other areas of the intermediate zone, axons may lose caliber and have decreased myelination. D = basement lamella, E = collagen fibers, F = endoneurial fibroblast.

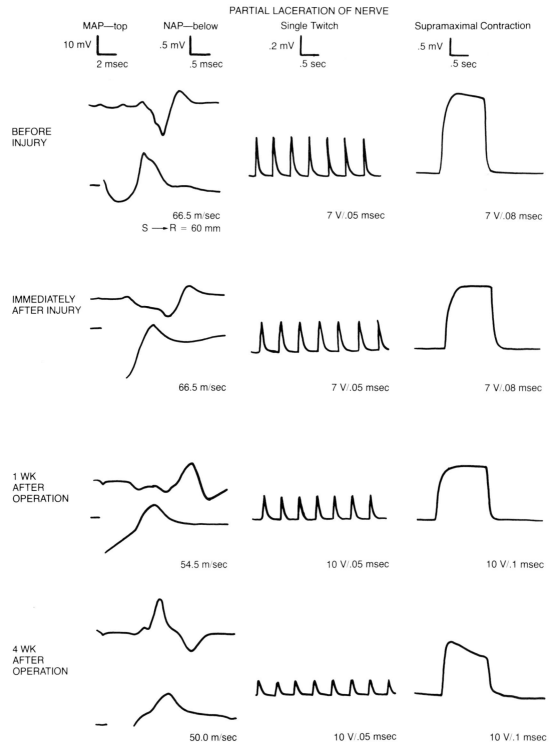

**Figure 1–4.** Progression of a partial nerve injury is documented by electrophysiologic studies. Baseline nerve action potential (NAP) and evoked muscle action potential (MAP), single twitch, and supramaximal contraction traces are at the top followed by traces made immediately after injury and recordings made at 1 and 4 weeks postoperatively. Settings for recordings were kept constant, but the amplitudes of the supramaximal single-twitch contraction as well as the tetanic contraction decreased with time. (From Kline D: Primate laboratory models for peripheral nerve repair. *In* Omer G and Spinner M, Eds. Management of Peripheral Nerve Injuries, WB Saunders, Philadelphia, 1980.)

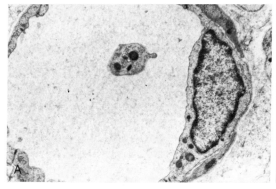

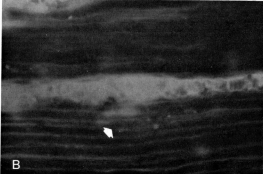

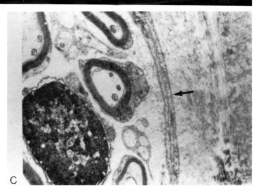

**Figure 1–5.** (*A*) Endoneurial microvessels have tight junctions. These intrafascicular microvessels are one of the sites of the blood-nerve barrier; the other is the perineurium. (*B*) Intrafascicular capillary in nerve whose blood supply was injected with a vital dye at the site at which the perineurium had been interrupted. Interruption of the perineurium can lead to leakage of serum from capillaries, as indicated by the extravascular dye in this study (*arrow*). (*C*) Electron micrograph showing perineurium (*arrow*); myelinated and unmyelinated axons and a Schwann cell are seen to the left.

along the axon alone, making for slower conduction.

A Schwann cell not only provides myelin and some guidance structure in terms of a basal membrane, but it is most likely the source of an as yet unidentified trophic or growth factor or factors.[24,25,39] Such trophic factors may originate from Schwann cells either proximal or distal to the injury site.[30,44,64,74] In any case, the growth cone, which is the tip of an advancing neurite, seems to depend on Schwann cell contact for elongation as well as guidance.[2,3,121,123] The local environment provides some adhesiveness and access to components such as laminin and

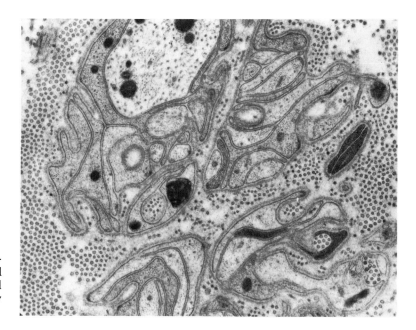

**Figure 1–6.** This electron micrograph shows unmyelinated fibers surrounded by basal lamina or endoneurium and by collagen fibrils.

fibronectin. These factors provide an optimal setting for the fiber's growth cone and, therefore, the advance of the neurite.[26–28,46,96] The local environment at the injury and regenerative site remains extremely important for the welfare of both the growth cone and the Schwann cell.[8,122]

During peripheral nerve neurite regeneration, ribonucleic acid (RNA) at a neuronal level increases, presumably to promote amino acid replenishment of axoplasm.[31,36] This increase in neuronal RNA persists until the regenerative process is finished.[37] Cytoskeletal proteins such as tubulin and neurofilament protein provide the building blocks for axonal regrowth.[29] Actin and probably myosin nourish the growth cone at the very tip of the advancing neurite.[120] The synthesized microtubules and neurofilaments form a network extending to the tip of the neurite.[12,13]

Axoplasm contains proteins and cytoskeletal elements, including microtubules and neurofilaments.[29] Axoplasm is continuously made and sustained by axonal transport mechanisms.[68]

There is a continuous bidirectional transport system for axoplasm in nerve which has both anterograde and retrograde slow and fast components. The slow components tend to carry more proteins, which are the building blocks for growth, than do the fast components. Slow transport at a rate of 1 to 2 mm per day moves the proteins from the neuron to the advancing neurite tip, but the local environment at the injury site may also provide important proteins for construction of the neurite tip.[15,82] Anterograde fast axonal transport of amino acids and proteins increases in response to injury but only provides some of the less major and smaller building blocks.[81] Retrograde fast axonal transport, which accelerates during the early phase of regeneration, may provide varying concentrations of trophic or signal protein to the neuron, but this remains to be conclusively proven.[57,88] Again, the local environment may provide a more immediate signal to the spatially close growth cone.[120]

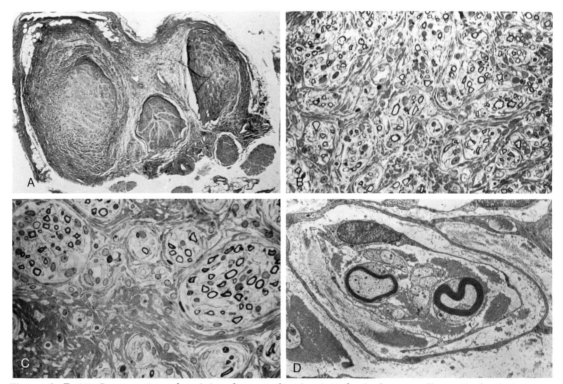

**Figure 1–7.** (*A*) Cross section of an injured nerve showing intrafascicular as well as extrafascicular scar. (*B*) Small, fine, regenerated axons are mixed in with endoneurial scar in this low-power, Masson stained, microscopic cross section. (*C*) Another area from the same cross section shows several areas of relatively heavy scar mixed in with clusters of relatively small, regenerating axons. (*D*) Electron micrographic preparation showing fibroblasts and scar around regenerating axons. See also color figure.

# PERIPHERAL NERVE REGENERATION

With serious injury to nerve, important connective tissue layers as well as their enclosed nerve fibers are injured. The connective tissue response to most injuries is a proliferative one.[47] This leads to a disorganized connective tissue skeleton which can thwart effective axonal regrowth[51,118] (Figure 1–7). Despite this, peripheral neurite regeneration is much more effective than that of axons or neurites in the CNS.[63] Peripheral nerve has a basal lamina provided by the Schwann cells and surrounding its axons, but the CNS does not. The basal lamina, although destroyed at the injury site, survives proximal and distal to it[52,76] (Figure 1–8). In the distal stump of an injured nerve, the lamina surrounds deposits of degenerating myelin and axoplasmic debris, which are gradually phagocytized.[6,87,124] The Schwann cells proliferate close to the growth cones and elongating neurites to form bands of Büngner.[90,129] As the neurites grow distally, the basal lamina tends to resist the expanding force of the growing neurite and to channel its advance within the sheath toward the "guidance system" of the distal stump (Figure 1–9). Trophic factors, which may exist in both the CNS and the peripheral nervous system, do help attract the new neurite. A proximal stump, separated by a distance from the distal stump, preferentially grows toward it rather than to non-neural tissue.[72] Nonetheless, the relatively structured tubular system of a nerve undergoing Wallerian degeneration and then regeneration helps also to direct axonal regrowth (Figures 1–10, 1–11, and 1–12).[53,90]

By comparison, in the CNS, where there is no basal laminar system, effective axonal regeneration may be poor because the expanding pressure of the neurite's terminal club is less restrained. This leads to rupture, loss of axoplasm, and release of lysosomal enzymes that can further damage the local environment.[123] Despite the relatively favorable circumstances for peripheral nerve regeneration, the growing neurite in higher animals such as monkeys and humans can be readily blocked. The nerve fiber is forced to change pathways or divide many times by the disorganized proliferation of both endoneurial and interfascicular epineurial connective tissues in response to injury[83] (Figure

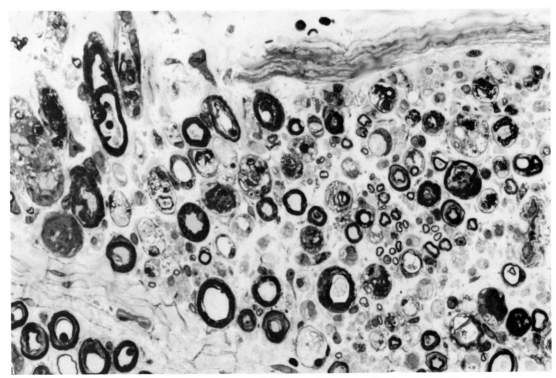

**Figure 1–8.** This photomicrograph shows areas of degenerating axons distal to a partial laceration to nerve.

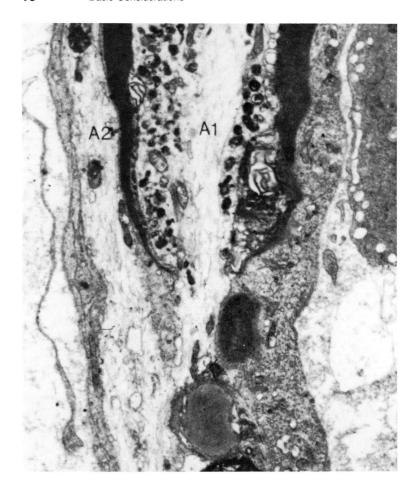

**Figure 1–9.** Process of axonal sprouting occurs in the proximal stump. A1 is a terminal sprout, and A2 is a collateral sprout. These sprouts are retained in the original basement lamella of the nerve fiber, and the regenerative unit thus formed crosses the suture line to reinnervate the distal stump or graft.

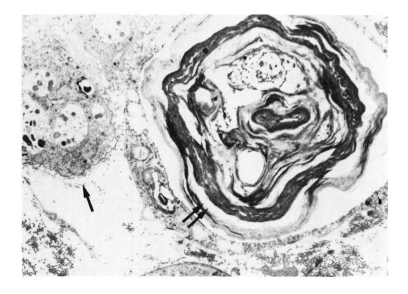

**Figure 1–10.** A regenerative unit (*single arrow*) invades the distal stump next to a fiber undergoing Wallerian degeneration (*double arrow*).

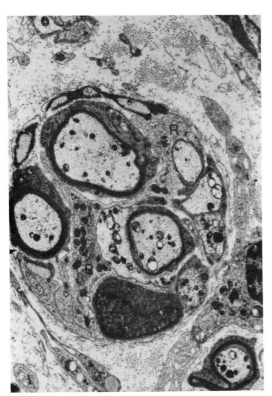

**Figure 1–11.** Axons of the regenerative unit start to myelinate as the regenerating fibers come into contact with the Schwann cells of the distal stump.

**TABLE 1–1**
Axonal Growth Characteristics

1. Initial delay while regenerating axons make up the area of retrograde degeneration.
2. Injury site delay while axons traverse injury site.
3. Distal delay as axons grow down the distal stump.
4. Terminal delay as axons both mature and reinnervate distal innervational sites.

spinal nerves and distal input connected with both motor and sensory branches.[11] Vessels travel not only in epineurium and interfascicular epineurium but also within the fascicles themselves.[70] There is a collateral blood supply that feeds into the epineurial longitudinal system through the mesoneurium[106] (Figure 1–15). These collateral vessels can be sacrificed during mobilization of a nerve without loss of function or decreased ability for the injured nerve to regenerate.[59] Longitudinal and intraneural vessels supply enough nourishment to maintain functional integrity and ability to regenerate.[7] Nonetheless, changes in blood flow to nerve can occur with various types of injuries.[83] In addition, the blood-nerve barrier can be disturbed by a variety of injuries and toxins.

1–13). This can result in distal stump axons of fine caliber and of relatively poor myelination. Of even greater consequence, axons may not regain their former sites of innervation or come close enough to them to mature and become functional. The factors responsible for such fibroblast proliferation and subsequent collagen alignment after injury are poorly understood[57,89,112] (Figure 1–14). Practical methods to ameliorate such changes biochemically are not as yet available.[23,77]

Adequate regeneration of a nerve fiber takes time, both for the fiber to reach a distal innervational site and for the fiber to mature. A series of delays are encountered, even if axonal regeneration is quite successful (Table 1–1).

## NEURAL BLOOD SUPPLY

Fortunately, the blood supply to nerve is a rich one.[1,84] It is predominantly longitudinal, with proximal input at the level of the roots or

## FASCICULAR STRUCTURE

Not as favorable for the surgeon is the next anatomic fact, which is that fascicular structure changes position along the longitudinal course of the nerve every few centimeters[111,114] (Figure 1–16). This makes fascicular matching difficult if there has been loss of neural substance.[112] Fascicles also trade fibers or sometimes bundles of fibers with neighboring fascicles as they travel down the course of the nerve.[111] In addition, the more centrally placed fascicles, especially in the proximal segment of a nerve, contain fibers serving a variety of distal functions. As the nerve approaches the more distal extremity, there is greater differentiation of function into specific fascicles, which then become predominantly motor or sensory. These fascicular positional changes and fascicular trade-offs are more dramatic in the proximal portions of a nerve than distally.[73] A fascicle may be at a 9-o'clock position at one level and,

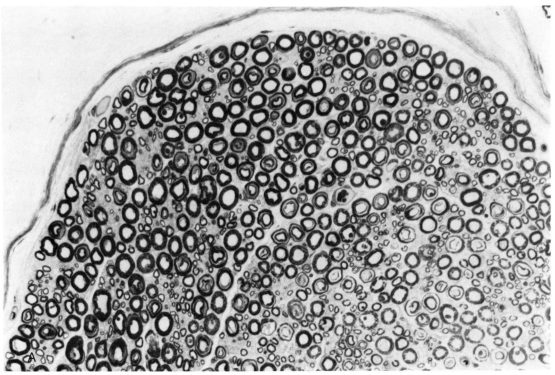

**Figure 1 – 12.** (*A*) With regeneration, fibers in the distal stump mature until a normal pattern of myelinated and unmyelinated fibers is seen.

*Illustration continued on opposite page*

within a few centimeters, be at a 12-o'clock or even 2-o'clock position.[114]

The final unit of function within a fascicle is the nerve fiber, composed of the axon and its attendant Schwann cells. The endoneurium surrounding the nerve fiber reacts to injury just as do the other connective tissue layers of the nerve. These nerve fibers and their fibrous coverings cannot be seen either by the naked eye or under the operating microscope; therefore, the structure that forms the subunit of various micro-operative procedures is the fascicle (Figure 1 – 17).

Microdissection of nerve at a fascicular level is difficult although not impossible.[40] Of equal importance, fascicular structure can appear to be intact, grossly or even under the operating microscope, and yet there may be severe axonal loss. The related endoneurial changes may be of such a nature as to prevent successful regeneration unless surgical repair is instituted.[55,111,127] This is particularly so with some contusive and many stretch injuries, in which, despite gross fascicular continuity, intrafascicular change is often neurotmetic.[101] Variability in this intrafa-

scicular pathology also makes intraoperative electrophysiologic assessment of an injury in continuity imperative (Figure 1 – 18). Electrical stimulation and stimulation and recording of nerve action potentials (NAPs) are, in our view, necessary intraoperative steps with most serious lesions in continuity.[55,78] This permits the assessment of the function of all the fascicles at the injury site regardless of the external appearance of the nerve or its fascicles.

Micro-operative technique is usually used to dissect fascicles within a nerve, and it should be stressed that such a dissection is along structural lines alone. A major assumption made by some clinicians during such procedures is that if the fascicle is grossly intact, the nerve fibers contained within that structure are probably normal or have the potential to become so. Although this may be true under some circumstances, it is far from universal. Intrafascicular neurotmetic changes can and often do occur despite the gross continuity of a fascicle.[55] This is particularly so if stretching forces are the primary mechanism of injury or if nerve has been injured by injection.[57] Unfortunately,

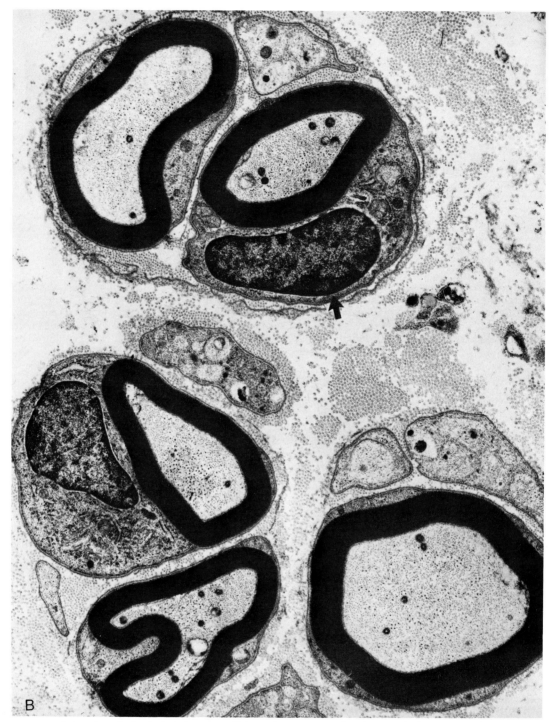

**Figure 1–12** *Continued.* (*B*) Each Schwann cell (*arrow*) is associated with a single large axon in the case of a myelinated fiber or with multiple small axons which remain either unmyelinated or poorly myelinated.

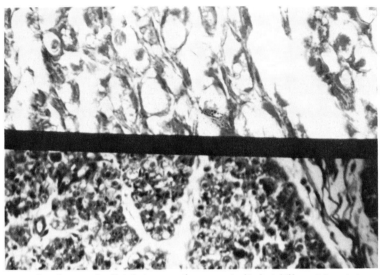

**Figure 1 – 13.** Degenerative changes in distal stumps of nerves studied at different time intervals. The top photograph shows degenerative axonal and myelin debris but with relatively open tubular system at 3 weeks after injury. The bottom photograph shows a distal cross section 3 months after more proximal injury. Endoneurial fibroblasts have proliferated, and the tubular system has been somewhat closed down by connective tissue. Despite this distal stump change, axons that eventually become functional can grow distally, depending on the local injury milieu more proximally. (Masson stain ×40.)

stretch is the leading cause or mechanism of serious nerve injury requiring operation; therefore, fascicular continuity by no means assures recovery unless the potential for such is shown by intraoperative electrical testing.[128]

Intrafascicular pathology can also vary from fascicle to fascicle at the same level in an injured nerve. This type of pathology cannot be ascertained by gross or microscopic operative inspection.

# BASIC RESPONSES TO INJURY

## The Neuron's Response

The cell body, which is located in the anterior horn of the spinal cord, in the posterior root ganglion, or in an autonomic ganglion, undergoes chromatolysis after an axon is interrupted.[100] Histologically, the neuronal swelling is accompanied by displacement of the Nissl

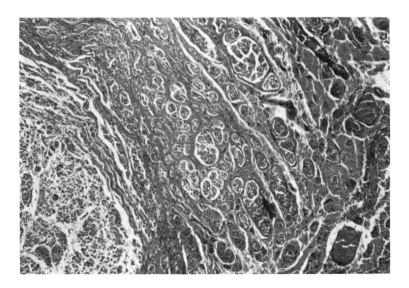

**Figure 1 – 14.** Fibroblast proliferation in graft. Despite this, small axons are seen at both intrafascicular and extrafascicular sites. (Masson stain ×35.)

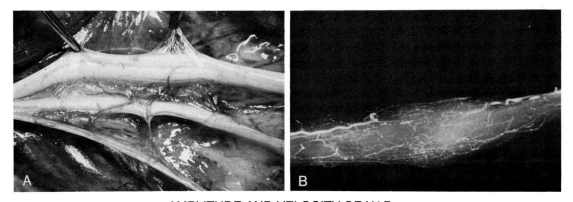

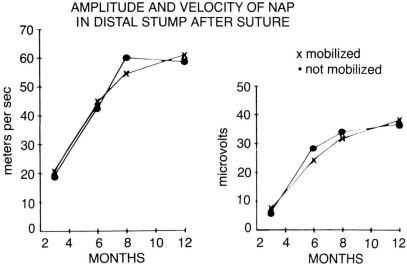

**Figure 1–15.** (*A*) Blood supply in the primate sciatic complex. Forceps are on the presumed mesoneurium. The longitudinal nature of the epineurial vessels is evident. Collateral vessels can be seen at several levels and reaching nerve via the mesoneurium. Tibial nerve is at the top, peroneal nerve is intermediate, and sural nerve is below. (From Kline D, Hackett E, Davis G, Myers B: Effect of mobilization on the blood supply and regeneration of injured nerves. J Surg Res 12:254–266, 1972. (*B*) Primate sciatic nerve injured by severance and then sutured together. Animal was perfused with contrast to demonstrate reconstitution of microvessels, especially at the injury site. (*C*) These two graphs depict distal stump nerve action potential (NAP) velocity and amplitude in primate nerves that were severed and sutured. Nerve on one side was mobilized from sciatic notch to calf levels before repair, whereas that on the other side was not mobilized. NAP velocities and amplitudes were relatively similar at each time interval up to 12 months after repair, whether or not nerve was mobilized. (Adapted by Gilliat RM (personal communication) from Kline D, Hackett E, Davis G, Myers B: Effects of mobilization on the blood supply and regeneration of injured nerves. J Surg Res, 1972.)

substance to the periphery of the cell.[9] Enlargement of a neuron after its axon has been injured is therefore usually regenerative rather than degenerative in nature.[17,65] Exceptions are found in severe proximal injury to neural elements, particularly the brachial plexus or the lumbosacral plexus, which can result in retrograde damage to the neuron serious enough to be incompatible with its survival.[45]

In neuronal chromatolysis that is regenerative in nature, the cytoplasm increases in volume, primarily because of an increase in RNA and associated enzymes.[36] RNA changes from large particles to submicroscopic particles, and this change results in an apparent loss of Nissl substance. From 4 days after injury until a peak is reached at 20 days, the amount of RNA increases, as does the cell's metabolic rate.[33] RNA appears to be necessary for the reconstruction of axons, and it provides the polypeptides and proteins necessary for replenishment of axoplasm, which is an extension of the neuron's cy-

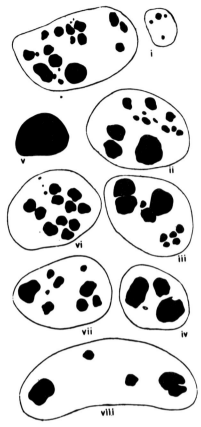

**Figure 1–16.** Change in fascicular pattern in radial nerve running from arm level (I) to forearm level (VIII). V represents the superficial sensory radial nerve, and VI and VII are the proximal and distal posterior interosseous nerves. (From Sunderland S: The intraneural topography of the radial, median, and ulnar nerves. Brain 68:243–299, 1945.

toplasm (Figure 1–19). Its role as the central ingredient in regeneration has, however, been questioned by some. The argument has been advanced that the increase occurs only if regeneration is already proceeding successfully.[37] The RNA may serve only as a marker for regeneration rather than heralding it. In any case, it has been clearly shown that increased RNA volume and activity persist until axonal regeneration and maturation cease. The closer the injury is to the spinal cord, the more hypertrophic are the neuronal changes, whereas with distal lesions, the changes are less marked. Given that a proximal injury requires a lengthier regeneration of the axon than a distal one, it is almost as if the neuron were able to anticipate the job ahead.

Methods for tracing axon connections back to the CNS have led to a number of interesting observations.[62] In a healthy axon-to-neuron relationship, metabolic building blocks for axoplasm are circulated from the nerve body down the axon and back up again (Figure 1–20). As specified earlier, the axoplasmic flow of these metabolites may be supplemented along the axon's course by local exchange of both metabolites and waste products. Some of the building blocks necessary for survival of the axon may be provided by the axon's local environment rather than by the neuron itself.[43,60]

Despite a number of neuronal, metabolic alterations, neurophysiologic markers such as resting potential and afterpotential spikes do

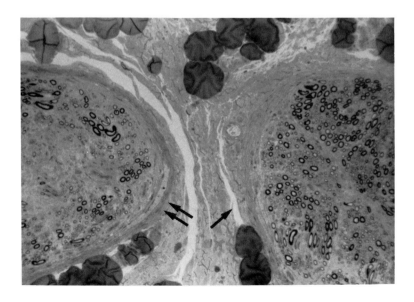

**Figure 1–17.** Elbow-level cross section of radial nerve in a patient with preganglionic injury of C7 and C8 spinal nerves. The superficial sensory radial part of the nerve, which is made up of sensory axons, is preserved to the right (*single arrow*) whereas most of the motor fascicle, seen to the left, is degenerated (*double arrow*). (Toluidine blue ×368.)

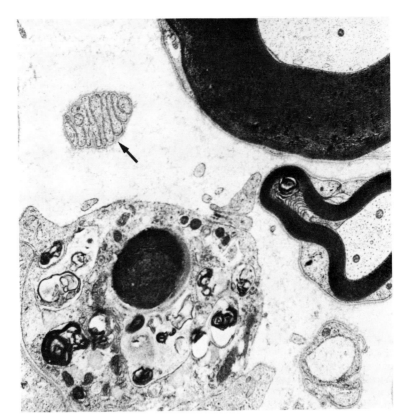

**Figure 1–18.** A large normal nerve fiber (*top right*) is adjacent to a smaller axon with a thinner myelin coating. At the lower left, a macrophage is digesting myelin debris. Above this is a band of Büngner (*arrow*) composed of a stack of Schwann cell profiles within a single basement lamella. Nerve fiber injury can be of a different degree within a single fascicle, and nerve fascicle injury can be of a different degree within a single peripheral nerve. The surgeon must be familiar with these concepts during evaluation of nerve lesions in continuity.

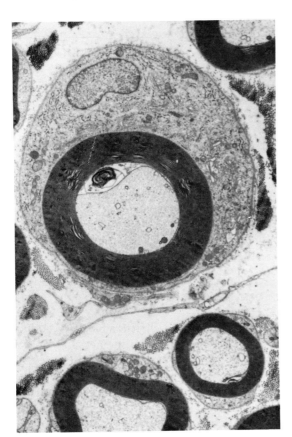

**Figure 1–19.** Axon is continuous with the nerve cell body in the spinal cord or posterior root ganglion. All protein synthesis occurs in the cell body and is transported down the axon. Surrounding the axon is the reduplicated surface membrane of the attendant Schwann cell—the myelin. By contrast, the cytoplasm of the Schwann cell is packed with organelles. A basement lamella coats the surface of the Schwann cell, and this forms a continuous structure along the length of the nerve fiber, made up of the continuous axon and a chain of discontinuous Schwann cells.

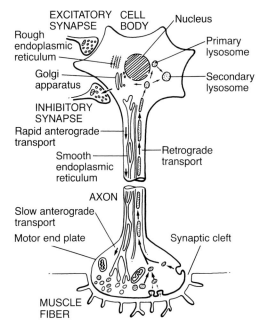

EXCITATORY CELL
SYNAPSE BODY
Rough
endoplasmic
reticulum
Golgi
apparatus
INHIBITORY
SYNAPSE
Rapid anterograde
transport
Smooth
endoplasmic
reticulum
AXON
Slow anterograde
transport
Motor end plate

Nucleus
Primary
lysosome
Secondary
lysosome

Retrograde
transport

Synaptic cleft

MUSCLE
FIBER

**Figure 1–20.** Diagram of a cell body with its supported axon and distal innervational site. The drawing shows some of the intraneuronal structures and the smooth endoplasmic reticulum, tubular structure, and microfilaments at the nerve level. Sites of metabolic exchange are noted. (Adapted from Lundborg G, Ed: Nerve Injury and Repair. Edinburgh, Churchill Livingstone, 1988.)

not change.[16,35] There is, however, a disturbance in the neuron's central synaptic function.[34] Longer latency and increased temporal dispersion of the reflex discharge evoked by the afferent stimulation of the neuron occur. Degenerative changes in synaptic vesicles have also been demonstrated by electron microscopy and may relate to interference in synaptic function.[93]

Experimental work suggests some expansion of the sensory neuronal field in response to distal axotomy and subsequent regeneration.[43,54] Neighboring neurons whose axons were not sectioned were found to branch and to grow into the neuronal zone of the axons that had been sectioned distally.[49,125] There is also some experimental evidence that the motor neuronal zone subtending a nerve's injury can increase in size or expand in terms of level.[20–22,42] How effective such expansion is in terms of useful regeneration remains to be shown, but it has been recorded, even in the primate.[58]

If the axon is freshly re-resected proximal to a previous transection site, new regenerative ac-

tivity on the part of the neuron results, and a new thrust of axoplasm occurs.[38] This has led to the suggestion that a possible way of accelerating axonal growth is to create a conditioning lesion or a second axotomy several weeks after the initial injury.[75] This presumes that regeneration by means of a nerve repair that is delayed for several weeks is augmented by the already increased (primed) metabolic activity of the neurons which resulted from the original injury.[75] It is unclear whether a second axotomy forces a completely new turnover of RNA or whether it changes the peak activity already achieved by the first axotomy. In any case, such conditioning may play a role in the usual surgical procedure to repair nerve. An important step in neural repair, either by suture or by grafts after any interval of time, is to trim or resect both distal and proximal stumps back to healthy tissue.[5] Thus, a second axotomy is universal in any repair of a serious nerve lesion; only the interval between the two axotomies and the nature of the axotomies may vary.

## Axonal Response to Injury

For clinical purposes, there are three basic ways in which nerve fibers can respond to trauma, and this has been nicely delineated by Seddon[102] and enlarged upon by Sunderland.[110] It must, however, be kept in mind that the thousands of axons making up each nerve are not only of variable size and disposition but also have different needs for nutrition and oxygenation. As a result, many nerve injuries are composed of mixed elements of neurapraxia, axonotmesis, and neurotmesis. Possible outcomes also relate to how complete the injury is to begin with. Thus, the amount of recovery from spontaneous regeneration is not always predictable (Figure 1–21).

## Neurapraxia

With neurapraxia, there is a block in conduction of the impulse down the nerve fiber, and recovery takes place without Wallerian degeneration. This is probably a biochemical lesion caused by a concussion or shock-like injury to the fiber. In the case of the whole nerve, neurapraxia is brought about by compression or by

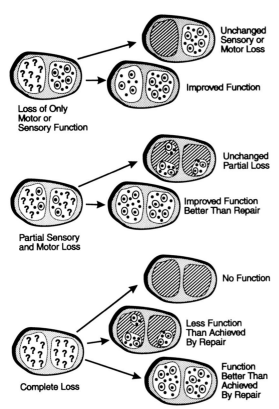

**Figure 1–21.** Various outcomes are shown for the three major types of injury to nerve. With loss of only motor or sensory function, the outcome can include either unchanged sensory or motor loss or improved function in both spheres. With time, the result with partial sensory and motor loss may be either unchanged partial loss or function that improves to a level better than repair would have given. With complete loss, there may be no functional return with time, less function than is achieved by repair, or better function than a repair might bring.

be generated by stimulating and recording below it. Segmental demyelination of some fibers may occur, and others may actually undergo axonotmesis, producing occasional fibrillations in muscle seen by electromyography (EMG) performed several weeks later. The overwhelming picture is, however, one of normal axons without Wallerian degeneration.[31,41] Such injury selectively affects the larger fibers serving muscle contraction as well as touch and position sense, whereas fine fibers subserving pain and sweating are spared.[109] Therefore, these injuries often have an element of pain. Because connective tissue elements as well as most of the microscopic anatomy of the axon and its coverings are preserved, recovery is assured, but it may require several days or even up to 5 to 6 weeks to occur.

## Axonotmesis

By comparison, axonotmesis involves loss of the relative continuity of the axon and its covering of myelin but preservation of the connective tissue framework of the nerve.[80] Because axonal continuity is lost, Wallerian degeneration occurs. EMG performed 2 to 3 weeks later shows

relatively mild, blunt blows, including some low-velocity missile injuries close to the nerve. Any injury in which there is the potential for compression or stretch can produce some element of neurapraxia[94] (Figure 1–22). Peroneal paralysis caused by a prolonged cross-legged position and radial or Saturday night paralysis caused by compression of the axilla are common examples of neurapraxic injuries. Stimulation proximal to such an injury fails to produce muscle function distally, but stimulation distal to the injury does produce muscle function. If the entire cross section of the nerve is affected, an NAP does not transmit across the lesion but can

Contusion radial (upper arm) - neurapraxia

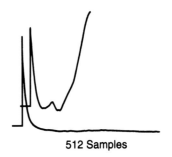

512 Samples

S→R 15 cm forearm to upper arm
100V / 0.2 msec

**Figure 1–22.** Recording made noninvasively at the skin level distal to an area of contusion 5 days after the onset of a complete radial palsy. Summated trace is above and single trace below. The summated trace shows a nerve action potential (NAP) after the stimulus artifact, and this is followed by the take-off of an evoked muscle action potential (MAP). Ability to stimulate both an NAP and an MAP by stimulation distal to the lesion provides evidence of the presence of neurapraxic lesion.

fibrillations and denervational potentials in musculature distal to the injury site.[40] Loss in both motor and sensory spheres is more complete with axonotmesis than with neurapraxia, and recovery occurs only through regeneration of the axons, a process requiring time (Figure 1–23). Axonotmesis is usually the result of a more severe crush or contusion injury than that producing neurapraxia. After the elapse of 2 to 3 days, stimulation either proximal or distal to such a lesion does not produce muscle contraction. An NAP cannot be evoked, either across the lesion or by recording from more distal nerve.

There is usually an element of retrograde proximal degeneration of the axon, and for re-generation to occur, this loss must first be overcome.[4] The regenerative fibers must cross the injury site and regenerate to the distal stump. In the human, spanning of the injury site and axonal regeneration through the proximal or retrograde area of degeneration may require several weeks. Then, the neurite tip progresses down the distal stump, at an average rate of only a millimeter per day.[113] This rate may be faster if the injury is closer to the CNS, as with an injury to a plexus trunk, or slower at a more distal site, such as the wrist or hand. Proximal lesions may grow distally as fast as 2 to 3 mm per day and distal lesions as slowly as 1.5 mm per day.[113]

After sufficient numbers of regenerating

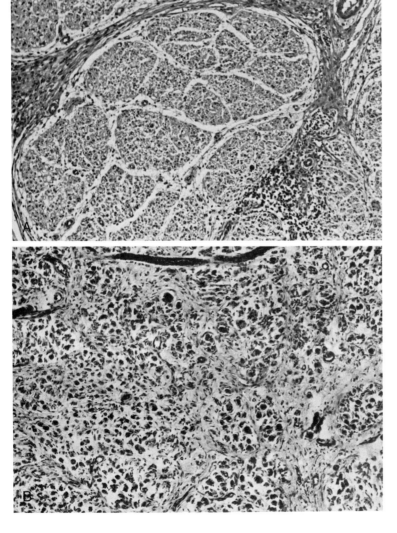

**Figure 1–23.** (*A*) Scarred distal stump with fine axons only. (*B*) Area of a distal stump with more adequate axonal regeneration than seen in *A*. Although the interval between injury and the making of these cross sections was the same, the mechanism of injury was different. Nerve injury in *B* was more axonotmetic than in *A*.

fibers have penetrated the injury site, there is restoration of an NAP recorded across it, but its amplitude is small and conduction velocity greatly reduced.[56] Such a distal stump response can be recorded long before a muscle action potential can be evoked or decrease in denervational change can be recorded from muscle distal to the lesion. There is then a substantial period of time during which regeneration can be satisfactory even without any further peripheral, clinical, or electrical evidence of improvement. As regeneration proceeds down the distal stump, this progress can be followed by NAP recordings. There is then a further delay after axons reach distal inputs during which the latter are reconstructed and their axons mature. At some point after axons reach muscle and before voluntary contraction can occur, stimulation of the regenerating nerve is able to produce muscle function. This finding may antedate clinical recovery by a number of weeks.[78] Despite these time requirements, regeneration with axonotmetic injury is superior to that with neurotmesis, even if the latter is corrected by surgical repair. With axonotmesis, the basement membrane system is relatively intact, and regenerating axon clusters are guided by Schwann cells or bands of Büngner enclosed within a relatively preserved endoneurium.

## Neurotmesis

More severe contusion, stretch, or laceration produces neurotmesis, in which not only axons but investing connective tissues lose their continuity. An obvious example of a neurotmetic injury to nerve is one that transects it, because both axonal and connective tissue continuity are lost. However, most neurotmetic injuries do not produce gross loss of continuity of the nerve but rather internal disruption of the architecture of the nerve sufficient to involve perineurium and endoneurium as well as axons and their coverings. Denervational changes recorded by EMG are the same as those seen with axonotmetic injury.[49] However, spontaneous reversal of these changes and recovery are unlikely to occur, because regenerating axons become mixed in a swirl of regenerating fibroblasts and collagen, producing a disorganized repair site or neuroma (Figure 1–24). Stimulation either above or distal to a neurotmetic segment of injury does not produce function, and

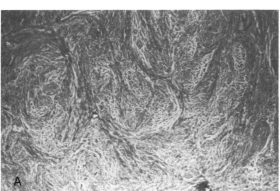
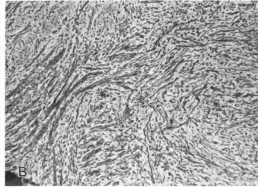
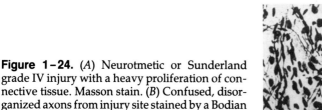
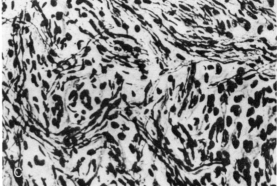

**Figure 1–24.** (*A*) Neurotmetic or Sunderland grade IV injury with a heavy proliferation of connective tissue. Masson stain. (*B*) Confused, disorganized axons from injury site stained by a Bodian technique. (*C*) Confused and disorganized axons from another injury site.

NAPs are not recordable across or distal to the lesion.[55] Furthermore, these abnormalities persist and do not improve as they do with neurapraxic and axonotmetic injuries. Although axons may reach the distal stump in great numbers in neurotmetic injuries, they often fail to find their preinjury pathways[127] (Figure 1–25). Most importantly, because of endoneurial proliferation and contraction of distal nerve sheaths, they may fail to regain sufficient axonal diameter and myelination to produce functional regeneration even if they do reach proper destinations.

In Sunderland's system, grade I or first-degree injury corresponds to a neurapraxic injury (Figure 1–26). Grade II injury involves loss of axon continuity with preservation of endoneurium and fascicular structure. Grade III is a mixed axonotmetic-neurotmetic injury with loss of both axons and endoneurium, but most of the perineurial and therefore some of the fascicular structure is maintained. Grade IV injury involves loss of axons, endoneurium, and perineurium, with absence of fascicular structure; continuity is maintained only by epineurium. This is a predominantly neurotmetic injury. Grade V injury involves a transected nerve and so is neurotmetic by definition.

In many partial lesions, there is a spectrum of injury to fibers. If function is preserved or partial recovery of function returns within 6 weeks, the injury permitted some axons to suffer only

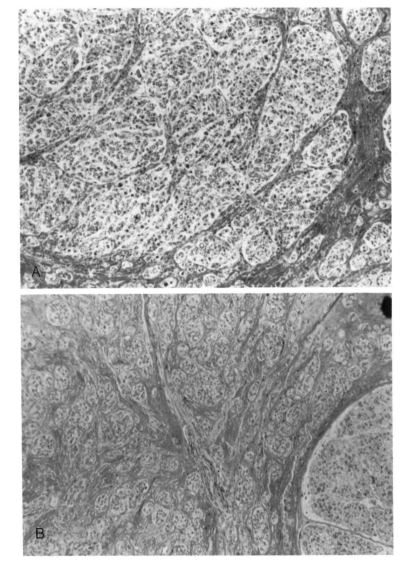

**Figure 1–25.** (*A*) Poor reinnervation of distal stump of nerve. The fibers are small, and those to the right are in an extrafascicular position. (*B*) Distal cross section through graft site. Some axons are within the graft at lower right, but many are in extrafascicular tissue.

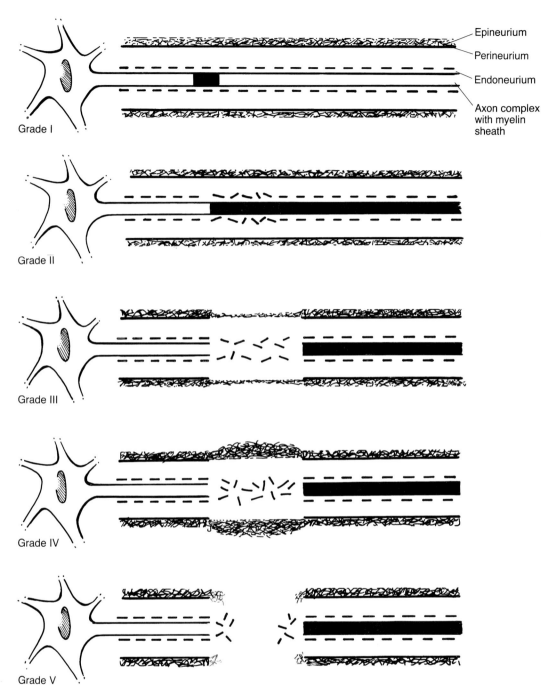

**Figure 1-26.** This drawing exhibits diagrammatically the five types of injury as described by Sunderland. Grade I is a neurapraxic injury with a block in conduction without Wallerian degeneration. Grade II is a pure axonotmetic injury with maintenance of the connective tissue framework and, thus, the potential for excellent regeneration. Grade III is a more severe lesion which usually has a mixture of axonotmetic and neurotmetic axons. Grade IV is a neurotmetic lesion in continuity in which endoneurial and perineurial connective tissue layers as well as axons are disrupted. Grade V is a transecting injury with, by definition, interruption of all connective tissue layers. (Adapted from Kline D, Hudson A: Acute injuries of peripheral nerves. *In* Youmans J, Ed. Neurological Surgery, 3rd Ed. Philadelphia, WB Saunders, 1990, pp. 2423–2510.)

neurapraxia and involved most of the remaining axonal population in axonotmesis, thus permitting their regeneration.[122] With no evidence of reversal of neurapraxia at 6 weeks, the proportion of axons involved by axonotmesis or neurotmesis remains undetermined. Predominance of injury type can be determined relatively early after injury only by combining operative inspection with intraoperative electrophysiologic testing.[56,60,78]

Depending on the time it takes for axons to reach a distal innervational site, the endoneurial pathways are expanded or decreased in diameter. Usually more than one fiber grows down a tube, but only those reaching a distal receptor and reinnervating it go on to mature and take on myelin; the others either degenerate or fail to mature[97] (Figure 1–27).

Regenerating axons may not function even after reaching distal end-organs unless they arrive close to their original site.[130] Regenerating fibers can induce some, but unfortunately not complete, change in end-organs not innervated by them before the injury.[105] Cutaneous fibers do not cross certain boundaries even for sensory reinnervation, and they are certainly not effective in reinnervating motor sites. In addition, regeneration of ulnar or median motor fibers into the fine hand muscles seldom produces even near normal muscle function.[50] The ability of the CNS to relate to new end-organ contact on the part of the axon is limited in both the sensory and the motor spheres. It does occur, but

usually with less than optimal results.[108] This is readily illustrated by the synkinesis seen with facial nerve regeneration, particularly that associated with hypoglossal-facial or accessory-facial anastomosis.[98] Many months to years may need to elapse before fiber number as well as maturity reaches a level where useful function is possible (Figure 1–28).

After denervation, the structure of muscle begins to change histologically by the third week. The muscle fibers kink, and their cross-striations decrease.[116] Atrophy or shrinkage of the muscle mass may be evident clinically within a few weeks, and it persists unless reinnervation occurs.[92] With continued denervation, particularly if this is accompanied by a lack of activity and movement, fibrosis replaces the muscle; by 2 to 3 years after denervation, the muscle can be totally replaced by scar tissue or fat.[48] For this reason, intervals of denervation beyond 2 to 3 years begin to impose major limitations on the motor function that can follow subsequent reinnervation, even by the most skillfully executed repair.

Function of the nerve must be assessed during operation by various electrophysiologic techniques, to be discussed in the following chapters. In most instances, these techniques are applied to the nerve trunk as a whole, and individual fascicular function is usually not measured during the course of standard peripheral nerve operations. Nonetheless, if it is necessary, fascicular function can be assessed in the

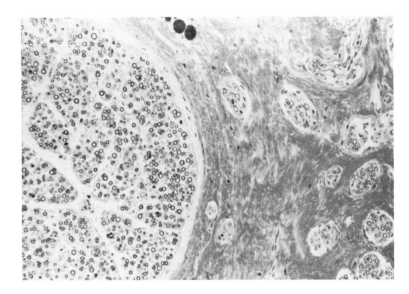

**Figure 1–27.** Fascicle of a distal stump on the left has been well-innervated by axons which are maturing and regaining myelin thickness. Several regenerative units have missed the distal fascicle at the suture line and have grown into the extrafascicular epineurial tissues, forming a suture line neuroma to the right.

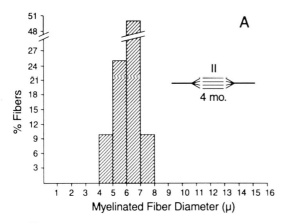

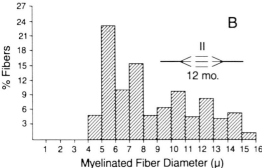

**Figure 1-28.** Composite graphs of myelinated axonal counts stratified by fiber size made 1 cm distal to a graft 2.54 cm in length at 4 months (*A*) and at 12 months (*B*). The majority of fibers are small and intermediate in size at 4 months. At 12 months, there are more larger fibers, but even after this period, their numbers are relatively small.

same way. Optimal appreciation of function and structure during the course of peripheral nerve surgery is gained by using electrophysiologic techniques and micro-operative techniques in a complementary fashion. Surgeons who treat disorders of peripheral nerves should be fully conversant with techniques that assess not only structure but also function intraoperatively. A combined anatomic and physiologic approach to nerve injuries is the major emphasis of this book.

## Bibliography

1. Adams WE: Blood supply of nerves. J Anat 76:323–341, 1942.
2. Aguayo A and Bray G: Cell interactions studied in the peripheral nerve of experimental animals. *In* Dyck P, Thomas P, Lambert E, Bunge R, Eds: Peripheral Neuropathy. Philadelphia, WB Saunders, 1984.
3. Aguayo A, Attiwell M, Trecarten J, et al.: Abnormal myelination in transplanted Trembler mouse Schwann cells. Nature 265:73–75, 1977.
4. Aitken JT and Thomas PK: Retrograde changes in fiber size following nerve section. J Anat 96:121–129, 1962.
5. Aleksavdrovskaya OV: Degeneration and regeneration of peripheral nerves in double injury. Tr Mosk Vet Akad 10:174–188, 1956.
6. Asbury A: The histogenesis of phagocytes during Wallerian degeneration procedures. Sixth International Congress of Neuropathology. Paris, Masson & Cie, 1970.
7. Bacsich P and Wyburn GM: The vascular pattern of peripheral nerve during repair after experimental crush. J Anat 79:9–14, 1945.
8. Baron-Van Evercooren A, Gansmüller A, Gumpel M, et al.: Schwann cell differentiation in vitro: Extracellular matrix deposition and interaction. Dev Neurosci 8:182–196, 1986.
9. Barr ML and Hamilton JD: A quantitative study of certain morphological changes in spinal motor neurons during axon reaction. J Comp Neurol 89:93–121, 1948.
10. Behrman I and Ackland R: Experimental study of the regenerative potential of perineurium at a site of nerve transection. J Neurosurg 54:79–83, 1981.
11. Bentley FH and Schlapp W: Experiments on blood supply of nerves. J Physiol (London) 102:62–71, 1943.
12. Bisby M: Changes in composition of labeled protein transported in motor axons during their regeneration. J Neurobiol 11:435–455, 1980.
13. Bisby MA: Synthesis of cytoskeletal proteins by axotomized and regenerating motoneurons. *In* Reier PJ, Bunge RP, and Seil FJ, Eds: Current Issues in Neural Regeneration. New York, Alan R Liss, 1988.
14. Bischoff A and Thomas PK: Microscopic anatomy of myelinated nerve fibers. *In* Dyck PJ, Thomas PK, and Lambert EH, Eds: Peripheral Neuropathy. Philadelphia, WB Saunders, 1975, pp. 104–130.
15. Black MM and Lasek RJ: Slow components of axonal transport: Two cytoskeletal networks. J Cell Biol 86:616–623, 1980.
16. Bradley K, Brock LG, and McIntyre AK: Effects of axon section on motoneuron function. Proc Univ Otago Med Sch 33:14–16, 1955.
17. Brattgård SO, Edström JE, and Hyden H: The productive capacity of the neuron in retrograde reaction. Exp Cell Res 5(Suppl):185, 1958.
18. Bray G and Aguayo AJ: Regeneration of peripheral unmyelinated nerves. Fate of the axonal sprouts which develop after injury. J Anat 117:517–529, 1974.
19. Bray GM, Raminsky M, and Aguayo AJ: Interactions between axons and their sheath cells. Ann Rev Neurosci 4:127–162, 1981.
20. Brushart TM and Mesulam MM: Alteration in connections between muscle and anterior horn motor neurons after peripheral nerve repair. Science 208:603–605, 1980.
21. Brushart TM and Seiler WA IV: Selective innervation of distal motor stumps by peripheral motor axons. Exp Neurol 97:289–300, 1987.
22. Brushart TM, Henry EW, and Mesulam MM: Reorganization of muscle afferent projections accompanies peripheral nerve regeneration. Neuroscience 6:2053–2061, 1981.
23. Bucko C, Joynt R, and Grabb W: Peripheral nerve regeneration in primates during D-penicillamine–

induced lathyrism. Plast Reconstr Surg 67:23–28, 1981.

24. Bunge M, Williams A, Wood P, et al.: Comparison of nerve cell plus Schwann cell cultures with particular emphasis on basal lamina and collagen formation. J Cell Biol 84:184–193, 1980.

25. Bunge RP and Bunge MB: Tissue culture in the study of peripheral nerve pathology. In Dyck PJ, Thomas PK, and Lambert EH, Eds: Peripheral Neuropathy. Philadelphia, WB Saunders, 1975, pp. 391–409.

26. Chang S, Rathjen FG, and Raper JA: Extension of neurites on axons is impaired by antibodies against specific neural cell surface glycoproteins. J Cell Biol 104:355–362, 1987.

27. Cunningham BA, Hemperly JJ, Murray BA, et al.: Neural cell adhesion molecule: Structure, immunoglobulin-like domains, cell surface modulation, and alternative RNA splicing. Science 236:799–806, 1987.

28. Daniloff JK, Levi G, Grumet M, et al.: Altered expression of neuronal cell adhesion molecules induced by nerve injury and repair. J Cell Biol 103:929–945, 1986.

29. Davison PF: Microtubules and neurofilaments: Possible implications in axoplasmic transport. Adv Biochem Psychopharmacol 2:168, 1970.

30. Dekker A, Gispen WH, and de Wied D: Axonal regeneration, growth factors and neuropeptides. Life Sci 41:1667–1678, 1987.

31. Denny-Brown D and Brenner C: Lesion in peripheral nerve resulting from compression by spring clip. Arch Neurol Psychiatry 52:120, 1944.

32. Ducker T, Kempe L, and Hayes G: The metabolic background for peripheral nerve surgery. J Neurosurg 30:270–280, 1969.

33. Ducker TB and Kaufmann FC: Metabolic factors in the surgery of peripheral nerves. Clin Neurosurg 24:406–424, 1977.

34. Eccles JC, Kryjevic K, and Miledi R: Delayed effects of peripheral severance of afferent nerve fibers on efficacy of their central synapses. J Physiol (London) 145:204–220, 1959.

35. Eccles JC, Libet B, and Young RR: The behavior of chromatolysed motoneurons studied by intracellular recording. J Physiol (London) 143:11–40, 1958.

36. Edstrom JE: Ribonucleic acid changes in motoneurons of frog during axon regeneration. J Neurochem 5:43–49, 1959.

37. Engh CA and Schofield BH: A review of the central response to peripheral nerve injury and its significance in nerve regeneration. J Neurosurg 37:198–203, 1972.

38. Forman D, McQuarrie I, Laborre F, et al.: Time course of the conditioning lesion effect on axonal regeneration. Brain Res 182:180–185, 1980.

39. Friedlander DR, Grumet M, and Edelman GM: Nerve growth factor enhances expression of neuron-glia cell adhesion molecule in PC12 cells. J Cell Biol 102:413–419, 1986.

40. Gilliatt R: Physical injury to peripheral nerves. Physiological and electrodiagnostic aspects. Mayo Clin Proc 56:361–370, 1981.

41. Gilliatt RW, Ochoa J, Ridge P, and Neary D: Cause of nerve damage in acute compression. Trans Am Neurol Assoc 99:71–574, 1974.

42. Gorio A, Marini P, and Zanoni R: Muscle reinnervation. III. Motoneuron sprouting capacity, enhancement by exogenous gangliosides. Neuroscience 8:417–429, 1983.

43. Gorio A, Millesi H, and Mingrino S, Eds: Post Traumatic Peripheral Nerve Regeneration: Experimental Basis and Clinical Implications. New York, Raven Press, 1981.

44. Grafstein B: Cellular mechanisms for recovery from nervous system injury. Surg Neurol 13:363–365, 1980.

45. Grafstein B and McQuarrie I: Role of the nerve cell body in axonal regneration. In Cotman CW, Ed: Neural Plasticity. New York, Raven Press, 1978.

46. Gunderson RW: Response of sensory neurites and growth cones to patterned substrata of laminin and fibronectin in vitro. Dev Biol 121:423–431, 1987.

47. Guth L: Regeneration in the mammalian peripheral nervous system. Physiol Rev 36:441–478, 1956.

48. Guttmann E and Young JZ: Reinnervation of muscle after various periods of atrophy. J Anat 78:15–43, 1944.

49. Horch KW: Central responses of cutaneous neurons to peripheral nerve crush in the cat. Brain Res 151:581–586, 1978.

50. Hubbard JI, Ed: The Peripheral Nervous System. New York, Plenum, 1974.

51. Huber CG: Experimental observations on peripheral nerve repair. In Medical Department, United States Army, Surgery in World War I: Vol. II, Part 1: Neurosurgery. Washington DC, US Government Printing Office, 1927.

52. Hudson A and Kline D: Progression of partial experimental injury to peripheral nerve. Part 2: Light and electron microscopic studies. J Neurosurg 42:15–22, 1975.

53. Hudson A, Morris J, and Weddell G: An electron microscope study of regeneration in sutured rat sciatic nerves. Surg Forum 21:451–453, 1970.

54. Jackson PC and Diamond J: Regenerating axons reclaim sensory targets from collateral nerve sprouts. Science 214:926–928, 1981.

55. Kline DG: Physiological and clinical factors contributing to timing of nerve repair. Clin Neurosurg 24:425–455, 1977.

56. Kline DG and DeJonge BR: Evoked potentials to evaluate peripheral nerve injuries. Surg Gynecol Obstet 127:1239–1250, 1968.

57. Kline DG and Hudson AR: Selected recent advances in peripheral nerve injury research. Surg Neurol 24:371–376, 1985.

58. Kline DG, Donner T, Happel L, et al. Intraforaminal repair of brachial plexus: Experimental study in primates. J Neurosurg 76:459–470, 1992.

59. Kline DG, Hackett E, Davis G, and Myers B: Effects of mobilization on the blood supply and regeneration of injured nerves. J Surg Res 12:254–266, 1972.

60. Kline DG, Hackett ER, and May P: Evaluation of nerve injuries by evoked potentials and electromyography. J Neurosurg 31:128–136, 1969.

61. Kline DG, Hudson AR, Hackett ER, et al.: Progression of partial experimental injury to peripheral nerve. Part 1: Periodic measurements of muscle contraction strength. J Neurosurg 42:1–14, 1975.

62. Kristensson K and Olsson Y: Retrograde transport of horseradish-peroxidase in transected axons. 3. Entry into injured axons and subsequent localization in perikaryon. Brain Res 126:154–159, 1977.

63. Lehman R and Hayes G: Degeneration and regeneration in peripheral nerve. Brain 90:285–296, 1967.

64. Levi-Montalcini R: The nerve growth factor 35 years later. Science 237:1154–1162, 1987.

65. Lieberman AR: The axon reaction: A review of principal features of perikaryal responses to axon injury. Int Rev Neurobiol 14:49–124, 1971.

66. Liu CT, Benda CF, and Lewey FH: Tensile strength of human nerves. Arch Neurol Psychiatry 59:322–336, 1948.
67. Low FN: The perineurium and connective tissue of peripheral nerve. *In* Landon DN, Ed: The Peripheral Nerve. New York, John Wiley and Sons, 1976, pp. 159–187.
68. Lubinska L: Mechanisms of neural regeneration. Axoplasmic streaming in regenerating and normal nerve fibers. Prog Brain Res 13:1–71, 1964.
69. Lundborg G: Intraneural microcirculation and peripheral nerve barriers: Technique for evaluation—clinical implications. *In* Omer GE and Spinner M, Eds: Management of Peripheral Nerve Problems. Philadelphia, WB Saunders, 1980.
70. Lundborg G: Structure and function of the intraneural microvessels as related to trauma, edema formation, and nerve function. J Bone Joint Surg 57A:938–948, 1975.
71. Lundborg G and Rydevik B: Effects of stretching the tibial nerve of the rabbit. A preliminary study of the intraneural circulation and the barrier function of the perineurium. J Bone Joint Surg 55B:390–401, 1973.
72. Lundborg G, Dahlin LB, Danielson N, et al.: Nerve regeneration across an extended gap: A neurobiological view of nerve repair and possible neuronotropic factors. J Hand Surg 7:580–587, 1982.
73. Mackinnon SE, Dellon AL, Hudson AR, and Hunter DA: Alteration of neuroma formation produced by manipulation of neural environment in primates. Plast Reconstr Surg 76:345–352, 1985.
74. Mackinnon SE, Dellon AL, Lundborg G, et al.: A study of neurotropism in a primate model. J Hand Surg 11A:888–894, 1986.
75. McQuarrie I: Acceleration of axonal regeneration of rat somatic motor neurons by using a conditioning lesion. *In* Gorio A, Millesi H, and Mingrino S, Eds: Post Traumatic Peripheral Nerve Regeneration. New York, Raven Press, 1981, pp. 49–58.
76. Morris JH, Hudson AR, and Weddell G: A study of degeneration and regeneration in the divided rat sciatic nerve based on electron microscopy. Z Zellforsch 124:76–203, 1972.
77. Nachemson A, Lundborg G, Myrhage R, et al.: Nerve regeneration after pharmacologic suppression of the scar resection of the suture site. An experimental study of the effects of estrogen-progesterone, methyl prednisolone acetate and *cis*-hydroxyproline in rat sciatic nerve. Scand J Plast Reconstr Surg 19:255–261, 1985.
78. Nulsen F and Lewey F: Intraneural bipolar stimulation: A new aid in assessment of nerve injuries. Science 106:301–303, 1947.
79. Ochoa J: Microscopic anatomy of unmyelinated nerve fibers. *In* Dyck PJ, Thomas PK, and Lambert EH, Eds: Peripheral Neuropathy. Philadelphia, WB Saunders, 1975, pp. 131–150.
80. Ochoa J, Fowler TJ, and Gilliatt RW: Anatomical changes in peripheral nerves compressed by a pneumatic tourniquet. J Anat 113:433–455, 1972.
81. Ochs S: Axoplasmic transport—a basis for neural pathology. *In* Dyck PJ, Thomas PK, and Lambert EH, Eds: Peripheral Neuropathy. Philadelphia, WB Saunders, 1975, pp. 213–230.
82. Ochs S: Axoplasmic transport—energy metabolism and mechanism. *In* Hubbard J, Ed: The Peripheral Nervous System. New York, Plenum 1974, pp. 47–67.
83. Ogata K and Naito M: Blood flow of peripheral nerve: Effects of dissection, stretching and compression. J Hand Surg [Br] 11:10–14, 1986.
84. Olsson Y: Vascular permeability in the peripheral nervous system. *In* Dyck PJ, Thomas PK, and Lambert EH, Eds: Peripheral Neuropathy. Philadelphia, WB Saunders, 1965, pp. 131–150.
85. Olsson Y and Reese T: Permeability of vasa nervorum and perineurium in mouse sciatic nerve studied by fluorescence and electron microscopy. J Neuropathol Exp Neurol 30:105, 1971.
86. Peale E, Luciano K, and Spitznos M: Freeze-fracture aspects of the perineurial sheath of rabbit sciatic nerve. J Neurocytol 5:385–392, 1976.
87. Pellegrino RG, Ritchie JM, and Spencer PS: The role of Schwann cell division in the clearance of nodal axolemma following nerve section in the cat. J Physiol (London) 334:68P, 1982.
88. Pleasure D: Axoplasmic transport. *In* Sumner A, Ed: The Physiology of Peripheral Nerve Disease. Philadelphia, WB Saunders, 1980, pp. 221–237.
89. Pleasure D, Bova F, Lane J, et al.: Regeneration after nerve transection. Effect of inhibition of collagen synthesis. Exp Neurol 45:72–79, 1974.
90. Ramon Y and Cajal S: Degeneration and Regeneration of the Nervous System. RM May, Trans. New York, Oxford University Press, 1928.
91. Ranvier M: Leçons sur l'Histologie du Système Nerveux. Paris, F Savy, 1878.
92. Richter H and Ketelsen U: Impairment of motor recovery after late nerve suture: Experimental study in the rabbit. II: Morphological findings. Neurosurgery 10:75–85, 1982.
93. Robertis E: Submicroscopic morphology and function of the synapse. Exp Cell Res Suppl 5:347–369, 1958.
94. Rudge P, Ochoa J, and Gilliatt RW: Acute peripheral nerve compression in the baboon. J Neurol Sci 23:403–420, 1974.
95. Rydevik B and Lundborg G: Permeability of intraneural microvessels and perineurium following acute, graded experimental nerve compression. Scand J Plast Reconstr Surg 11:179–187, 1977.
96. Salonen V, Peltonen J, Röyttä M, et al.: Laminin in traumatized nerve: Basement membrane changes during degeneration and regeneration. J Neurocytol 16:713–720, 1987.
97. Sanders FK and Young JZ: The influence of peripheral connections on the diameter of regenerating nerve fibers. J Exp Biol 22:203–212, 1946.
98. Schemm GW: The pattern of cortical localization following cranial nerve cross anastomosis. J Neurosurg 18:593–596, 1961.
99. Schwann T: Microscopic Researches into the Accordance in the Structure and Growth of Animals and Plants. H Smith, Trans. London, Sydenham Society, 1847.
100. Sears TA: Structural changes in motoneurons following axotomy. J Exp Biol 132:93–109, 1987.
101. Seddon H: Degeneration and regeneration. *In* Seddon H: Surgical Disorders of the Peripheral Nerves. Edinburgh, E & S Livingstone, 1972, pp. 9–31.
102. Seddon H: Three types of nerve injury. Brain 66:237–288, 1943.
103. Shantaveerappa TR and Bourne GH: Perineurial epithelium: A new concept of its role in the integrity of the peripheral nervous system. Science 154:1464–1467, 1966.
104. Shantaveerappa TR and Bourne GH: The "perineurial epithelium," a metabolically active continuous proto-

plasmic cell barrier surrounding peripheral nerve fasciculi. J Anat 96:527–536, 1962.

105. Simpson SA and Young JS: Regeneration of fiber diameter after cross-unions of visceral and somatic nerves. J Anat 79:48, 1945.

106. Smith JW: Factors influencing nerve repair. II: Collateral circulation of peripheral nerves. Arch Surg 93:433–437, 1966.

107. Spencer PS, Weinberg HJ, and Paine CS: The perineurial window—a new model of focal demyelination and remyelination. Brain Res 96:923–929, 1975.

108. Sperry RW: The problem of central nervous reorganization after nerve regeneration and muscle transposition. Q Rev Biol 20:311, 1945.

109. Strain R and Olson W: Selective damage of large diameter peripheral nerve fibers by compression: An application of Laplace's law. Exp Neurol 47:68–80, 1975.

110. Sunderland S: A classification of peripheral nerve injuries producing loss of function. Brain 74:491, 1951.

111. Sunderland S: Nerve and Nerve Injuries. Baltimore, Williams & Wilkins, 1968.

112. Sunderland S: Nerve Injuries and Their Repair: A Critical Appraisal. Edinburgh, Churchill Livingstone, 1991.

113. Sunderland S: Rate of regeneration in human peripheral nerves. Arch Neurol Psychiatry 58:251–295, 1947.

114. Sunderland S: The intraneural topography of the radial, median, and ulnar nerves. Brain 68:243–299, 1945.

115. Sunderland S and Bradley K: The cross-sectional area of peripheral nerve trunks devoted to nerve fibers. Brain 72:428–439, 1949.

116. Sunderland S and Ray LJ: Denervation changes in muscle. J Neurol Neurosurg Psychiatry 13:159–177, 1950.

117. Thomas PK and Jones DG: The cellular response to nerve injury. II: Regeneration of the perineurium after nerve section. J Anat 101:45–55, 1967.

118. Thomas PK and Jones DG: The cellular response to nerve injury. III: The effect of repeated crush injuries. J Anat 106:463–470, 1970.

119. Thomas PK and Olsson Y: Microscopic anatomy and function of the connective tissue components of peripheral nerve. *In* Dyck PJ, Thomas PK, Lambert EH, and Bunge R, Eds: Peripheral Neuropathy, 2nd Ed., Vol. 1. Philadelphia, WB Saunders, 1984, pp. 97–120.

120. Uzman B, Snyder S, and Villegas G: Status of peripheral nerve regeneration. *In* Neural Regeneration and Transplantation. New York, Alan R Liss, 1989.

121. Varon S and Adler R: Trophic and specifying factors directed to neuronal cells. Adv Cell Neurobiol 2:115–163, 1981.

122. Varon R and Bunge R: Tropic mechanisms in the peripheral nervous system. Ann Rev Neurosci 1:327–361, 1978.

123. Veraa R and Grafstein B: Cellular mechanisms for recovery from nervous system injury. A conference report. Exp Neurol 71:6–75, 1981.

124. Waller A: Experiments on the section of the glossopharyngeal and hypoglossal nerves of the frog. Phil Trans R Soc (London) 140:423–429, 1850.

125. Weddell G, Guttmann L, and Guttmann E: The local extension of nerve fibers into denervated areas of skin. J Neurol Neurosurg Psychiatry 4:206, 1941.

126. Weiss P: Neuronal dynamics and neuroplastic flow. *In* Schmidt F, Ed: The Neurosciences (2nd Study Program). New York, The Rockefeller Press, 1970, pp. 840–850.

127. Weiss P: Technology of nerve regeneration. A review. J Neurosurg 1:400–450, 1944.

128. Williams HB, Terzis JK: Single fascicular recordings: An intraoperative diagnostic tool for the management of peripheral nerve lesions. Plast Reconstr Surg 57:562–569, 1976.

129. Yamada KM, Spooner BS, and Wessells NK: Ultrastructure and function of the growth cones and axons of cultured nerve cells. J Cell Biol 49:614–635, 1971.

130. Zalewski A: Effects of neuromuscular reinnervation on denervated skeletal muscle by axons of motor, sensory, and sympathetic neurons. Am J Physiol 219:1675–1679, 1970.

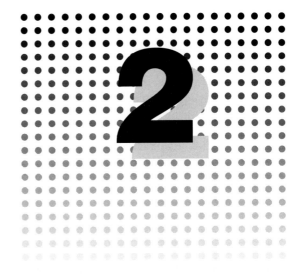

# Mechanisms and
# Pathology of Injury

## SUMMARY

The serious student of nerve must understand the diversity of surgical lesions affecting major nerves and how these differing mechanisms shape outcome. For example, the bluntly or contusively transected nerve does not do well with acute repair, but the sharply and neatly transected nerve does. Lesions in continuity caused by gunshot wounds, contusion, or stretch may or may not need surgery and are usually operated on after some delay. There are important exceptions, however, and sometimes acute operation is in order. On the other hand, not all such lesions can be helped by surgery. The behavior of an acutely compressed nerve differs from that of nerve more chronically and spontaneously entrapped. Electrical and thermal injuries share some similarities but differ greatly from chemical injuries caused by injection or those resulting from ischemic damage to a limb. As the differences in injury response according to mechanisms are understood, a more rational approach for timing and selection of operation can be developed.

## TRANSECTION

Soft tissue lacerations have the potential to transect nerves, and these are usually favorable injuries for surgical repair. Unfortunately, only 30% of serious nerve injuries in our series are caused by transection associated with soft tissue laceration[10] (Figure 2–1). The remainder result from contusive and stretching mechanisms that are more likely to leave the nerve in continuity and provide intraneural damage of variable severity.[65] Knives, glass, propeller and fan blades, chain saws, auto metal, surgical instruments, and other relatively sharp objects can partially or totally transect nerve, or they can bruise and stretch it without cutting (Figures 2–2 and 2–3).

Almost 15% of nerve injuries associated with a potentially transecting mechanism leave the nerve in some continuity.[36] Loss of function results from a variable amount of neurotmesis, axonotmesis, and neurapraxia, but the nerve or a portion of it still runs along. With time, this bruised and stretched segment of nerve thickens, and, depending on the severity of internal disruption, it may become a neuroma in continuity. This can be found even though functional loss distal to the soft tissue laceration is complete.

If nerve is partially transected, the injury to those fibers cut is by definition neurotmetic or Sunderland grade V. On the other hand, those fibers not directly transected can have a variable degree of injury and be Sunderland grade II, III, or IV. Functional loss can vary from that which

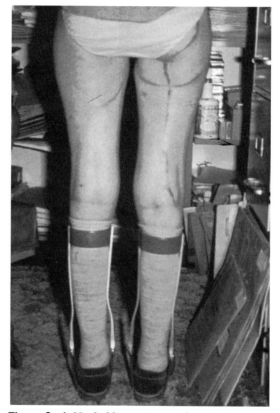

**Figure 2–1.** Healed lacerations and surgical scars in a teenager with bilateral sciatic lacerations from glass. Left side was primarily repaired by the referring surgeon. When the proximal stump on the right could not be found through the transverse transecting laceration, the patient was sent for a secondary repair. Proximal stump had retracted to the level of the buttocks and required a lengthy up-and-down exposure to gain enough length for an end-to-end repair.

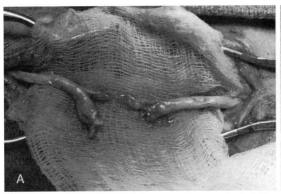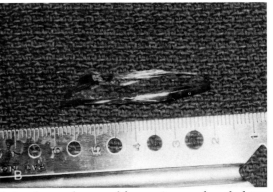

**Figure 2–2.** (*A*) Ulnar nerve severed somewhat obliquely by glass and exposed for repair several weeks later. Note slightly bulbous but minimally neuromatous proximal and distal stumps. This lesion probably could have been repaired primarily within the first day or two after injury. (*B*) A shard of glass responsible for a transecting injury to nerve.

is mild and incomplete to that which is severe and total. In addition, ability to recover is quite variable, as is the time required for recovery.[30] Serial electrical studies on partially lacerated and initially quantified functional loss in primates indicate some extension of loss within the first few hours.[39] This is presumably a result of loss of the perineurial nerve barriers provided by the various fascicles' perineurial envelopes and by intrafascicular as well as extrafascicular swelling[29] (Figure 2–4). Some of the progressive portion of the loss reverses through regeneration, but much does not. In the human, the partially transected portion of a nerve seldom regenerates well enough spontaneously to restore function. What does return in some cases can be attributed to reversal of neurapraxia or regeneration in the bruised and stretched portion of the nerve rather than in the transected portion.

The physical appearance of a totally transected nerve varies acutely and with time and is related to the sharpness of the laceration. With sharp transection, the epineurium is cleanly cut, and there is minimal contusive change or hemorrhage in either stump. With time and even

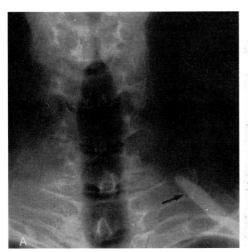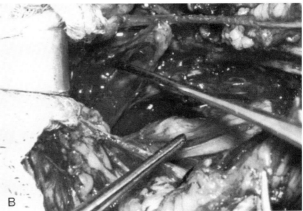

**Figure 2–3.** (*A*) Shard of glass (*arrow*) in neck and partially beneath the clavicle. This patient had sustained multiple head and neck lacerations from flying glass in a factory explosion. (*B*) Large piece of glass being extracted from beneath the left clavicle. It was resting on top of the lower trunk of the plexus, which it had contused but not lacerated. Middle trunk and upper trunk were mobilized somewhat laterally to make this exposure.

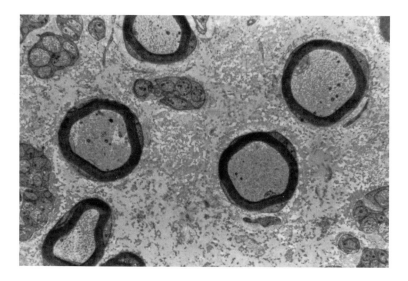

**Figure 2-4.** Electron micrograph showing area adjacent to partial nerve injury site at which perineurium had been disrupted. Axons have decreased myelin thickness, and there is increased ground substance between them.

with sharp division, the stumps retract and also become enveloped in scar. The amount of proximal and distal neuroma formed on either stump is minimal compared with that formed in a more contusive or blunt transection.

Blunt transection is associated with a ragged tear of the epineurium acutely and an irregular, up-and-down length of damage to a segment of the nerve. Bruising and hemorrhage can extend for several centimeters up or down either stump. With time, sizable proximal and distal neuromas develop (Figure 2-5). Retraction and proliferative scars around the stumps are often more severe than those that are seen with sharp transection.[11]

If the object penetrating the limb takes an oblique course through the soft tissues, the actual site of injury to the nerve may be at a distance from the entrance site (Figure 2-6). Any laceration serious enough to damage a nerve can also cut or bruise muscle, tendons, or vessels, and function of these structures also requires evaluation and sometimes repair.[45]

Operative iatrogenic transection may be sharp, as with scalpel injury, or blunt and rending, as with severe stretch during excessive retraction or manipulation of the limb or wound site. Nerve can also be inadvertently divided during surgery by cautery or by laser.

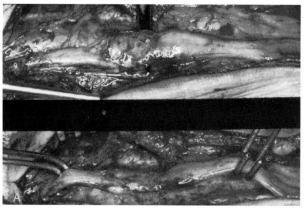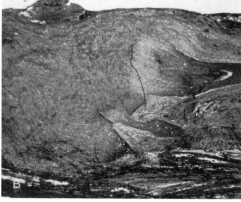

**Figure 2-5.** (A) Relatively sharp lesion to median nerve transecting most of it, exposed 5 weeks after injury (*top photograph*). Despite some physical continuity, there was no conducted nerve action potential (*lower photograph*). Lesion in continuity was resected, and an end-to-end epineurial repair was done. (B) Large neuroma caused by a blunt, transecting injury. Axons from the fasciculi to the right have attempted to grow to the left but are greatly disorganized and mixed with relatively heavy scar tissue. (Masson stain ×40.)

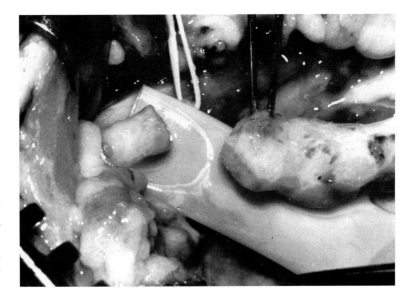

**Figure 2–6.** C5 spinal nerve transected by a knife at its junction with the upper trunk of the plexus. The wound of entrance was above the clavicle in the posterolateral neck and reached C5 in an oblique fashion.

## LESIONS (NEUROMAS) IN CONTINUITY

The majority of serious nerve injuries that lead to more than transient distal dysfunction do not transect or distract nerve but leave it in gross continuity. Depending on the series reported and the practice pattern of the clinician, this figure can vary between 60 and 70% of serious nerve injuries. If loss is partial in the distal distribution of such an injury, improvement is more likely to occur, but this is not always the case. Even with incomplete loss, predictability of outcome is limited. Prognosis is especially complicated if loss distal to a lesion in continuity is complete (Table 2–1). In this case, good recovery may occur spontaneously with time, or recovery may be partial and less than that which a good repair would achieve, or, surprisingly often, very little significant spontaneous return of function may occur. This makes prediction of outcome with lesions in continuity very difficult.[36]

Lesions in continuity can be either focal or diffuse, and can even have skipped areas of damage depending on the mechanism of injury. In most cases, the entire cross section of the nerve has the same extent of damage.[38] In some cases, however, one or more fascicles may be

**TABLE 2–1**
Management of Neuroma in Continuity

---

**Incomplete Loss With Significant Distal Sparing**

---

Most cases improve with conservative treatment. Follow-up by serial clinical and electromyographic (EMG) examinations.
Operation may still be required:
    Partial lesions associated with expanding masses caused by hematoma, aneurysm, or arteriovenous fistula usually require urgent operation.
    Partial lesions near or in areas of potential entrapment may require relatively early operation.
    Lesions in which distal loss is partial but significant may require later operation.
    Neural pain not amenable to medications and physical therapy may require later operation.

**Complete or Almost Complete Loss With Little or no Distal Sparing**

---

Relatively focal lesions in continuity caused by fracture or gunshot wound:
    Follow by clinical and EMG examinations for 2 to 3 months.
    If no clinical or electrical improvement, explore.
    Use intraoperative stimulation and nerve action potential (NAP) studies to decide for or against resection.
Relatively lengthy lesions in continuity caused by stretch/contusion or shotgun wound:
    Follow by clinical and EMG examinations for 4 to 5 months.
    If no significant clinical or electrical improvement, explore.
    If no response to stimulation and no NAP across lesion, resect and repair by suture or graft.
Intraoperative evoked cortical or somatosensory studies may be necessary to evaluate reparability of proximal spinal nerves.

---

partially or completely spared. This results in partial deficit distal to the lesion. In a few cases, all or a portion of the fibers are concussed and have a temporary neurapraxic injury, resulting in a reversible deficit. In other cases, there is a spectrum of fiber injury types involving not only neurapraxic block in conduction but also axonotmesis and neurotmesis.[57] With serious loss of function, axonotmesis and neurotmesis predominate. Effective spontaneous regeneration depends on minimal connective tissue damage. Unfortunately, with many stretch-contusive injuries, injury to perineurial and endoneurial layers is severe, connective tissue proliferation occurs, and effective axonal regeneration is minimal.[56]

With the usual lesion in continuity, the nerve is acutely swollen, with extravasation of serum and blood elements, necrosis of axons with loss of their myelin coverings, and some disruption of the connective tissue elements.[59,80] Wallerian degeneration occurs, and axonal and myelin debris is phagocytized from both the injury site and more distal nerve. The Schwann cells and also the basal lamina and distal connective tissue elements survive, and they are ready for new axonal downgrowth. Unfortunately, the endoneurial and perineurial elements at the injury site rapidly proliferate and lay down poorly structured collagen, interfering with organized and properly directed axonal regeneration. Because there is some retrograde damage proximal to the injury site with most nerve injuries, clusters of regenerating axons must first make up this area of loss and then struggle through the injury site disorganized by the poorly restructured collagen.[34] Axons are forced to branch many times as they traverse the site of injury. Such axonal branching in the human may occur several hundred times.[79] Other axons may be deflected into peripheral connective tissue layers at the injury site as well as distally. Axons reaching distal stump are thin, poorly myelinated, and less likely to reach prior distal end inputs than with a more axonotmetic injury. Many serious lesions in continuity are therefore not capable of regeneration of a quality to lead to recovery of useful distal function.

If connective tissue disorganization is severe, regenerating axons, although penetrating the injury site by the thousands, are poor in caliber and misdirected.[80] On the other hand, if connective tissue involvement is mild with relative preservation of not only perineurial tissues but a proportion of the endoneurial pathways across the injury site, axons regenerate well, regenerative units reach distal structures after minimal branching, and individual axons come close to prior innervational inputs and eventually regain an adequate degree of caliber and myelination. This is the type of spontaneous regeneration that can lead to restoration of useful function.

Predicting which lesion in continuity will recover adequate distal function spontaneously is difficult. A less severe compressive or contusive injury, a very mild stretch injury, or, surprisingly some gunshot wounds (GSW) are more likely to spare some internal connective tissue architecture and permit a structured axonal response. The patient presenting with brachial plexitis usually recovers function over a period of time, but there are also exceptions with this disorder of unknown cause.[49,72] Those injuries resulting from the more contusive and stretching forces associated with high-speed land, water, and air accidents are less likely to regenerate in a fashion leading to useful distal function. *Despite these generalizations, it is difficult to predict outcome, and most lesions in continuity have an uncertain future.*[70] For these reasons, most lesions in continuity are clinically followed and re-evaluated at intervals for several months before surgical exploration, intraoperative recordings, and repair are undertaken.

A nerve that has been sutured or repaired by grafts also becomes a lesion or neuroma in continuity.[79] The size, firmness, and histologic appearance of such a lesion depends on the interval since repair, the thoroughness of resection of damaged tissue before suture, the accuracy with which the stumps and their fascicular structures were opposed, and the degree of tension on the repair site.[68] Variable proportions of the suture neuroma in continuity are derived from epineurial and from interfascicular epineurial connective tissue proliferation, but the scar that usually thwarts successful regeneration is derived from the endoneurial fibroblasts. Even with an excellent repair, the new lesion in continuity produced by the suture or grafts shows swirls of connective tissue and a variable number of misdirected axons. Some axons reach more distal fascicular structure, but others are directed by the repair site scar into extrafascicular sites within the interfascicular epineurium or even the epineurium itself. Even with a poor repair, however, a large number of axons reach the distal stump of the nerve, because the neuronal thrust for regeneration of axons is great. Depending on the number of times they must divide to reach this level and the scar at the repair site, axons may or may not take on enough caliber to be functional.

Another factor affecting function is whether regenerating fibers reach or come close to previously innervated sites for sensation and motor function. Even if the fibers are successful in reaching distal innervational sites and maturing at the level of the distal stump, they remain slender and relatively poorly myelinated for many years at the repair site.[79,80] With a poor repair, connective tissue proliferation is great. Axons are forced by the scar to divide many more times to traverse this barrier, distal extrafascicular placement is more likely, and maturity of fibers at the repair site and also more distally is less complete than with a successful repair.

## NEUROPHYSIOLOGY OF LESIONS IN CONTINUITY

Because most lesions or neuromas in continuity have lost axonal continuity, the Wallerian process occurs. This takes time, and stimulation distal to the injury site can produce muscular contraction for 1 to 3 days even though the patient cannot contract those muscles voluntarily. In the experimental setting, early regenerating fine fibers can be stimulated and recorded from across a lesion in continuity. This requires direct stimulation and recording from the nerve. To record such nerve action potentials (NAPs) in the early days after injury, summation is necessary, as is a computer to average, integrate, and take the small potentials generated off the slope of the trace descending from the stimulus artifact peak. This is interesting but not clinically predictive because almost all lesions in continuity have such fine fibers penetrating the injury site. These fibers may or may not mature enough to become functional with time.

Intraoperative recording can produce reliable information about regeneration by 6 to 8 weeks after injury in relatively focal lesions in continuity caused by fractures and some contusions and

GSWs.[37,69] Less focal lesions require more time for adequate regeneration to occur through the lesion in continuity and to be picked up by even direct operative NAP recording. Several thousand fibers greater than 6 $\mu$m in diameter are required to produce such an NAP. In an adequately regenerating lesion in continuity, such a response can be traced through the injury site and into the distal stump. Amplification used is similar to that provided by an oscilloscope with a differential amplifier, and a computer is not necessary to integrate or summate such responses.

With further time, adequate regeneration is heralded by reversal of distal denervational change in muscle and presence of nascent or early reinnervation potentials.[24] Insertional activity and eventually a muscle action potential (MAP or MUAP) can be evoked on electromyography (EMG).[32] In addition, at some time before recovery of voluntary function, stimulation of the successfully regrowing nerve is able to produce muscular contraction. These more distally related regenerative changes take many months to occur, particularly in sciatic injuries, in proximal arm-level radial, median, and ulnar injuries, and in most brachial plexus injuries.

Conduction velocity determinations, which are usually dependent on recording from distal reinnervational sites, remain slow, and this may be true for many months. Conduction across the injury site also remains slow for years and sometimes forever because, despite more distal axonal maturation, fiber diameter and myelination remain poor at the injury site. Velocity values assess large fibers only, whereas NAP amplitude and the area beneath the NAP curve give a rough estimate of the fiber spectrum involved. There are relative variables such as interelectrode distance, electrode contact, wound temperature, and moisture, and these factors must be assessed before final interpretation of NAP amplitudes is completed.[14]

## STRETCH, TRACTION, AND CONTUSION

The largest category of serious injuries to nerve is stretch, traction, and contusion. This relates to the fact that the majority of forces injurious to nerve are blunt or tractive in nature.[34] Such forces can occasionally distract a nerve, pulling it totally apart, but more commonly leave it in continuity. If distracted by such forces, nerve is frayed, and both stumps are damaged over many centimeters. Retraction and scar about both stumps are severe. If nerve is left in continuity, as is more likely, the degree of intraneural damage is variable and may, on occasion, present as a spectrum of fiber change including axonotmesis and neurotmesis as well as neurapraxia.

Mechanisms responsible for a relatively mild degree of stretch may be associated with forces producing fractures or those related to lesser degrees of surgical retraction[60] (Figure 2–7). More commonly, traction forces are sufficient to tear apart intraneural connective tissue structure as well as disconnect axons[62] (Figure 2–8). Such lesions are Sunderland grade IV and are neurotmetic despite physical continuity of the nerve.[28] Less frequently, such forces result in a more axonotmetic or Sunderland grade II or III lesion which may have the potential for effective regeneration because of less connective tissue destruction.

Brachial plexus stretch injury is a common disorder resulting in blunt damage. Stretch or traction injuries to the plexus most commonly result from extremes of movement at the shoulder joint, with or without actual dislocation or fracture of the humerus or the clavicle. With blunt or traction forces, scapular, rib, or cervical spine fractures, or any combination of these, can also occur. A clavicular fracture attests to the disruptive force applied to the shoulder joint but may or may not imply a focal injury to the underlying plexus.[67] Either upper or lower elements of the plexus may suffer the predominant injury, or, with severe traction forces, all elements may be involved in addition to phrenic nerve and even subclavian vessels (Figure 2–9). All grades of damage are possible. Spinal nerves and roots can be avulsed from the spinal cord or more laterally from truncal or more distal outflows. The stretched elements may be left in continuity and have a mixture of neurapraxia and axonotmesis. More commonly, only neurotmesis or, less frequently, a combination of neurapraxia, axonotmesis, and neurotmesis may coexist.

Most traction injuries do not avulse or pull apart the plexus elements. Instead, the elements are left in some continuity but have a severe degree of internal disruption such as a neurotmetic or Sunderland grade IV injury. Each plexus element may have a different grade of damage within the same injury site. In such cases, the

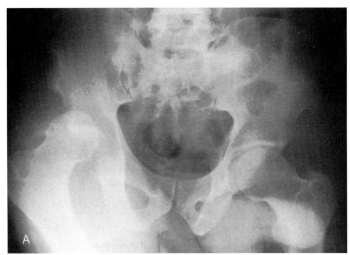
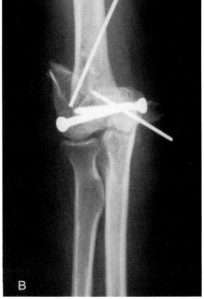

**Figure 2–7.** (*A*) Right hip dislocation resulted in a sciatic nerve injury. (*B*) Distal humeral fracture associated with ulnar nerve injury. Fracture was fixed by pins and screws.

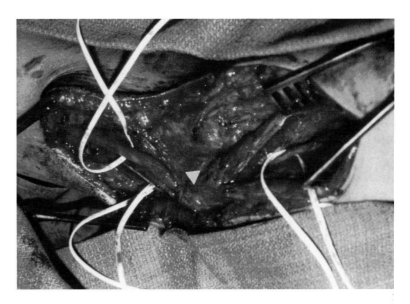

**Figure 2-8.** Median nerve entrapped at a fracture site (*arrowhead*).

lesion is not focal but extends over 5 to 6 cm or more of nerve. The effect of stretch on peripheral nerve is similar throughout the body, but specific anatomic relationships contribute to characteristic patterns of injury in the case of brachial plexus stretch.[65]

The attachment of the rootlets to the spinal cord is best appreciated by examination of an anatomic specimen. A surgeon can observe the delicate rootlets during spinal operations, and the radiologist can demonstrate these structures effectively by the use of water-soluble contrast material, provided sufficient concentration is maintained in the cervical area (Figure 2-10).

Magnetic resonance imaging (MRI) can on occasion delineate the actual root itself, but such noninvasive visualization is difficult to obtain in a consistent fashion for the entire length of one root, let alone for each root making up the brachial plexus. Traction along the axis of the brachial plexus can literally tear these roots out of the spinal cord. Subsequent observation at open operation during a dorsal root entry zone procedure for pain reveals the absence of any dorsal proximal stumps and the presence of brownish staining of the pia in a line with unaffected rootlets above and below the primary lesion, as well as some cord atrophy on that side.[19]

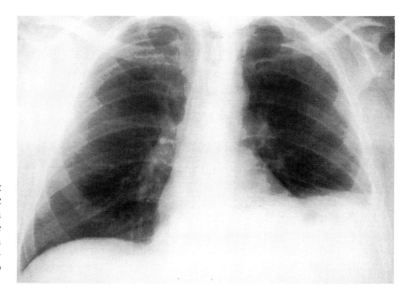

**Figure 2-9.** Elevation of left diaphragm because of phrenic nerve injury associated with a severe stretch injury to the plexus. When seen with a closed injury, this finding implies very proximal damage to L5.

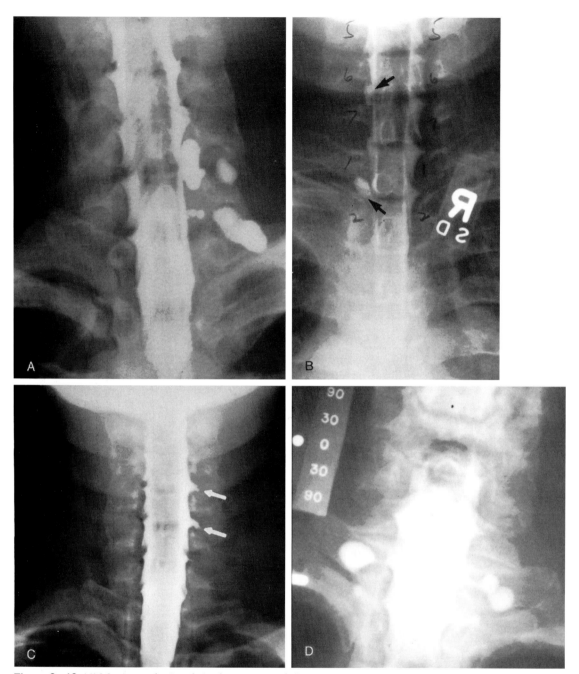

**Figure 2–10.** (*A*) Meningoceles involving lower roots of plexus associated with a stretch injury. (*B*) More subtle meningoceles associated with left C7 and T1 spinal nerves (*arrows*). (*C*) Small meningoceles (*arrows*) associated with the C5 and C6 spinal nerves on the left. (*D*) Tarlov cysts involving the T1 roots bilaterally.

Avulsion of rootlets subtended by a single spinal nerve does not imply avulsion of all the rootlets of the brachial plexus; likewise, rootlet avulsion may coexist with brachial plexus injuries more peripherally placed and affecting other elements of the plexus.

After the roots penetrate dura, they become spinal nerves. The spinal nerves run in the gutters of the foramina in the vertebrae for which they are named. At this intraforaminal level, the nerves are relatively tethered by mesoneurial-like connections to the gutters. The spinal nerves then angle inferiorly to appear between the scalenus anticus and scalenus medius muscles and thus gain the posterior triangle of the neck. Spinal nerves are often injured in a characteristic fashion just as they run off the lip of the gutter of the transverse process. Forces here may distract spinal nerve from trunk or, more commonly, produce severe intraneural damage resulting in lengthy lesions in continuity that involve not only spinal nerves and trunks but also more distal elements.

The clavicle, padded by the subclavius, has an important relation to the plexus, but common clavicular fracture rarely involves the brachial plexus. However, the entire plexus may be tethered at this point, and abduction and adduction of the arm at operation may show acute angulation of the nerve structures below the clavicle if they cannot move freely in a normal fashion.

A very common finding with severe stretch injuries is to see cords pulled away from more proximal elements of the plexus such as roots and trunks. Unfortunately, under these circumstances, intraneural damage on these proximal elements often extends close to, if not all the way to, the spinal theca or cord.[66] Callus from a healing clavicular fracture may, on occasion, impinge directly on the plexus, where it may cause a brachial plexus palsy by compression or prolong or aggravate underlying nerve injury. More distal infraclavicular stretch injury is not uncommon and frequently involves the axillary nerve (Figure 2–11).

Occasionally, even the lumbosacral plexus may sustain a stretch injury. This results in a lengthy lesion in continuity or distraction of lumbosacral roots, as suggested by meningoceles on myelography. Distal intraneural damage to the lumbar or sacral plexus can occur in association with some extensive pelvic fractures or, more rarely, with severe hyperextension of the thigh.

Birth palsies from difficult deliveries are less common now because of improved obstetrical training and practice, but they still occur. The most common is Erb's palsy, involving the upper and middle trunk, which is usually caused by forcible depression of the shoulder and arm during delivery of the infant. Klumpke paralysis involves damage to the lower trunk, roots, or spinal nerves and occurs because the arm remains caught in the pelvis and is held abducted while traction is applied to the body. Like stretch injuries in adults, some injuries in children improve and some do not, but unlike the adult injuries, which are usually caused by greater forces, those associated with delivery have a greater chance for spontaneous recovery.

The peroneal nerve can be stretched in association with a variety of knee injuries and sometimes with fracture or avulsion of the fibular head.[77] Peroneal components of the sciatic nerve at the level of the sciatic notch and buttocks can be stretched with hip dislocation or fracture. A stretch mechanism is also responsible for segments of damage to nerve dis-

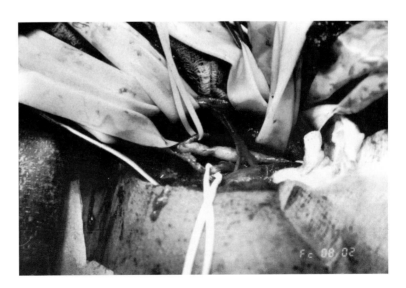

**Figure 2–11.** A very focal stretch injury involving the axillary nerve. Subscapular branches are encircled with the white plastic loops. (Reprinted with permission from Dubuisson A, Kline D: Indications for peripheral nerve and brachial plexus surgery. Neurol Clin North Am 10:935–951, 1992.)

placed by high-velocity missiles, especially with GSWs.

The important point with stretch injuries is that, although some may improve, there may be no definitive operative answer for those that do not. If the major injury is neurotmetic, it can involve such a long segment of the neural complex that the only operative method for replacing the resulting extensive neuroma is use of lengthy grafts, which may fail at the proximal levels where many stretch injuries begin.

## GUNSHOT WOUNDS TO NERVE

A frequent source of contusion and stretch to nerve is GSW (Figure 2–12). In some parts of the world, this is a common source of nerve injury even in a peacetime, civilian setting. Most

such injuries are not caused by direct hit of the nerve by the missile or its fragments. This does occur about 15% of the time and can result in physical, albeit blunt, partial or complete transection of the nerve. In a few other cases, particularly shotgun blast, pellets can embed in nerve even though its continuity is maintained. In an equally small number of cases, missile fragments can strike adjacent bone and secondarily drive bone fragments into nerve, once again partially or completely transecting it.

In the majority of cases, nerve injured by GSW is left in physical continuity.[33] Such lesions have a variable degree of intraneural derangement. This is because most (85%) of missile trajectories associated with neural injury do not directly strike nerve, but instead provide a near miss, but one which can be as destructive as a direct hit.[64] As the missile approaches nerve, the latter explodes away from its trajec-

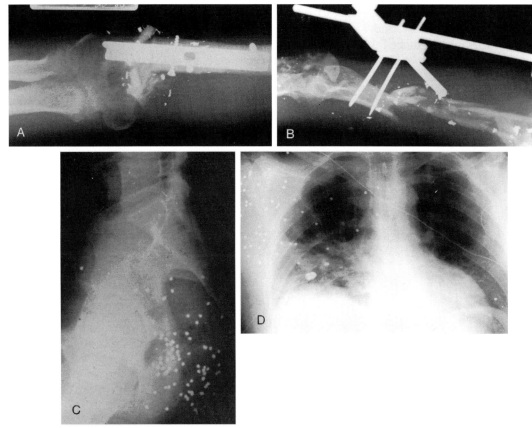

**Figure 2–12.** Various gunshot wounds (GSW) involving nerves. (A) Severe GSW fractured distal humerus and required repair by plate and screws. Injury also involved median nerve. (B) Forearm fractures caused by a GSW required external fixation. Both median and ulnar nerves were injured. (C) Shotgun injury to buttocks involved sciatic nerve. (D) Shotgun injury involving right chest and infraclavicular brachial plexus.

tory and then implodes back as the missile passes by.[54] These dual stretchings as well as contusive forces can result in a neurapraxic block in conduction, axonotmesis, neurotmesis, or a mixture of two or even three of these injury types. All too frequently, the contusive and stretching forces associated with GSW pull apart not only axons but also their connective tissue investments and even intraneural vasculature. Such damage extends over a length of the nerve. Acutely, it produces a swollen, somewhat hemorrhagic neural segment. With time, as connective tissue proliferates and sprouts divide many times, a neuroma in continuity is produced. This lesion may or may not have the potential for useful regeneration, depending on the proportion of axonotmetic to neurotmetic changes.

If missiles transect or partially lacerate nerve, the lesion is a blunt and not a sharp injury. Acutely, the nerve end tends to be shredded and irregular, with hemorrhagic contusive changes in both stumps.[76] With time, a bulbous proximal neuroma and less swollen distal neuroma form, as with other blunt transecting mechanisms such as auto metal, fan blades, propellers, and chain saws. Embedded shell fragments or spicules of bone may be associated with localized edema or hemorrhage. With time, intraneural connective tissue elements may proliferate around these foreign objects.

Because it takes time to determine the extent of tissue change, whether nerve is transected or stretched but left in continuity, delay in exploration and repair is usually indicated.[37] Associated vascular, osseous, pulmonary, or abdominal wounds may require more acute surgical intervention. Acute hematoma, traumatic aneurysm, arteriovenous fistula, and neural injury close to areas of potential entrapment may also require relatively early operation. Some pain syndromes such as true causalgia require early sympathetic blocks and, in many cases, sympathectomy. On occasion, shell fragments embedded in nerve or intraneural pellets produce a severe dysesthetic pain. Manipulation of the nerve associated with their relatively early removal can sometimes help such pain.

An excellent example of the role of an associated injury is provided by vascular injury. Pseudoaneurysm is usually secondary to a relatively small hole or laceration in a major artery caused by a penetrating missile or a knife or other sharp instrument (Figure 2–13). Blood under pressure dissects into and around the wall of the vessel. This produces an expanding mass which can compress adjacent nerves. This is especially true with pseudoaneurysms of the axillary, femoral, and popliteal arteries, sites at which vessels are in close juxtaposition to nerves. An axillary artery aneurysm, for example, may compress lateral, posterior, or medial cord and its peripheral outflows, since plexus elements are incorporated in the wall of the false aneurysm. Such compression as well as stretching often further compounds partial or incomplete injury to these elements, leading to a progressive loss of function.[35]

Few lesions produce progression of peripheral nerve loss after the first few hours have passed. Pseudoaneurysm, arteriovenous fistula, and hematomas are the exceptions. On the other hand, some progression of damage may very well occur in the early hours after wounding. Serial electrical studies on partially lacerated nerves with initially documented loss indicate some extension of loss within the first few hours.[39] This is presumably caused by loss of the perineurial nerve barriers provided by the various fascicles' perineurial envelopes and by intrafascicular as well as extrafascicular swelling. Some of the progressive portion of the loss reverses with regeneration, but much does not.

## ISCHEMIA AND COMPRESSION

### Ischemia

Peripheral nerve, like other neural tissues, is critically dependent on blood flow. Because it is rarely possible to compress a nerve segment without simultaneously affecting its blood supply, the relative roles of ischemia and physical deformation in compression lesions remain unsettled.[8] Recent evidence suggests that although ischemia may be primarily responsible for a mild type of rapidly reversible nerve lesion, direct mechanical distortion is the major factor underlying more severe, long-lasting forms of pressure palsy such as Saturday night palsy or tourniquet paralysis.[75] Nevertheless, it is likely

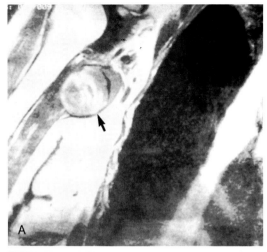

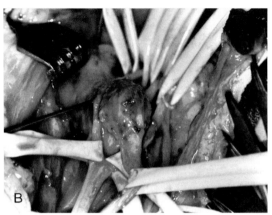

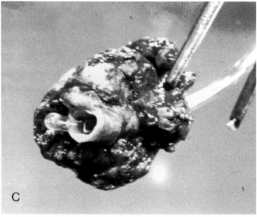

**Figure 2–13.** (*A*) Magnetic resonance scan of an axillary pseudoaneurysm (*arrow*) caused by a penetrating wound. (*B*) Exposure of pseudoaneurysm. Lateral and medial cord contributions to the median nerve were stretched and deformed by this lesion. (*C*) Another pseudoaneurysm which required resection of a segment of axillary artery for repair. Note that the artery is patent. Preoperative arteriogram was normal.

that in most compressive lesions, including chronic entrapment neuropathies, localized ischemia at the site of deformation plays some role.[12,78] Ischemia can produce a wide range of nerve fiber lesions and, if severe and prolonged, results in widespread axonal loss and Wallerian degeneration.[18]

In less severe degrees of ischemia, reduction in nerve fiber density is characteristically the result of early dropout of large myelinated fibers.[42] Although damage to a nutrient artery may lead to ischemic injury of a peripheral nerve, pure, isolated ischemic neurogenic lesions are uncommon in humans. An example is occasionally provided by a midforearm-level injury or by some vascular diseases affecting median nerve with its dominant median artery. Here, necrosis of the distal stump of the nerve may occur. More commonly, nerve trunks are involved along with other soft tissue structures of the limbs such as muscle and major vessels,

and the severity of the nerve injury depends on the degree and duration of ischemia and compression. Studies on limb ischemia suggest that there is a critical period of approximately 8 hours, after which irreversible nerve injury ensues.[43]

The vascular anatomy of peripheral nerves, with rich anastomoses between longitudinal vessels in the epineurium, perineurium, and endoneurium and the regional segmental supply, allows the surgeon to mobilize long segments of nerve without producing ischemia. Nevertheless, extensive intraneural dissection by an inexperienced surgeon can jeopardize the microcirculation and result in ischemic damage.[44] Evidence also suggests that a transected nerve or one under tension is more sensitive to ischemia.[61] The surgeon should minimize interruption of both regional and segmental longitudinal vascular supply and also avoid tension at the suture site.

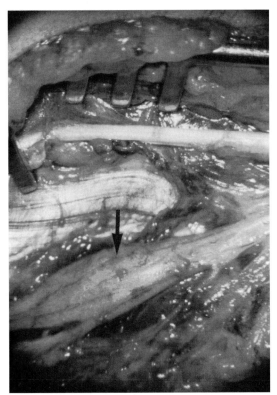

**Figure 2–14.** Enlargement of posterior interosseous nerve (*arrow*) just proximal to entrapment site at arcade of Frohse. Superficial sensory radial nerve is seen at the top.

## Compression

The sequential pathology of nerve fiber injury is rather stereotyped and occurs regardless of the compressive agent[1] (Figure 2–14). An ex-ception to this rule appears to be the nerve fiber pathology that results from more minor forms of compression.[26] Compression of nerve fibers appears to produce myelinated nerve fiber changes that are peculiar to this mechanism.[2,50] These include alterations in paranodal myelination, axonal thinning, and segmental demyelination.[15,16,17,55] Wallerian degeneration results from more severe degrees of compression.

The degree of recovery after compression or ischemic injury may be accurately predicted in some clinical situations. The characteristic Saturday night palsy results from compression of the radial nerve against the humerus. Total radial nerve palsy often results, but return of motor and sensory function occurs in the majority of cases without any need for surgical intervention. Most palsies associated with unconsciousness due to anesthesia and poor positioning or pressure during operation as well as those related to improper application of plaster casts carry a good prognosis for spontaneous recovery.[45] There are, however, important exceptions. Sometimes the compression or crushing injury has been severe enough or prolonged enough to cause damage that is irreversible unless operative repair is done (Figure 2–15). The brachial plexus and the ulnar, sciatic, and peroneal nerves are most commonly affected.[52] On the other hand, restoration of function after acute compression and ischemic injury may be less certain in other circumstances. It may be difficult, for example, to predict the degree of recovery that follows evacuation of hematomas

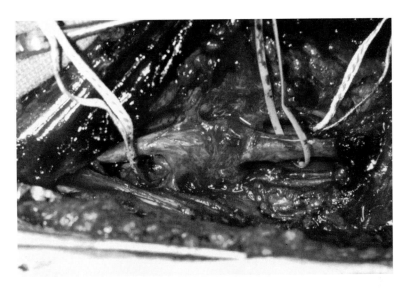

**Figure 2–15.** Crushing injury to lateral cord of the brachial plexus.

or relief of aneurysmal compression of such structures as the brachial plexus and the femoral or sciatic nerves.[23] There are also circumstances in which two levels of compression may exist.[74] The patient with cervical spondylolysis or relatively mild disc disease affecting a root or spinal nerve may be more likely to become symptomatic with an otherwise mild degree of compression of the median nerve at the wrist or ulnar nerve at the elbow. In these circumstances, multiple factors exist that affect the outcome of peripheral nerve surgery, including the identity and level of the nerve involved, the age of the patient, the extent of the precompression injury to nerve, and the timing of the corrective surgery.

Severe crushing injury, skeletal fracture with vascular compromise, and anticoagulant administration can lead to increased pressure within a fascial compartment, and severe compression and ischemic damage to peripheral nerves as well as other soft tissues can result. A closed compartment syndrome with impending ischemic paralysis requires immediate decompression with properly placed and usually extensive, longitudinal fasciotomies.[63] Delay in treatment results in ischemic infarction of muscle, nerve, and other tissues, leading to contractures and other crippling deformities.

## Compartment Syndromes

Volkmann contracture is a serious example of ischemic compression. Paralysis can follow manipulation with or without casting and immobilization of a closed fracture near the elbow that is associated with severe muscle swelling and hemorrhage into the anterior compartment of the forearm.[25] This type of ischemic injury is most frequently associated with supracondylar fracture of the humerus and dislocation of the elbow and can occur even before manipulation or casting is done. Actual infarction of the volar forearm musculature can occur. Blunt but contusive injury to the forearm, such as from a pool cue or baseball bat, can also result in enough swelling to compress nerves secondarily even though arterial injury or spasm may not be present. Two patients seen by us had been injured by pool cue blows to the forearm, and

swelling led to both radial and median nerve palsies even though there was no fracture of the radius or ulna.

In the usual Volkmann case, there is injury to the brachial artery along with diffuse segmental damage to the median nerve and volar forearm muscles. The large median and sometimes radial nerve fibers serving motor and proprioceptive function are more severely involved than the smaller pain fibers. The EMG may aid in diagnosis by showing temporary but repetitive and spontaneous motor discharges from muscles most distal to the injury site.[32] Swelling of the forearm resulting in a painful paresthetic hand must alert the physician to a tight-space syndrome long before more obvious signs of vascular compromise are apparent.

Ischemia of sufficient magnitude to produce Volkmann's contracture results in severe endoneurial scarring over so long a segment of the median nerve as to make spontaneous regeneration unlikely (Figure 2–16). Bunnell believed that Volkmann's contracture was sufficiently explained by closed-space compression of the brachial vessel between the fracture and the lacertus fibrosus at the level of the elbow.[65] In any case, spasm of the artery results in ischemia and sometimes in actual infarction of soft tissues of the volar forearm compartment.

Section and repair of the damaged segment of the brachial artery may be necessary.[58] Anticoagulation alone may not suffice and may even be deleterious. We have seen one patient whose syndrome progressed shortly after heparinization, probably because of hemorrhage into already ischemic musculature.

In addition to the median nerve, the radial and even occasionally the ulnar nerve may be involved because of a severely swollen elbow and forearm, particularly if the contracture was initially associated with multiple contusive injuries at these levels. Immediate fasciotomy is in order because remedial operation for the more severe degrees of Volkmann's contracture, although possible, is disappointing.[73] Compression of the median nerve must be relieved by operation, especially in the region of the pronator teres and flexor digitorum sublimis muscles. Closed-space swelling of this type can be aggravated by a tight-fitting cast or by fixation of the elbow in acute flexion. Emergency treatment is

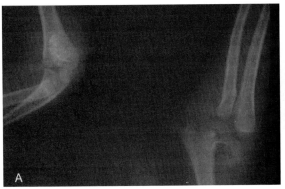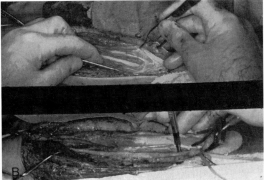

**Figure 2–16.** (*A*) Distal humeral fracture-dislocation that resulted in brachial arterial damage and Volkmann's ischemia. (*B*) Long-standing Volkmann's contracture caused by intra-arterial morphine injection. Pronator over median has been replaced by both scar and fat and is being pulled away from median nerve in top photograph. Lengthy ischemic as well as acutely compressed segment of median is shown in lower photograph. Area to the right in the lower photograph looks like a finger but is caused by a bloodied stockinette. See also color figure.

necessary at the first signs of ischemia if irreversible neural damage and contractures of the extremity are to be prevented.

A related condition is the anterior compartment syndrome involving the lower leg, which results in a progressive peroneal palsy or foot drop. A fracture or fractures of the tibia and fibula may or may not be a concomitant finding, but soft-tissue swelling is always present. Early fasciotomy is indicated, just as with Volkmann's contracture. Tissue pressure can be readily measured by placing a needle in the swollen limb and attaching it to a saline-filled tube and manometer. If the difference between arterial pressure measured by cuff and tissue pressure measured by manometer is less than 40 mm Hg, ischemic infarction is likely to occur.

In summary, extension of neural injury by compression and ischemia is a serious possibility if enough soft tissue swelling or an aneurysm, fistula, hematoma, or arterial insufficiency occurs in a relatively closed or confined neurovascular compartment. These lesions are particularly apt to occur with perforating wounds that involve arteries and with fractures but can also be caused by blunt or contusive trauma. Neural damage usually is preventable, but it becomes irreversible if severe ischemia involves a long segment of nerve and/or persists for too long a period of time.

## ELECTRICAL INJURY

Electrical injury by passage of a large current through a peripheral nerve usually results from accidental contact of the extremity with a high-tension wire.[9] If the individual does not succumb to respiratory or cardiac arrest, diffuse nerve and muscle damage results.[3] Pathologic reports of peripheral nerve damage caused by this mechanism are sparse, and guidelines for treatment are controversial.[13] Conservative management of the nerve injury itself and early orthopedic reconstruction of the extremity seem to be best.[27] Operative experience with seven such cases involving one or more peripheral nerves indicates that only a few of these lesions improve spontaneously with time. Resection of a lengthy segment of damaged nerve and repair by grafts is usually necessary. Histologically, the segment of the nerve is virtually replaced, first with necrosis and then with connective tissue reaction, including a severe degree of both perineurial and endoneurial scar tissue. Fascicular outline may be preserved, but intrafascicular damage can be severe enough to prevent any but fine axon regeneration. The accompanying severe skin burns and necrosis of bone and other soft tissues frequently thwart reconstructive efforts.[41] The muscle in the extremity often is extensively coagulated, leading to severe contractures, which further decreases the likelihood of useful reinnervation.

## THERMAL INJURY

Although not a common mechanism of peripheral nerve injury, thermal injury by flame, steam, or hot elements can result in neural damage ranging from a transient neurapraxia to severe neurotmesis with extensive necrosis of nerve as well as adjacent tissues. In patients with circumferential burns, neural damage may be related to delayed constrictive fibrosis, resulting in a tourniquet effect. Patients with severe burns involving nerve present with complete motor and sensory loss. The clinical examination is often difficult because of associated soft tissue injuries, extensive skin loss, and often a massively swollen extremity. The degree of tissue necrosis, the extent of bacterial contamination, and the need for an adequate soft tissue bed make immediate reconstruction of nerve rarely feasible. Proper attention to the wound with repeated escharectomy, if indicated, increases the success of secondary repairs. In thermal injury, whether by direct effect or secondary to constrictive fibrosis, long lengths of nerves are often involved, necessitating nerve grafts. The prognosis for functional recovery is poor in such cases, especially if there is also extensive involvement of muscle and other soft tissues.

Serious surface burns caused by thermal agents can lead to coagulation necrosis of underlying nerves. Like electrical injuries, the more serious burns can affect a length of nerve. Experience with four patients who required graft replacement of both median and ulnar nerves at the wrist demonstrated the difficulty in providing useful recovery. Although all four had undergone prior skin grafts or other soft tissue transfers to provide coverage, tendon grafts were also necessary in two of these patients. In one of these cases, burn involved the palmar surface of the hand, and severe contractures were present despite extensive prior soft tissue operations. Infection can complicate any soft tissue wound involving nerve (Figure 2–17). It is more likely to do so if the injury mechanism has produced necrosis of soft tissue, and thus it is often seen with thermal and electrical burns and some compartment syndromes. The nerve's epineurial and interfascicular connective tissue layers usually resist invasion unless they are extensively injured. There are, however, exceptions, and then infection can lead to an extensive segment of intraneural necrosis and a lengthy lesion that is difficult to repair with any success.

## INJECTION INJURY

Injection injury, a surprisingly common category of neural injury, deserves special attention.

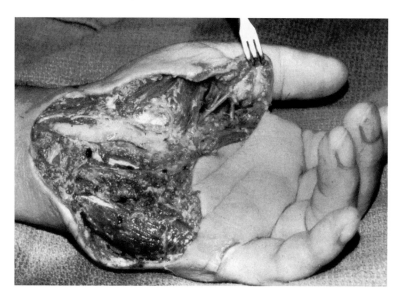

**Figure 2–17.** Severe infection of the palm of the hand after carpal tunnel release. Despite this, most of the median as well as ulnar hand function was maintained in this case, the nerve being somewhat resistant to infection.

It is caused by a needle placed into or close to nerve, and damage results from neurotoxic chemicals in the agent injected. The extent of damage varies, depending not only on the agent injected but whether the needle and therefore the toxic agent were placed in or close to nerve. There are cases in which some or all of the injury relates to the damage done by the needle placement itself. Experimentally, damage from injection seems to require placement of the agent either within the epineurium or, for more serious damage, at an intraneural locus, either intrafascicular or in the connective tissue layers between the fascicles.[20] In the human, however, about 10% of patients subsequently found to have an injection injury have a delay of hours or even days before the onset of symptoms. This suggests either a purely epineurial locus for deposition of the agent in these cases, place-

ment of medication close to but not in the nerve, or placement in a tissue plane from which the agent can gravitate to and bathe the nerve and thus possibly damage the nerve.

Pathology of injection injuries also varies depending on the injection site and the agent injected.[4] With the unfortunately more common intraneural locus, there is acute edema and inflammatory change, often with necrosis, which usually includes connective tissue elements as well as axons and their coverings[46] (Figure 2–18). With time, connective tissue elements may proliferate, producing intraneural scar, and this can thwart effective axonal regeneration.[53] The blood-nerve barriers at both the perineurial and endoneurial levels are severely affected.[21] This may occur despite maintenance of fascicular outlines. The principal pathogenetic mechanism is necrosis.[40] After the first few days, the

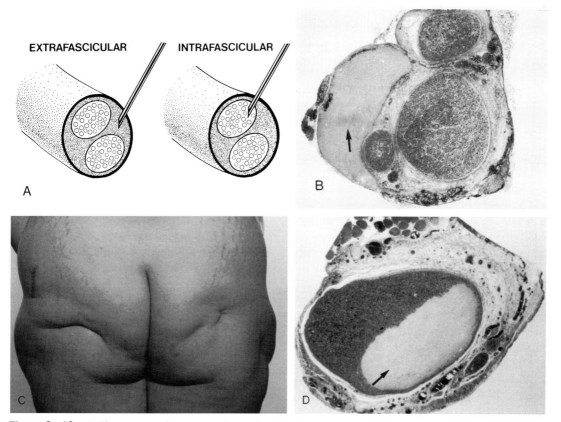

**Figure 2–18.** (A) The two usual intraneural sites for injection injuries. (B) Nerve injected at an extrafascicular site (*arrow*). (C) Buttocks of a patient who had multiple buttocks-level injections and received a sciatic palsy on the right. (D) Example of intrafascicular injection (*arrow*), in this case produced by direct injection of collagen in a primate nerve. (C) Reproduced with permission from Hudson A: Nerve injection injuries. Terzis J, Ed: Microreconstruction of Nerve Injuries. Philadelphia, WB Saunders, 1987.

injected segment is no longer swollen and may with further time appear shrunken or even as a segment of nerve with normal diameter. On gross inspection with or without magnification, the nerve usually appears to have excellent physical continuity. Even intraneural dissection may reveal good fascicular continuity despite intrafascicular damage that is quite neurotmetic. Some agents injected into epineurium or adjacent to nerve produce more proliferation of inflammatory tissue and scar than at an intraneural locus, but the necrosis at the latter locus is especially damaging and difficult for the regenerative process to overcome spontaneously.

In the usual clinical setting, needle placement results in an electric-like shock down the extremity, followed by or concomitant with a severe radicular burning pain and paresthesias as the agent is injected. Acute symptoms are variously described but are usually severe. Pain associated with the injection is described as searing, burning, electrical, or numbing, and with serious injection injury the sensation usually travels down the limb and in the distribution of the nerve injected.[51] With delayed onset, which seems to occur in about 10% of patients with injection injuries, the symptoms are less dramatic but nonetheless bothersome.[31] These include a burning pain, paresthesias, and radiation of a deep discomfort down the limbs and in the distribution of the less directly involved nerve.

Initial loss may be complete or incomplete in the distribution of the injected nerve. There can be a variable degree of sensory and motor loss. Sometimes, fiber dropout is mild, and although the lesion is painful, sensory or motor loss may be minimal. Occasionally, absence of reflexes or conductive abnormalities in the distribution of the injured nerve are the only clinical findings. More often, clinical loss is more dramatic and more severe, including complete sensory or motor loss or both. Initial loss may improve with time, but all too often severe loss persists with the more severe injection injuries. Initial loss may therefore persist depending on the severity of the injection injury. Denervational changes by EMG as well as clinical loss can be severe. Many such injuries do not regenerate adequately or at all, and, despite maintenance of physical continuity, clinical loss remains complete or severe unless corrected by surgical intervention.

The most common neural injection sites are the sciatic nerve at the buttock level and the radial nerve in the lateral upper arm.[40] Nonetheless, we have seen injection injuries involving almost every major nerve in the body (Figure 2–19). Included have been injection injuries to femoral and lateral femoral cutaneous nerves as well as ulnar and median nerves at wrist, elbow, and upper arm levels. Although quite unusual, injection injuries of musculocutaneous and antebrachial cutaneous nerves and even portions of the brachial plexus have been seen. The most common site is sciatic at the buttock or proximal thigh level.[5] Classically, this is most likely to occur if the injection is not made in the upper outer quadrant of the buttock.[7] However, from the histories given, even this may not always be a safe site. If the patient is lying on one side or bent over while standing, the relation of the presumed upper outer buttock quadrant to the sciatic nerve can change. Another factor making sciatic injection more likely to cause injury is a thinly constructed buttock, which is more likely in a cachectic, chronically ill patient or a constitutionally thin individual.

The length of the needle used and the angle at which the needle penetrates soft tissues are factors, but the force with which the injection is given is also a factor. If the hub of the needle inverts skin and underlying soft tissue with enough force during injection, the tip of the needle can penetrate to a level deeper than surmised. This may be compounded if the needle penetrates soft tissue at an angle headed toward nerve rather than at a right angle to a horizontal plane through the body. Other factors, such as movement of the patient as the injection is being made, can sometimes play a role. If the patient shrugs or jerks up the shoulder, perhaps in anticipation of the pain connected with the event, an injection intended for the deltoid can injure the radial nerve. Injection injury of radial nerve at the midhumeral level is the second most frequent site of injection injury. Infusions or needles intended for veins can also be inadvertently placed in nerves. This is more likely to occur to median or ulnar nerve, the former either at the wrist or elbow and the latter at the wrist. Infusion complications have, however, been also seen involving the brachial plexus, the femoral nerve, and the posterior tibial nerve at the ankle.

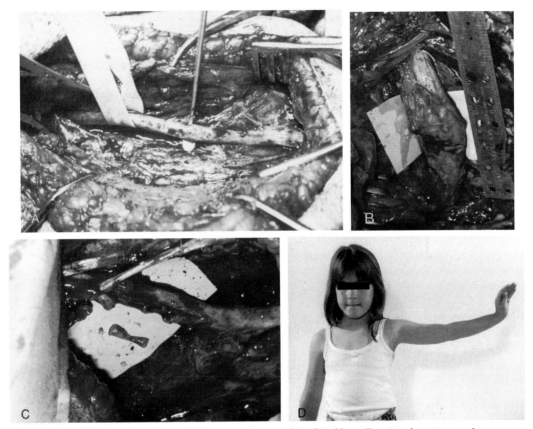

**Figure 2–19.** (*A*) Injection injury to radial nerve with complete distal loss. Despite almost normal gross appearance, it did not transmit a nerve action potential and required resection and repair 4.5 months after injury. (*B*) Severe, granulomatous injection injury involving sciatic nerve at a buttocks level. (*C*) Injection injury resulting in partial loss of function is in the process of a split repair. (*D*) Recovery of radial function after repair of a radial injection injury.

The sciatic nerve lies in a trough beneath the piriformis muscle and on top of the gemellus, quadratus, and obturator internus muscles, between the bony boundaries of the ischial tuberosity and the greater trochanter. Drugs not injected directly into the nerve may pool in this trough and bathe the nerve to produce neuritis. Intraneural damage is similar to the changes seen with antibiotic injection into the brain. Although the deficit in neural function usually is caused by intraneural neuritis and scar tissue rather than extraneural scarring, some authors believe that external neurolysis for this complication can reverse loss of function.[48] We do not agree with this; however, a lesion with partial loss of function and severe pain not responding to analgesics may be helped by internal neurolysis. An occasional patient may have a true causalgia after injection, and they may benefit from sympathectomy, especially if recurrent sympathetic blocks have provided temporary relief.

Sedatives and narcotics as well as antibiotics and steroids can cause injection neuropathy. If the complication is noticed immediately, 50 to 100 mL of normal saline can be placed in the region of the injection site in the hope of diluting the drug and avoiding permanent neuropathy. Open operative irrigation might be even more logical, but because such patients are not usually seen acutely, experience with either approach is lacking. If the nerve deficit is partial, expectant treatment is best, provided pain is not a severe problem, but if the deficit is complete after several months of observation, exploration becomes warranted. In this regard, if an injection injury to the sciatic nerve spares either the peroneal or tibial division but is complete in the other division, it is a complete lesion of one division, and this division may need resection and repair if function is to be regained.

Our policy with injection injuries has been to expose the nerve that shows little or no function after 8 to 16 weeks and attempt to evoke an NAP through the injury. If no response is recorded, the lesion must be resected. With sciatic palsies, one division may require resection and the other only neurolysis. The gross appearance of the nerve lesion is deceiving in many of these injuries. Segments that appear to inspection and palpation to be minimally injured may have such extensive axonal and endoneurial disruption as to preclude useful functional regeneration. In these cases, only resection and repair can provide hope for recovery. As a result, a severe palsy secondary to injection injury usually should be followed for only 2 to 4 months. If there is then no significant recovery, electrically or clinically, the nerve should be explored so that direct stimulation and evoked NAP studies can be made. The final caveat is that neuropathy from drug injections must be prevented by proper education of nurses and ancillary personnel as well as physicians.

## IRRADIATION INJURY

An iatrogenic cause of nerve damage less common than injection is irradiation.[6,71] This usually affects the brachial plexus but can also occur at the level of the pelvic plexus.[22] Extensive fibrosis to surrounding soft tissues and severe intraneural changes can result.[47] Management of these difficult cases is addressed in subsequent chapters.

## IATROGENIC INJURY

Accidental injury to a peripheral nerve creates a situation that is distressing to both the physician and the patient. It is essential that the patient be managed with great care so that the situation is not subsequently aggravated by inappropriate actions.

In the majority of iatrogenic cases we have seen, the originating physician was unaware that the nerve had been accidentally injured. The nerve may have been injured by inap-propriate retractor pressure or more directly by cautery, incision, or suture (Figure 2–20). Nerves may be injured by pressure while they are immobilized in the operating room or subsequently by plaster casts. Inappropriate operative management of peripheral nerves may also result in complete or partial nerve injury.

## Diagnosis

The iatrogenic nerve injury is diagnosed in exactly the same manner as any other nerve injury, that is, by a very careful motor and sensory clinical examination supplemented by electrophysiologic studies. The true diagnosis may not be apparent for a few days if the patient is immobilized postoperatively or is suffering from postoperative pain and is under sedation. For example, it is not unusual for sciatic or femoral nerve palsy complicating hip surgery to be diagnosed a few days after the operation (Figure 2–21). The local discomfort after a cervical

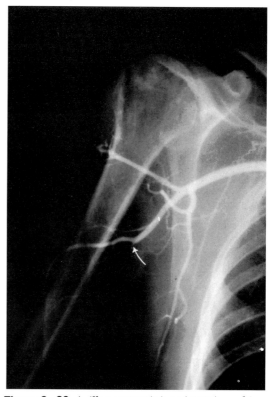

**Figure 2–20.** Axillary artery injury (*arrow*) resulting from a transaxillary first rib resection. The medial cord of the plexus was also severely injured.

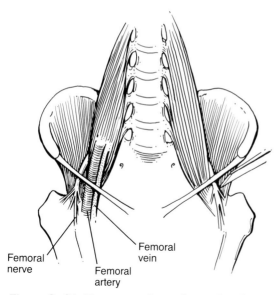

**Figure 2-21.** Damage to femoral complex during the course of a hip joint repair. In this case a periosteal dissector slipped medially on the anterior ileum and damaged the left femoral nerve.

Femoral nerve
Femoral vein
Femoral artery

lymph node biopsy may confuse the patient, but the symptoms resulting from trapezius palsy attendant on accessory nerve injury are usually reported by the patient within a few weeks of operation.

Record keeping should be of the highest order. It is totally inappropriate to redictate the original operative note after an iatrogenic injury is discovered postoperatively. Similarly, the chart should be carefully guarded so that it or portions of it are not lost. Any alteration or loss of records is liable to be interpreted as evidence of lack of honesty by the surgeon, even if this is not the case. Notes should be appropriate to the problem. Lengthy treatises concerning irrelevant issues, although accurate in themselves, may be subsequently interpreted as attempts to confuse rather than illuminate the clinical problem. It is most appropriate to consult an expert on nerve who records on the chart that such a consultation has occurred and its results.

## Management

In the majority of instances, the assumption is made that a lesion in continuity is present. The patient is therefore managed appropriately for 3 to 4 months while evidence of spontaneous regeneration is sought by repeated clinical examinations supplemented by electrical studies. Patients may require appropriate splints and other orthotic devices as well as physical therapy during this time of waiting (Figure 2-22).

If a sharp cut is made in a nerve and it is recognized at surgery, the appropriate management is to reconstitute the nerve using standard suture technique at the same operation. This allows end-to-end apposition. There is no requirement to trim the stumps, and retraction of nerve stumps will not have occurred.

If there is a strong probability that blunt transection has occurred at operation, then it may be

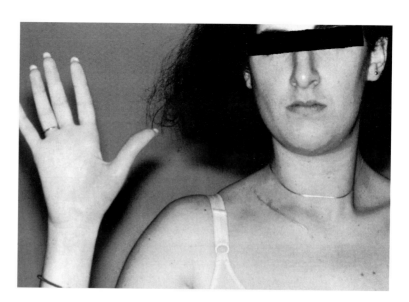

**Figure 2-22.** Supraclavicular sympathectomy for presumed reflex sympathetic dystrophy led to the loss of hand intrinsic function because of a lower trunk injury.

appropriate to reoperate several weeks after the iatrogenic injury, just as with noniatrogenic blunt lacerations. Concern about legal consequences of iatrogenic injury may alter a physician's usual pattern of practice. The attending physician must be extremely careful that any alteration of normal practice does not compromise the end result. We strongly advise that patients should be managed according to the usual clinical guidelines for each type of injury, whether it be sharp transection or a focal or lengthy lesion in continuity.

As in every nerve injury case, every effort must be made to reduce the final disability by appropriate care of the limb after the second operation.

## Bibliography

1. Aguayo A: Neuropathy due to compression and entrapment. *In* Dyck PJ, Thomas PK, and Lambert EH, Eds: Peripheral Neuropathy. Philadelphia, WB Saunders, 1975, pp. 688–713.
2. Aguayo A, Nair C, and Midgely R: Experimental progressive compression neuropathy in the rabbit. Arch Neurol 24:358–364, 1971.
3. Aita JA: Neurologic manifestations of electrical injury. Nebr Med J 40:530–533, 1965.
4. Broadbent TR, Odom GL, and Woodhall B: Peripheral nerve injuries from administration of penicillin: Report of four clinical cases. JAMA 140:1008–1010, 1949.
5. Clark K, Williams P, Willis W, and McGavran WL: Injection injuries of sciatic nerve. Clin Neurosurg 17:111–125, 1970.
6. Clodius L, Uhlschmid G, and Hess K: Irradiation plexitis of the brachial plexus. Clin Plast Surg 11:161–165, 1984.
7. Coombes MA, Clark WK, Gregory CF, and James JA: Sciatic nerve injury in infants. Recognition and prevention of impairment resulting from intragluteal injections. JAMA 173:1336, 1960.
8. Denny-Brown D and Brenner C: Paralysis of nerve induced by direct pressure and tourniquet. Arch Neurol Psychiatry 51:1–26, 1944.
9. DiVincenti FC, Moncrief JA, and Pruitt BA: Electrical injuries: A review of 65 cases. J Trauma 9:497–507, 1969.
10. Ducker T and Garrison W: Surgical aspects of peripheral nerve trauma. Curr Probl Surg Sept:1–62, 1974.
11. Ducker TB: Pathophysiology of peripheral nerve trauma. *In* Omer GE and Spinner M, Eds: Management of Peripheral Nerve Problems. Philadelphia, WB Saunders, 1980.
12. Eames RA and Lange LS: Clinical and pathological study of ischemic neuropathy. J Neurol Neurosurg Psychiatry 30:215–226, 1967.
13. Fischer H: Pathologic effects and sequelae of electrical accidents. J Occup Med 7:564–571, 1965.
14. Friedman W: The electrophysiology of nerve injuries Neurosurg Clin North Am 2:43–56, 1991.
15. Fullerton PM: The effect of ischemia on nerve conduction in the carpal tunnel syndrome. J Neurol Neurosurg Psychiatry 26:385–397, 1963.
16. Fullerton PM and Gilliatt RW: Median and ulnar neu-

ropathy in the guinea-pig. J Neurol Neurosurg Psychiatry 30:393–402, 1967.
17. Fullerton PM and Gilliatt RW: Pressure neuropathy in the hind foot of the guinea-pig. J Neurol Neurosurg Psychiatry 30:18–25, 1967.
18. Gelberman RH: Operative Nerve Repair and Reconstruction. Philadelphia, JB Lippincott, 1991.
19. Gentilli F and Hudson A: Peripheral nerve injuries: Types, causes, grading. *In* Williams R, Rengachary S, Eds: Neurosurgery. New York, McGraw-Hill, 1985.
20. Gentilli F, Hudson AR, and Hunter D: Clinical and experimental aspects of injection injuries of peripheral nerves. Can J Neurol Sci 7:143–151, 1980.
21. Gentilli F, Hudson A, Kline D, and Hunter D: Nerve injection injury with local anesthetic agents, fluorescent, microscopic and horseradish peroxidase study. Neurosurgery 6:34–73, 1980.
22. Gilbert H and Kagan AR, Eds: Radiation Damage to the Nervous System. New York, Raven Press, 1980.
23. Gilden D and Eisner J: Lumbar plexopathy caused by disseminated intravascular coagulation. JAMA 237:2846–2847, 1977.
24. Gilliatt R: Physical injury to peripheral nerves, physiological and electrodiagnostic aspects. Mayo Clin Proc 56:361–370, 1981.
25. Goldner JL and Goldner RD: Volkmann's ischemia and ischemic contractures. *In* Jupiter J, Ed: Flynn's Hand Surgery. Baltimore, Williams & Wilkins, 1991.
26. Granit R, Leksell L, and Skoglund CR: Fiber interaction in injured or compressed region of nerve. Brain 67:125–140, 1944.
27. Grube BJ: Neurologic consequences of electrical burns. J Trauma 30:254–258, 1990.
28. Highet J: Effect of stretch on peripheral nerve. Br J Surg 30:355–369, 1942.
29. Hudson A, Hunter D, and Kline D: Progression of partial injury to peripheral nerve II: Light and electron microscope studies. J Neurosurg 42:15–22, 1975.
30. Hudson AR and Hunter D: Timing of peripheral nerve repair: Important local neuropathologic factors. Clin Neurosurg 24:391–405, 1977.
31. Hudson AR, Kline DG, and Gentilli F: Peripheral nerve injection injury. *In* Omer GE and Spinner M, Eds: Management of Peripheral Nerve Problems. Philadelphia, WB Saunders, 1980.
32. Kimura J: Electrodiagnosis in Diseases of Nerves and Muscles: Principles and Practices. Philadelphia, FA Davis, 1983.
33. Kline DG: Civilian gunshot wounds to the brachial plexus. J Neurosurg 70:166–174, 1989.
34. Kline DG: Macroscopic and microscopic concomitants of nerve repair. Clin Neurosurg 26:582–606, 1979.
35. Kline DG: Peripheral nerve injuries observed or incurred during vascular operation. Semin Vasc Surg 41:20–25, 1991.
36. Kline DG: Physiological and clinical factors contributing to timing of nerve repair. Clin Neurosurg 24:425–455, 1977.
37. Kline DG and Hackett E: Reappraisal of timing for exploration of civilian peripheral nerve injuries. Surgery 78:54–65, 1975.
38. Kline DG and Hudson AR: Acute injuries of peripheral nerves. *In* Youmans J, Ed: Neurological Surgery. Philadelphia, WB Saunders, 1990.
39. Kline DG, Hudson AR, and Bratton BR: Progression of partial injury to peripheral nerve I: Periodic measurements of muscle contraction strength. J Neurosurg 42:1–15, 1975.
40. Kolb LC and Gray SJ: Peripheral neuritis as a complication of penicillin therapy. JAMA 132:323–326, 1946.

41. Lewis GK: Trauma resulting from electricity. J Int Coll Surg 28:724–738, 1957.

42. Lundborg G: Intraneural microcirculation and peripheral nerve barriers. Techniques for evaluation — clinical implications. *In* Omer GE Jr and Spinner M, Eds: Management of Peripheral Nerve Problems. Philadelphia, WB Saunders, 1980, pp. 903–916.

43. Lundborg G: Ischemic nerve injury: Experimental studies on intraneural microvascular pathophysiology and nerve function in a limb subjected to temporary circulatory arrest. Scand J Plast Reconstr Surg (Suppl) 6: 1–113, 1970.

44. Lundborg G: Structure and function of the intraneural microvessels as related to trauma, edema, formation and nerve function. J Bone Joint Surg 57A:938–948, 1975.

45. Mackinnon SE and Dellon AL: Surgery of the Peripheral Nerve. New York, Thieme Medical Publishers, 1988.

46. Mackinnon SE, Hudson A, Gentilli F, Kline DG, and Hunter D: Peripheral nerve injection injury with steroid agents. Plast Recontr Surg 69:482–490, 1983.

47. Match RM: Radiation-induced brachial plexus paralysis. Arch Surg 110:384–391, 1975.

48. Matson DD: Early neurolysis in treatment of injury of peripheral nerves due to faulty injection of antibiotics. New Engl J Med 242:973–975, 1950.

49. Mumentholer M: Brachial plexus neuropathies. *In* Dyck PJ, Thomas PK, Lambert EH, and Bunge R, Eds: Peripheral Neuropathy, 2nd Ed. Philadelphia, WB Saunders, 1984, pp. 1383–1394.

50. Ochoa J and Marotte L: The nature of the nerve lesion caused by chronic entrapment in the guinea pig. J Neurol Sci 19:491–495, 1973.

51. Ochs G: Painful dysesthesias following peripheral nerve injury: A clinical and electrophysiological study. Brain Res 4:228–240, 1989.

52. Parks B: Postoperative peripheral neuropathies. Surgery 74:348–357, 1973.

53. Pizzolato P and Mannheimei W: Histopathologic Effects of Local Anesthetic Drugs and Related Substances. Springfield, IL, Charles C Thomas, 1961.

54. Puckett WO, Grundfest H, McElroy W, and McMillen J: Damage to peripheral nerves by high velocity missiles without direct hit. J Neurosurg 3:294–299, 1946.

55. Rudge P, Ochoa J, and Gilliatt R: Acute peripheral nerve compression in the baboon. J Neurol Sci 23: 403–420, 1974.

56. Samii M: Fascicular peripheral nerve repair. *In* Ranshoff J, Ed: Modern Techniques in Surgery: Neurosurgery. Mt. Kisco, NY, Futura, 1980, pp. 1–17.

57. Seddon HJ: Three types of nerve injury. Brain 66: 238–288, 1943.

58. Seddon HJ, Ed: Peripheral Nerve Injuries. Medical Research Council Special Report Series No. 282. London, Her Majesty's Stationery Office, 1954.

59. Seddon HJ, Ed: Surgical Disorders of the Peripheral Nerves. Baltimore, Williams & Wilkins, 1972.

60. Seletz E: Surgery of Peripheral Nerves. Springfield, IL, Charles C Thomas, 1951, pp. 119–137.

61. Smith JW: Factors influencing nerve repair II: Collateral circulation of peripheral nerves. Arch Surg 93: 433–437, 1966.

62. Speed JS and Knight RA, Eds: Peripheral Nerve Injuries. *In* Campbell's Operative Orthopaedics, Vol. 1. St. Louis, CV Mosby, 1956, pp. 947–1014.

63. Spinner M: Injuries to the Major Branches of Peripheral Nerves of the Forearm, 2nd Ed. Philadelphia, WB Saunders, 1978.

64. Spurling RG and Woodhall B, Eds: Medical Department, United States Army, Surgery in World War II: Neurosurgery, Vol. 2. Washington, DC, US Government Printing Office, 1959.

65. Sunderland S: Nerve and Nerve Injuries, 1st Ed. Baltimore, Williams & Wilkins, 1968.

66. Sunderland S: Nerves and Nerve Injuries, 2nd Ed. Edinburgh, Churchill Livingstone, 1978, pp. 133–141.

67. Sunderland S: Nerve Injuries and Their Repair: A Critical Approach. Edinburgh, Churchill Livingstone, 1991.

68. Tarlov IM: How long should an extremity be immobilized after nerve suture? Ann Surg 126:336–376, 1947.

69. Terzis J and Dykes R: Electrophysiological recordings in peripheral nerve surgery: A review. J Hand Surg 1: 52–66, 1976.

70. Tindall S: Painful neuromas. *In* Williams R and Regachary S, Eds: Neurosurgery. New York, McGraw-Hill, 1985, pp. 1884–1886.

71. Thomas JE and Colby MY: Radiation-induced or metastatic brachial plexopathy? A diagnostic dilemma. JAMA 222:1392–1397, 1972.

72. Tsairis P, Dyck PJ, and Muldner DW: Natural history of brachial plexus neuropathy: Report on 99 patients. Arch Neurol 27:109–117, 1972.

73. Tsuge K: Treatment of established Volkmann's contracture. J Bone Joint Surg 57A:925–929, 1975.

74. Upton ARM and McComas AJ: Double crush in nerve-entrapment syndromes. Lancet 2:359–361, 1973.

75. Weisl H and Osborne GV: The pathological changes in rat nerves subject to moderate compression. J Bone Joint Surg 46B:297–306, 1964.

76. Whitcomb BB: Techniques of peripheral nerve repair. *In* Spurling RG and Woodhall B, Eds: Medical Department, United States Army, Surgery in World War II: Neurosurgery, Vol. 2. Part 2: Peripheral Nerve Injuries. Washington, DC, US Government Printing Office, 1959.

77. White JC: The results of traction injuries to the common peroneal nerve. J Bone Joint Surg 40B:346–351, 1968.

78. Williams IR, Jefferson D, and Gilliatt RW: Acute nerve compression during limb ischemia: An experimental study. J Neurol Sci 46:199–207, 1980.

79. Woodhall B, Nulsen FE, White JC, and Davis L: Neurosurgical implications. *In* Peripheral Nerve Regeneration. Veterans Administration Monograph. Washington, DC, US Government Printing Office, 1957, pp. 569–638.

80. Zachary RB and Roaf R: Lesions in continuity. *In* Seddon HJ, Ed: Peripheral Nerve Injuries. Medical Research Council Special Report Series No. 282. London, Her Majesty's Stationery Office, 1954.

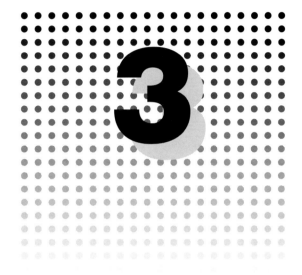

# Clinical and Electrical Evaluation

# SUMMARY

With a little practice, even the busy physician can learn much about nerve function by a careful physical examination of the limb. This is also the case in the acute or emergent setting, where even if the patient's cooperation is lacking, much can be observed. Despite the importance of the sensory and autonomic territories for the median, ulnar, and tibial nerves, motor function and its accurate evaluation is of even greater importance for most major nerves. Substitute and trick movements need to be recognized, and lack of function caused by tendinous or bony injury must be differentiated from neural loss. It is important not only to identify the nerve involved and the injury level in the limb but also to ascertain whether loss, especially motor loss, is complete or, if incomplete, the distribution and severity of the loss. Although this text is not intended to replace a more thorough exposition of electrophysiologic evaluation of nerve and muscle, a selected exposure to electromyography, conductive studies, nerve action potential recording, and somatosensory studies is important. It is most important to understand how such studies can evaluate a lesion and also to appreciate some of their limitations. Likewise, the contributions of various radiologic studies to the field of nerve injury need to be not only understood but, in some cases, weighted appropriately to realize their limitations.

Important clinical questions associated with nerve lesions include the nerve involved, the level of the injury, and the severity of the injury.[30] It is especially important to determine how complete the loss is distal to the level of the injury, because incomplete loss may improve with time but complete loss often does not. To do this well requires intimate knowledge of the anatomic distribution of the nerve in question[20] and how to test the muscles and sensory distribution usually innervated by that nerve.[45] It is also important to know the tricks or substitutive motions used by patients to provide movement despite paralysis, as well as the areas of skin where nerves have sensory as well as autonomic overlap.[16,59] Experience in examining the limb with paralysis is paramount.[28] Knowledge of innervational anatomy and variation in patterns is useless unless complemented by the ability to examine the limb in a comprehensive fashion.[24,55] Practice in examination is the key; documentation of the severity of the loss becomes easier with time and patience. Clinical evaluation is especially useful if one learns to grade the severity of the injury, not only for the important individual motor and sensory sites, but for the nerve as a whole. Others have attempted to standardize some of the nomenclature concerned with nerve, but, unfortunately, there is not as yet a clearly acceptable set of criteria for grading clinical function.[11,46,62] As a re-sult, the next chapter is devoted to methods of grading and changes we have found useful in these methods.

# EVALUATION IN THE EMERGENCY SETTING

There are few surgeons of experience who have not discovered paralysis denoting peripheral nerve injury some time after suturing a lacerated wound or treating a fracture of an extremity by open or closed methods. This oversight applies even more to inexperienced individuals such as senior medical students or interns working in busy emergency rooms. The question then arises as to whether the paralysis was present at the time of admission or whether it arose from what the patient or someone else thought was poor treatment. It should be an ironclad rule that an examination for peripheral nerve injury be made and recorded in every patient suffering from a severe closed injury, fracture, dislocation, or lacerating wound of an extremity, whether the patient is conscious or unconscious. Most of the necessary acute observations and tests for distal motor function are quite simple. In addition, absence of a median or ulnar nerve injury can even be established in an unconscious patient, merely by the direct observation of presence of sweating on the forefinger or little finger or wrinkling of the skin of these digits after immersion in water.

Before one can exclude a lesion of a peripheral nerve, one must be certain that the most distal portion of that nerve is functioning.[25] Strong extension of the wrist does not preclude an injury to the posterior interosseous branch of the radial. This nerve innvervates finger and thumb extensors after some but not all extensors to the wrist have received branches. Furthermore, flexing of the fingers does not preclude a distal median nerve paralysis. A lesion of the median nerve at the wrist can still give an opponens pollicis and abductor pollicis brevis paralysis, and more importantly, anesthesia of the palmar surface of the thumb and first three fingers. A test worth remembering, then, must be one that establishes clearly the presence or absence of the most distal function of the nerve being tested.

For the upper limb, one method of grossly reviewing innervation consists of making a five-fingered cone with the tips of the fingers and then extending the thumb[56] (Figure 3–1). The intact ulnar nerve bunches the fingers into a cone by the action of the intrinsic hand muscles, the opponens pollicis muscle innervated by the median nerve opposes the palmar surface of the thumb to the pads of the terminal phalanges, and the radial nerve extends the thumb. The test is a good one, but the disadvantage is that a patient with an acute injury of an extremity may not move the fingers because of pain or fear of causing pain by movement. The test, moreover, is difficult to carry out with the arm in a cast extending to the metacarpophalangeal junctions. Nevertheless, if the test can be well executed, one can be quite certain that there is not a severe lesion of the median, ulnar, or radial nerves. If the great toe can be extended, the peroneal portion of the sciatic nerve is not divided; if the great toe can be actively flexed, the same may be said for the tibial portion of this nerve; and if the great toe can be extended and flexed, there cannot be a complete lesion of the sciatic nerve.

Kenneth Livingston has reported a simple method for the testing of the most commonly injured nerves of the upper extremity.[61] In testing the median nerve, perception of pinprick over the palmar surface of the distal phalanx of the index finger is observed. If there is good sensation there, complete interruption of the

Cone Test

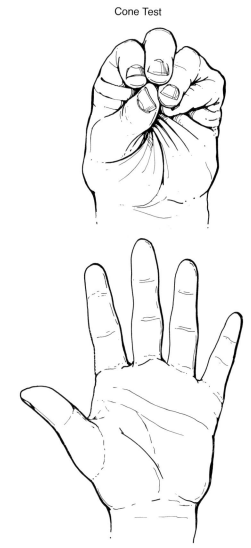

**Figure 3–1.** A rapid and relatively simple test of the distal function of median, ulnar, and radial nerves. Fingers and thumb are brought together by opponens pollicis (median) and opponens digiti quinti minimi (ulnar) as well as finger flexors (median and ulnar). Fingers are then opened up and extended by radial-innervated extensor muscles. This is called the cone test.

median nerve is excluded. For the ulnar nerve, the palmar surface of the distal phalanx of the little finger is tested for sensation. In testing the radial nerve, the ability to extend the distal phalange of the thumb with force rules out a serious lesion of that nerve. Sensory tests of the radial nerve are, as a rule, not sufficiently diagnostic. There can be objections to the use of sensory examinations in testing median and ulnar nerve functions because they do not exclude hysterical or malingered anesthesia. In children, because of fear and lack of cooperation, both sensory and motor examinations may be impossible to carry out.

## AUTONOMIC FUNCTION

Although careful sensory and motor evaluation is the key to the diagnosis of nerve lesions, a surprising amount of information can be gained from assessing autonomic function. Sweating results from stimulation of the sympathetic components of a peripheral nerve. The sympathetic fibers run in the peripheral nerve and do not extend significantly along peripheral major vessels. The area of skin to which these sympathetic components are distributed thus corresponds to the sensory distribution of a peripheral nerve. After division of a nerve, the region in which sweating is lost corresponds to the area of anesthesia. Loss of sweating can be demonstrated by complicated methods such as Minor's starch-iodine method or quinizarine, or by the use of paper impregnated with an iron solution that changes color after moisture comes in contact with it.[2] These methods are not always available, but sweating or its absence can be observed directly with the plus or minus 20 lens of the ophthalmoscope or some other source of light.[23] This illuminates the highly refractile droplets of sweat under magnification as they appear on the papillary ridges of the finger.

The ophthalmoscope lens gives a magnification of only approximately 5 times, but this is sufficient to demonstrate the individual droplets as they appear at the mouths of the sweat ducts on the papillary ridges. The observation is most easily made in somewhat subdued surrounding light (Figure 3–2). The droplets appear as highly refractile, rounded points of light. One may at first mistake sebaceous material for sweat. There are no sebaceous glands on the palmar surfaces of the hands, but sebaceous material commonly appears there from contact with the face or backs of the hands. The sebum is seen through the ophthalmoscope as a fine, scale-like, silver substance. With a little practice or by removing the sebum with ether, it can be readily differentiated from sweat. The secretion of the sebaceous glands is the end product of cellular disruption and, in contradistinction to the secretion of sweat glands, is not under control of the sympathetic nervous system.

Palpation of a denervated area may reveal a

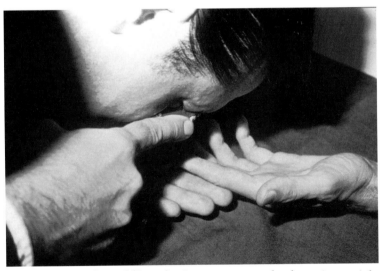

**Figure 3–2.** The cholinergic unmyelinated fibers that innervate sweat glands run in a peripheral nerve. Therefore, sweating is abolished in the peripheral nerve distribution of a transected nerve. This results in a very characteristic dryness and change in resistance when the fingers of the examiner slide over the affected area. Return of sweating to a previously denervated area is an early sign of nerve regeneration. The ophthalmoscope is a source of both illumination and magnification, and beads of sweat can be seen glistening on the dermal ridges. Unfortunately, return of sweating, like a positive Tinel sign, does not guarantee a successful result.

characteristic dry sensation, and there is limited resistance to the examiner's fingers gliding over the skin. If sweating can be demonstrated in the autonomous zones of the median and ulnar nerves, there cannot be a complete lesion of either of these nerves, and surgical exploration in the near future, at least, is contraindicated.

When sweating occurs in normal individuals, it is, in general, symmetrical in intensity. The absence of sweating is only of significance, therefore, if it is unilateral. If sweat particles are seen in the autonomous zone of the ulnar nerve, complete division of that nerve cannot be present. The absence of sweat here, however, is only of importance if there is visible sweating in the corresponding area of the other hand. In another sense, the presence of sweating in the distribution of the nerve being tested is of more real value if evident than if absent.

Return of sweating may antedate sensory or motor return by weeks to months, but a return of sweating does not necessarily mean that sensory or motor function will follow. The regeneration of a few unmyelinated autonomic fibers does not, unfortunately, guarantee regeneration of motor or sensory fibers. Another test that is probably related to the presence or absence of autonomic function is the O'Rian wrinkle test.[54] Normally, innervated fingers, immersed in tepid water, wrinkle after 5 to 10 minutes. With denervation, the fingers no longer wrinkle, but, with reinnervation, wrinkles can once again be seen.

Autonomic dysfunction resulting in discoloration of the skin and changes in skin temperature, in addition to changes in sweating pattern, is usually associated with pain such as true causalgia or reflex sympathetic dystrophy;[12] this is discussed in succeeding chapters.

## SENSORY FUNCTION

Sensory testing is important, but can be difficult and at times misleading. One must be certain that observations are made in autonomous zones where the likelihood of overlapping innervation from adjacent uninjured nerves is minimal. The autonomous zone for the median nerve includes the volar and distal dorsal surfaces of the forefinger and the volar surface of the thumb (Figure 3–3). The ulnar nerve has a comparable zone which includes the volar and distal dorsal surface of the little finger and the distal and volar surface of the ring finger. The radial nerve does not have a reliable autonomous zone, but if there is any sensory loss at all, it is usually found over the region of the anatomic snuffbox.[53] Autonomous zones for the tibial nerve include the heel and a portion of the sole of the foot (Figure 3–4), while a less autonomous zone for the peroneal nerve exists over the dorsum of the foot.

Sensory return in nonautonomous areas usually precedes motor return. Sensory return in an autonomous area is usually a later development that follows the earliest motor return. In the case of median nerve injury, sensory recovery can be the primary concern from the standpoint of practical function (Figure 3–5). The arrival of new sensory axons in the hand proximal to the autonomous zone at the fingertips can be recognized by sensory displacement.[38] With initial testing, the patient localizes the stimulus to another point within the median sensory area that is removed from the actual stimulus site. This is not a result of overlapping innervation by neighboring nerves or recovery from neurapraxia. Sensory displacement indicates that a regenerating axon has strayed into a sensory receptor that is remote from the one that the brain is accustomed to having it supply.

Two-point discrimination in the normal adult finger pad should span 3 to 5 mm. This can be tested simply with a bent paper clip or a pair of calipers. Values for return of good two-point discrimination for the palm of the hand and the sole of the foot are usually 6 to 10 mm, and those for the dorsal surfaces of the hand and foot are 7 to 12 mm.[47] In our opinion, it is of greater functional significance to test for relative decreases in response to touch and pinprick than to test two-point discrimination. In other words, sensation in the involved limb is best compared to that in the uninvolved limb. Of practical significance also is the ability of the patient to localize both touch and pinprick sensation to the specific area being stimulated (Figure 3–6).

Definite sensory recovery in autonomous zones, even with sensory displacement, can be important early evidence of regeneration in distal lesions of major sensory nerves such as the median and tibial nerves. On the other hand,

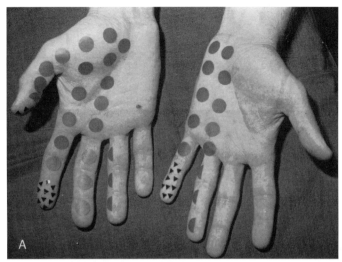

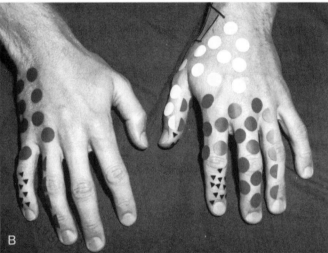

**Figure 3–3.** (*A*) Usual sensory zones of the hand for median (hand to the left in the photograph) and ulnar (hand to the right in the photograph) nerves. Small triangles indicate autonomous zones where loss can be due only to median or ulnar nerve loss. Conversely, recovery in an autonomous zone means that nerve has regenerated and reversal is not caused by overlap from an adjacent nerve. (*B*) White circles on the dorsum of the hand to the right indicate the usual sensory territory of the radial nerve. Boxed area on wrist indicates the "anatomic snuffbox," the area in which radial sensory loss, if present, will be found. Dark circles on the hand to the right in the photograph outline the usual median distribution; those on the hand to the left indicate the usual ulnar distribution. Small triangles indicate the dorsal surface autonomous zones for median and ulnar nerves, respectively.

**Figure 3–4.** The sensory examination of the sole of the foot must be performed with care because the peripheral nerve supply is complex. The calcaneal branches of the posterior tibial nerve are given off before the tarsal tunnel in many cases, so the heel may escape sensory disturbance in true tarsal tunnel syndrome in which compression is closer to the sole of the foot. The sensory distributions of the medial and lateral plantar nerves in the foot are roughly analogous to those of the median and ulnar nerves in the hand. However, the sural nerve clearly supplies the outer border of the foot. The femoral nerve contributes the saphenous branch, which usually supplies a strip of sensation to skin as far as the medial malleolus and instep. The circles on the heel of the foot indicate the usual autonomous zone for the tibial nerve.

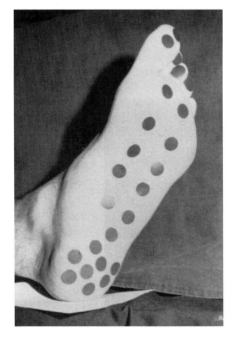

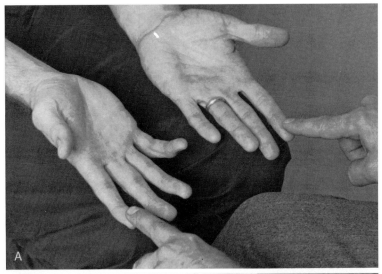

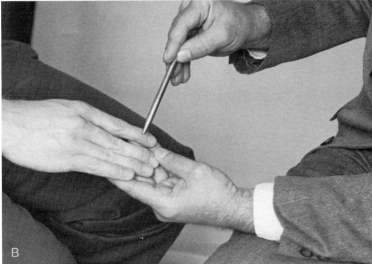

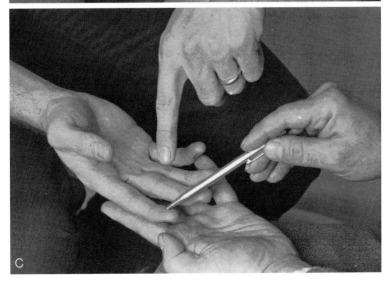

**Figure 3–5.** (*A*) In testing touch in median autonomous zones, the examiner modulates touch bilaterally on the volar surfaces of the forefingers, using his own forefingers as the stimuli. (*B*) Autonomous zone on dorsum of forefinger is tested for localization by touching it with a pen while the patient's eyes are closed. (*C*) Testing for localization on the volar surface of the forefinger. With eyes closed, the patient is able to point out accurately the area being stimulated.

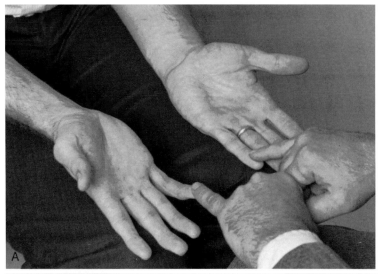

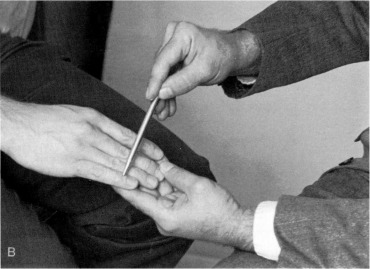

**Figure 3–6.** (*A*) In this photograph, the patient's response to touch is being compared by modulating touch, using the examiner's own little fingers on the patient's little fingers. (*B*) Here, ability to localize the pressure from the examiner's pen in an autonomous zone of the ulnar nerve is being assessed.

sensory recovery usually occurs relatively late and can be very misleading as an indicator of eventual useful motor recovery, particularly in the case of radial and peroneal nerves (Figure 3–7).

For the majority of serious nerve lesions, and especially those proximal to the wrist or knee levels, sensation can be tested for relative perception and localization by having the patient compare responses, with closed eyes, to stroking of the patient's fingers or foot areas bilaterally. Response to pinprick can be tested in the same comparative fashion. At the same time, the patient's ability to localize both touch and pinprick can be tested. Sensory responses can be graded for each nerve tested (see next chapter, Grading Results).

The area of sensory supply of a peripheral nerve should not be confused with the area of sensory supply of a segmental spinal nerve (dermatomal pattern). On occasion, the maps of the dermatomal and peripheral nerve distribution overlap (Figure 3–8).

The spinal nerve is derived from a single spinal segment and supplies a specific skin area of the embryo. The limb bud grows and drags the dermatomes to the periphery, leaving a gap in the body sequence, with a sudden jump from the level of the fourth cervical to the second thoracic.

The peripheral nerve surgeon should be aware of the map for peripheral nerve distribution and areas of confusion that may arise in attempting to differentiate a radicular from a pe-

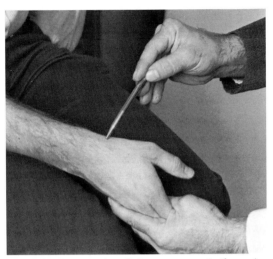

**Figure 3–7.** Patient's radial sensory area in the region of the anatomic snuffbox is tested for localization by using the tip of the pen. There may not, however, be sensory loss even in this area despite a complete radial injury.

ripheral nerve lesion. On sensory examination of the shoulder, it may be difficult to distinguish a C5 from an axillary nerve injury. The C6 dermatome may be confused with the median nerve sensory distribution so that a C5-C6 disc may be removed instead of releasing the carpal tunnel. Sensory loss in the C8-T1 distribution may be confused with ulnar nerve pathology, and the surgeon must appreciate the peripheral sensory distribution of ulnar nerve, medial antebrachial cutaneous and medial cutaneous nerves of the arm, so as to avoid confusion between radicular and peripheral nerve pathology.

The information required for accurate clinical diagnosis can be determined by using simple stimuli applied with cotton wool, a pin and paper clip, or the examiner's touch. The examiner should not be deterred by absence of very specialized methods of sensory study because

**Figure 3–8.** A dermatome is the area of skin supplied by a single spinal nerve. Patterns vary from patient to patient, but usually the inner aspect of the leg is supplied by L4, the outer leg by L5, and the lateral aspect of the foot by S1. The map of a peripheral nerve distribution differs from that for nerve roots or spinal nerves. It is imperative that the differential diagnosis between spinal and peripheral conditions be made with care. Loss in the dermatome for L5 may mimic a peroneal nerve sensory loss; both L5 radicular pathology and peroneal nerve palsy can give rise to a foot drop. Likewise, radicular pathology involving the L2 root could be confused with meralgia paraesthetica. The lower dorsal or thoracic dermatomes and those of the sacral roots are close posteriorly and yet separate anteriorly. These dermatomes are usually tested to assess the level of a spinal cord injury. (By comparison, sensory testing in the groin and area of the genitalia is used to assess ilioinguinal and genitofemoral nerve pathology.) A perianal target-like area of sensory loss is a reliable indicator of sacral root pathology. For completeness' sake, the surgeon should review the peripheral pathways subtending both perianal and perivaginal sensation, as well as the peripheral supply of the rectal sphincters. The clinician must be a master of both the dermatomal and peripheral maps of both the lower and upper limbs. In most cases, the history can guide the examiner as to which of these two maps to consult in a given patient. Both authors have several examples of patients who underwent spinal surgery (often on the basis of a slightly abnormal scanning study or myelogram) even though the pathology was at a peripheral nerve level.

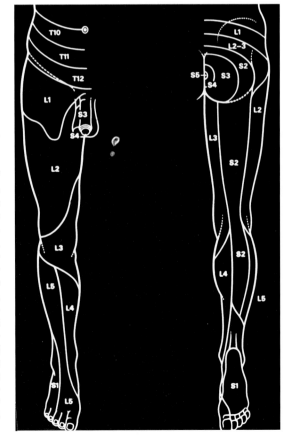

those techniques add little to the examination conducted by an experienced and thorough clinician. Special techniques such as laser beams are used by those studying pain or the physiology of sensation but are not necessary for practical diagnostic accuracy at the bedside or in the office.

## MOTOR FUNCTION

There is no substitute for a thorough motor examination if major nerve injury is suspected. To do this well requires patience and perseverance as well as some experience (Figure 3–9). Each major peripheral nerve innervates a cascade of muscles. After the physician learns these patterns and gains experience in testing them, his or her ability to localize spinal cord and spine-related nerve root problems, as well as neuropathies, is increased greatly. A good beginning is provided by the MRC handbook on peripheral nerve examination as well as a number of other texts.[6,24,45] Study of these and similar texts also gives the examiner an idea of

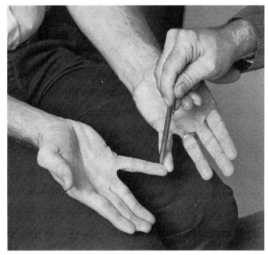

**Figure 3–9.** The abductor of the small finger is supplied by short twigs derived from the ulnar nerve in Guyon's canal, whereas the flexor of the terminal phalanx of the small finger is supplied by the ulnar nerve in the proximal forearm. Thus, abductor digiti quinti minimi and flexor profundus to the ring finger are useful muscles to test to determine the level of injury to the ulnar nerve. The examiner is asking the subject to resist the passage of the pencil between the little fingers. The slightly atrophied hypothenar eminence of the patient's right hand gave way, demonstrating impairment of ulnar input on that side.

the more common anomalies in innervation.[11,49] Photographs of various tests for muscle function are included throughout this book and in the appendix (Figure 3–10).

A common error in clinical examination is to assume injury at a specific level and neglect examination of muscles innervated above this level[52] (Figure 3–11). Another frequent error is failure to examine muscles innervated by other nerves in the limb. Muscles in the distribution of noninjured nerves can sometimes substitute for loss and make the injury appear partial or even nonexistent. For example, abduction of the fingers, a function supplied by the ulnar nerve, can be mistaken for radial-innervated finger extension (Figure 3–12A). The reverse can be true for ulnar palsy, in which extension of the fingers by radial-innervated extensor communis may provide some abduction of the little finger (Figure 3–12B). The classic example of substitutive movement is illustrated by a wrist-level median palsy in which opponens pollicis is paralyzed. Extensor pollicis, which is radial-innervated, pulls the thumb away from the palm; ulnar-innervated adductor pollicis displaces the thumb toward and across the palm; and flexor pollicis longus, which is innervated above the wrist by the median, pulls the tip of the thumb toward opposing fingers, completing the thumb's opposition-like motion.

The patient with a complete radial palsy can sometimes provide some dorsiflexion of the wrist by flexing the fingers and making a fist. Extensor tendons shortened by the palsy force the hand backward, even though they are not innervated.

Substitution can mislead the examiner. For example, despite complete palsy of biceps/brachialis, the forearm can be readily flexed on the upper arm by the brachioradialis, which is supplied by the radial nerve (Figure 3–13). This further highlights the need for a thorough examination of all the major muscles in a limb in which nerve injury is suspected.

In some patients with paralysis of the deltoid, a good deal of abduction can be gained by use of the supraspinatus to initiate abduction, and then use of the long head of the biceps to provide forward abduction (Figures 3–14 through 3–16). These substitutes for deltoid can be aided by scapular rotation and elevation of the shoulder by the serratus anterior and trapezius.

**Figure 3–10.** (*A*) The adductor of the thumb is supplied by the terminal branch of the ulnar nerve. Having passed around the hook of the hamate, the ulnar nerve crosses the hand to supply the intrinsic muscles and terminates in the adductor pollicis. This muscle is useful to test in assessing ulnar nerve function, because its power is reduced by a lesion at any level along the course of the nerve. The patient is asked to maintain the card as the examiner attempts to pull the card away. The subject is instructed to keep the thumb straight. Because the ulnar-supplied adductor is weak, the card starts slipping out, so the patient responds by using his median-supplied flexor pollicis longus to supplement his effort (the Froment sign). (*B*) The extensor surfaces of the three bones of the thumb each have a tendon attached. All three of the muscles for these tendons are supplied by the posterior interosseous nerve (PIN) in the proximal forearm. The median-nerve–innervated muscles flex and oppose the thumb, but the function of the three PIN-supplied muscles is to retrieve the thumb from the flexed position, allowing subsequent grasping motions. In this photograph, the patient is attempting to extend the thumb against resistance, and the long (EPL) tendon is easily seen. The power is compared with thumb extension in the contralateral limb.

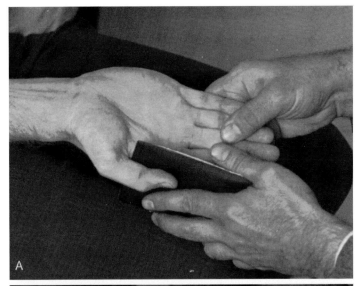

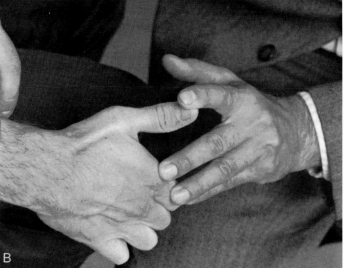

This misleading set of circumstances can be obviated if the examiner passively elevates the patient's limb to the horizontal. The examiner then palpates the patient's deltoid with the other hand and asks the patient to sustain the abduction. Minor degrees of deltoid contraction can be readily appreciated in this manner. Gravity can also supplement or replace in part muscles providing function such as forearm extension, knee flexion, and plantar flexion. Testing of muscles serving these functions has to take this into account. Evaluation for completeness of injury or, conversely, return of function, can be difficult for injuries involving neural input to either the shoulder or to the fine muscles of the hand. In these areas especially, experience is the only effective teacher.

Anomalous innervation can trick the examiner into erroneously concluding that either a partial or a complete lesion of a nerve exists. Some knowledge of the common anomalies helps avoid these misperceptions.[24,49,55,58]

With penetrating injuries, loss of function can result from tendon transection, but usually if this is the case, the soft tissue injury is much too distal to account for loss of function on a neural basis alone. For example, the patient who has a wrist-level laceration and inability to flex the

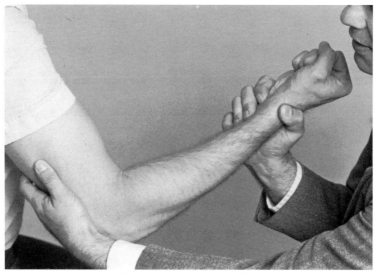

**Figure 3–11.** Triceps is primarily supplied by C7 through the middle trunk, the latter's posterior division, and the posterior cord to radial nerve. The initial branches to the three heads of this muscle arise in the axilla, and injuries to the radial nerve at a lateral humeral level, such as Saturday night palsy, are not accompanied by paralysis of triceps. Testing of this proximal muscle is therefore critical in determining the level of radial nerve injury. The examiner is resisting the patient's attempt to extend the elbow while inspecting and palpating the triceps. Loss of triceps function is not nearly as important to the patient as loss of elbow flexion because gravity extends the previously flexed elbow.

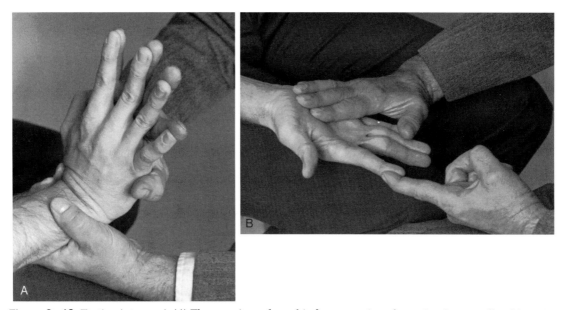

**Figure 3–12.** Testing interossei. (*A*) The examiner places his fingers against the patient's, extending his wrist. He asks the patient to spread or abduct the fingers and then bring them back together or adduct them. In this fashion, the examiner takes away any ability for the patient to use the radial-innervated extensors to simulate a true abduction motion of the fingers. (*B*) The first dorsal interosseous is being tested by asking the patient to abduct the forefinger against the examiner's forefinger, which is placed above the plane of the palm so that interosseous and not extensor communis to forefinger is tested.

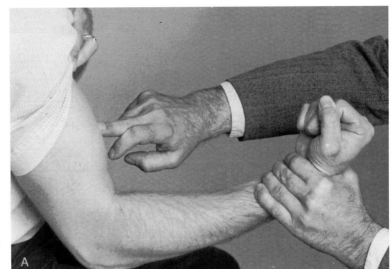

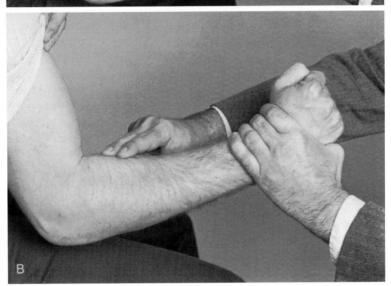

**Figure 3–13.** (*A*) Biceps is primarily supplied by the sixth cervical nerve through the upper trunk, the latter's anterior division, the lateral cord, and the musculocutaneous nerve. This muscle is both a powerful flexor of the elbow and supinator of the forearm. (*B*) Brachioradialis is primarily supplied by C6 through the upper trunk, the latter's posterior division, the posterior cord, and the radial nerve. It is a modest flexor of the elbow but can hypertrophy in cases of biceps paralysis so as to flex the elbow more strongly. The examiner is testing elbow flexion against resistance in full supination (biceps) and with wrist partially pronated (brachioradialis). Biceps examination is key to the diagnosis of proximal upper element plexus injury or musculocutaneous nerve injury. Brachioradialis function is key to assessing progress after radial nerve injury.

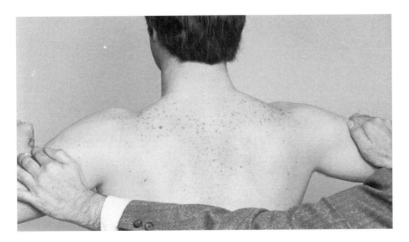

**Figure 3–14.** This patient is resisting the examiner's attempt to adduct or push the shoulders down and to the patient's side. The function of trapezius (cranial nerve XI) and deltoid (spinal nerve C5 through the upper trunk, the latter's posterior division, the posterior cord, and the axillary nerve) can be seen, palpated, and compared.

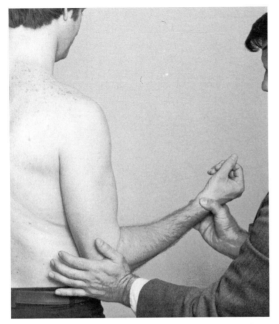

**Figure 3–15.** Internal and external rotation of the shoulder is checked against resistance. External rotation is accomplished by the infraspinatus supplied by the suprascapular nerve with input primarily from C5. Every effort should be made to regain external shoulder rotation during surgery on upper plexus elements, in addition to providing outflow for elbow flexion and shoulder abduction. Internal rotation is primarily accomplished by the pectoralis major, which has a very widespread innervation from the roots of the brachial plexus through the lateral and medial pectoral nerves (named for their cords of origin).

distal phalanx of the thumb or forefinger has such loss because of transection of the flexor pollicis longus or the flexor profundus and not because of median nerve laceration. This is because these muscles receive their innervation quite proximal to the wrist. Few serious injuries of an extremity involve only nerve without muscle, tendon, vascular, or bone injuries. Evidence of these as well as nerve injury should always be sought[69] (Figure 3–17).

## SIMULATED MUSCLE AND SENSORY ABNORMALITY

As one attempts to grade muscle strength, lack of effort (LOE) on the part of the patient can usually be detected by an experienced examiner. LOE may result because motion is painful to the patient, because of lack of confidence to move the involved limb, or sometimes because of a need for secondary gain.[12] One can be suspicious of LOE if the patient does not fully contract nearby muscles that are not at all related to the nerve injury in question, for example, if the patient does not give full effort to wrist extension (radial nerve) or to flexion of the tip of the thumb (median nerve) when loss of hand intrinsics is suspected because of an elbow-level ulnar injury. A similar example for the lower extremity would be lack of full plantar flexion,

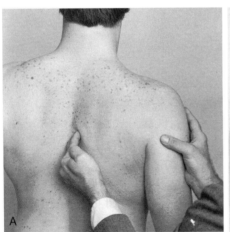
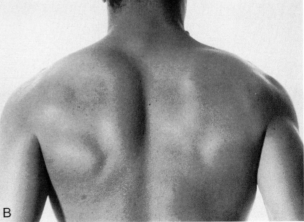

**Figure 3–16.** (A) Rhomboids on the patient's right side are palpated by the examiner's finger. The patient was asked to brace his shoulders backward as if "at attention." (B) This patient's right rhomboid was paralyzed as a result of a stab wound. The nerve to rhomboids was cut as it departed the C5 spinal nerve. In brachial plexus stretch cases, paralysis of rhomboid or electrophysiologic evidence of denervation in that muscle indicates a very proximal C5 lesion.

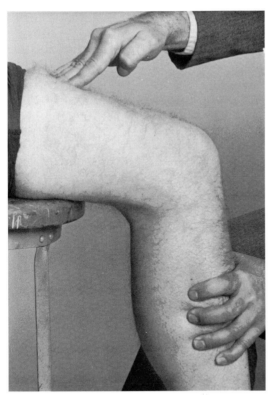

**Figure 3 – 17.** The usually massive quadriceps is supplied by the femoral nerve, which has both an extraperitoneal intra-abdominal course in the pelvis and a branching appearance in the proximal thigh. The examiner is palpating the anterior thigh and also inspecting the lateral aspect of the thigh so as not to be misled by any concomitant contraction of tensor fascia lata (supplied by superior gluteal nerve.) The obturator nerve is tested by attempting to force the knees apart against an adducting motion of the thighs by the patient. This nerve has the same spinal nerve origin (L2, L3, L4) as the femoral. The presence of hip adduction in the absence of knee extension implies that the spinal nerves are intact and that the lesion is therefore in the femoral nerve itself. Femoral palsy due to injury may be accompanied by serious vascular and/or abdominal injury.

foot inversion, and toe flexion in a patient with a fibular-level peroneal nerve lesion. One always has to be careful not to overlook a partial or mild palsy associated with a severe one, but well-selected electrical tests usually provide evidence for the former as well as document the latter.

Another sign of LOE is a tendency for the tested function to have a staccato or give-and-take contraction of the muscle concerned. An example of this behavioral aberration is sometimes seen if the flexor profundus of the forefin-

ger is tested in a patient with a median palsy. The patient may provide only slight flexion, then extension, then a little more flexion, then once again extension. This provides a back-and-forth or give-and-take type of motion rather than the sustained attempt at contraction that the examiner is asking for. This type of contraction could be caused by severe paresis but more than likely is a result of either LOE or lack of concentration on the patient's part. Sometimes, with repeated exhortation on the part of the examiner, the patient can correct the aberration and provide a sustained and more complete contraction of the muscle in question.

A more obvious sign of LOE is give-way weakness, wherein the patient starts out with good contraction of a muscle but in the midst of contraction the strength of the muscle seems to suddenly give way or fade.

Patients with significant somatization may also show characteristic sensory findings. The reported sensory loss will not, under these circumstances, be in a normal anatomic distribution. Frequently, there is a sharp cut-off between areas of reported anesthesia or hypesthesia and normalcy, and these borders do not coincide with known peripheral or dermatomal sensation. These patients may be highly suggestible and can sometimes be talked into or out of sensory abnormalities by the examiner. Nonorganic loss or loss of functional origin needs early diagnosis and input from the surgeon, physical therapist, and sometimes psychiatrist so that stiffness, pain, and secondary autonomic dysfunction, all related to disuse, can be minimized. It is, of course, possible that psychological overlay has been added to a real organic deficit and/or real and not imagined pain. This type of complex presentation requires experience to sort out. Thus, the diagnoses of "malingering, anxiety, compensation neurosis, or frank hysteria" are not easy to make.

Nerve injuries can be painful, and the patient may blame lack of limb movement on the pain, something that is difficult for the examiner to prove or disprove. Once the secondary effects of disuse have set in, it may be quite difficult to break the cycle as well as to correctly weigh the organic versus the functional portion. It is essential, therefore, to assess the psychological components early and to institute early and vigorous physical therapy. Unfortunately, in some cases, compensation for disability can prolong symptoms and this can be to the patient's disadvantage.

## TINEL SIGN

Presence of a Tinel sign provides some evidence favoring axonal regeneration. If paresthesias are obtained by percussion over the course of the nerve distal to the injury site (Tinel sign), some continuity of sensory axons from the point percussed through the lesion to the central nervous system is suggested. If the response moves distally with time, and particularly if progression down the extremity is associated with diminished paresthesias in response to tapping over the injury site, evidence for continued sensory-fiber regeneration down the distal stump is present (Figure 3-18). A positive Tinel sign implies only fine-fiber regeneration, however, and tells the examiner nothing about

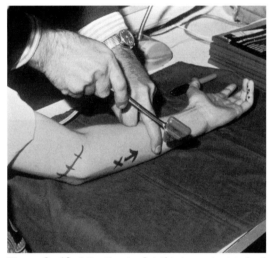

**Figure 3-18.** Attention to detail is important to both elicit and interpret a Tinel sign. The level of a left ulnar nerve injury is shown by the dotted line proximal to the elbow. Sharp percussion of the nerve at site "X" on a previous visit had elicited paresthesias, and the examiner is now attempting to elicit them at a more distal site on a subsequent visit. An advancing Tinel sign indicates that at least some fine fibers are growing down the nerve but does not guarantee a good clinical result. The absence of advance, however, indicates a poor chance of recovery. Note that the nerve is not percussed at the point of injury. Any focal nerve injury will respond with local paresthesias if directly percussed.

the quantity or eventual quality of the new fibers. More than 50 percent of the World War II soldiers who ultimately required resection and suture of nerve injuries had earlier shown an advancing Tinel sign. Henderson studied a large group of patients with nerve injuries in a concentration camp in which operation was not permitted.[17] He found the Tinel sign to be useful as long as it advanced rapidly along the distal stump and was not confined to the injury alone. Even so, the majority of the patients who had a Tinel sign advancing down the limb and distal to the lesion had not regained significant useful function on follow-up after the war.

On the other hand, if no Tinel response is obtained and sufficient time has elapsed for fine-fiber regeneration to occur (4-6 weeks), the absence of a Tinel sign distal to a lesion is such strong evidence against regeneration as to constitute a significant negative finding.[68] In other words, a positive Tinel sign is comparable to the finding of paresthesias on electrical stimulation of the distal nerve. Such a finding has no quantitative significance. On the other hand, an absent sensory response on tapping distal to the injury after an appropriate time lapse strongly suggests total neural interruption or extremely poor axonal regrowth to the level of the nerve being tapped.

## OTHER FINDINGS ASSOCIATED WITH NERVE LESIONS

Because of autonomic fiber loss, skin in the distribution of the injured nerve and sometimes beyond it feels dry and cool. Loss of sympathetic input to skin, sweat glands, and vasodilatory fibers to small skin arterioles presumably leads to these changes. With time, the skin can seem shiny in appearance and texture as it becomes less coarse or wrinkled. If a digit with sensory and autonomic loss is immersed in water for several minutes, it fails to wrinkle as a normally innervated finger or toe would. More chronic deinnervation makes the skin appear shiny or glossy.

Proximal involvement of the C8 or T1 spinal nerves may also produce a Horner syndrome, which is caused by loss of sympathetic fiber input to both the iris and the levator palpebrae superioris (Figure 3–19).

Patients frequently report a tendency for the denervated portion of an extremity to bruise easily. Skin and underlying soft tissues seem not only to bruise more readily than normal tissues but also to heal more slowly. Soft tissue hemorrhage seems to take longer to mobilize, and skin lacerations or scratches take longer to heal than usual. Osteoporosis and actual shrinkage of bone architecture can occur, especially to the fingers, with a long-standing palsy. Denervated digits tend to narrow in diameter and taper down at their tips. This may be accompanied by what appears to be excessive and abnormal nail growth; the latter not only elongates more rapidly than normal, but also becomes thickened and at times ridged or discolored. Some patients, especially children or those with dementia who have median or ulnar injury, may repetitively suck or chew on their anesthetic fingers (Figure 3–20). Occasionally, such individuals

even autocannibalize their fingers or hand. Skin and nail changes from such behavior should be obvious but can be overlooked or not appreciated unless the nature of the responsible neuropathy is appreciated.

All or any of these changes can occur without the patient having either reflex sympathetic dystrophy (RSD) or causalgia.[39] Nonetheless, with these sympathetically-related disorders, the onset of such findings may be accelerated and accentuated.[11,64] For example, the patient with RSD affecting the hand frequently does not trim his or her nails because this activity is too painful. As a result, such a patient can present with long, often curved, talon-like nails. Early in the course of the disorder, hyperhidrosis and vasodilation can predominate.[40] The sine qua non for both of these disorders is a burning-like pain and a hand or foot that cannot be manipulated, even if the patient's attention is distracted from the examination.

The limb with disuse atrophy, or one immo-

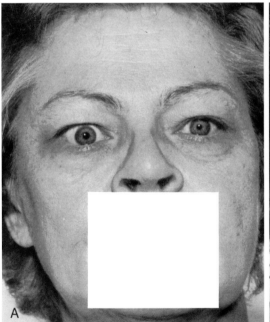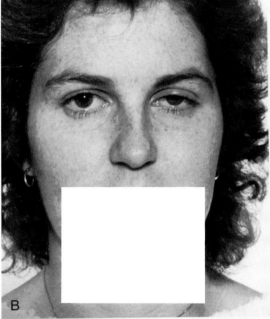

**Figure 3–19.** The examiner should automatically look for a Horner syndrome while taking the patient's history, particularly if there is any complaint of hand weakness. (*A*) This patient's small left pupil is obvious, but if there is any doubt, the lights should be dimmed—the normal contralateral pupil will then dilate, making the inequality of pupil size more obvious. This patient suffered from a breast carcinoma with invasion of C8 and T1 spinal nerves. (*B*) The difference in size of the palpebral fissure may be obvious initially, and this lady's ptosis accompanied an avulsion injury of C8 and T1 spinal nerves. This physical sign signals a proximal injury to the spinal nerve in this setting and is hence an unwelcome sign usually observed immediately when the patient enters the examining room. The ptosis rarely interferes with vision and frequently becomes much less severe with the passage of a few weeks. The relatively small pupil, however, remains.

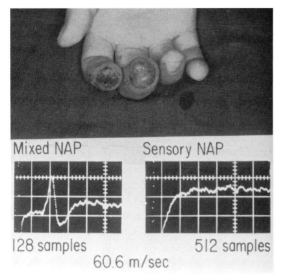

Mixed NAP          Sensory NAP

128 samples              512 samples

60.6 m/sec

**Figure 3–20.** Hand of a child who sustained a laceration to the wrist and presented with a mutilated forefinger and long finger caused by sucking and chewing on them. The noninvasive, positive tracing to the left was recorded by stimulating median nerve at wrist and recording over the course of the median at the elbow. The flat trace to the right was obtained by stimulating over forefinger digital nerves and recording over median nerve just above the wrist.

bilized too long by a cast or rigid splint, usually has severe distal changes affecting skin and other soft tissue as well as bone.[7] The easy tendency of the shiny, fragile skin and tapered fingers to bruise or slough can be reduced somewhat, although not eliminated, by early vigorous and repetitive physical therapy.

Unusual symptoms can occur with nerve lesions or their regrowth. These are not always painful and may consist of tingling or a sharpened awareness of touch. For example, itchiness of the palm and fingers of the hand can be associated with carpal tunnel syndrome.

## TIME AND DISTANCE IN AXONAL REGENERATION

The time-honored rule of thumb for rate of regeneration is 1 mm per day or 1 inch per month.[56] The rate is faster at more proximal levels of the nerve and slower at more distal levels. However, this rule of thumb is applicable primarily to new fibers after they have reached the distal stump, and it does not take into ac-

count the time necessary to traverse injury or repair sites or to mature and form meaningful distal connections. The overall rate of significant regrowth is much slower than is generally held.[62] As a result, the regenerative process extends and continues over a greater period of time than is usually recognized or acknowledged. Figure 3–21 depicts the usual steps in the regenerative process.

There are several steps in this process:

1. There is a variable extent of retrograde degenerative change after injury. The more blunt or stretching the force, the lengthier this zone of injury. New neurites must first overcome this defect, which may be a few millimeters up to several centimeters proximal to the site of primary impact.
2. Axons must penetrate the original injury or repair site. Progress here is especially slow and requires much more time than studies in the rat or lower animals suggest.[72] This is especially so if grafts have to be interposed between the stumps of a nerve to make up a gap. Here, axons traversing the graft repair site may require weeks of growth rather than days.
3. After the new axons have reached the distal stump, they grow at a rate of 1 mm per day for the average nerve at midlimb level. Rate of growth down the distal stump tends to be faster for lesions of proximal limb and much slower for those in distal limb. Rate may also be slow if substantial endoneurial proliferation has had time to occur before axons reach the distal stump.
4. On reaching distal target sites, further time, which can be several weeks or even a month, may be necessary before axonal-to-endplate motor functions are reconstituted or significant sensory reinput occurs.
5. Fiber maturation with recovery of axonal volume and myelin thickness takes further time.

The regenerative process for a proximal plexus element or a long nerve such as the sciatic nerve may take 5 to 6 years for completion. Total time for maximal recovery for a median nerve injured at the wrist may be only 2 to 3 years, but the same nerve injured at the elbow level may require an additional year or so. Predictions of recovery based on measurements be-

Steps in Regeneration of Nerve

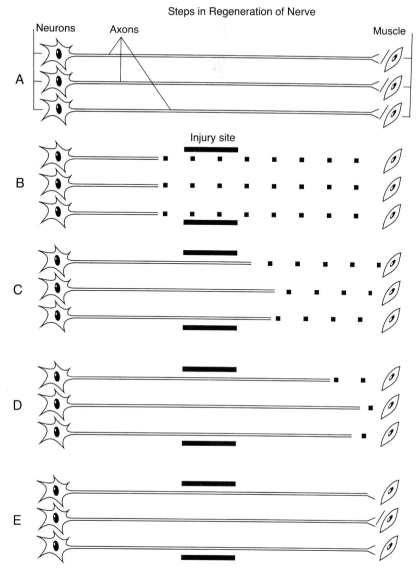

**Figure 3–21.** (*A*) The top drawing shows neurons, their axonal extensions, and their distal input, in this case to muscle. (*B*) After an injury that parts axons, there is a segment of retrograde degeneration and, over the ensuing weeks, Wallerian degeneration of the distal nerve. (*C*) Over a period of several weeks, axons of variable number and size traverse the injury site, reach the distal stump, and begin to descend in it. There is no spontaneous clinical function, nerve cannot be stimulated to produce distal function, and electromyography (EMG) shows a severe denervational pattern. Two to three months after injury, a nerve action potential (NAP) may be recordable by stimulating proximally and recording distally. Months may be required for axons to proceed on down the distal stump. (*D*) Axons begin to reach end inputs, but not enough time has passed or reconstruction occurred to permit spontaneous function. At this point, an NAP can be recorded, sometimes nerve can be stimulated, and some distal muscle may contract. EMG may show some reversal of denervational change and signs of reinnervation such as nascent potentials. (*E*) More of the motor end plates have been reconstructed, and reinnervational changes by EMG are more pronounced. Time between D and E varies but may be weeks to a month or two.

tween the lesion or repair site and muscles expected to be reinnervated, applying the millimeter-per-day or inch-per-month rule, must be tempered by the above factors.[32]

It is also important to realize whether the time for useful recovery by spontaneous regeneration has passed after injury. Nerve repair may have little to offer beyond such a time.[21,37] If 24 or more months of total muscle denervation have elapsed, many muscles cannot recover sufficient function even after regaining neural fiber input.[6,36] Atrophy can be so advanced, or muscle actually replaced by fibrotic change or fat, that even the arrival of very healthy axons cannot restore function in the muscle.[15] This is less likely to be the case for relatively large, bulky muscles such as the biceps/brachialis or gastrocnemius-soleus than for smaller muscles such as thenar and hypothenar intrinsics, interossei, or lumbricals. An exception referable to size appears to be the facial muscles, which may benefit from late reinnervation by facial nerve repair or by neurotization procedures.

Other exceptions to this "24-month rule" may occur in a few lesions in continuity that have maintained or restored some distal continuity even though it is not enough to produce useful distal function. Sometimes, presence of distal fibers may keep enough of the distal stump and end-input architecture preserved or accessible so that very late repair after resection of the original lesion can, on occasion, produce function.

Implications of these observations referable to management are important. Distance from the injury site to the functional unit desired for reinnervation tempers the timing for surgical repair: the longer the distance, the earlier surgical intervention should be considered.[9] This is especially so with brachial plexus and proximal sciatic lesions. Relatively early timing for exploration and, if indicated, repair also plays a role in upper-arm median, ulnar, and some radial injuries. There is no place for a "wait and see" attitude. If the physician waits for recovery based on a millimeter per day or inch per month rule and it does not occur, it will be too late for nerve repair to be effective.

In some cases, the distance between the injury site and the function desired is such that early or late repair or even spontaneous regen-

eration can achieve little.[19] This is especially so for proximal ulnar lesions or their origins such as C8, T1, lower trunk, or medial cord. These proximal elements supply ulnar nerve and thus input to the very small and very distal intrinsic hand muscles. Lesions of the proximal peroneal division of the sciatic nerve have similar limitations in time. Peroneal-innervated muscles have a complex innervational and firing pattern for function. Input for these relatively lengthy muscles most likely occurs at multiple levels in a specific pattern. This complex input must be reinstituted to achieve recovery of useful dorsiflexion of the foot or toes. This is a difficult regenerative task even if circumstances are ideal.

Sensory and autonomic recovery is not subject to as severe limitations in time as motor function.[61,72] This is an important consideration favoring median nerve repair at an axillary level even though it may contribute little to recovery of median-innervated hand function. Repair of the tibial division of the sciatic nerve may be useful even at a buttock level despite the great distance and time involved for regrowth to that level. Some recovery of at least protective sensation on the sole of the foot usually results even from graft repairs at this level. In addition, some degree of plantar flexion usually results even though inversion of the foot and toe flexion may be poor.

## ELECTROPHYSIOLOGIC TESTING

Electrical tests are not only invaluable in working up the patient with injury and documenting recovery but are also important for entrapments and, at times, for nerve tumors.[27,35] Electrical tests need to be well selected and thorough, and they should be done by individuals not only well versed in these techniques but also interested in patients suffering from nerve injury. Although a thorough electromyogram (EMG) helps localize the level of the lesion and the nerve involved, this should never substitute for a thorough physical examination.[5] Specific electrophysiologic findings are emphasized in subsequent chapters. From the point of view of the surgeon, the following initial observations may be of value.

# Electromyography

Acutely and for the first few days after injury, nerve distal to the injury site can be stimulated to produce distal muscle function. This is so even though axons have lost their continuity proximal to the stimulating site. Response to stimulation occurs because Wallerian degeneration takes time to proceed down the distal stump of a nerve. After 48 to 72 hours, the distal stump no longer responds to stimulation, but sampling of muscle shows no denervational change. Such change takes several more weeks to come about. At 2 to 3 weeks, the electromyographer can help the clinician by documenting the extent of denervation as well as its distribution (Figure 3–22). With time and on repeat EMG study, denervational changes may reverse, or there may be nascent activity, indicating reinnervation, especially in proximal muscles. Unfortunately, such physiologic evidence of fiber return to muscle does not promise effective function, but at the least it does indicate some nerve fiber regrowth to those sites where it is recorded.[29,34] EMG should never substitute for clinical examination, however, because even a muscle with extensive denervation may still contract if a portion of its input has been spared or has recovered.[27,66] Conversely, a few fibers may penetrate an injury site and reverse denervational change in a portion of a muscle, yet without sufficient regrowth through the remainder of the injury site to reverse poor distal function.

There are three phases or steps to performing an EMG (Figure 3–23). The first phase is a brief burst of electrical or insertional activity in response to a needle being placed into muscle. The second phase occurs when the muscle is at rest; in healthy, well-innervated muscle, the trace should be flat. The third phase is the electrical response as the patient attempts to contract muscle or the electromyographer stimulates nerve supplying it. With good innervation, this produces an evoked muscle action potential, or MAP (MUAP). The patient should be able to recruit or increase the firing of these MAPs.

With serious denervation, there is loss or severe reduction in insertional activity. With the muscle at rest, instead of a flat trace, spontane-

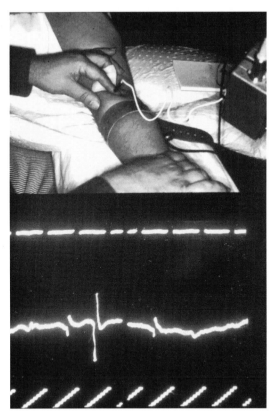

**Figure 3–22.** In the upper photograph, the electromyographer is recording from the pronator muscle in a patient who had sustained a more proximal gunshot wound involving the median nerve 4 months previously. The lower photograph shows recorded fibrillations and a denervational potential. A similar pattern was seen in other muscles sampled, including flexor superficialis, flexor profundus, and flexor pollicis longus, indicating a complete median lesion.

ous firing of rapid biphasic, low-amplitude, sharp waves or fibrillations occurs. On attempted muscle contraction, there is no MAP or a poorly formed one, and recruitment is poor. With reinnervation, these changes begin to reverse, especially in muscle closest to the injury site. The intensity or frequency of fibrillations and denervational potentials decreases. There may also be nascent potentials that are broader based and higher in amplitude than fibrillations. Insertional activity is partially restored, and some restoration of an MAP becomes evident with time, especially if nerve going to that muscle is stimulated. Eventually, even ability to recruit begins to occur.

EMG can suggest reinnervation only after axons have regrown all the way to muscle.[13] A

Three Phases of Electromyographic Testing of Muscle

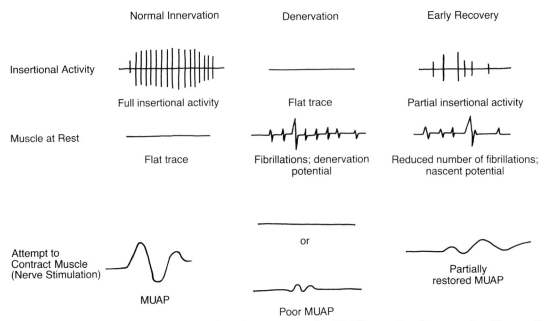

**Figure 3–23.** The three phases usually used on electromyography (EMG) recording from muscle with a needle, coaxially placed in muscle. Traces on EMG with normal innervation, denervation, and early recovery of innervation. The test further delineates these findings. MUAP = evoked muscle action potential.

nerve can be regenerating well beyond an injury and on down the distal stump for months before reversal of denervation changes or regenerative changes is noted by EMG.[31,67] In these earlier weeks to months, only nerve action potential (NAP) recording will indicate regeneration.[29,65,73] Usually, we obtain a baseline EMG on any serious nerve lesion at 3 weeks or so after injury and repeat this after 1 to 2 months in those lesions suspected to be in continuity. These lesions are thus monitored for a period to determine if surgery is necessary.

EMG results must be weighed carefully, taking into account the individual nerve, the level of the injury, time required for regrowth to the proximal muscles tested, and the clinical findings, especially those on motor examination. Unfortunately, finding a decrease in denervation activity and even nascent activity favors but does not guarantee eventual regeneration that is functionally significant.[42,68] Conversely, denervational activity can persist for some time even after muscle is observed to contract, so clinical muscle testing remains paramount. After repair, EMG is only predictive and then only after axons are estimated to have reached muscle based on the assumed rate of regenera-

tion.[44] In an adult with a buttock-level sciatic nerve repair that is regenerating well, a decrease in denervation or reinnervational activity may not begin to occur for a year. On the other hand, EMG signs of regeneration may occur by 3 months in brachioradialis muscle in cases involving a midhumeral-level radial lesion that is axonotmetic.

The other facet of EMG testing involves conduction studies on nerves (Figure 3–24). These tests are of greatest value for suspected entrapments of nerve. They are of less predictive value for the seriously injured nerve, because no conduction will occur beyond the lesion for many, many months. In addition, when conduction does return, it remains slow even years after restoration of function.

## Nerve Stimulation

Nerve stimulation below the level of a neurapraxic injury produces motor function, but stimulation proximal to the injury does not. In addition, simple stimulation of a nerve that is regenerating can evoke muscle contractions several weeks before the patient can do so vol-

D. W.

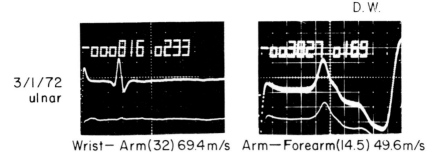

3/1/72
ulnar

Wrist— Arm(32) 69.4 m/s   Arm—Forearm(14.5) 49.6 m/s

**Figure 3-24.** Noninvasively recorded nerve action potentials on whole ulnar nerve in a patient with an elbow-level entrapment. Response from stimulus over ulnar nerve at the wrist was recorded from distal upper arm (left tracing). Conduction is normal over this length because the more normal conduction on distal nerve is averaged with that which is abnormal across the elbow. Right tracing was recorded distal to the elbow-level lesion. Top trace in each inset is summated recording; bottom trace is a single nonsummated trace. Wrist to arm recording (to the left) was over a 32 cm distance with conduction at 69.4 meters per second, whereas that to the right was over a 14.5 cm distance and conducted at 49.6 meters per second.

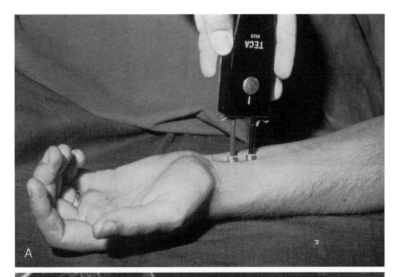

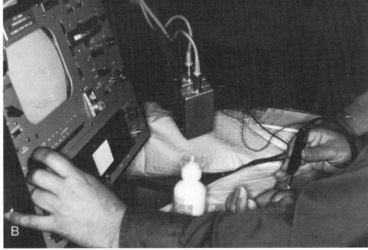

**Figure 3-25.** (*A*) Skin-level nerve stimulation by handheld electrode. Stimuli were delivered to the median nerve proximal to a wrist-level lesion to see if thenar intrinsics, and especially abductor pollicis brevis, would contract. (*B*) Electromyographer is varying stimulus voltage amplitude and duration to determine a threshold for distal muscle contraction in response to median stimulation.

untarily[51] (Figure 3–25). This simple observation may be a useful prognosticator of good clinical recovery and suggest further conservative management. Of course, stimulation of a nerve that has undergone Wallerian degeneration fails to give muscle contraction. This is therefore a valuable observation in the early weeks after injury. After that, however, regeneration may be progressing down the distal stump quite well and yet not have reached muscle, so that stimulation could not be expected to make it contract.[32] On the other hand, there is a delay of weeks to several months after new fibers reach muscle before they mature enough and reinnervate enough motor units for voluntary contraction to occur.[67] Stimulation can produce muscle contraction at some point between the time when fibers first begin to reinnervate muscle and the time at which recovery of voluntary function occurs.

Simple nerve stimulation is especially helpful in early recognition of adequate peroneal recovery, and this can sometimes obviate need for operation.[68] With milder degrees of peroneal injury, stimulation at the head of the fibula 4 or 5 months after injury may produce eversion (peroneus) or even foot dorsiflexion (anterior tibialis). The same could be said for an adequately recovering radial nerve injured at a midhumeral level. Under these circumstances, distal radial nerve stimulation may produce brachioradialis contraction 2 to 6 weeks before this is observable clinically. Depending on the injury mechanism and the extent of radial injury, this may be somewhere between 2 and 3.5 months after injury. Care must be taken not to interpret muscle contraction in response to stimulation of adjacent uninjured nerves or contraction of muscles proximal to the injury site as contraction from muscles below or distal to the lesion.

NAP recording across the lesion provides earlier and also more reliable information about regeneration than stimulation alone but usually requires operative exposure of the nerve (Figure 3–26).

## Sensory Conduction Studies

Sensory nerve action potential (sNAP) studies are of major use for brachial plexus stretch injuries.[34] They can sometimes differentiate preganglionic from postganglionic sites of injury. Lesions at a root or spinal nerve level restricted to the preganglionic region and not extending through the dorsal root ganglion or into the postganglionic area produce complete distal sensory loss but also preserve distal sensory conduction. Injury of preganglionic fibers between the dorsal root ganglion and the spinal cord does not cause degeneration of the distal postganglionic fibers. Unfortunately, if the lesion is both pre- and postganglionic, the trace is flat, so a negative study is not as helpful diagnostically as a positive one.[27] Sensory studies can be done by stimulating the hand in the C6 (thumb and index finger), C6-C7 (index and long finger), or C8-T1 (little and ring finger) areas and recording from median, radial, or ulnar nerves more proximally. If the area stimulated is anesthetic to touch, then recording of an sNAP indicates a preganglionic injury in the distribution of one or more roots.

Because distal sensory distributions of roots overlap, even at a finger level, it can be difficult to be certain which root or roots have preganglionic injury.[32] Stimulation of an anesthetic forefinger or even thumb can produce an sNAP if C6, C7, or both are damaged at a preganglionic level. This makes it difficult to be certain whether C6 has preganglionic injury. For C5, there are no specific stimulation or recording sites for noninvasive sNAP studies.[32] It is difficult to evaluate the upper roots with this technique, and yet these are the very roots one would like to know the most about. On the other hand, sNAP studies may provide useful information about the lower roots, especially C8 and T1. Such studies have replaced axon-response testing by histamine injection.[5] With preganglionic injury, injection of histamine into an anesthetic area of skin produces a wheal much like normally innervated skin. Sensory conduction studies are also of great value for some entrapments. For example, sNAPs across the wrist are abnormal relatively early in patients with carpal tunnel syndrome (Figure 3–27). On the other hand, sensory radial responses are normal in a patient with posterior interosseous nerve entrapment. This is because the point of entrapment is distal to the origin of the uninvolved superficial sensory radial nerve.

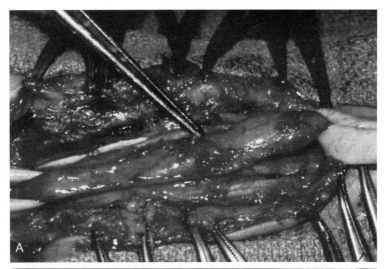

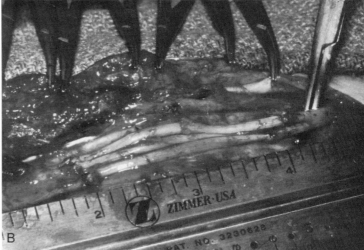

**Figure 3-26.** (*A*) Forearm-level lesion in continuity to the median nerve. Proximal and elbow level is to the right, and distal and hand level is to the left. There was no distal muscle contraction when either the proximal or distal stump was stimulated. (*B*) This lesion also did not transmit a nerve action potential and required a graft repair. Grafts were approximately 6 cm in length.

## Somatosensory Studies

These tests involve peripheral stimulation and more central spinal cord or cortical recordings.[71] Recording sites include those over the spine, or spinal-evoked potentials (SEP) and those over the cerebral cortex at a scalp level, or evoked cortical responses (ECR).[63] Somatosensory studies are primarily used in plexus injuries and, like sensory conduction studies (sNAPs), can be helpful in differentiating preganglionic from postganglionic lesions.[22,33] Recording an SEP or ECR requires only a few hundred intact fibers between point stimulated and that recorded from, so a positive response ensures only minimal continuity of sensory spinal nerve

or root, and a negative study may be more important than a positive one.[74] Such studies when recorded from the CNS do not provide information about the motor root. If done in the early months after severe plexus injury, and if distal sites are used for stimulation, as is the usual case, information provided about regeneration is also minimal. Fibers will not have grown enough to reach most of the distal sites used for stimulation; this requires many more months after injury or repair. On the other hand, intraoperative somatosensory studies, particularly if spinal nerves or roots are directly stimulated close to or in their foramina, can be very valuable.[32,60]

For a given nerve injury, a combination of

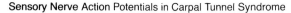

Sensory Nerve Action Potentials in Carpal Tunnel Syndrome

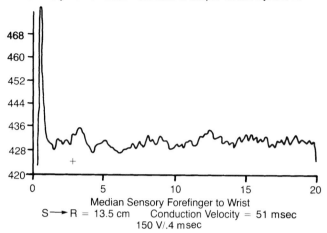

Median Sensory Forefinger to Wrist
S——►R = 13.5 cm     Conduction Velocity = 51 msec
150 V/.4 msec

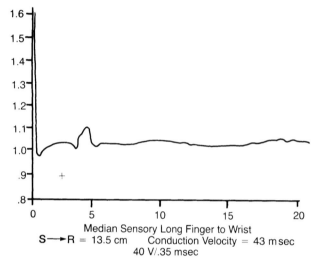

Median Sensory Long Finger to Wrist
S——►R = 13.5 cm     Conduction Velocity = 43 msec
40 V/.35 msec

**Figure 3-27.** Noninvasively recorded sensory potentials in a patient recovering from carpal tunnel syndrome after carpal tunnel release. Amplification necessary to record forefinger to wrist response (top graph) was much greater than that required for response from long finger to wrist (bottom graph) even though velocity was greater. Conduction velocity is in meters per second (m/sec) and stimulus intensity is in volts and milliseconds (v/m/sec).

electrophysiologic tests is often necessary to provide an optimal level of information about denervation and regeneration (Figure 3-28). This is especially so with brachial plexus lesions, in which multiple electrical tests can provide a thorough work-up of the variety of lesions seen.

A combination of clinical and electrical tests can be used to determine whether loss from injury is complete and how complete deinnervation is (see Tables 3-1 and 3-2). Such a determination is of great importance because complete loss in the distribution of a nerve does not usually recover spontaneously. On the other hand, loss that is partial to begin with or that improves either clinically or electrically is usually associated with spontaneous recovery.

## RADIOLOGIC STUDIES

### Radiographs

Fractures can be associated with nerve injury, so radiographs of the traumatized limb with palsy are usually indicated[43,58] (Figure 3-29). Midhumeral fractures are associated with radial nerve injuries. Incidence of serious radial palsy increases if humeral fracture is comminuted or compound or if operation is necessary for fixation. Ulna or radius fractures, especially if comminuted, can be associated with a combined median and ulnar nerve injury or, on occasion, with posterior interosseous palsy. Hip dislocation or fracture has an incidence of sciatic palsy

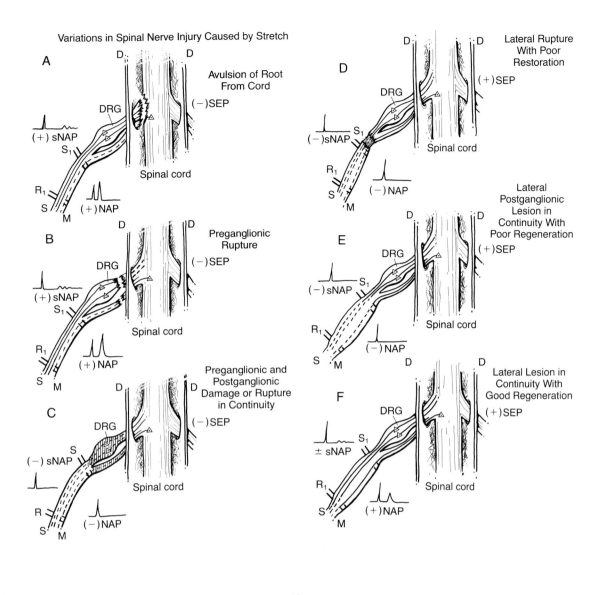
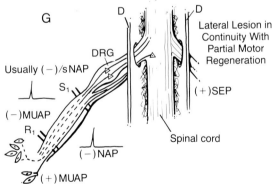

**Figure 3–28.** Variations in spinal nerve injury caused by stretch and their usual electrophysiologic findings. Injuries are progressively depicted from medial or proximal sites to more lateral or distal sites. Parts E, F, and G depict several sets of findings that are not uncommon with stretch injury to the plexus but not as widely known as A, B, C, and D. In G, a few hundred fibers have regenerated or were spared to distal muscle. Thus, the muscle has some contraction when the plexus element is stimulated but does not have an NAP because it does not have 4000 or more fibers greater in size than 5 microns. D = dura mater; DRG = dorsal root ganglion; M = muscle; MUAP = muscle action potential recorded by electromyography; NAP = nerve action potential; $R_1$ = recording electrode; $S_1$ = stimulating electrode; SEP = somatosensory-evoked potential recorded after stimulation of spinal nerve near spine; sNAP = sensory nerve action potential.

**TABLE 3−1**
Evidence Favoring Complete Injury With Deinnervation

1. Complete sensory and sweating loss, especially in autonomous zones
2. No voluntary muscle function on full effort
3. No motor responses on stimulation of nerve below lesion site
4. No electrical activity on electromyographic needle insertion, fibrillations and deinnervation potentials, no muscle action potentials on voluntary effort (samples must be thorough)
5. No nerve action potential past lesion, provided enough time for regeneration has elapsed

associated with it, as do operations to restore hip function. More distal fractures of the femur can involve either the tibial or peroneal divisions of the sciatic nerve, or both. At times, a midshaft fracture of the femur can be related to a more proximal stretch injury to the sciatic nerve at a buttock level. The level of the nerve lesion does not always relate to the level of the fracture, and localization hinges on good clinical and electrodiagnostic evaluation.

Cervical spine fractures can be associated with severe and irreparable proximal stretch injuries to the plexus, especially at the root or spinal nerve level of the involved vertebra.[3] Fractures of the humerus, clavicle, scapula, or ribs may provide rough estimates of the forces brought to bear on the neck, shoulder, and arm, as well as brachial plexus, but do not necessarily help to localize the level or document the extent of injury. Plexus damage is usually more proximal than such fractures would indicate, and it is usually at a root or spinal nerve level.[34,58] Occasionally, excessive callus formation from a fracture of the clavicle, midlevel humerus, elbow, hip, or head of fibula entraps nerve or complicates partial neural injury at these levels.

## Myelography

This radiologic study is still an important test for supraclavicular brachial plexus injuries.[26,41,49] It is true that the myelogram can be falsely negative, so meningoceles can be absent at levels where damage to the spinal nerve has extended to the spinal cord.[18,57] It is also true that meningoceles can be present on roots that function normally or have the potential for recovery, resulting in a false-positive study.[42,50] More commonly, in our experience, a meningocele means that either the root is avulsed or it is in gross continuity but has severe internal damage extending to a very proximal level.[75] In either case, the root at this level is usually not reparable. Presence of a meningocele usually means there was enough force to produce an arachnoidal tear and, if the root is not functional, that damage has extended proximally.[62] Such a finding suggests but does not prove that other roots without a meningocele also have been damaged proximally.[70] Fortunately, this is not always the case. A number of our patients with meningoceles at some (usually lower) levels but not all levels have had successful repair of one or more spinal nerves at an upper level.

Other myelographic findings of importance with stretch injuries include subdural or extradural extravasation of contrast, evidence of cord swelling acutely, or, after a few weeks, spinal cord atrophy.[10] To date, neither computed tomography (CT) scan with metrizamide nor magnetic resonance imaging (MRI) with or without contrast substitutes for a well-done myelogram using concentrated water-soluble contrast with good anteroposterior, lateral, and oblique views. With CT scans, even close transverse cuts may miss root-level changes. At the present time, it is also difficult to visualize enough or all of the roots and spinal nerves with MRI to exclude proximal damage.

Tumors involving plexus roots can also be

**TABLE 3−2**
Evidence Favoring Partial Injury or Functional Regeneration

1. Preservation of or recovery of sensation or sweating in autonomous zones of nerve concerned
2. Voluntary muscle function, especially against resistance in injured nerve's motor distribution
3. Motor response on stimulation of nerve (must be discrete for nerve stimulated)
4. Ability to evoke and record nerve action potentials across and distal to injury site

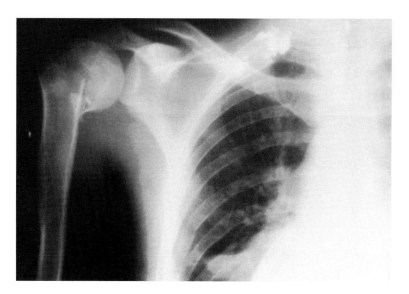

**Figure 3–29.** Shoulder radiograph showing fractured humeral neck associated with a stretch injury to the brachial plexus.

partially evaluated by myelogram, which may show deformity of one or more root sleeves or compression or deformity of the lateral contrast column.[10]

## CT Scan and MRI

A CT scan with metrizamide can miss one or more meningoceles because the cuts may not be fine enough to cover the entire course of the nerve root. CT scans, however, are valuable for tumors, as is the MRI scan.[1] Nonetheless, either study confined to the cervical spine can miss tumors in the neck or shoulder. In an injury setting, MRI can show a nerve root,[1] but it seldom provides enough detail for all roots to preclude the need for a myelogram.[14] As the technology involved with MRI studies develops further, there will be the potential for the MRI to show all of each root. MRI can also confirm degeneration of a nerve, but is not discriminating enough as yet to document regeneration into a previously degenerated site.[43] MRI has been shown by recent studies to depict denervated muscle, which will appear "whitish or dense" (Figure 3–30). The MRI is also being explored as a tool to depict actual degeneration and regeneration in nerve.[10a,54a] These changes on MRI gradually reverse as muscle is reinnervated. On the other hand, the MRI's forte in this field is in depicting tumor impinging on or arising from nerve, particularly the brachial plexus or pelvic plexus,

where inspection and palpation may not delineate the size and extent of the mass.

## Angiography

The use of arteriography and venography is discussed in detail in the sections dealing with gunshot wounds and other penetrating wounds, stretch/contusions to the brachial plexus, and thoracic outlet syndrome. In some

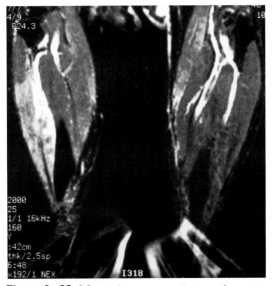

**Figure 3–30.** Magnetic resonance image of anterior and posterior compartment muscle in a patient with a severe peroneal palsy caused by a large intraneural ganglion cyst. T2 phase shows a "whitish-like density" of muscle characteristic of denervation.

centers, it is probably overused with blunt injury but not done enough in cases of penetrating injury or a suspected compartment syndrome. Occasionally, angiography is useful for certain tumors involving nerves or plexus and for an entrapment such as that involving axillary nerve with arm abduction.[8]

In most instances, the working clinical diagnosis is obvious after history and physical examination are recorded and selected electrical and radiographic studies are obtained. Occasionally, difficulty may be experienced. For example, both authors have seen C5-C6 discectomies performed in patients with median nerve pathology and L4-L5 discectomies performed in patients with peroneal nerve palsies.

## Bibliography

1. Armington W, Harnsberger H, Osborn A, et al.: Radiographic evaluation of brachial plexopathy. Am J Neurorad 8:361–367, 1987.
2. Aschan W and Moberg E: Ninhydrin fiber printing test used to map out partial lesions to nerves of hand. Acta Chir Scand 123:365–370, 1962.
3. Bateman JE: The Shoulder and Neck, 2nd Ed. Philadelphia, WB Saunders, 1978, pp. 565–616.
4. Bauwens P: Electrodiagnostic definition of the site and nature of peripheral nerve lesions. Ann Phys Med 5:149–152, 1960.
5. Bonney G: The value of axon responses in determining the site of lesion in traction injuries of the brachial plexus. Brain 77:588–609, 1954.
6. Brown P: Factors influencing the success of surgical repair of peripheral nerves. Surg Clin North Am 52:1137–1155, 1972.
7. Bunnell S: Active splinting of the hand. J Bone Joint Surg 28:732–736, 1946.
8. Cahill BR: Quadrilateral space syndrome. In Omer GE Jr and Spinner M, Eds: Management of Peripheral Nerve Problems. Philadelphia, WB Saunders, 1980, pp. 602–606.
9. Campbell JB: Peripheral nerve repair. Clin Neurosurg 17:77–98, 1970.
10. Drake CG: Diagnosis and treatment of lesions of the brachial plexus and adjacent structures. Clin Neurosurg 11:110–127, 1964.
10a. Filler A, Howe F, Hayes C, et al: Magnetic resonance neurography. Lancet 341:659–661, 1993.
11. Gelberman RH: Operative Nerve Repair and Reconstruction. Philadelphia, JB Lippincott, 1991.
12. Goldner JL: Pain: Extremities and spine—evaluation and differential diagnosis. In Omer GE Jr and Spinner M, Eds: Management of Peripheral Nerve Problems. Philadelphia, WB Saunders, 1980, pp. 602–606.
13. Grundfest H, Oester YT, and Beebe GW: Electrical evidence of regeneration. In Peripheral Nerve Regeneration. Veteran Administration Monograph. Washington, DC, US Government Printing Office, 1957, pp. 203–240.
14. Gupta RK, Mehta VS, and Banerj AK: MRI evaluation of brachial plexus injuries. Neuroradiology 31:377, 1989.
15. Guttman E and Young JZ: Reinnervation of muscle after various periods of atrophy. J Anat 78:15–43, 1944.
16. Haymaker W and Woodhall B: Peripheral Nerve Injuries: Principles of Diagnosis, 2nd Ed. Philadelphia, WB Saunders, 1953.
17. Henderson WR: Clinical assessment of peripheral nerve injuries. Tinel's test. Lancet 2:801–804, 1948.
18. Heon M: Myelogram: A questionable aid in diagnosis and prognosis of brachial plexus components in traction injuries. Conn Med 22:260–262, 1965.
19. Hubbard J: The quality of nerve regeneration. Factors independent of the most skillful repair. Surg Clin North Am 52:1099–1108, 1972.
20. Hudson A, Berry H, and Mayfield F: Chronic injuries of peripheral nerves by entrapment. In Youmans J, Ed: Neurological Surgery: A Comprehensive Reference Guide to the Diagnosis and Management of Neurosurgical Problems, 2nd Ed. Philadelphia, WB Saunders, 1982.
21. Hudson AR and Hunter D: Timing of peripheral nerve repair: Important local neuropathologic factors. Clin Neurosurg 24:391–405, 1977.
22. Jones SJ: Diagnostic use of peripheral and spinal somatosensory evoked potentials in traction lesions of the brachial plexus. Clin Plast Surg 11:167–172, 1984.
23. Kahn EA: Direct observation of sweating in peripheral nerve lesions. Surg Gynecol Obstet 92:22–26, 1951.
24. Kaplan EB and Spinner MB: Normal and anomalous innervation patterns in the upper extremity. In Omer G and Spinner M, Eds: Management of Peripheral Nerve Problems. Philadelphia, WB Saunders, 1980.
25. Kempe L: Operative Neurosurgery, Vol 2. New York, Springer, 1970.
26. Kewalramani L and Taylor R: Brachial plexus root avulsion: Role of myelography. J Trauma 15:603–608, 1975.
27. Kimura J: Electrodiagnosis in Diseases of Nerves and Muscles: Principles and Practices. Philadelphia, FA Davis, 1983.
28. Kline DG: Diagnostic approach to individual nerve injuries. In Wilkins R, Rengachary S, Eds: Neurosurgery. New York, McGraw-Hill, 1985.
29. Kline DG: Evaluating the neuroma in continuity. In Omer GE and Spinner M, Eds: Management of Peripheral Nerve Problems. Philadelphia, WB Saunders, 1980.
30. Kline DG: Macroscopic and microscopic concomitants of nerve repair. Clin Neurosurg 26:582–606, 1979.
31. Kline DG: Operative experience with major lower extremity nerve lesions, including the lumbosacral plexus and the sciatic nerve. In Omer GE Jr and Spinner M, Eds: Management of Peripheral Nerve Problems. Philadelphia, WB Saunders, 1980, pp. 607–625.
32. Kline DG and Hudson AR: Acute injuries of peripheral nerves. In Youmans J, Ed: Neurological Surgery, 3rd Ed. Philadelphia, WB Saunders, 1990.
33. Landi A, Copeland SA, Wynn-Parry CB, et al.: The role of somatosensory evoked potentials and nerve conduction studies in the surgical management of brachial plexus injuries. J Bone Joint Surg 62B:9–22, 1980.
34. Leffert RD: Clinical diagnosis, testing, and electromyographic study in brachial plexus traction injuries. Clin Orthop Rel Res 237:24–31, 1988.

35. Licht S, Ed: Electrodiagnosis and Electromyography. New Haven, CT, E Licht, 1961.

36. Liu CT and Lewey FH: The effect of surging currents of low frequency in man on atrophy of denervated muscles. J Nerv Ment Dis 105:571–581, 1947.

37. Lundborg G: Nerve Injury and Repair. Edinburgh, Churchill Livingstone, 1988.

38. Mackinnon S and Dellon A: Surgery of the Peripheral Nerve. New York, Thieme Medical Publishers, 1988.

39. Mayfield F: Causalgia. Springfield, IL, Charles C Thomas, 1951.

40. Mayfield F: Reflex dystrophies of the hand. In Flynn JE, Ed: Hand Surgery. Baltimore, Williams & Wilkins, 1966, pp. 738–750; 1095.

41. McGillicuddy J: Clinical decision-making in brachial plexus injuries. Neurosurg Clin North Am 2:137–150, 1991.

42. McQuarrie I: Clinical signs of peripheral nerve regeneration. In Wilkins R and Rengachary S, Eds: Neurosurgery. New York, McGraw-Hill, 1985.

43. McQuarrie I: Peripheral nerve surgery–today and looking ahead. Clin Plast Surg 13:255–268, 1986.

44. McQuarrie I and Idzikowski C: Injuries to peripheral nerves. In Miller T and Rowlands B, Eds: Physiologic Basis of Modern Surgical Care. St. Louis, CV Mosby, 1988, pp. 802–815.

45. Medical Research Council, Nerve Injuries Committee: Aids to Investigation of Peripheral Nerve Injuries. MRC War Memorandum No. 7. London, His Majesty's Stationery Office, 1943. London, Balliere Tindall, 1986.

46. Millesi H and Terzis JK: Nomenclature in peripheral nerve surgery. Clin Plast Surg 11:3–8, 1984.

47. Moberg E: Objective methods for determining the functional value of sensibility in the hand. J Bone Joint Surg 40B:454–475, 1958.

48. Murphey F, Hartung W, and Kirklin JW: Myelographic demonstration of avulsing injury of brachial plexus. AJR Am J Roentgenol 58:102–105, 1947.

49. Murphey F, Kirklin J, and Finlaysan AI: Anomalous innervation of the intrinsic muscles of the hand. Surg Gynecol Obstet 83:15–23, 1946.

50. Narakas A: The surgical treatment of traumatic brachial plexus injuries. Int Surg 65:521–527, 1980.

51. Nulsen FE and Lewey FH: Intraneural bipolar stimulation: A new aid in the assessment of nerve injuries. Science 106:301–304, 1947.

52. Omer G: The evaluation of clinical results following peripheral nerve suture. In Omer G and Spinner M, Eds: Management of Peripheral Nerve Problems. Philadelphia, WB Saunders, 1980, pp. 431–438.

53. Omer GE and Spinner M: Peripheral nerve testing and suture techniques. American Academy of Orthopaedic Surgons Instructional Course Lectures, Vol. 24. St. Louis, CV Mosby, 1975, pp. 122–143.

54. O'Rian S: New and simple test of nerve function in the hand. Br Med J 3:615, 1973.

54a. Polak J, Jolesz F, Adams D: Magnetic resonance imaging of skeletal muscle prolongation of T1 and T2 subsequent to denervation. Invest Radiol 23:365–369, 1988.

55. Prutkin L: Normal and anomalous innervation patterns in the lower extremities. In Omer G and Spinner M, Eds: Management of Peripheral Nerve Problems. Philadelphia, WB Saunders, 1980.

56. Seddon HJ: Surgical Disorders of the Peripheral Nerves. Baltimore, Williams & Wilkins, 1972.

57. Simard J and Sypert G: Closed traction avulsion injuries of the brachial plexus. Contemp Neurosurg 50:1–6, 1983.

58. Spinner M: The anterior interosseus-nerve syndrome with special attention to its variations. J Bone Joint Surg 52A:84, 1970.

59. Spurling RG and Woodhall B, Eds: Medical Department, United States Army, Surgery in World War II: Neurosurgery, Vol. 2. Washington DC, US Government Printing Office, 1959.

60. Sugioka H, Tsuyama N, Hara T, et al: Investigation of brachial plexus injuries by intraoperative cortical somatosensory evoked potentials. Arch Orthop Trauma Surg 99:143–151, 1982.

61. Sunderland S: Nerve and Nerve Injuries, 1st Ed. Baltimore, Williams & Wilkins, 1968.

62. Sunderland S: Nerves and Nerve Injuries, 2nd Ed. Edinburgh, Churchill Livingstone, 1978.

63. Syneck V and Cowan J: Somatosensory evoked potentials in patients with supraclavicular brachial plexus injuries. Neurology 32:1347–1352, 1982.

64. Ulmer JL and Mayfield FH: Causalgia: A study of 75 cases. Surg Gynecol Obstet 83:789–796, 1946.

65. Van Beek A, Hubble B, and Kinkead L: Clinical use of nerve stimulation and recording. Plast Reconstr Surg 71:225–232, 1983.

66. Wilbourn A: Electrodiagnosis of plexopathies. Neurol Clin 3:511–529, 1985.

67. Williams H and Terzis J: Single fascicular recordings: An intraoperative diagnostic tool for the management of peripheral nerve lesions. Plast Reconstr Surg 57:562–569, 1976.

68. Woodhall B, Nulsen FE, White JC, and Davis L: Neurosurgical implications. In: Peripheral Nerve Regeneration. Veterans Administration Monograph. Washington, DC, US Government Printing Office, 1957, pp. 569–638.

69. Wynn-Perry CB: Rehabilitation of the Hand. London, Butterworths, 1966.

70. Yeoman P: Cervical myelography in traction injuries of the brachial plexus. J Bone Joint Surg 50B:253–257, 1968.

71. Yiannikas C, Chahani BT, and Young RR: The investigation of traumatic lesions of the brachial plexus by electromyography and short latency somatosensory potentials evoked by stimulation of multiple peripheral nerves. J Neurol Neurosurg Psychiatry 46:1014–1022, 1983.

72. Zachary RB and Roaf R: Lesions in continuity. In Seddon HJ, Ed: Peripheral Nerve Injuries. Med Res Council Spec Report Series No. 282. London, Her Majesty's Stationery Office, 1954.

73. Zalis A, Rodriquez A, Oester Y, and Mains D: Evaluation of nerve regeneration by means of evoked potentials. J Bone Joint Surg 54A:1246–1253, 1972.

74. Zhao S, Kim D, Kline D, et al.: Somatosensory evolved potentials induced by stimulating a variable number of nerve fibers in rat. Muscle Nerve 16:1220–1227, 1993.

75. Zorub D, Nashold BS Jr, and Cook WA Jr: Avulsion of the brachial plexus, I. A review with implications on the therapy of intractable pain. Surg Neurol 2:347–353, 1974.

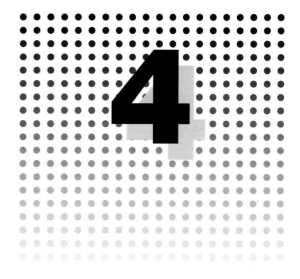

# Grading Results

## SUMMARY

If results of management are to be used to formulate future therapy, they must not only be graded for motor and important sensory function but individualized for different nerves and different anatomic levels. There are always potential criticisms of a grading system. Most of the grading systems used in the past were developed from criteria used to grade function in patients with polio, in whom a trace of either retained function or recovery of function, even short of ability to overcome gravity, had great predictive importance. Grading such small amounts of function, although sometimes important for nerve injuries, pales in comparison to grading contraction against gravity and against mild, moderate, and great resistance. For this reason, the Louisiana State University Medical Center system goes from 0 = no function, to 1 = trace, to 2 = contraction against gravity, to 3 = contraction against gravity and mild resistance, to 4 = contraction against gravity and moderate resistance, to 5 = contraction against considerable or full resistance.

It is also important to be able to grade a whole nerve's function level by level. For the results reported in this text, this has been done by comparatively grading function for the proximal or closest muscles to the level of a given nerve's injury and for those in the nerve's more distal distribution. Individual grading tables have thus been developed for most major nerves at their more important levels.

The system is presented only to be enlarged upon, changed, or redirected. Clearly, the older British and American systems, although valuable, do not provide quite as much information as that proposed here. Conversely, the grading system presented has not addressed use of the limb for activities of daily living or employment, although the case summaries provided in later chapters often provide some insight in this regard.

One of the central themes of this book is the use of data concerning results of management. Difficulties in obtaining these data have, on several occasions, delayed publication of this book. Nevertheless, a useful system for grading loss and recovery of sensory and motor function has always been paramount. Moreover, a system is needed not only for grading individual muscle and sensory responses but for evaluating function in the distribution of an entire nerve or plexus element. Most nerves and plexus elements innervate one or more proximal muscles, a group of more distal muscles, and also a distal sensory field of variable functional importance. There are a number of useful publications that have used or reported on various grading systems.[1-8,12-26] Discussion of the reasons for selection of the grading systems in use, however, has been difficult to find. In this book, the grading system used to evaluate recovery — the Louisiana State University Medical Center (LSUMC) system — is based on earlier British and American systems but includes some important changes.[9-11]

Both the British Medical Research Council (MRC) and the American systems for grading loss or return of motor function after nerve injury and repair were originally based on grading systems developed to evaluate paralysis associated with poliomyelitis (Tables 4-1 through 4-3). In the polio patient, retention or return of a very small amount of function held important prognostic and often therapeutic value. Grades 1, 2, and 3 in those systems took the muscle

**TABLE 4-1**
Muscle Power Grading (British System)

| Grade | Description |
| --- | --- |
| 0 — None | No palpable muscle contraction |
| 1 — Trace | Palpable muscle contraction, detectable by examiner |
| 2 — Poor | Active joint motion present with gravity eliminated |
| 3 — Fair | Muscle can move joint through full range of motion against gravity |
| 4 — Good | Full range of motion against gravity and some resistance |
| 5 — Normal | Full range of motion with a maximum force that is normal for that muscle |

## TABLE 4–2
### Grading of Entire Nerve (British MRC System)

M5— Complete recovery
M4— All synergetic and independent movements are possible
M3— All important muscles contract against resistance
M2— Return of perceptible contraction in both proximal and distal muscles
M1— Return of perceptible contraction in proximal muscles
M0— No contraction any muscle

(Seddon H: Peripheral Nerve Injuries. Medical Research Council Special Report Series No. 282. London, Her Majesty's Stationery Office, 1954.)

## TABLE 4–3
### Grading of Entire Nerve (American System)

M6— Complete recovery
M5— Some synergetic and isolated movements possible
M4— All important muscles have sufficient power to act against resistance
M3— Proximal muscles act against gravity; perceptible contraction in intrinsic muscles
M2— Proximal muscles act against gravity; no return of power in intrinsic muscles
M1— Return of perceptible contraction in the proximal muscles
M0— No contraction

(Woodhall B, Beebe G, Eds: Peripheral nerve regeneration: A follow-up study of 3656 W W II injuries. VA Medical Monograph, US Government Printing Office, Washington, DC, 1956.)

function only to the point of overcoming gravity, and function after that point received limited gradation. With nerve injury, small amounts of recovery are also important, but so is a gradual gradation after recovery of contraction against gravity. As a result, these systems were modified to rate contraction against gravity alone a 2, and to provide a grade of 3 for contraction against gravity and mild resistance. The LSUMC modified system also provides a 4 for contraction against moderate resistance and, finally, a 5 for contraction against maximal resistance (Table 4–4; Figure 4–1). Sensory grades were also changed to accommodate a more practical and readily carried out examination, concentrating on ability to localize various stimuli.

For grading whole nerve function, we began

with the MRC system, which takes into account proximal as well as distal muscle function. A similar but altered scheme was devised (Table 4–5), again expanding grades between 2 and 5. The designation of independent and synergetic movements, used for grade 4 in the MRC system and grade 5 in the American system, was eliminated even though this was a potentially valuable observation. Instead, grade 4 for whole nerve was made to include contraction of proximal and distal muscles against gravity and some resistance. It was determined that full recovery of function was unlikely with most serious injuries to major nerves, so grade 5 includes contraction of proximal and distal muscles against gravity and moderate rather than full re-

## TABLE 4–4
### Louisiana State University Medical Center Grading System for Motor and Sensory Function

**Individual Muscle Grades**

| Grade | Evaluation | Description |
|---|---|---|
| 0 | Absent | No contraction |
| 1 | Poor | Trace contraction |
| 2 | Fair | Movement against gravity only |
| 3 | Moderate | Movement against gravity and some (mild) resistance |
| 4 | Good | Movement against moderate resistance |
| 5 | Excellent | Movement against maximal resistance |

**Sensory Grades**

| Grade | Evaluation | Description |
|---|---|---|
| 0 | Absent | No response to touch, pin, or pressure |
| 1 | Bad | Testing gives hyperesthesia or paresthesia; deep pain recovery in autonomous zones |
| 2 | Poor | Sensory response sufficient for grip and slow protection; sensory stimuli mislocalized with over-response |
| 3 | Moderate | Response to touch and pin in autonomous zones; sensation mislocalized and not normal with some over-response |
| 4 | Good | Response to touch and pin in autonomous zones; response localized but sensation not normal; no over-response |
| 5 | Excellent | Near normal response to touch and pin in entire field including autonomous zones |

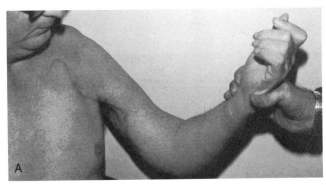
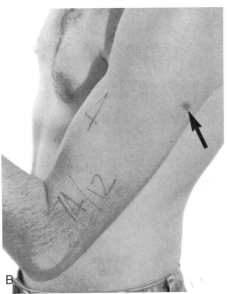

**Figure 4–1.** (A) Grading biceps in a patient who sustained lateral cord to musculocutaneous nerve and lateral cord to median nerve injuries as a result of stretch/contusion. (B) Recovery of biceps 14 months after a gunshot wound (arrow shows entry site) and 12 months after a suture repair of the musculocutaneous nerve.

sistance. These changes in the British and American systems for grading whole nerve function resulted in the system shown in Table 4–5.

## GRADING UPPER AND LOWER EXTREMITY NERVE INJURIES

A severe high or proximal injury to radial nerve results in loss of triceps, brachioradialis, supinator, extensor carpi ulnaris (ECU) and radialis (ECR), extensor communis (EC), and extensor pollicis longus (EPL) function (see Figure 4–1). Sensory loss on the dorsum of the hand and over the anatomic snuffbox area is variable. For grading purposes, proximal muscles

for a proximal radial lesion would be triceps and brachioradialis, and distal muscles would be ECR, ECU, EC, and EPL (Figure 4–2). Sensory loss is less important and more variable with a radial lesion than with a median or ulnar lesion. Therefore, sensory grading is not included when function for the whole radial nerve is graded.

For a proximal radial lesion, the grading scale is as follows:

0 = Absent radial motor function.
1 = Some contraction of triceps; if brachioradialis contracts, it does so against gravity only.
2 = Triceps and brachioradialis contract against force, but there is little or no supination and no wrist extension.

**TABLE 4–5**
Louisiana State University Medical Center Criteria for Grading Whole Nerve Injury

| Grade | Evaluation | Description |
|---|---|---|
| 0 | Absent | No muscle contraction, absent sensation |
| 1 | Poor | Proximal muscles contract but not against gravity; sensory grade 1 or 0 |
| 2 | Fair | Proximal muscles contract against gravity; distal muscles do not contract; sensory grade if applicable is usually 2 or lower |
| 3 | Moderate | Proximal muscles contract against gravity and some resistance; some distal muscles contract against at least gravity; sensory grade is usually 3 |
| 4 | Good | All proximal and some distal muscles contract against gravity and some resistance; sensory grade is 3 or better |
| 5 | Excellent | All muscles contract against moderate resistance; sensory grade is 4 or better |

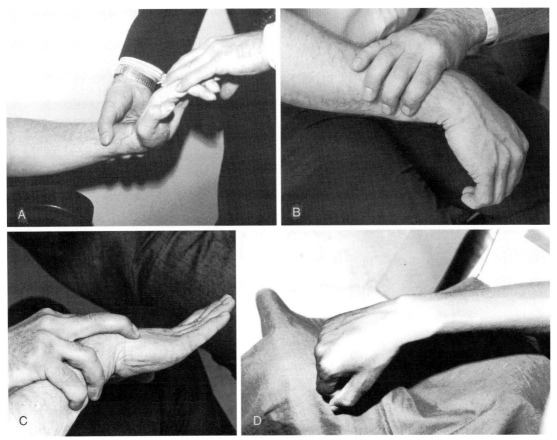

**Figure 4-2.** *(A)* Grading wrist extension in a patient with a posterior cord to radial nerve lesion. *(B)* Trace contraction of wrist extension. *(C)* Extension of wrist against gravity and some pressure. *(D)* Partial extension of wrist despite total radial palsy. Extensor tendons had shortened owing to denervation, and when this patient made a fist, the wrist cocked back.

3 = Triceps and brachioradialis contract against force; supination and wrist extension against at least gravity. There may be a trace of finger or thumb extension, or this may be absent.

4 = Triceps and brachioradialis contract against force; supination and wrist extension are present against force. There is usually a trace or better finger and thumb extension.

5 = Good triceps and brachioradialis function as well as supination and wrist extension; finger and thumb extension against at least gravity and some resistance.

Construction of a grading paradigm for a more distal radial lesion involving posterior interosseous nerve (PIN) would include the following criteria:

0 = No ECU, EC, or EPL muscle function.

1 = Either trace function or contraction against gravity only for ECU; absent EC and EPL muscle function.

2 = Recovery of ECU function; absent or trace only of EC or EPL muscle function, or both.

3 = Recovery of ECU, some EC, weak or absent EPL muscle function.

4 = Recovery of moderate strength of EC and EPL; full strength in ECU muscle function.

5 = Recovery of full strength of EPL, EC, and ECU muscle function.

For grading of the more common midarm radial lesion, such as that caused by a fracture at a midhumeral level, the brachioradialis, supinator, and ECR are the proximal muscles, and the ECU, EC, and EPL are the distal muscles. By comparison, for a posterior cord lesion, the proximal muscles would be latissimus dorsi, deltoid, and triceps, and the more distal muscles would be brachioradialis, supinator, and ECR.

Such a template is easier for a femoral nerve lesion and somewhat more complex for a median or ulnar nerve lesion. For a proximal pelvic level femoral lesion:

0 = Absence of iliacus as well as quadriceps muscle function.

1 = Contraction of iliacus against gravity but not pressure.

2 = Contraction of iliacus against gravity and some pressure; usually a trace of quadriceps function is present.

3 = Good iliacus contraction, and quadriceps contracts against gravity.

4 = Good iliacus function, and contraction of quadriceps against gravity plus some force.

5 = Contraction of both iliacus and quadriceps against considerable force.

By comparison, grading a proximal median lesion would include more detail because of its important distal sensory as well as motor input (Figure 4–3). For a proximal median lesion:

0 = No median-innervated pronation or wrist or finger or thumb flexion, no thenar intrinsic function (abductor pollicis brevis and opponens pollicis); absent to poor median sensation.

1 = Pronation present but quite weak, median-innervated wrist and finger flexors contract, but not against gravity; sensory grade, if present, is 1.

2 = Pronation and wrist and finger flexion against gravity; more distal muscles either do not contract or have trace function only; sensory grade is 2 or lower.

3 = Pronation as well as wrist and finger flexion against gravity and some resistance; some distal muscles such as flexor pollicis longus and even thenar intrinsics contract against gravity; sensory grade is usually 3.

4 = Pronators, wrist and finger flexors, flexor pollicis longus muscles, and even thenar intrinsics contract against some resistance; sensory grade is 3 or better.

5 = All median-innervated muscles contract against considerable force; sensory grade is 4 or better.

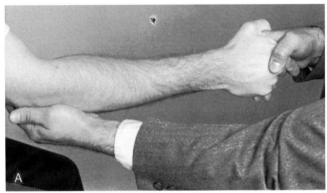

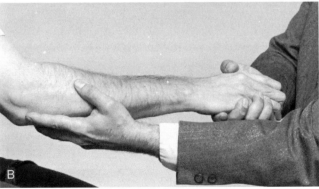

**Figure 4–3.** Steps in grading pronator. Hand and forearm are partially pronated in (A) and fully pronated against resistance in (B).

A similar system can be devised for the ulnar nerve, which also has a sensory field. A grading system for portions of the brachial plexus that eventually go to either the median or ulnar nerve also has design similarities to that used for the median nerve.

Grading systems for the sciatic nerve once again depend on both proximal and distal muscles but also work best if the tibial half of that nerve's function is evaluated separately from the peroneal half. For proximal tibial lesions:

0 = No gastrocnemius-soleus function, no inversion, no toe flexion, little or no sensation on the plantar surface of the foot.

1 = Trace gastrocnemius but no other tibial muscle function; trace to poor plantar sensation.

2 = Gastrocnemius contracts against gravity only; plantar surface usually has a sensory grade of 2 or less.

3 = Gastrocnemius-soleus contracts against gravity and some force; trace or better inversion; plantar sensory grade of 3 or better.

4 = Gastrocnemius contracts against moderate resistance, inversion grades 3 or better, either a trace or no toe flexion; sensation grades 4 or better.

5 = Gastrocnemius has full function, inversion grades 4 or better, toe flexion present; plantar sensation grades 4 or better.

For a proximal peroneal division lesion, grading includes a thigh muscle but excludes a less important sensory field:

0 = No or little short head of biceps function, no peronei, no anterior tibialis (AT), no extensor hallucis longus (EHL) or EC function.

1 = Short head of biceps contracts, no distal peroneal-innervated motor function.

2 = Short head of biceps contracts, peronei contract against gravity or better; no AT or more distal motor function.

3 = Short head of biceps contracts, peronei grade 3 or better; AT contracts against gravity, but function of EHL and EC for toes is usually absent.

4 = Short head of biceps and peronei contract, as does AT, which is grade 3 or better; EHL and EC may have trace function.

5 = Short head of biceps and peronei contract, AT grades 4 or better, and EHL and EC contract against at least gravity.

## GRADING C5-C6 OR UPPER TRUNK LESIONS

Loss in this distribution involves supraspinatus, infraspinatus, deltoid, latissimus dorsi, biceps/brachialis, brachioradialis, and supinator muscle (Figure 4–4). Although deltoid is more proximal than biceps/brachialis or brachioradialis, it often recovers later than these muscles because it requires a very complex innervation to work even against gravity. Infraspinatus seldom recovers after severe proximal plexus injury. These variations are reflected in the following grading scale:

0 = No function in the C5-C6 or upper trunk distribution.

1 = Some supraspinatus contraction, trace of biceps/brachialis, no deltoid.

2 = Supraspinatus contraction, but no deltoid contraction or trace only; contraction of biceps against gravity only.

3 = Supraspinatus contraction, trace only deltoid, contraction of biceps/brachialis or brachioradialis against gravity and some force.

4 = Supraspinatus contraction is against gravity or more, deltoid contracts against gravity or more, biceps/brachialis or brachioradialis contracts against moderate resistance; infraspinatus may or may not contract.

5 = Good recovery of supraspinatus function; deltoid contracts against gravity and at least mild resistance; biceps/brachialis or brachioradialis against great resistance; some recovery of supination; infraspinatus may or may not contract.

## GRADING C5, C6, AND C7 LESIONS OR UPPER PLUS MIDDLE TRUNK LESIONS

Loss in this distribution includes supraspinatus, infraspinatus, supinator, deltoid, latissimus dorsi, biceps/brachialis, brachioradialis, and

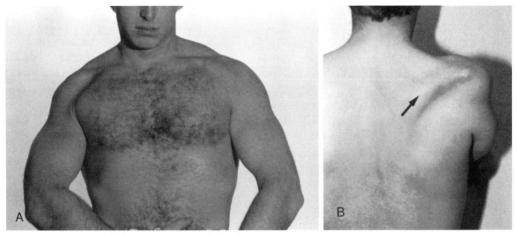

**Figure 4–4.** *(A)* Absence of the patient's right deltoid in an otherwise muscular young man. The only abduction of the arm was provided by supraspinatus, so deltoid (and thus axillary) function was 0. *(B)* In this patient, there was loss of not only deltoid but supraspinatus and infraspinatus function. Note the muscular atrophy on either side of the scapula's spinous process *(arrow)*. Supraspinatus function was trace only, as was that of deltoid; infraspinatus function was absent (0). This gave an overall grade for C5 function of 1. See also color figure.

usually latissimus dorsi and triceps loss (Figure 4–5). There is often some weakness in pronation. There may or may not be weakness or loss of wrist extension and finger and thumb extension. Less frequent is weakness in wrist and finger flexion. There may also be some sensory loss in the median distribution. The grading system is as follows:

0 = No function in the C5, C6, and C7 distribution.
1 = Some supraspinatus contraction, trace contraction of biceps/brachialis, but absent deltoid function and also no function in the more distal C7-innervated muscles.

2 = Supraspinatus contraction, trace contraction of deltoid, and contraction of biceps/brachialis against gravity only; no function of triceps or other distal C6- or C7-innervated muscles.
3 = Supraspinatus contraction; deltoid contracts against gravity, biceps/brachioradialis or brachioradialis against gravity and some resistance, triceps trace or better.
4 = Supraspinatus contraction, deltoid contracts against gravity or better, biceps/ brachialis or brachioradialis against gravity and at least moderate resistance, and triceps against gravity; some true supination, some return of wrist, finger,

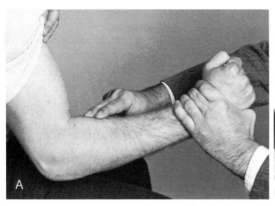
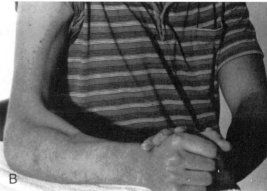

**Figure 4–5.** Grading brachioradialis. *(A)* Muscle contraction is palpated, and resistance is applied by the examiner as the patient flexes forearm that is partially pronated. *(B)* In this patient, biceps function was absent, but brachioradialis contracted against gravity and mild pressure (grade 3).

and thumb extension or flexion if these functions were absent before operation.

5 = Supraspinatus contraction, deltoid against some resistance, biceps/brachioradialis and brachioradialis against moderate or more resistance, some supination, triceps against gravity, and some resistance and some contraction of wrist, finger and thumb extensors or flexors if they were absent preoperatively.

## GRADING C8-T1 LESIONS

Complete loss in this distribution always includes hand intrinsic muscle loss. This includes muscles in the ulnar distribution, which are hypothenars, interossei, lumbricals, and adductor pollicis (Figure 4–6). There is also weakness of flexor pollicis brevis and sensory loss in the ulnar distribution. In the median distribution, function of thenar intrinsics, including abductor pollicis brevis and opponens pollicis, is lost; flexor pollicis brevis function is also lost because both distal median and ulnar outflows supply this muscle with dual innervation. There may or may not be further loss, including decreased extension of the fingers, which is sometimes worse in little and ring fingers than in forefinger and long finger but occasionally occurs the other way around. In other patients, the flexor profundus muscles may be weak, and again the distribution of this loss varies from patient to patient, so that in some it affects fingers on the ulnar side of the hand more than on the radial side, and in other cases the other way around. On occasion, even wrist and finger extensors and/or flexor profundus muscles may be weak or totally paralyzed. Shoulder, upper arm, and usually forearm muscle functions are excellent, but the hand is severely affected (Figure 4–7). The grading system is as follows:

0 = No function in C8-T1 distribution.

1 = Some but usually poor (grade 2 or less) sensation in ulnar distribution of hand; some recovery of finger extensor or finger flexor function if that had been absent previously (grade 2).

2 = Finger extensors or flexors functional if function was lost before (grade 3); ulnar sensation is grade 3 or better; hypothenars contract and are grade 2 or better; function of other intrinsics is trace or absent.

3 = Ulnar sensation is grade 3 or better; finger extensors or flexors, if function was lost before, grade 3 or better; hypothenar muscles grade 3 or better; most other hand intrinsics contract against gravity only.

4 = Ulnar sensation grade 3 or better; finger extensors or flexors, if function was lost before, grade 3 or better; hypothenars

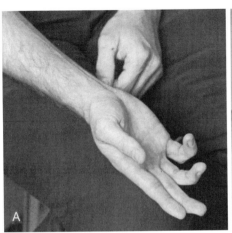
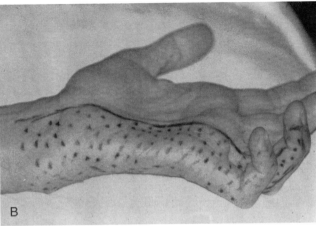

**Figure 4–6.** *(A)* Clawing associated with loss of function of lumbrical to little and ring fingers in an ulnar palsy. After flexor carpi ulnaris is tested, flexor profundus function in the little and ring fingers is assessed. Then, the hand intrinsic muscles are examined. *(B)* In this case of severe ulnar palsy caused by an elbow-level injury, loss was complete below the level of the flexor carpi ulnaris. Only a trace of abductor digiti minimi and opponens digiti minimi function was present (grade 1). Typical sensory loss with a proximal ulnar injury is evident.

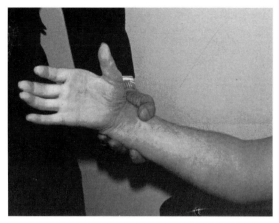

**Figure 4–7.** Interossei in this patient could contract, but not against resistance. This gave overall grade 2 function.

grade 3 or better; most other intrinsics contract against gravity and some resistance.

5 = Ulnar sensation grade 4 or 5; return of any lost finger extension or flexion; all intrinsics contract against at least moderate pressure or resistance.

## GRADING C5-T1 LOSS

Complete loss of function in this distribution produces a flail arm. In the usual injury, rhomboids and serratus anterior still contract because of very proximal origin from spinal nerve branches to these muscles. Diaphragm functions, and there is a variable amount of paraspinal denervation. There is no other function preserved in the arm with a complete lesion in this distribution, so shoulder movement, other than that provided by trapezius, is absent, as is elbow, wrist, and finger motion. Sensory loss is complete in median and ulnar distributions of the hand and even in the radial distribution on the back of the hand. Usually there is no significant sensory perception below the elbow. Because of widespread autonomic loss, there is absence of sweating on all fingers. The grading scale is as follows:

0 = No sensory or motor function in the arm.
1 = Supraspinatus contracts against gravity;

trace contraction of biceps/brachialis or brachioradialis.

2 = Supraspinatus contracts against gravity and some pressure; biceps/brachialis or brachioradialis contract against gravity.

3 = Supraspinatus is good, biceps/brachialis or brachioradialis contract against gravity and some pressure; contraction of deltoid usually trace to against gravity; there may be a trace of triceps function.

4 = In addition to findings for grade 3 above, triceps contracts against at least gravity; deltoid contracts against at least gravity; there may be a trace of wrist and/or finger function.

5 = In addition to recovery of shoulder and arm muscle contraction against gravity and at least some resistance, there is either wrist flexion or extension, and there is some finger flexion.

## GRADING LATERAL CORD LOSS

Loss in this distribution includes biceps/brachialis loss and sensory loss in the median distribution. Pronation is weak or absent, and wrist and finger flexion, including thumb flexion, may be weak. The grading system is as follows:

0 = No motor or sensory function.
1 = Trace of biceps/brachialis function with or without slight return of some sensation in median distribution (sensory grade 1).
2 = Biceps/brachialis contract against gravity; sensation in the median distribution is grade 1 or higher.
3 = Biceps/brachialis contract against gravity and some pressure; sensation is grade 2 or higher; any wrist or finger flexion weakness has improved.
4 = Biceps/brachialis contract against gravity and moderate pressure; sensation is grade 3 or higher.
5 = Biceps/brachialis contract against gravity and considerable pressure; sensation grades 3 or higher.

## GRADING MEDIAL CORD LOSS

In addition to severe hand intrinsic muscle function loss and ulnar distribution sensory loss, there is a variable amount of forearm-level, median-innervated motor loss. This usually involves wrist and finger flexion weakness (see Figure 4–7). Grading is as follows:

0 = No sensory or motor function.

1 = Return of wrist and finger flexion if absent or paretic previously.

2 = Some sensation in ulnar distribution (grade 2); weak (trace) hypothenar function.

3 = Return of contraction of hypothenars against gravity and some pressure. Sensation in ulnar distribution grades 3; trace or better function of interossei, lumbricales, and adductor pollicis.

4 = Hypothenars contract against gravity and mild pressure, as do interossei and lumbricales.

5 = Return of motor function of hypothenars, interossei, and lumbricales to grade 4 or better. Thenar intrinsics and adductor pollicis contract against at least gravity. Ulnar sensation is grade 4 or better.

## GRADING PAIN

Some interesting attempts have been made to grade pain (Table 4–6). Various investigators have devised questionnaires and body diagrams for patients on which patients are requested to describe their pain. Attempts have

**TABLE 4–6**

Pain Grades

| Grade | Description |
|---|---|
| P4 (100%)— | Severe enough to prevent all activity and causes distress |
| P3 (75%) — | Prevents some activity |
| P2 (50%) — | Interferes with activity |
| P1 (25%) — | Annoying |

(Omer GE and Spinner M, Eds: Management of Peripheral Nerve Problems. Philadelphia, WB Saunders, 1980, p. 434.)

**TABLE 4–7**

Upper Extremity Nerve Injuries: In Continuity Cases Studied 1965–1990

| | No. With (+) NAP/Result After Neurolysis | No. With (−) NAP/Result After Repair |
|---|---|---|
| Median | | |
| Upper arm | 23/22 | 16/11* |
| Elbow, forearm | 25/24 | 16/12* |
| Wrist | 24/24 | 17/14 |
| | 72/70 | 49/37 |
| Radial | | |
| Upper arm | 30/28 | 62/42† |
| Elbow | 10/09 | 08/07 |
| Posterior interosseous | 05/05 | 04/04 |
| Forearm | 01/01 | 04/02 |
| Superficial sensory radial | 03/03 | 06/06 |
| | 49/46 | 84/61 |
| Totals | 121/117 (97%) | 123/98 (79%) |

Result = number achieving an LSUMC whole nerve grade 3 or better result. Repair was either by end-to-end suture or grafts.
*1 split repair.
†2 split repairs.
(Adapted from Kline D, Happel L: A quarter century's experience with intraoperative nerve action potential recording. Can J Neurol Sci 20:3–10, 1993.)

also been made to quantify or grade such systems. All investigators agree, however, that grading of pain is very difficult to achieve in a satisfactory fashion. For purposes of this text, we have tried to describe the pain pattern whenever possible rather than attempting to grade this response or outcome.

## OUTCOME STUDIES

Tables 4–7 through 4–10 summarize outcomes of lesions in continuity studied intraoperatively by nerve action potential (NAP) recordings. *For these tabulations, a good result was viewed as recovery of whole nerve function to an LSUMC grade of at least 3.* This meant that recovery included contraction of proximal muscles against gravity and some resistance, contraction of some distal muscles against gravity, and a sensory grade of 3 or better, if applicable to the nerve in question. These particular tables cover

**TABLE 4–8**

In Continuity Case Studies (1965–1990),
Upper Extremity Nerves

| | No. With (+) NAP/Result After Neurolysis | No. With (−) NAP/Result After Repair |
|---|---|---|
| Ulnar | | |
| Upper arm | 17/16 | 16/07* |
| Elbow, forearm | 45/43 | 14/10* |
| Wrist | 08/08 | 08/05† |
| Combined median-ulnar | 40/36 | 48/30* |
| Combined median-radial | 11/08 | 05/04 |
| Combined median-ulnar-radial | 04/04 | 08/06 |
| Totals | 125/118 (93%) | 99/62 (61%) |

Result = number achieving an LSUMC whole nerve grade 3 or better result.
*1 split repair.
†2 split repairs.

**TABLE 4–9**

In Continuity Case Studies (1965–1990),
Lower Extremity Nerves

| | No. With (+) NAP/Result After Neurolysis | No. With (−) NAP/Result After Repair |
|---|---|---|
| Sciatic | | |
| Buttock | | |
| Tibial | 30/28 | 23/20* |
| Peroneal | 28/23 | 19/06* |
| Thigh | | |
| Tibial | 38/36 | 37/33† |
| Peroneal | 34/31 | 43/19* |
| Tibial | 13/12 | 11/10* |
| Peroneal | 34/30 | 69/15† |
| Femoral | 15/13 | 14/07 |
| Totals | 193/173 (90%) | 216/110 (51%) |

Result = number achieving an LSUMC whole nerve grade 3 or better result.
*1 split repair.
†2 split repairs.
(Adapted from Kline D, Hoppel L: A quarter century's experience with intraoperative nerve action potential recording. Can J Neurol Sci 20:3–10, 1993.)

a 25-year period of clinical work and include only those cases in which lesions were in continuity, NAP recording was done, and follow-up was available. The tabulations provide some idea of the use of whole nerve grading to provide one type of outcome analysis. Because grade 3 or better was used as the determinant for relative success, the tabulation does not tell us how many patients reached a level of grade 4 or 5. These tabulations are provided in some of the subsequent chapters, not only by nerve involved but also by mechanism of injury or type of operation done. If reliable nonoperative spontaneous recovery data were available, this information has also been included in separate tables.

**TABLE 4–10**

In Continuity Element Studies (1965–1990), Brachial Plexus

| | No. With (+) NAP/Result After Neurolysis | | No. With (−) NAP/Result After Repair | |
|---|---|---|---|---|
| Injury Mechanism | Complete | Incomplete | Complete | Incomplete |
| Lesion in continuity | 10/09 | 18/17 | 15/10 | 04/03 |
| Gunshot wound | 41/40 | 47/44 | 116/64* | 08/08† |
| Iatrogenic | 18/17 | 17/17 | 32/23† | 06/04 |
| Stretch/contusion | 93/84 | 102/96 | 336/150† | 45/28‡ |
| Totals | 162/150 | 184/174 | 499/247 | 63/42 |

Result = number achieving an LSUMC grade 3 or better result for various plexus elements; Complete = complete loss in the distribution of one or more major elements preoperatively; Incomplete = incomplete loss of function in the distribution of element tested.
*1 split repair.
†2 split repairs.
‡5 split repairs.
(Adapted from Kline D, Hoppel L: A quarter century's experience with intraoperative nerve action potential recording. Can J Neurol Sci 20:3–10, 1993.)

## How to Interpret Outcome Tables

If the reader looks at Table 4 – 7, in 39 patients with arm level median palsies caused by lesions in continuity, 23 had a confirmed NAP ( + ) and underwent neurolysis and 22 recovered to a grade 3 or better level. Sixteen patients underwent resection and repair because of an absent NAP ( − ), and 11 of these recovered to grade 3 or better function. In one of the 11 cases with recovery, a split repair was done—i.e., one portion of the lesion had a neurolysis and the rest a repair.

## Bibliography

1. Bateman JE: Results and assessment of disability in iatrogenic nerve injuries. *In* Bateman JE: Trauma to Nerves in Limbs. Philadelphia, WB Saunders, 1962, pp. 285 – 305.
2. Bowsen RE and Napier JR: The assessment of hand function after peripheral nerve injuries. J Bone Joint Surg 43B:481, 1961.
3. Daniels L and Worthingham C: Muscle Testing, 3rd Ed. Philadelphia, WB Saunders, 1972.
4. Dellon AL: Results of nerve repair in the hand. *In* Dellon AL: Evaluation of Sensibility and Re-education of Sensation in the Hand. Baltimore, Williams & Wilkins, 1981, pp. 193 – 201.
5. Evarts CM: Examination of the musculoskeletal patient. *In* Evarts CM, Ed: Surgery of the Musculoskeletal System. New York, Churchill Livingstone, 1983, pp. 9 – 17.
6. Groff RA and Houtz SJ: Recovery and regeneration. *In* Manual of Diagnosis and Management of Peripheral Nerve Injuries. Philadelphia, JB Lippincott, 1945, pp. 33 – 35.
7. Haymaker W and Woodhall B: Peripheral Nerve Injuries, Principles of Diagnosis, 2nd Ed. Philadelphia, WB Saunders, 1953.
8. Highet WB: Grading of motor and sensory recovery in nerve injuries. Report to the Medical Research Council. London, Her Majesty's Stationery Office, 1954.
9. Kline DG and Hurst J: Prediction of recovery from peripheral nerve injury. Neurol Neurosurg Updated Series, 5:2 – 8, 1984.
10. Kline DG and Judice D: Operative management of selected brachial plexus lesions. J Neurosurg 58:631, 1983.
11. Kline DG and Nulsen F: Acute injuries of peripheral nerves. *In* Youmans J, Ed: Neurological Surgery, 2nd Ed. Philadelphia, WB Saunders, 1981.
12. Mannerfelt L: Motor function testing. *In* Omer GE and Spinner M, Eds: Management of Peripheral Nerve Problems. Philadelphia, WB Saunders, 1980, pp. 16 – 29.
13. Mannerfelt L: Studies on the hand in ulnar nerve paralysis. Acta Orthop Scand Suppl 87:1 – 176, 1966.
14. McNamara MJ, Garrett WE, Seaber AV, and Goldner JL: Neurorrhaphy, nerve grafting and neurotization: A functional comparison of nerve reconstruction techniques. J Hand Surg 12A:354 – 360, 1987.
15. Medical Research Council: Aids to the Examination of the Peripheral Nervous System. Memorandum No. 45. London, Her Majesty's Stationery Office, 1976.
16. Miller RG: Injury to peripheral motor nerves. AAEE Mimeograph No. 28. Muscle Nerve, 10:698 – 710, 1987.
17. Millesi H: Brachial plexus injuries—management and results. Clin Plast Surg 11:115 – 120, 1984.
18. Mumenthaler M and Schliak H: Läsionen peripherer Nerven, Diagnostik und Therapie. Stuttgart, George Thieme Verlag, 1977.
19. Omer G: Results of untreated peripheral nerve injuries. Clin Orthop Rel Res 163:15 – 19, 1982.
20. Omer G: The evaluation of clinical results following peripheral nerve suture. *In* Omer G and Spinner M, Eds: Management of Peripheral Nerve Problems. Philadelphia, WB Saunders, 1980.
21. Pollock LJ and Davis L: The results of peripheral nerve surgery. *In* Peripheral Nerve Injuries. New York, Paul B Hoeber, 1933, pp. 545 – 561.
22. Seddon HJ: Results of repair of nerves. *In* Seddon HJ: Surgical Disorders of the Peripheral Nerves. Baltimore, Williams & Wilkins, 1972, pp. 299 – 315.
23. Spinner M: Factors affecting return of function following nerve injury. *In* Spinner M: Injuries to the Major Branches of Peripheral Nerves of the Forearm, 2nd Ed. Philadelphia, WB Saunders, 1978, pp. 42 – 51.
24. Sunderland S: Nerves and Nerve Injuries. Baltimore, Williams & Wilkins, 1968.
25. Tinel J: Prognosis and treatment of peripheral nerve lesions. *In* Joll CA, Ed: Nerve Wounds. London, Bailliere, Tindall and Cox, 1917, pp. 297 – 299.
26. Woodhall B and Beebe GW, Eds: Peripheral nerve regeneration: A follow-up study of 3656 World War II injuries. Washington, DC, US Government Printing Office, 1956, pp. 115 – 201.

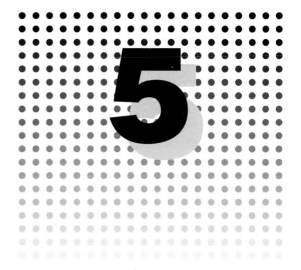

# Nerve Action Potential Recordings

# SUMMARY

The majority of serious injuries affecting nerve leave the nerve in continuity. If a lesion does not recover enough function in the early months after injury to make intervention unnecessary, then the operative decision of whether to resect the lesion can be difficult. Inspection and palpation can be misleading. Simple stimulation may provide contraction in muscles with relatively early innervation distal to the lesion, but with serious injuries to most major nerves, this cannot be expected for many months. Furthermore, a lesion with an injury site that has primarily poor regenerative potential may nevertheless permit a few hundred axons to reach a distal muscle site and respond to stimulation, whereas an adequately regenerating nerve can have thousands of axons extending into the distal stump by 2 to 3 months after injury and yet not have enough distal muscular input to reverse denervational change or to respond to simple stimulation.

One way to measure regeneration into the distal nerve is to stimulate and record across the injury site. This is nerve action potential (NAP) recording. Because presence or absence of an operative NAP has helped direct the operative management for almost all the lesions in continuity reported in this text, the rationale for this operative approach, the techniques and equipment used for such recordings, and the overall results with a variety of lesions in various nerves are summarized in this chapter. Presence or absence of a response is emphasized, rather than its configuration, latency, or velocity.

If an NAP was present in this series, the lesion usually was treated with an external neurolysis if it was unassociated with pain, or an internal neurolysis if severe and neuritic pain was a problem. Some lesions in continuity having an NAP had more obvious severe injury to one portion of the nerve than to another. In these cases, the nerve was split into groups of fascicles and differentially evaluated by NAP recordings. A split repair was then usually done. Those lesions in continuity not transmitting an NAP two or more months after injury were resected and proved to be neurotmetic or Sunderland Grade IV histologically. NAP recording was also used as an investigative tool for entrapments such as those involving ulnar, posterior interosseous, or peroneal nerves and for tumors arising from or affecting nerve.

Evaluation of lesions in continuity is challenging because preoperative studies, at least in the early months after injury, cannot prove the need for resection and repair, and even intraoperative inspection can be misleading (Figure 5–1).[8,10,35,36] Whenever possible, we have evaluated lesions in continuity by stimulation and recording studies of the whole injured peripheral nerve by nerve action potential (NAP) or compound nerve action potential (cNAP) recordings. If such studies led to resection of a lesion in continuity, the resected segment was evaluated histologically. Excellent correlation between negative NAP recordings and neurotmetic lesions has been demonstrated in many hundreds of resected nerve specimens. The intraoperative electrical studies have also been correlated with the preoperative severity of clinical loss, with electromyographic (EMG) findings, and usually with the subsequent clinical course of the patient.[19-22] Similar clinical studies using NAP recording have also been reported by a number of other investigators.[7,13,15,16,25,30-32,37] A number of laboratory studies in primates have also been done[18,23] in which NAP studies could be correlated with the histology at the recording site. In the primate, an NAP could be recorded distal to a successfully regenerating injury or repair site many weeks to months before there was EMG evidence of recovery.

Because NAP recordings and results are frequently referred to in subsequent chapters, a review of basic considerations and instrumentation is given here, partially abstracted from Happel and Kline (1991).[12] Results with record-

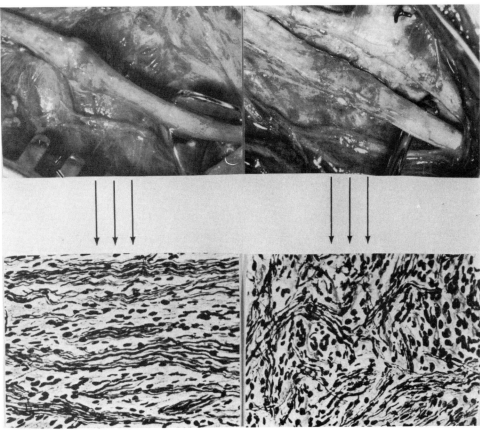

**Figure 5 – 1.** The usual problem encountered in evaluating a lesion in continuity intraoperatively without electrical recordings. The lesion at the top left appeared irregular and felt firm, but had a very structured and relatively mature axonal pattern at the regenerative site (*bottom left*). The lesion at the top right appeared relatively non-neuromatous but had a very disorganized regenerative pattern composed of fine axons (*bottom right*).

ing for various categories of lesions will be found in Chapter 4, in Tables 5 – 1 and 5 – 2, and in subsequent chapters on individual nerves.

## BASIC CONSIDERATIONS FOR NAP RECORDING

In healthy nerve, stimulation of a nerve fiber membrane produces a conducted impulse or NAP if stimulus intensity exceeds the fiber's threshold.[6,14] Various axons which respond to lower intensity stimuli do so because of their membrane properties.[33] The medium-sized fibers have the lowest threshold, the large fibers have the intermediate threshold, and the fine or small fibers have the highest threshold.[4,5] NAP amplitude can vary depending on the intensity of the stimulus applied to the whole nerve and, consequently, the number of fibers stimulated.[9]

If the stimulus is supramaximal in intensity, then NAP amplitude and its integral (area covered by the NAP) will be maximal[17,28] (Figures 5 – 2 and 5 – 3).

Threshold for stimulation and therefore ability to evoke an NAP depends on both the duration of applied current and the intensity of the stimulus. If the duration is decreased too much, then the intensity must be increased to reach threshold. An injured but regenerating nerve has a spectrum or range of various-sized fibers reaching the distal stump.[1,11] This spectrum of fiber sizes alters with length of time after injury or repair.[24,36] Small axons, including regenerating fibers, have a much higher threshold and may require substantially greater stimulation to cause an NAP.[33] In some abnormal fibers, even maximal stimulus intensity may not evoke a response unless stimulus duration is also in-

**TABLE 5–1**
Upper and Lower Extremity Nerves With Serious Lesions in Continuity

| Nerve | No. With (+) NAP/Result After Neurolysis | No. With (+) NAP/Result After Split Repair | No. With (−) NAP/Result After Repair |
|---|---|---|---|
| Median | 72/70 | 2/2 | 47/35 |
| Radial | 49/46 | 2/2 | 82/59 |
| Ulnar | 70/67 | 4/4 | 34/18 |
| Combined Nerves | 55/48 | 4/4 | 57/36 |
| Sciatic Nerve: | | | |
|   Tibial Division | 68/64 | 3/3 | 57/50 |
|   Peroneal Division | 62/54 | 2/2 | 60/13 |
| Tibial Nerve | 13/12 | 1/1 | 10/9 |
| Peroneal Nerve | 34/30 | 2/2 | 67/13 |
| Femoral Nerve | 15/13 | 0/0 | 14/07 |
| Totals | 438/404 (92%) | 20/20 (100%) | 428/240 (56%) |

Result = Number gaining a grade 3 or better outcome. Complete = complete preoperative loss in distribution of element tested operatively; Incomplete = incomplete preoperative loss in distribution of element tested operatively.

Numbers in parentheses under Injury Mechanism are cases operated on. Number (No.) with ( + ) or ( − ) NAP are plexus elements studied.

creased. This fact is useful for clinical recording because the relatively short stimulus used to reduce stimulus artifact as seen on the oscilloscope screen is also less likely to stimulate small, fine fibers. This helps because the surgeon needs to evaluate the status of medium-sized or larger fibers between the site of stimulation and that of recording.[20] It is important to be able to assess regenerating fiber populations and numbers that are different from those in healthy nerve[3,12] (see Tables 5–3 and 5–4).

Nerve fibers embedded in scar or within tumor require higher currents for stimulation because both the capacitance and resistance of such tissue tend to shunt stimuli away from the neural tissue.[12] Connective tissue surrounding nerve can also shunt current away from electrodes used for recording. Recording from a regenerating nerve may require not only more intense stimuli to evoke a response but also higher amplification and very low background noise level for adequate recordings. Surrounding tissues can reduce NAP amplitude and distort its form. Computer averaging may improve noise level and help make the evoked response look better or larger, but it does not reflect the activity required for intraoperative decision making as accurately as a single trace (Figure 5–4).[31]

In a myelinated axon, impulse conduction occurs when a region of active membrane, usually involving several nodes of Ranvier, excites adjacent nodes. Distance between nodes and the number of nodes responding determine the

**TABLE 5–2**
Brachial Plexus Lesions in Continuity

| Injury Mechanism | No. With (+) NAP/Result After Neurolysis | | No. With (−) NAP/Result After Repair | |
|---|---|---|---|---|
| | Complete | Incomplete | Complete | Incomplete |
| Stretch/Contusion (300) | 93/84 | 102/96 | 336/150* | 45/28† |
| Gunshot Wound (90) | 41/40 | 47/44 | 116/64‡ | 8/7* |
| Iatrogenic (30) | 18/17 | 17/17 | 32/23* | 6/4 |
| Laceration in Continuity (12) | 10/09 | 18/17 | 15/10 | 4/3 |
| Totals | 162/150 (93%) | 184/174 (95%) | 499/247 (49%) | 63/42 (67%) |

Result = Number gaining a grade 3 or better outcome. Complete = complete preoperative loss in distribution of element tested operatively; Incomplete = incomplete preoperative loss in distribution of element tested operatively.

*1 split repair.
†2 split repairs.
‡5 split repairs.
Numbers in parentheses under Injury Mechanism are cases operated on. Number (No.) with ( + ) or ( − ) NAP are plexus elements studied.

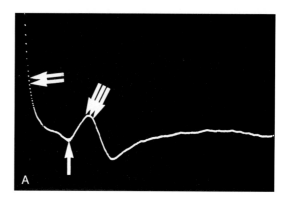

**Figure 5-2.** (A) Healthy nerve action potential (NAP) recorded from median nerve. NAP onset is marked by arrow. Downsweep of stimulus artifact is marked by double arrow and peak of NAP amplitude by triple arrow. (B) Drawing to show the important features of an evoked NAP. In this instance, the onset of a muscle action potential, or MAP, is also shown. The size of the stimulus artifact will vary according to stimulus intensity.

axon's conduction velocity.[2] Another factor in determining velocity is the time required to produce the action potential at each node.[28] Distribution of conduction velocities among myelinated axons is related to both fiber diameter and distance between nodes. The axonal diameter affects the flow of electrical current down the length of an axon and helps determine how many nodes of Ranvier act as a unit.[33] Distribution studies of conduction velocities provide a relation between NAP tracing shape and axon composition in the whole nerve.

The presence of a compound nerve action potential, or cNAP, indicates viable axons (Figures 5-5 and 5-6). At the recording site in primates, a cNAP seems to require at least 4000 moderate or larger-sized fibers with some degree of myelination.[18,23] If this requirement is met in vivo, direct recording does not require excessive amplification or summation.

Ability to record such an NAP distal to a nerve's injury site correlates with a good eventual clinical outcome due to spontaneous regeneration. On the other hand, resection and repair of such a lesion would usually give a less satisfactory outcome.

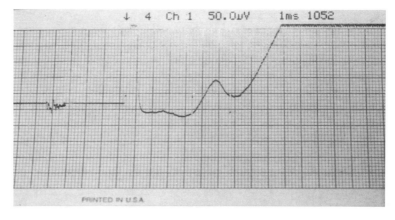

**Figure 5-3.** Nerve action potential recorded distal to an injured upper trunk of the plexus, indicating regeneration across the lesion. This plexus element underwent neurolysis rather than resection and repair. Amplitude is set on 50 μV and timebase on 1 millisecond per division.

**TABLE 5–3**
## Rationale for NAP Recording

Sixty percent or more of nerve injuries have some degree of continuity.

*If exploration is determined by failure of anticipated recovery, repair, if needed, will be too late.*

Operative inspection and palpation of a neuroma in continuity can be misleading.

Operative stimulation and recording (NAPs) can provide early information about significant recovery by 8 weeks after injury.

To transmit an NAP through an area of injury requires at least 4000 axons greater than 5 $\mu$ in diameter at the recording site.

Presence of an NAP recorded distal to a lesion in continuity in the early months after injury promises recovery without resection and repair.

In an occasional case, one portion of the cross section of the nerve is more severely injured than the remainder and, despite an NAP recorded distal to the injury, the lesion requires a split repair.

**TABLE 5–4**
## Timing for NAP Recording

Two to 4 months for relatively focal contusions caused by fractures and gunshot wounds and for lacerations in continuity

Four to 5 months for stretch injuries, especially those involving plexus

At any time for partial injuries and entrapments and other compressive lesions and tumors

In the acute setting, to identify an area of conduction block, although lesion may result from neurapraxia, axonotmesis, or neurotmesis.

# ELECTRODES USED FOR NAP STIMULATION AND RECORDING

Electrodes are made of either a noble metal such as platinum or medical grade stainless steel in order to minimize electrolysis associated with metal in contact with the nerve during stimulation. Eighteen-gauge wire is bent like a shepherd's crook on one end so that nerve can be suspended in the crook and gently lifted away from other tissues. The other end of each wire is placed through the center of a drilled-out Delrin or Teflon rod and soldered to a lead for attachment to instrumentation used for simulating and recording. The drilled-out center of the rod is then sealed with a surgical epoxy cement. With carefully selected materials, the electrodes can withstand autoclaving, gas sterilization, and water absorption (Figure 5–7).

The ends of the two active electrodes used for

simulation are separated by at least 3 mm (Figure 5–8). Electrode tips are separated by a longer distance (5–7 mm) for stimulation of big nerves such as sciatic or some brachial plexus elements because a larger volume of tissue is involved (Figure 5–9). If electrode tips are spaced too closely, not all fibers are stimulated. Stimulation of a nerve both in continuity and in situ differs from the classic physiologic recording in vitro with one or both nerve ends killed. Accordingly, some small but important alterations in electrode configuration are necessary.

If two stimulating electrode tips are used, not only is a current generated in the gap between the two but also a current flowing away from the electrodes through nerve and other body tissues and back again to nerve. This shock is almost instantaneous but still tends to give a large stimulus artifact. If stimulating and recording electrodes are relatively close, as they must be in some clinical situations, the after-slope of this stimulus artifact can obscure the evoked NAP. One way to minimize this is to use three tips for the stimulating electrode.[12,22] The outermost two tips form a common anode and are connected to each other, and the middle tip is the cathode. Application of a potential difference between the outermost and innermost active electrodes still produces two current paths, but

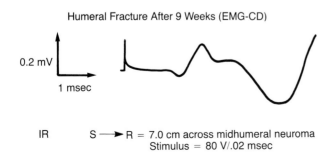

Humeral Fracture After 9 Weeks (EMG-CD)

0.2 mV

1 msec

IR      S ——► R = 7.0 cm across midhumeral neuroma
Stimulus = 80 V/.02 msec

**Figure 5–4.** Recording made across neuroma involving radial nerve in humeral groove secondary to fracture 9 weeks before. Loss was complete below triceps clinically and by electromyography (EMG). CD = complete denervation; IR = invasive recording; R = recording; S = stimulus. The NAP indicates excellent early regeneration, and as a result only a neurolysis was done. Overall radial recovery was grade 4/5 by 3 years postoperatively.

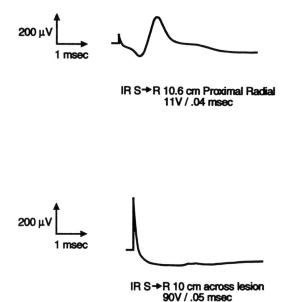

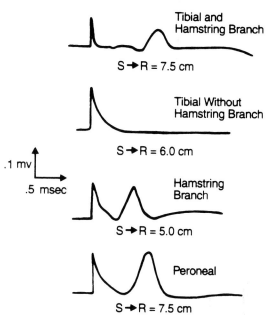

**Figure 5–5.** Operative nerve action potential (NAP) recordings proximal to a radial lesion *(top trace)* and across it *(bottom trace)*. Only a tiny NAP is seen in the lower trace. Lesion was resected and was largely neurotmetic or Sunderland grade IV histologically. Stimulus parameters were 11.0 V at 0.04 msec for proximal trace and 90 V at 0.05 msec for lower trace. IR = invasive recording; S → R = stimulus to recording (distance).

**Figure 5–6.** Recordings made operatively in a patient with lesions in continuity involving both divisions of the sciatic nerve. Recording made from the tibial and hamstring branches together was positive *(top)*. When the hamstring branch was dissected away, tracing from tibial alone was flat and that from the hamstring branch was positive. Thus, the tibial nerve had a neurotmetic injury while the hamstring branch was viable. Nerve action potential recorded from peroneal nerve is seen at the bottom. This patient had a graft repair of the tibial division and only a neurolysis of the peroneal division. Stimulus artifacts in this series of traces have the same amplitude since stimulus intensity was relatively constant.

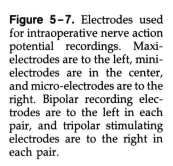

**Figure 5–7.** Electrodes used for intraoperative nerve action potential recordings. Maxi-electrodes are to the left, mini-electrodes are in the center, and micro-electrodes are to the right. Bipolar recording electrodes are to the left in each pair, and tripolar stimulating electrodes are to the right in each pair.

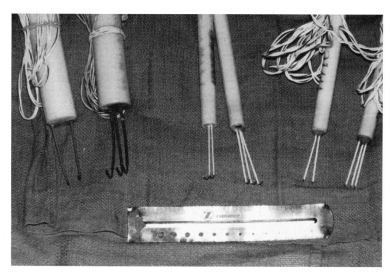

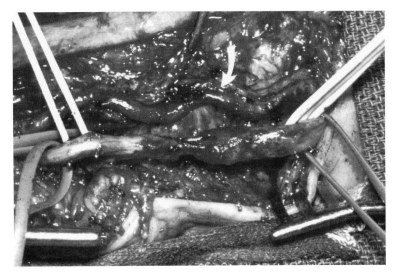

**Figure 5-8.** Recording from ulnar nerve injury in the region of Guyon's canal. Tripolar stimulating electrodes are to the right and bipolar recording electrodes are to the left. There was no transmission in this complete lesion, so a resection and repair were necessary. Ulnar artery has been mobilized away from ulnar nerve and is seen at the top *(arrow).*

neither involves the whole nerve, and thus the stimulus artifact is reduced. The tripolar stimulation electrode also limits the spread of the stimulating current along a longitudinal course in the nerve, making for a more precise and somewhat isolated site of stimulation.

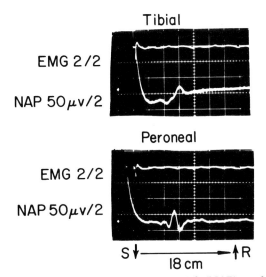

**Figure 5-9.** Nerve action potential (NAP) and evoked electromyographic (EMG) recordings made on tibial and peroneal nerves after evacuation of an old popliteal blood clot and neurolysis of nerves involved by scar. Despite presence of an NAP (lower trace on each graph), no muscle action potential could be recorded from gastrocnemius (EMG trace for tibial nerve) or anterior tibialis (EMG trace for peroneal nerve). It was concluded that the NAPs, which conducted at 30 m/sec, were regenerative but that not enough fibers had yet reached musculature to produce an evoked muscle action potential.

Recording electrode configuration is also important. The electrodes are bipolar, and each wire or tip at the recording site is separated by 3 to 5 mm, so that one electrode is recording from an active and the other from a relatively inactive portion of the nerve. If these two recording tips are too close together on the nerve, amplitude of the evoked NAP can be reduced, or the NAP can be eliminated altogether. If the distance between stimulating and recording electrodes is large, there is a need to separate the two recording electrode tips by a greater distance. There is a larger length of active nerve because of greater temporal dispersion in conduction if recordings are made over a long distance. The time of arrival of responses at the recording site is quite variable. This temporal dispersion is caused by differences in conduction velocities among different-sized myelinated axons.

Distance between stimulating and recording electrode sets is also important. If they are too close, the stimulus artifact can still be extensive despite use of a tripolar stimulating electrode. These technical points are important because the surgeon must have faith in the equipment used. Poor equipment could give tracings that are difficult to interpret and lead to incorrect surgical decisions.

Fine electroencephalographic needles can also be placed in nerve to both stimulate and record NAPs.[15] Done carefully, this is not damaging even to intact nerve. Needle recordings are especially useful if the surgical exposure of nerve is limited or at a deep level. Usually, two needles are placed in the nerve or element to be evaluated, several millimeters apart, for stimulation proximally, as well as two needles, also separated by several millimeters, for recording more distally.

Lead-in and lead-out wires from the stimulating and recording electrodes should be separated by several inches, if possible; otherwise, capacitance between the wires can further increase stimulus artifact and also produce other electrical noise.[34] Shielding is usually used for lead-out wires because isolation needs to be maximized. Electrode-to-wire connections and integrity of the wire can be readily checked by use of an amp meter.

Grounding is provided by attaching the lead-out from a Bovie pad affixed to the patient's skin to the grounding portion of the recording machine. The electrosurgical unit is turned off to provide safe grounding and to reduce unwanted electrical noise. Operating room equipment, either battery-operated or motor-driven, and fluorescent lights should be turned off or, better yet, disconnected by having their outlets removed from nearby wall sockets. This reduces the possibility of 60-cycle interference. A single wave isolated from a 60-cycle recording may be misinterpreted as a positive NAP by an inexperienced observer. The surgeon should learn to recognize this and not misinterpret it as a positive NAP.

## STIMULATING AND RECORDING EQUIPMENT

Most EMG machines manufactured within the last 15 years have the necessary built-in stimulating and recording parameters for satisfactory NAP recording.[17,28] We have found it convenient to use the TECA, model TD 20, which is self-contained and provides some degree of flexibility[20,22] (Figure 5–10). One can also construct a system using a Grass model stimulator (S-44) with a stimulus isolation unit (SIU-6) to provide stimulation.[21] Recording can be done using an oscilloscope with a differential amplifier, as is available for the Tektronix 7000 series. A trigger wire can be led from the stimulator to the oscilloscope so that a trace is prompted with each stimulus delivered to the stimulating electrodes.

Whether a compact EMG machine such as the TECA TD 20 or a larger system is used, attention must be paid to both the high- and low-frequency filters. The low-frequency filter setting is usually placed in the 5 to 10 Hz range or lower and the high-frequency setting at 2500 Hz or higher. These settings tend to decrease stimulus artifact and noise without filtering out the evoked NAP response. If the response is overfiltered, the stimulus artifact is greater and the amplitude and integral of the NAP are less. If a 60-Hz notch filter is built into the recording

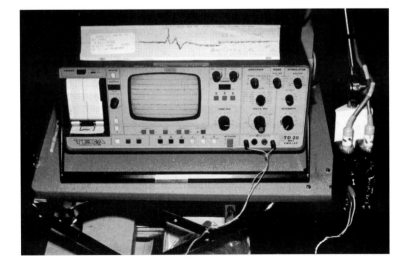

**Figure 5–10.** TECA TD 20 electromyography instrument used for stimulation and recording. Stimulating electrodes are led out of the stimulating portion of the instrument at the bottom and recording electrodes into differential amplifier to the right of the photograph. Tracing propped on top of the instrument is of a nerve action potential recorded at a site distal to a stretch injury involving an axillary nerve.

instrument, it is usually better not to use it for NAP recording. The filter device itself can generate a wave resembling an NAP.

## TECHNIQUE FOR STIMULATING AND RECORDING NAPs

Short-duration stimuli are used both to decrease stimulus artifact and to decrease stimulation of fine fibers, which may or may not mature with time and lead to useful function. Typical settings range between 0.05 and 0.1 msec in duration (Table 5–5). This requires increased voltage for adequate stimulation. Although healthy nerves require voltages between 3 and 15 V, regenerating nerve may need 100 V or more. Frequency of stimulation should be kept at 2 per second or less to prevent damage to nerve with these short-duration, high-voltage stimuli.

**TABLE 5–5**
Intraoperative NAP Recording Settings

| Stimulus | Setting |
| --- | --- |
| Duration | 0.05 to 0.1 msec |
| Intensity | 1 to 12.5 volts |
| Frequency | 1 to 2 per second |
| Recording Amplification | 50 $\mu$V to 5 mV per division |
| Time Frame | 0.5 to 2.0 msec per division |
| Frequency Filters | 1 to 3 Hz |

msec = milliseconds; mV = millivolts; Hz = Hertz.

NAPs are recorded with the oscilloscope set between 50 $\mu$V and 5 mV per division on the oscilloscope face. The time base is set at 0.5 to 2 msec per division. Because the limb must be available for inspection and palpation throughout the operation, appropriate draping at the start is essential. We usually begin recording the NAP proximal to the injury site by both stimulating and recording above it[19] (Figure 5–11,

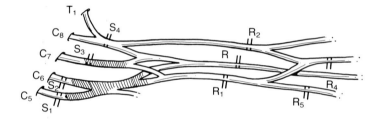

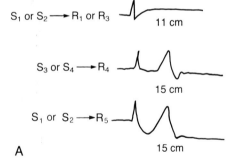

A

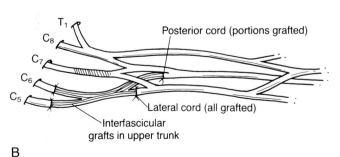

B

**Figure 5–11.** Use of nerve action potential (NAP) recording to sort out a stretch injury involving right C5, C6, and C7 spinal nerves and their more distal outflows as viewed from the side. In this case, recordings proximal to the injury sites were not possible. Stimulation of C5 and C6 and recording from upper trunk divisions as well as lateral and posterior cords gave no NAPs. Stimulation of C7 to middle trunk and posterior cord gave an NAP, as did stimulation and recording from the lower plexus elements. A graft repair extending from proximal C5 and C6 to lateral and posterior cords was carried out. It would have been difficult to make the correct intraoperative decisions regarding resection without the use of NAP recordings.

## TABLE 5-6
### Intraoperative NAP Recording Steps

If possible, place both stimulating and recording electrodes proximal to the injury site, separated by 3 to 4 cm, and record a proximal NAP. An adjacent less involved element or nerve can be tested to check the equipment if proximal nerve is not available.

If stimulation of an intact nerve produces muscle contraction but no NAP is recorded, then the various hookups for recording need to be rechecked.

Keeping stimulus duration brief, gradually increase stimulus intensity until NAP is evoked. Gradually increase amplification. Try different low- and high-frequency filters to optimize the evoked response.

Move distal recording electrodes into or onto the injury site to see if an NAP response is maintained.

Amplification setting may have to be increased or filters further adjusted.

Move recording electrodes distal to the injury site to see if NAP response can be evoked to that level and, if so, how far down the distal stump it can be recorded.

Observe muscles distal to stimulus site for contraction.

Table 5–6). If electrodes and stimulating and recording equipment are working and 3 to 4 or more centimeters of nerve can be exposed proximal to the lesion in continuity, an NAP response should be recordable. If the recordings are suboptimal, all equipment is checked in a systematic way before any attempt is made to record from the injured nerve. Recording electrodes are then moved onto the lesion site and beyond to see whether an NAP can be recorded and, if so, how far distal to the injury site (Figure 5–12).

If a proximal segment of the injured nerve is not available for a baseline recording, then an adjacent uninvolved nerve may be used to check the electrodes and the stimulation and recording settings. These settings can then be used as a starting point to stimulate and record

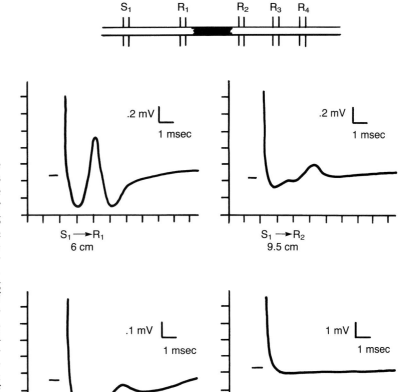

**Figure 5-12.** Operative nerve action potential (NAP) studies on an injection injury of the ulnar nerve at 3 months after injury. $S_1$ to $R_1$ is a recording proximal to the lesion. $S_1$ to $R_2$ is a recording across the lesion, and $S_1$ to $R_3$ and $S_1$ to $R_4$ are recordings made more distally. This nerve was regenerating well despite complete loss of function clinically, and electrically, more distally. Therefore, only neurolysis was performed and the lesion was not resected. (From Kline D: Microsurgery of peripheral nerves: Selection for and timing of operation. *In* Bunke H., Furnas D, (Eds): Symposium on Clinical Frontiers in Reconstructive Microsurgery. St. Louis, CV Mosby Co, 1984, pp 341–349.

from the injured nerve (Figure 5–13). Intensity of stimulation and, if need be, duration can be increased, as well as amplification used for recording. There are cases, particularly severe plexus stretch injuries studied intraoperatively, in which one cannot record from nerve proximal to injury site or even from other uninvolved or less involved nerves.[22] One must then be content with stimulating at the lesion site or even distal to it and recording below or distally.

Response of distal muscle to stimulation of nerve proximal to a lesion usually indicates good regeneration, not only through the lesion but to that muscle.[26,27] Such a response is usually an indication of excellent spontaneous recovery. In the early months after injury, such obvious evidence of sparing or recovery is usually not present unless the lesion was partial to begin with. *The objective in operative recording is to measure an NAP distal to the lesion. In the initial 9 months after injury, the NAP's amplitude and conduction velocity are not as important as the simple presence or absence of a response. Presence of an NAP indicates axons of sufficient number, caliber, and maturation to presage useful recovery of function for at least a portion of the injured cross section of nerve. Absence of an NAP indicates that recovery will not occur without resection and repair.*

In some cases, an NAP is present but visual inspection of the conducting segment suggests that one portion of the lesion's cross section is more severely injured than another. Then, the lesion can be split into groups of fascicles, and groups of fascicles or individual fascicles can be tested separately.[34] Usually, some fascicles conduct and others do not. This leads to a split repair, in which a portion of the nerve is repaired by direct suture or graft and a portion by neurolysis alone.

As stimulation and recording begin, the stimulus intensity (voltage) is gradually increased, and the amplification for recording is also increased until an NAP is seen. Different filter settings can also be tried. The stimulating electrodes are usually placed proximally and the recording ones distally. A proximal stimulation site ensures activation of a maximal number of fibers.[29] If a stimulus site proximal to an injured but regenerating nerve is accessible, more normal fibers can be stimulated proximally than distally.[12] This decreases the need for a high-in-

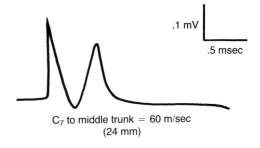

C₇ to middle trunk = 60 m/sec
(24 mm)

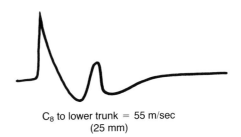

C₈ to lower trunk = 55 m/sec
(25 mm)

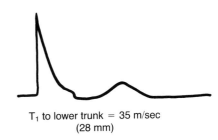

T₁ to lower trunk = 35 m/sec
(28 mm)

**Figure 5–13.** Operative nerve action potential recordings from a patient suspected of thoracic outlet syndrome. T1 to lower trunk trace is reduced in amplitude, has a broad base, and is relatively slow at 35 m/sec. This indicates an irritative and/or compressive lesion involving T1 to lower trunk. A neurolysis of the lower elements of the plexus was done. C7 to middle trunk recordings were normal by comparison.

tensity stimulus and, as a result, decreases the stimulus artifact recorded distally. Stimulating and recording electrode tips are used to lift and hold the nerve away from other tissues or tissue fluids (Figures 5–14, 5–15, and 5–16).

More distant evoked muscle action potentials (MAPs) can be picked up by the recording electrodes placed on nerve. These responses, however, are quite delayed compared to NAPs. Their calculated velocities are slow, usually less than 20 m/sec. They are also larger in amplitude than NAPs and more likely to be polyphasic.

With a plexus lesion in which roots are injured at a preganglionic level but are intact post-

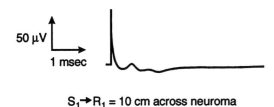

50 µV

1 msec

$S_1 \rightarrow R_1$ = 10 cm across neuroma

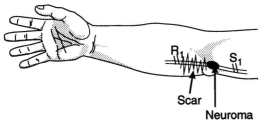

R₁

Scar

S₁

Neuroma

**Figure 5–14.** Ulnar neuroma caused by fracture and contusion at the level of the elbow. Despite complete clinical loss below flexor carpi ulnaris and complete denervation as confirmed by electromyography, a nerve action potential could be recorded to a point 6 cm distal to the neuroma. As a result, a neurolysis, transposition, and submuscular burial were done.

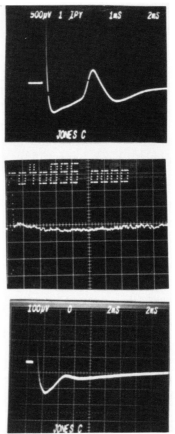

ganglionically, rapidly conducting (60–80 m/sec) and relatively large-amplitude NAPs can be recorded. The large and well-myelinated sensory fibers have been spared Wallerian degeneration because they remain continuous with their cell bodies in the posterior root ganglion; therefore, they conduct a rapid and large response to stimulation. These responses differ from the slower, lower-amplitude regenerative NAPs and may even be faster and larger than those seen when recording from an intact plexus element.[9,18] If there is doubt, the proximal part of the spinal nerve can be stimulated and an attempt made to record somatosensory

**Figure 5–16.** A series of electrical traces recorded from an injured median nerve at a forearm level with complete loss distal to the injury. Top trace was an operative trace made proximal to the injury site. Bottom trace was recorded operatively across the injury site at 3.5 months, indicating early but adequate regeneration through the lesion. Middle trace was an attempt to evoke a response across the lesion noninvasively and at a skin level. However, even with summation, the small potential seen in the bottom trace could not be recorded noninvasively. This nerve did well with only a neurolysis.

**Figure 5–15.** Large ulnar lesion in continuity caused by contusion associated with a fracture, which conducted a nerve action potential, much to our surprise. The patient recovered a good deal of function after neurolysis and transposition beneath pronator teres and flexor carpi ulnaris.

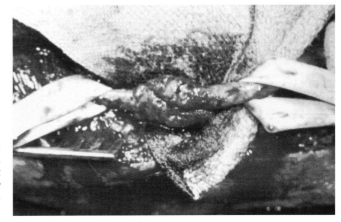

evoked potentials through cutaneous electrodes previously placed over upper and posterior cervical spine. With preganglionic injury, these evoked responses are absent.

If an extremity is operated on under tourniquet and the latter is inflated for 60 minutes or longer, the tourniquet should be left down for 20 or more minutes before NAP recording is tried (Table 5–7). Ischemia and low wound temperature can block successful recordings.[29] In several earlier cases in which recording was done under tourniquet, NAP traces were flat, and yet regeneration, as shown by either histologic study of resected segment or subsequent clinical course, was adequate.[19] Local anesthetic use may also temporarily block conduction. Because the block can persist for many hours, absence of an NAP under these circumstances may not indicate a need for resection. On the other hand, muscle paralysis by curare-like drugs does not interfere with NAP recording. These drugs do, of course, prevent muscle contraction in response to nerve stimulation if regeneration has advanced to that degree.

Noninvasive recording of whole or cNAPs is possible for some nerve lesions but has a definite incidence of false-negative traces, as subsequently shown by intraoperative NAP studies. Such recordings are more readily achieved with nerves distal in the extremity and close to skin, such as median or ulnar nerves near the wrist. Occasionally, stimulation of a nerve close to but uninvolved by the injury produces a falsely positive study, so patients must be carefully selected for such a noninvasive approach.

Discussion with the anesthetist preoperatively can ensure an anesthetic technique in which the neuromuscular blockade used in induction wears off by the time the surgeon has dissected the area of injury. The surgeon is then able to stimulate normal or injured nerve, observe the effect of appropriate muscle contraction, and elicit NAPs from nerves that give no response to direct stimulation. After the NAP recording phase of the operation is concluded, the anesthetist can use whatever anesthetic technique is appropriate.

## Bibliography

1. Collins W, O'Leary J, Hunt W, and Schwartz H: An electrophysiological study of nerve regeneration in the cat. J Neurosurg 12:39–46, 1955.
2. Cragg BG and Thomas PK: Changes in conduction velocity and fiber size proximal to peripheral nerve lesions. J Physiol (London) 157:315–327, 1961.
3. Cragg BG and Thomas PK: The conduction velocity of regenerated peripheral nerve fibres. J Physiol (London) 171:164–175, 1964.
4. Dawson GD: The relative excitability and conduction velocity of sensory and motor nerve fibers in man. J Physiol (London) 131:436–451, 1956.
5. Dorfman L, et al.: Conduction Velocity Distributions: A Population Approach to Electrophysiology of Nerve. New York, Alan R Liss, 1981.
6. Erlanger J, Gasser H: Electrical Signs of Nervous Activity. Philadelphia, University of Pennsylvania Press, 1937.
7. Friedman W: The electrophysiology of peripheral nerve injuries. Neurosurg Clin North Am 2:43–56, 1991.
8. Gilliatt R: Physical injury to peripheral nerves: Physiologic and electrodiagnostic aspects. Mayo Clin Proc 56:361–370, 1981.
9. Gilliatt RW and Sears TA: Sensory nerve action potentials in patients with peripheral nerve lesions. J Neurol Neurosurg Psychiatry 21:109–118, 1958.
10. Grundfest H, Oester YT, and Beebe GW: Electrical evidence of regeneration. In Woodhall B and Beebe GW, Eds: Peripheral Nerve Regeneration. VA Monograph. Washington, DC, US Government Printing Office, 1956.
11. Gutmann E and Sanders F: Recovery of fiber numbers and diameters in the regeneration of peripheral nerves. J Physiol (London) 101:489–518, 1943.
12. Happel L and Kline D: Nerve lesions in continuity. In Gelberman R, Ed: Operative Nerve Repair and Reconstruction. Philadelphia, JB Lippincott, 1991.
13. Hudson A and Hunter D: Timing of peripheral nerve repair: Important local neuropathologic factors. Clin Neurosurg 24:392–405, 1977.
14. Hodgkin A and Huxley A: Currents carried by sodium and potassium ions through the membrane of the giant axon of Loglio. J Physiol (London) 116:449, 1952.
15. Hudson AR and Trammer B: Brachial plexus injuries. In Wilkins R and Rengachary S, Eds: Neurosurgery. New York, McGraw-Hill, 1985.

**TABLE 5–7**
## Trouble Shooting for NAP Recording

1. Electrode connection or wire break. *Amp meter testing will resolve.*
2. Operating room noise, especially from fluorescent lighting or 60 cycle interference from other instruments. *Shut off other electrical sources, try different wall outlets, ground the machine.*
3. Local anesthetic block or ischemic (tourniquet) block. *Can record only when effects have worn off* (usually 30 to 40 minutes).
4. Poor electrode contact, excessive blood or serum around electrodes, wound and thus nerve cool. *Readjust electrode position; irrigate with warm saline.*
5. A proximal NAP should be recordable in most settings; then it is important to record directly across the lesion.
6. Preganglionic injury may give a high amplitude, rapidly conducting response that is not regenerative. A muscle action potential (MAP) has a longer latency, higher amplitude, and more rounded peak than a regenerative NAP.

16. Kaplan B, Friedman W, and Gravenstein D: Intraoperative electrophysiology in treatment of peripheral nerve injuries. J Fla Med Assoc 71:400–403, 1984.
17. Kimura J: Electrodiagnosis in Diseases of Nerve and Muscle: Principles and Practice. Philadelphia, FA Davis, 1983.
18. Kline DG and DeJonge BR: Evoked potentials to evaluate peripheral nerve injuries. Surg Gynecol Obstet 127:1239–1250, 1968.
19. Kline DG and Hackett ER: Reappraisal of timing for exploration of civilian peripheral nerve injuries. Surgery 78:54–65, 1975.
20. Kline DG and Hackett ER: The neuroma-in-continuity: A management problem. In Wilkins RH and Rengachary S, Eds: Neurosurgery. New York, McGraw-Hill, 1984.
21. Kline DG and Nulsen FE: The neuroma-in-continuity: Its preoperative and operative management. Surg Clin North Am 52:1189–1209, 1972.
22. Kline DG, Hackett ER, and Happel L: Review of surgical lesions of the brachial plexus. Arch Neurol 43: 170–181, 1985.
23. Kline DG, Hackett ER, and May PR: Evaluation of nerve injuries by evoked potentials and electromyography. J Neurosurg 31:128–136, 1969.
24. Lyons W and Woodhall B: Atlas of Peripheral Nerve Injuries. Philadelphia, WB Saunders, 1949.
25. McGillicuddy J: Clinical decision-making in brachial plexus injuries. Neurosurg Clin North Am 2: 137–150, 1991.
26. Nulsen FE and Lewey FH: Intraneural bipolar stimulation: A new aid in the assessment of nerve injuries. Science 106:301, 1947.
27. Seddon HJ: Surgical Disorders of the Peripheral Nerves. Baltimore, Williams & Wilkins, 1972.
28. Sumner A: The Physiology of Peripheral Nerve Disease. Philadelphia, WB Saunders, 1980.
29. Sunderland S: Nerves and Nerve Injuries, 2nd Ed. Edinburgh, Churchill Livingstone, 1978.
30. Terzis J, Dykes R: Electrophysiological recordings in peripheral nerve surgery: A review. J Hand Surg 1:52–66, 1976.
31. Van Beek A, Hubble B, and Kinkead L: Clinical use of nerve stimulation and recording. Plast Reconstr Surg 71:225–232, 1983.
32. Vanderark G, Meyer G, Kline D, and Kempe L: Peripheral nerve injuries studied by evoked potential recordings. Milit Med 135:2:90–94, 1970.
33. Waxman SG: Physiology and Pathobiology of Axons. New York, Raven Press, 1978.
34. Williams HB and Terzis JK: Single fascicular recordings: An intraoperative diagnostic tool for the management of peripheral nerve lesions. Plast Reconstr Surg 57: 562–569, 1976.
35. Woodhall B, Nulsen F, White J, and Davis L: Neurosurgical implications. In Peripheral Nerve Regeneration. VA Monograph. Washington, DC, US Government Printing Office, 1957.
36. Zachary R, Roaf R: Lesions in continuity. In Seddon H, Ed: Peripheral Nerve Injuries. Medical Research Council Special Report Series No. 282. London, Her Majesty's Stationery Office, 1954.
37. Zalis A, Rodriguez A, Oester Y, and Maius D: Evaluation of nerve regeneration by means of evoked potentials. J Bone Joint Surg 54A:1246–1253, 1972.

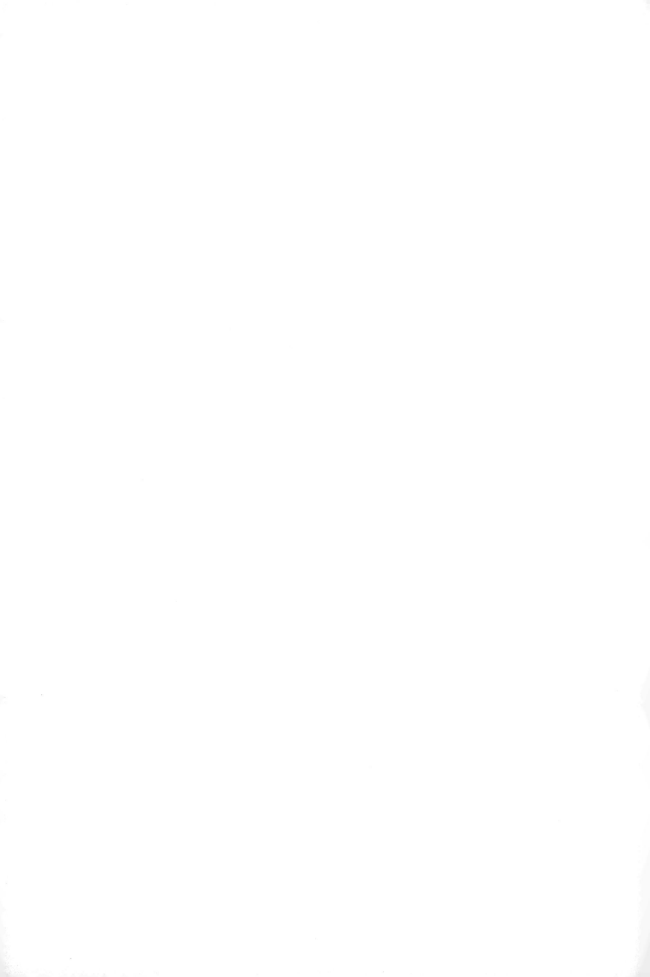

# Operative Care
# and Techniques

# SUMMARY

A successful operation hinges on an intimate knowledge of the anatomy of the involved limb, shoulder, neck, or pelvis. Exposure must be generous and whenever possible should include more normal proximal and distal nerve so that the injury site is worked out by dissecting from normal to abnormal. An appreciation of related structures such as vessels, tendons, and other nerves is necessary, as well as skill in dissecting those out and retracting them gently in order to preserve them. Great attention must be given to hemostasis and as gentle handling of tissues as possible. There is not only a spectrum but a flow of procedures or repair strategies. These include, usually in this order, external neurolysis, nerve action potential recording for lesions in continuity, internal neurolysis for selected circumstances such as severe neuritic pain or split repair, and then either epineurial end-to-end repair or interfascicular graft repair. A rational and well-reasoned program for preoperative and postoperative care as well as careful instruction of the patient and family is equally important. A reasoned and well-balanced prognosis and outline of expectations and limits of recovery must be shared with the patient and family.

Specific operative approaches are covered in some detail under each major nerve or neural complex. Nonetheless, some general comments are in order.

# PREOPERATIVE CARE

Preoperative care of the patient's injured limb is extremely important. The most neglected aspect of this is provision of active or passive motion on a frequent, repetitive basis. Injured nerves do not recover by being put to rest. Immobilized joints rapidly stiffen. Provision of physical therapy once a day during the work week does not suffice to keep the limb with severe paralysis mobile. The patient and his or her family must be shown how to provide range of motion (ROM) not only to joints subtended by the paralysis but also to those above and below. Such home ROM must be done many times a day. All too often, a patient presents with a stiff and painful shoulder, elbow, or wrist whose neuropathy originated weeks earlier. A similar scenario can affect the lower extremity. Hip, knee, or ankle stiffness can readily occur if non–weight-bearing has been (wrongly) advised after nerve injury. There are admittedly clinical settings in which concomitant bony, vascular, or tendinous injury requires a period of immobilization. Even in these settings, though, structured therapy directed toward shoulder, fingers, hip, or foot helps to maintain the limb as optimally as possible. From the outset, the patient must assume responsibility for the denervated limb. A passive attitude, in which the patient assumes the physical thera-

pist will do the work, is associated with bad clinical outcomes.

In addition to securing a thorough clinical and, if possible, electrophysiologic preoperative evaluation of the limb, the surgeon has the responsibility of pointing out to the patient and the family not only the possible complications of the proposed procedure but also some estimation of its limits in terms of restoring function and decreasing or removing pain. Recovery of significant function cannot always be promised, and because of the severity of the lesion, the nerve involved, or concomitant injuries, failure can result. The patient and the patient's family must be made to understand that the operation may not work (Table 6–1). In addition, restoration of useful function after major injuries often takes years rather than weeks or months to occur. Patients are usually unaware of these time frames and may expect immediate postoperative recovery.

The patient's psychologic state during both the preoperative and postoperative periods is of the utmost importance. This factor alone may be the single most important determinant of outcome. Depression and anxiety are common concomitants of significant nerve injury. These emotional responses to physical trauma should be explored with the patient and managed appropriately. A depressed patient who does not initially obey the surgeon's postoperative in-

**TABLE 6-1**
Preoperative Care

1. Initial wound or injury care for soft tissue damage and arteries, tendons, bones, chest, abdomen, etc.
2. Appropriate radiographs and, on occasion, scanning studies
3. Early clinical grading of both motor and sensory function
4. Baseline electromyogram at 2 to 3 weeks
5. Institution of early range of motion and, if possible, strengthening exercises of spared or potentially injured functional units
6. Several visits for clinical examination and electromyographic evaluation if delayed surgery is indicated
7. Realistic appraisal of possible outcomes for the patient and the patient's family
8. Preoperative clearance by medical and anesthesia services; perioperative antibiotic administration

structions and who subsequently fails to maintain a vigorous home physical therapy program may also complain bitterly of dysesthesias and pain. Such a psychologic state can defeat the results that could have been realized after successful surgery. Conversely, a patient who optimizes residual and returning function rather than complaining of the deficit is more likely to regain a useful functioning limb, even if perfection is not achieved. The patient must be aware that sometimes the paresthesias associated with even successful regeneration are painful. There must also be a commitment to long-term self-care of the limb and completion of a certain number of follow-up visits. Despite advance preparations, some patients still awaken from their operation disappointed that their limb movement has not been magically restored and with the belated realization that they face a lengthy period of waiting and hard work on their part to optimize any recovery that may occur.

A more precise prognosis hinges on the operative findings. Preoperatively, the surgeon should try to provide a description of the possible procedures to be done, such as neurolysis, suture, grafts, and split repair, and give the patient some idea of results with each. Postoperatively, the surgeon has a feel for the procedure's possible success and can usually provide a more accurate estimate of expected recovery or lack thereof.

In our practice we have developed pamphlets describing some of these factors in relatively simple language for patient use.

# OPERATIONS

## Scheduling

Duration of surgery varies considerably. A brachial plexus procedure may be concluded in 3 to 12 hours, depending on the pathology revealed. On occasion, operations may be performed in two stages, with total duration well in excess of 12 hours. If bone, vascular, or tendon work is required, this is best accomplished before nerve surgery, either at the same or in a separate operation. In this way, nothing in subsequent procedures will disturb a delicate nerve repair. Electrophysiologists or technicians should be scheduled to be available for nerve action potential (NAP) recordings. Usually, a single surgical assistant suffices, but segments of complex operations may necessitate additional help, and appropriate individuals should be available to simultaneously harvest sural nerves and close multiple operative wounds. The scheduled anesthetist should understand the sequence of nerve stimulation and NAP recording and the absolute necessity of patient immobility at the conclusion of the procedure, while dressings and casts are being applied. On occasion, quick sections may be required during the operation, and the scheduled pathologist should have reviewed any slides obtained from any previous biopsy before the new specimens are examined. Biopsies may be of single fascicles, and the pathologist must be comfortable handling small specimens.

The operating room nurse is an important

member of the team. It helps if the scrub nurse is interested in and has some knowledge of the basic anatomy, physiology, and pathology of nerve injuries and tumors. This person should be in charge of the sterilization, packaging, and subsequent arrangement of the various surgical instruments, as well as the electrodes and other equipment needed for operative recordings.

## Positioning

The patient should be positioned so as to avoid pressure palsies. Limbs must be available for inspection during surgery. The legs must be available for potential sural nerve donation. Limbs may need to be moved during surgery, and draping should accommodate this. Drapes at the root of limbs should not be so snug as to cause a venous tourniquet effect. Surface electrodes for somatosensory-evoked potential recording should be checked immediately before skin preparation to ensure they have not moved during patient positioning.

The initial approach in most nerve operations is without magnification. Dissection of nerve and attendant scar, as well as preservation of adjacent structures, is aided by the use of loupes. If an operating microscope is to be used later in the procedure, it helps to position and sometimes drape it before the procedure begins. Trial positioning of the microscope should ensure that, if the instrument is subsequently used, both surgeon and assistant can work in comfort for prolonged periods without cervical or lumbar strain. The lens and eyepiece can be partially focused and positioned for the surgeon and the surgeon's assistant. In addition, this "dry run" will help place the scrub nurse and the instrument table(s).

## Instrumentation

There is no set position for the instrument tray; adaptation and innovation are necessary according to potential access required for graft donation, positioning of the surgeon and assistant, and location of the anesthetic equipment. The operating technician or instrument nurse should have comfortable access during potentially prolonged operations.

We prefer a variety of scalpels including a long-handled plastic knife holder with a No. 15 blade and long-handled Metzenbaum scissors for most dissections (Figure 6–1). Cushing or similar forceps are used for much of the dissection, and ophthalmic forceps are used for fascicular work. Penrose drains and fine plastic loops (Vasoloops) are helpful for neural retraction. A variety of hemostats, Munyons, and self-retaining retractors are necessary, as is an assortment of microinstruments, including several types of bipolar forceps, microscissors, and microforceps. Instruments are conveniently separated into macro and micro sets.

Variable-caliber, pressure-controlled suction tubes are needed during the macro and micro stages of the operation. Large-caliber, high-pressure suction tubes tend to injure the sites of nerve surgery. A cell saver may be helpful for large operations or those in which blood loss is predicted to be high. Provision of both the Bovie and a good bipolar coagulator is necessary.

## Initial (Macro) Exposure

The first steps of the operation, such as skin incision and soft tissue dissection to reach the nerve, are usually done without magnification. To do this well, the operator should have a detailed and profound knowledge of the immediate and surrounding anatomy of the site of nerve injury. The surgeon should operate with confidence and reasonable speed during exposure of the area, based on a sound knowledge of key anatomic landmarks and structures (Figure 6–2). Use of a microscope too early in the dissection will unnecessarily prolong it. The pace of progress subsequently slows when painstaking dissection of complex injuries and attendant scar is required. Here, magnification by loupes or microscope may be necessary. Exposure should also be generous because the surgeon must control bleeding from vessels above and below the site of injury. Normal nerve above and below the injury should also be exposed to allow identification of discrete nerve elements with injury, particularly in plexus cases. Great care must be exercised in placing self-retaining retractors so that adjacent structures are not injured during prolonged surgery.

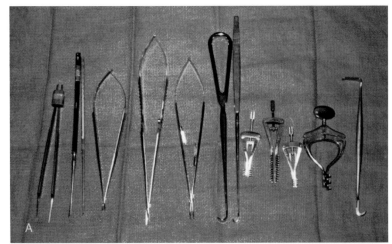

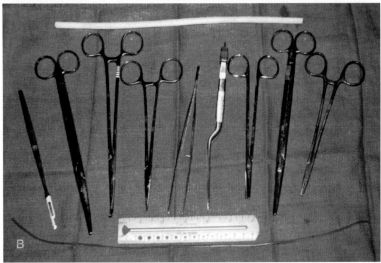

**Figure 6–1.** Display on operating table of some of the instruments more commonly used. (*A*) Fine bipolar forceps, microscissors, and right-angled dissector for passing drains beneath nerves, vein retractors, and a variety of small Alm and mastoid retractors as well as a small plastic rake. (*B*) No. 15 scalpel blade on a long-handled knife, a variety of Metzenbaum scissors, a Cushing-Gerald forceps with teeth, bayonet-shaped bipolar forceps with relatively broad tips, a Penrose drain (*top*), and a ruler and a plastic loop (*bottom*).

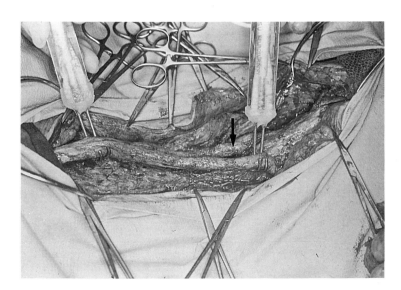

**Figure 6–2.** Exposure and neurolysis of contused sciatic complex. Sciatic nerve and its tibial and peroneal branches have been exposed completely with a 360-degree dissection around each element. Electrodes to the left are around the whole sciatic nerve and those to the right are hooked around the peroneal nerve, while the black arrow points to the tibial nerve.

## Closure

It is best to close all wounds except the main access wound before nerve grafting. This ensures minimal disturbances after the nerve repair has been made. Careless application of sponges during closure can cause grafts to adhere to gauze so that suture lines are disrupted. Careless removal of self-retaining retractors can disrupt suture lines. Closed compartment syndromes should be avoided, so tight fascial closure around repaired nerve(s) should not be attempted. Skin closure should be meticulous because scars tend to spread badly if care is not given to this end stage of the operation (Figure 6–3). Suction drains should be placed well away from graft sites and should not damage the nerve repair when they are subsequently removed. Vigorous cleaning of skin near the site of nerve repair must be avoided, and a senior member of the team must supervise application of dressings, slings, or casts. The tired operating team must maintain vigilance during the closure phase, or all their good work may be undone in a single careless moment.

## OPERATIONS COMMONLY DONE

### External Neurolysis

This procedure is the cornerstone for almost all peripheral nerve surgery. Neurolysis is done before intraoperative electrical recordings and is necessary before suture or graft repair. External neurolysis involves cleaning the nerve of investing tissues including scar. As used in this text, neurolysis means freeing up the nerve in a full, circumferential fashion and over some length. For the injured nerve, this includes resection of epineurial scar tissue. Simple exposure or unroofing of a nerve, such as might be done by section of the transverse carpal ligament for uncomplicated carpal tunnel syndrome, does not constitute external neurolysis.

External neurolysis, if injury is present, is usually done by freeing up more normal nerve proximal and distal to the site of scarring and alternatively working toward this site and in a circumferential fashion around the nerve. This can usually be done with a No. 15 scalpel blade on a long-handled plastic knife holder or sometimes more readily by a pair of Metzenbaum scissors. This portion of the dissection can be helped by gently displacing the nerve to one side or the other by use of a 4 × 4-inch moistened sponge or by traction on adjacent tissues with Gerald forceps.

Nerve proximal and distal to the injury site can be encircled with Penrose drains (Figure 6–4). These drains can be used to elevate and shift the nerve to ensure dissection along its epineural surface. Finer loops such as Vasoloops can be used on smaller nerves or branches of larger nerves, but if used on a larger nerve, they unduly constrict it. At times, epineurial bands or constrictive circles of mesoneurium can be ob-

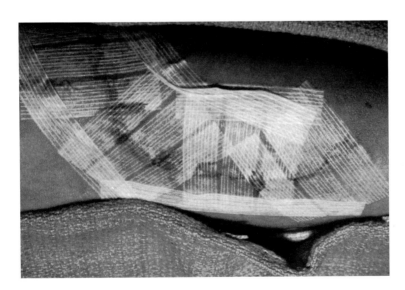

**Figure 6–3.** Steri-Strips applied to wound closed subcutaneously after exploration of the radial nerve at the level of the elbow.

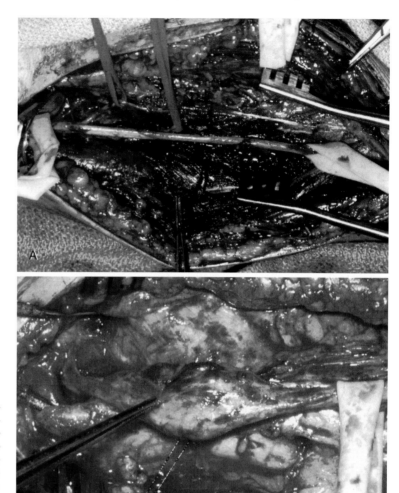

**Figure 6–4.** (*A*) Complete external neurolysis and 360-degree circumferential exposure of a stretch injury site. Penrose drains encircle proximal nerve to the left and distal nerve to the right. (*B*) Exposure of a more severe lesion in continuity. Penrose drain encircles distal nerve to the right.

served. These should be sharply lysed without injuring underlying nerve. Exposure of more healthy nerve proximal to the injury site is a luxury not available to the surgeon for many supraclavicular plexus injuries or with lesions of the sciatic nerve close to the sciatic notch. In those settings, exposure of more distal elements or nerve with dissection proximally helps, as does careful attention to surrounding anatomic details or landmarks.

Resection of epineurial scar may require use of fine dissection scissors or microscissors, but sometimes it can be done by scalpel blade (Figure 6–5). As much fascicular tissue is spared as possible. Bleeding points at an epineurial or subepineurial level are coagulated using fine-

tipped bipolar forceps while the surgical assistant irrigates the area with saline.

External neurolysis is the first step preparatory to intraoperative electrical evaluation of any lesion in continuity. There are those who believe that close microscopic inspection of the nerve after external neurolysis or use of internal neurolysis and attempts to trace fascicles through the injury site are the only operative observations necessary in order to make decisions about the need for complete or partial resection. By comparison, we favor use of intraoperative stimulation and recording studies to evaluate such lesions. After external neurolysis has been completed, stimulating and recording electrodes are placed on the nerve, proximal to

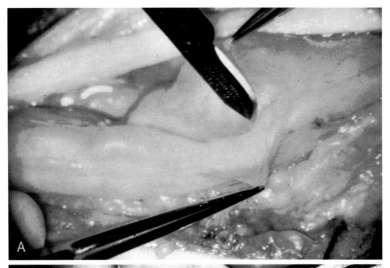

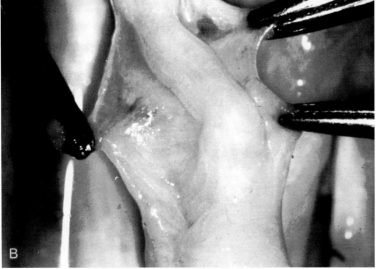

**Figure 6–5.** (*A*) Resection of epineurial scar. (*B*) Epineurium and scar teased away from main nerve trunk. Forceps grasp the epineurium, which has been dissected away from the fascicles.

the level of the lesion if possible. Stimulation should produce a recordable NAP above or proximal to the lesion. The recording electrodes are then moved into the region of the injury, and changes in the evoked NAP are noted. Recording electrodes are then moved distally to see if a response is transmitted beyond the lesion in continuity. If there is an NAP, the time interval since injury is 9 months or less, and severe pain in the distribution of the nerve or element is not a problem, then one can be content with the external neurolysis alone and be confident of recovery of function. If, on the other hand, there is no NAP transmitted across the lesion, resection and repair are usually indicated.

Sometimes inspection of the injury site suggests severe involvement of a portion of the cross section and relative maintenance of continuity of the rest. This finding should lead to internal neurolysis, fascicular-level NAP recordings, and what is termed split repair.

## Internal Neurolysis

Internal neurolysis involves the careful splitting of nerve into its individual fascicles or bundles of fascicles. Internal neurolysis requires magnification and, usually, use of microinstruments as well. It is more easily accomplished on nerves in the distal portion of the extremity than proximally, where there are more fascicular trade-offs or interconnections. An indication for internal neurolysis is an injury which is more severe to one portion of nerve than another and which, despite presence of a transmitted NAP across the lesion, requires a split or partial repair. Another indication is pain of a severe, neuritic nature for which conservative pharmacologic management has failed and in which the pain pattern is associated with partial or no major anatomic dysfunction. Both of these situations can sometimes be helped by internal neurolysis, but there may be a price paid in terms of further decrease of function, even if the procedure is carefully done. Fascicles or groups of fascicles are isolated over a length by sharp dissection and elevated by Vasoloops or fine drains (Figure 6–6). It usually helps to split apart the fascicles proximal and distal to the injury site, and then to trace them through the re-

gion of injury. Sometimes, maintenance of a group or groups of fascicles is preferential to splitting the nerve apart fascicle by fascicle, and this is left to the judgment of the individual surgeon, based on the fascicular pattern of that particular nerve at that level (Figure 6–7). Fascicular groups or individual fascicles should then be cleaned of interfascicular epineurium or scar. It is then important to test each fascicle or group of fascicles by NAP recordings, for it is pointless to leave behind functionless and nonrepaired tissue. The remaining bundles or fascicles are thoroughly irrigated with sterile saline, and bleeding points are coagulated with the bipolar forceps. Occasionally, interfascicular repair without interposition of grafts is indicated, and then an internal neurolysis of each

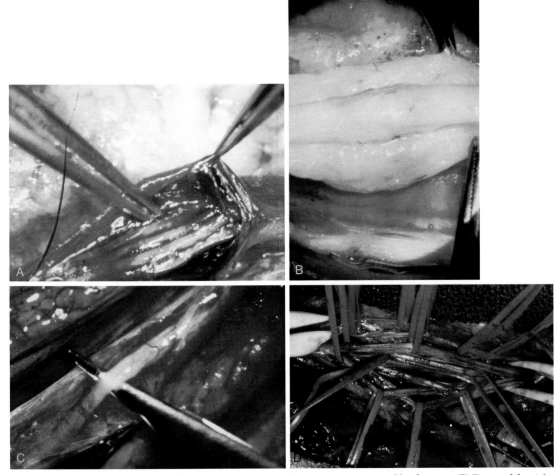

**Figure 6–6.** (*A*) Internal neurolysis showing a portion of epineurium retracted by forceps. (*B*) Exposed fascicles before separation by sharp dissection. (*C*) Dissection of a single fascicle shown beneath fine Metzenbaum scissors. (*D*) Extensive internal neurolysis of a sciatic nerve lesion. Fascicles were split apart both by sharp dissection with a scalpel and by use of fine Metzenbaum scissors and microscissors.

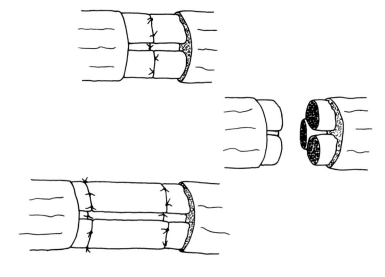

**Figure 6-7.** Groups of fascicles have been dissected out in a nerve with a defect (*right center*). This nerve may be repaired by a fascicular repair (*top*) or by a grouped interfascicular repair (*bottom*).

stump (if the lesion is caused by transection) or of whole nerve (if the lesion is blunt) is performed (Figure 6-8).

## End-to-End Suture Repair

If nerve has been transected or lesions in continuity that are relatively short are resected, end-to-end epineurial repair can sometimes be achieved. If transection is present, dissection should proceed whenever possible from more normal proximal and distal nerves toward their neuromas. Sharp dissection is usually necessary to free stumps from adjacent and scarred soft tissues. Stumps are then trimmed back to healthy epineurium and fascicular structure. Structure of the proximal stumps is readily evident because the freshened fascicles pout from beneath the trimmed epineurium (Figure 6-9). Depending on the time interval between the occurrence of the nerve injury and the operation for repair, distal stump fascicles may be surrounded by a variable amount of scar. Distal neuroma is resected back to a discernible fascicular pattern and one which is relatively soft to palpation with a double-ended dissector or with the handle of the scalpel. It helps to section these stumps after placing them on a piece of sterile tongue blade or similar firm surface. We prefer a fresh scalpel blade mounted on a scalpel handle so that the orientation of the cuts can be readily controlled, and so that nerve at the site of section is not unduly squashed or squeezed. Nerve beyond the neuroma can be

**INTERFASCICULAR REPAIR**

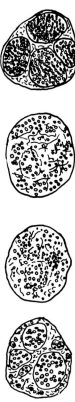

**Figure 6-8.** Usual histologic result of an interfascicular repair without grafts. More normal fascicular pattern is present at top. Proximal to distal extent of scar mixed with axons (*middle two drawings*) tends to be longer than in an end-to-end repair. Many axons have reached distal stump fascicles (*bottom*), but some are at extrafascicular loci. (Adapted from Hudson A, Hunter D, Kline D, Bratton B: Histological studies of experimental interfascicular graft repairs. J Neurosurgery 51:333–340, 1979.)

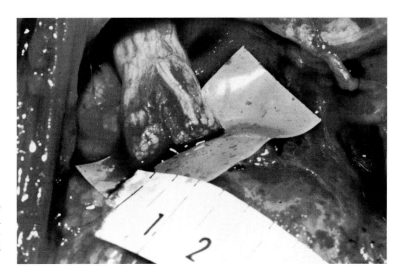

**Figure 6–9.** Several large groups of fascicles trimmed back to healthy tissue are evident on this freshly prepared proximal stump.

steadied by the gloved thumb and forefinger or can be held on top of the cutting surface by fine-toothed forceps grasping the epineurium.

Blood from either sectioned stump is irrigated away. Sometimes such bleeding, if caused by oozing from multiple small vessels, can be diminished by placing a piece of muscle or Gelfoam beneath a cotton pad and against the stump. This is held in place for a few minutes to tamponade the bleeding source. If bleeding is arterial, the bleeding point in the stump may have to be searched out and coagulated by the fine-tipped bipolars. Under these circumstances, it helps if the surgeon's assistant irrigates away the blood as the bleeding vessel is sought out.

After bleeding is controlled and the stumps are as fresh as possible, the suture repair is carried out (Figure 6–10). Preparatory to this, the stumps are mobilized, usually both proximally and distally, to provide a repair with mild tension only. This may be aided by transposition anterior to the elbow for an ulnar repair, partial fibulectomy for a peroneal repair, or transposition of distal radial beneath biceps/brachialis for arm-level radial repair. Mild flexion of the elbow helps gain length for most nerve repairs of the arm. Flexion at the knee helps gain length for most sciatic nerve repairs but delays weight bearing for weeks. The value of transposition and of limb positioning in making up length therefore varies from nerve to nerve and for various lengths of gaps. We do not believe that some tension with an end-to-end repair is bad

or deleterious, but certainly that tension which could lead to distraction is to be avoided. In this series, gap after resection of a neuroma or of a lesion in continuity was often lengthy, so grafts were often used for repair. In general, if there is debate about the integrity or possibility of distraction of an end-to-end repair, it is better to resort to grafts. If a completed end-to-end repair distracts with slight movement of the limb despite mobilization of the nerve stumps and provision of some joint flexion, it is better to take down the repair and replace it with grafts than to risk distraction in the postoperative period.

Repair is done by first placing two lateral sutures, usually 6-0 in caliber, at the 3 o'clock and 9-o'clock positions (Figures 6–11 and 6–12). Sites for these sutures may be close to longitudinally oriented vessels at an epineurial level or in relationship to major fascicles or bundles seen on the face of both stumps. This helps the surgeon to align the fascicular structure as much as possible. As the surgeon and the assistant tie these laterally placed sutures, it is helpful to make the first tie a surgeon's knot, especially if there is any tension on the repair. After the lateral sutures are tied, their ends are clamped with a fine hemostat and the lateral edges are spread somewhat so that there is a clear delineation of the proximal and distal intervening epineurial edges. These are approximated by interrupted sutures to appose the two stumps rather than "accordion" them together. The lateral sutures are then rotated to expose the back side of the repair site. This side is then closed by a number

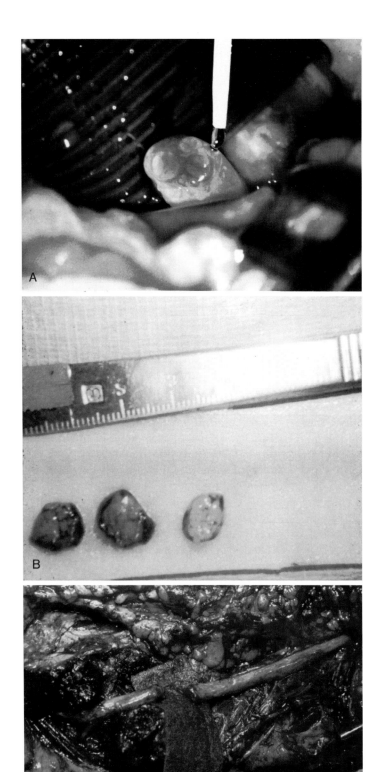

**Figure 6–10.** (*A*) Sectioning back to healthy-appearing fascicular tissue. The freshly sectioned end is being irrigated by heparinized saline. (*B*) Segments or sections of scarred nerve removed from a lesion in continuity. Note the absence of a healthy fascicular pattern, as seen in *A*. (*C*) Freshly trimmed nerve stumps after resection of an injection injury involving arm-level radial nerve. An end-to-end repair was then done.

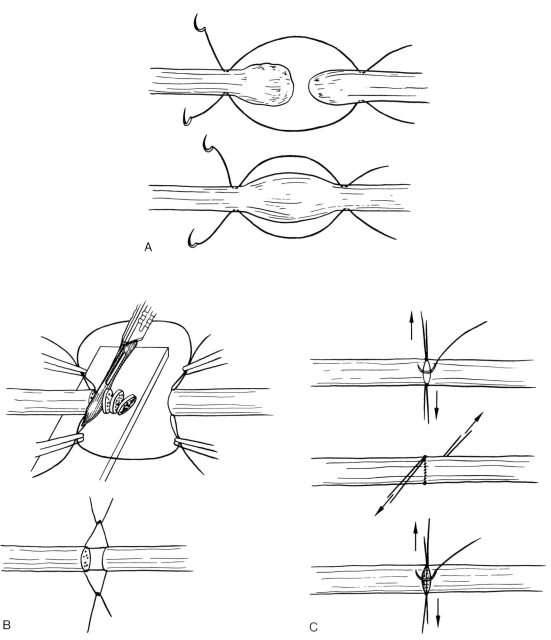

**Figure 6–11.** (*A*) Preplacement of lateral sutures on both a transected nerve (*top*) and a lesion in continuity (*bottom*). (*B*) Sectioning back to healthy proximal stump tissue and pulling together the preplaced lateral sutures. (*C*) Placement of epineurial sutures on uppermost epineurial borders, rotation of the nerve using lateral sutures, and placement of apposite epineurial sutures.

of finely spaced sutures. Epineurium should be reapposed within reason, but this should not be overdone. Thus, the number of epineurial sutures placed should permit accurate coaptation and no more. Excess suture will result in additional scarring.

The caliber of the suture used varies with the size of the nerve to be sutured and the degree of tension predicted for the repair site. As the suture needle traverses the epineurium, a little of the deeper structure is usually included so that fascicular coaptation is maintained. Most polyfascicular nerves are repaired when possible by an epineurial end-to-end technique. We have

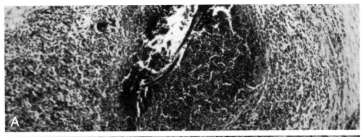

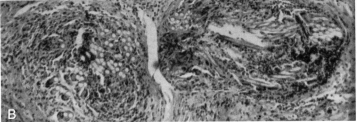

**Figure 6–12.** Histologic comparison of two different types of suture used to repair nerve. The top photograph (*A*) shows a heavy inflammatory response to silk, whereas the lower photograph (*B*) shows less response to Mersilene. Sections were taken 6 weeks after sutures were placed. (H & E, × 40.)

repaired some oligofascicular nerves using fascicular suture. The latter becomes more useful for some distal median and ulnar repairs in which mixed motor-sensory fascicles can sometimes be defined well.

Sometimes, there is disparity between the stump sizes, with usually the proximal being greater in caliber than the distal stump. If this is the case, sutures can be placed at the 12-o'clock and 6-o'clock positions after the lateral sutures are tied. Then, a suture is placed midway between each of these sutures, and this is repeated again until the epineurium is reapposed circumferentially in a symmetric fashion.

After the epineurium is closed, the repair site is gently grasped by the moistened tips of the gloved thumb and forefinger. The suture site is then rolled back and forth between the fingertips several times to align the stumps and their fascicular structure as well as possible, and to make sure the sutures are securely tied and that distraction with slight movement does not occur.

Two important points demand special emphasis. The leading cause for failure of repair is inadequate resection of injured nerve back to healthy tissue. The second leading cause is distraction of the repair site at some time postoperatively. Both of these complications can be avoided if individual lesions are well selected for end-to-end repair. Nonetheless, graft repair should be used if gaps are long or tension is great, for in these cases, inadequate resection and subsequent distraction of the repair are risks. If a gap is small (a few centimeters or less in length), end-to-end suture works well and, in our experience, gives better results than grafts (Figure 6–13). If a gap is larger and cannot be readily made up by mobilization or mild positioning of the extremity without significant tension on the repair site, then grafts are in order and should give results superior to suture.

## Grafts

We prefer to narrow the interstump gap somewhat before placement of grafts. This is done after trimming of the neuromas or after resection of a lengthy lesion in continuity by mobilization of both stumps and mild flexion of an extremity, especially an arm, that can be readily placed in a sling for a few weeks. However, if grafts less than 5 cm in length are possible, positioning the extremity to further shorten the gap provides little extra advantage. After grafts have been decided on, epineurium from each stump is trimmed, and then each stump end is split into multiple bundles or fingers of fasciculi (Figure 6–14). This is usually done by microscissors after visualizing the fascicular pattern on each stump. Sometimes, the nerve end is placed on a firm surface such as a tongue blade and split into quarters or fifths lengthwise by use of a scalpel. Similarly disposed ends or

## EPINEURIAL REPAIR

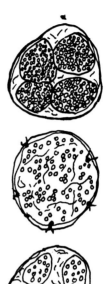

**Figure 6–13.** Usual histologic picture of an epineurial or end-to-end repair several months after operation. Normal proximal stump morphology is seen at the top. Axons mixed with scar are seen in the middle at the center of the repair site, and some restoration of distal stump fascicular structure is seen at the bottom. (Adapted from Hudson A, Hunter D, Kline D, Bratton B: Histologic studies of experimental interfascicular graft repairs. J Neurosurg 51:333–340, 1979.)

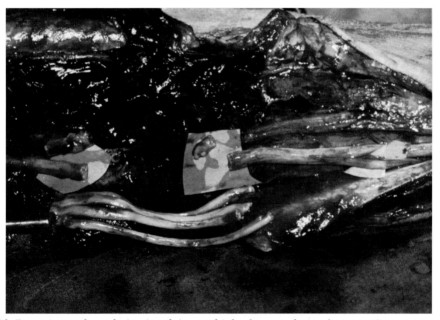

**Figure 6–14.** Preparing a plexus lesion involving multiple elements for graft repair. Grouped interfascicular grafts are about to be sewn in place at the bottom of the photograph; at the top, elements have been sectioned back to healthy tissue. Note that the grafts are somewhat longer than the gap to be bridged.

tails are then created on the opposite stump. Interfascicular epineurial tissue or scar is then trimmed from between the fasciculi or groups of fasciculi.

The gap is then measured, and the number of grafts necessary to close it is calculated. Individual graft length, which should be a little longer than the gap to account for retraction and shrinkage, is then multiplied times the number of grafts needed. This gives the length of donor nerve to be harvested. The majority of grafts are fashioned from the sural nerve. Antebrachial cutaneous nerves can be used for infraclavicular arm injuries to nerves requiring grafts, especially if these potential donor nerves are uninvolved by injury themselves. Their integrity can be tested by intraoperative NAP recordings. Some distal radial and particularly posterior interosseous gaps needing grafts can be closed by harvest of the superficial sensory radial branch, because this goes to a relatively unimportant sensory zone on the dorsum of the hand, where sensation can be sacrificed.

Sural grafts are usually harvested through a mildly curvilinear incision on the posterolateral calf. Nerve can be most reliably located lateral to the Achilles tendon and an inch or so above the lateral malleolus. It usually lies beneath vein and is slightly adherent to it. A segment can be readily dissected free, elevated by a Vasoloop, and then traced proximally. If significantly large branches are encountered, they are traced back down the limb distally and, if necessary, used as graft material too. Any large proximal branches can be traced beneath gastrocnemius soleus fascia to their origin from peroneal divisions of the sciatic nerve or sometimes peroneal and tibial nerves themselves. Care should be taken not to cause a traction injury to the nerve during harvesting. Sural nerve is then sectioned proximally and distally after the desired length is dissected free. The bipolar forceps tip is usually used to attempt to seal shut the ends of the proximal fascicles. Whether this is done or not, it is important to leave the proximal stump buried beneath muscle, especially if shorter grafts are harvested farther down the leg. If only a short segment is needed, it is probably better to take a longer length of sural nerve than necessary. This ensures that the proximal sural end lies beneath some muscle or fascia rather than remaining relatively exposed farther down the limb and beneath skin only.

Antebrachial cutaneous nerve can be harvested from the medial arm. If used for distal plexus or proximal nerve injuries, these nerves can be located as they originate from medial cord. They can then be located distally and dissected free from brachial vessels and other soft tissues. As with sural nerve harvest, the fascicles of the proximal ends are coagulated by the bipolar forceps after removal of a segment of nerve.

After donor nerve has been harvested, it is handled gently, kept moist in isotonic saline, and then moved to the graft site. Excessive mesoneurial or other tissue is removed from the nerve by sharp dissection. Donor nerve is then divided into segments about 10% longer than the gap to be closed.

Grafts are sewn in place to proximal and distal fascicular groups of the stumps by two lateral sutures (Figure 6–15). Because donor graft caliber is usually smaller than what is sewn to, the lateral sutures are used to spread or "fishmouth" the end of the graft segment to cover as much of the fascicular structure as possible (Figure 6–16). Sometimes a third or even a fourth suture is used. In some settings, such as placement of intraforaminal-level spinal nerve grafts, only one suture can be accurately placed, usually running through the center of the proximal stump of the spinal nerve as well as the center of the end of the donor nerve. Usually, 7-0 or 8-0 nylon or Prolene suture is used. Finer suture is difficult to handle even with magnification, and a larger caliber suture takes up too much of the intraneural space.

Depending on the setting, all of the grafts can be sutured first proximally and then distally, or each graft can be sewn in one at a time. The former is a useful tack if one or both graft ends need to be sewn to plexus elements close to the clavicle. Clavicle can be mobilized by the surgeon and retracted by the assistant so that one set of graft ends can be sewn in, and then traction on the clavicle relaxed or retracted in the opposite direction as the other set of ends is sutured in place.

It is important to reinspect the graft anastomoses at the completion of the repair because graft ends can be easily distracted as other grafts are being sutured in place (Figure 6–17). The graft site is then irrigated and bleeding points are coagulated with the bipolar forceps. As with end-to-end repair, it is important to

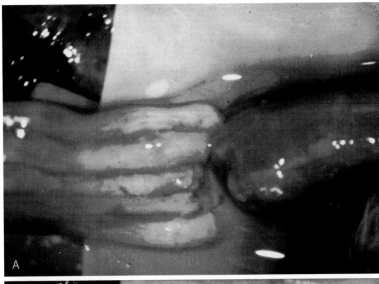

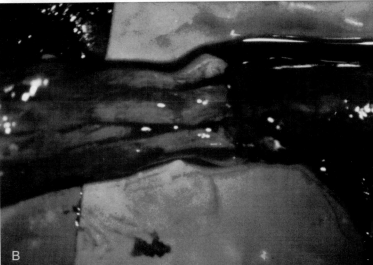

**Figure 6-15.** (*A*) Grafts have been led out of groups of proximal stump fascicles to the left (out of picture). They lie next to the distal stump, which is ready to be split into groups of fascicles to receive the grafts. (*B*) Grafts have been sewn to groups of fascicles on the right without tension. Only a few sutures are necessary to coapt each graft to each group of fascicles.

place the grafts in a bed as free of scar tissue as possible.

At the present time, there does not seem to be any indication for entubulation of either a graft site or an end-to-end suture site. Nonresorbable materials such as Silastic usually have to be removed at a secondary operation, while resorbable materials or autologous tissues fashioned into wrappers or tubes tend to lead to more scar than they prevent. In any case, the scar that seems to prevent or diminish useful axonal regeneration is from intraneural and endoneurial levels and interfascicular epineurial sources rather than extraneural sites. Wrapping or entubulation in humans does not modify intraneural scarring. On the other hand, much research in

recent years has concentrated on use of small tubes lined with laminin or other attractant agents as a potential replacement for grafts. There has been much experimental and some clinical interest in vascularized nerve grafts, but, to date, the potential advantages and reported results do not seem to warrant this more extensive procedure.

After placement of grafts, we usually place the upper limb in a sling, particularly for plexus cases. We do prohibit abduction of the shoulder above the horizontal for about 3 weeks but still encourage circular motions and partial shoulder abduction until then. Figure 6-18 shows the usual histologic appearance several months after repair.

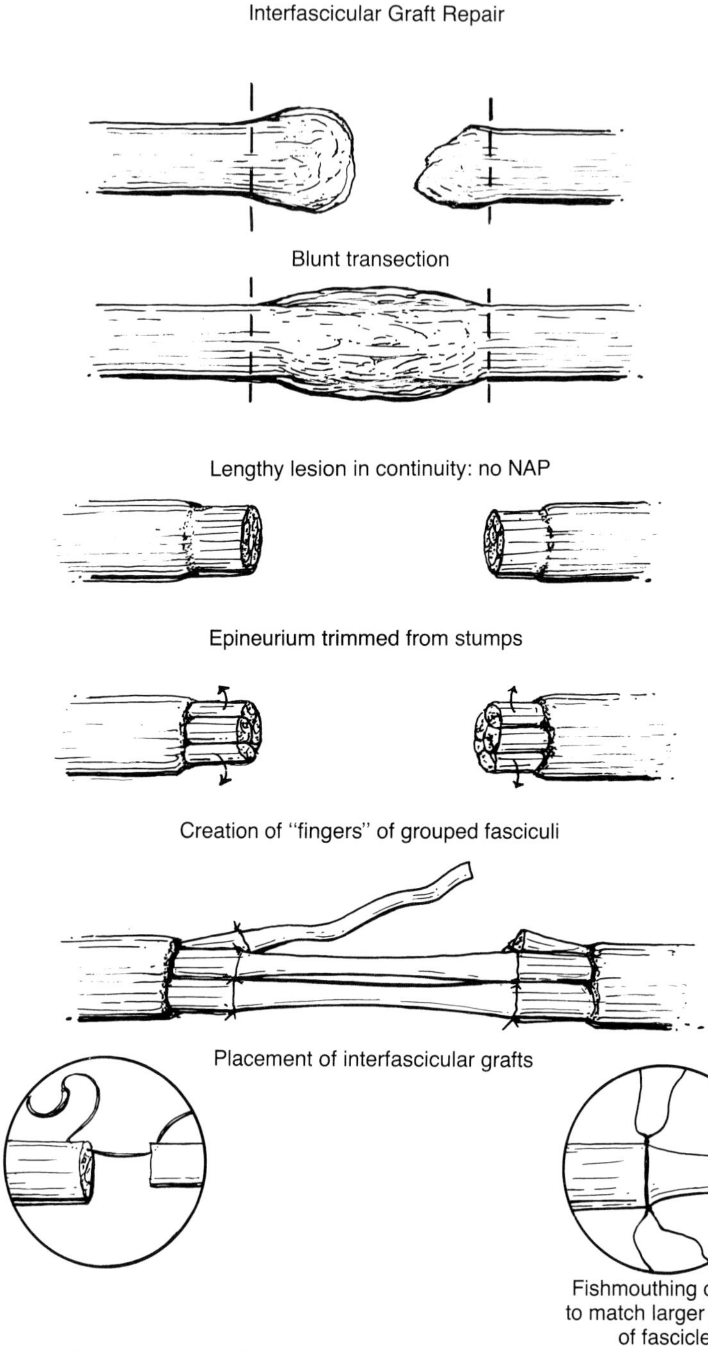

Interfascicular Graft Repair

Blunt transection

Lengthy lesion in continuity: no NAP

Epineurium trimmed from stumps

Creation of "fingers" of grouped fasciculi

Placement of interfascicular grafts

Fishmouthing of graft
to match larger groups
of fascicles

**Figure 6–16.** Drawing of steps necessary for the usual interfascicular graft repair done either for a blunt transection with retraction of neuromatous stumps or for a lengthy lesion in continuity requiring resection. Epineurium is trimmed from both stumps after they have been sectioned back to healthy tissue. Groups or "fingers" of fasciculi are fashioned and then bridged with grafts. Note how the end of each graft has been spread or "fishmouthed" to cover stump fascicular structure.

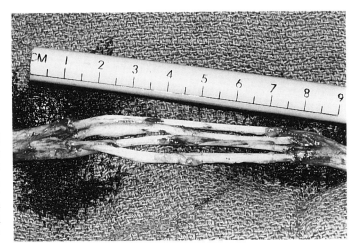

**Figure 6–17.** A completed grouped interfascicular repair using 4 sural grafts 7 cm in length. (From Dubuisson A, Kline D: Indications for peripheral nerve and brachial plexus surgery. Neurol Clin North Am 10:935–951, 1992 with permission.)

## INTERFASCICULAR GRAFT REPAIR

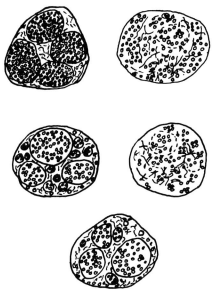

**Figure 6–18.** Usual histologic picture of a grouped interfascicular graft repair using multiple grafts several months after repair. More normal fascicular pattern is seen at top left. Site of scar, axons, and disorganization are seen at interface between proximal stump and proximal grafts (*top right*). At the mid-segment of the grafts, some of their fascicular structure is still evident, with regenerated axons within but also external to fascicles (*middle left*). In the more distal portion of the grafted segment, more disorganization is evident, especially close to and at the level of the anastomosis of the graft to the distal stump's groups of fascicles (*middle right*). At the bottom center is the distal stump morphology; regenerated axons are both intrafascicular and extrafascicular. (Adapted from Hudson A, Hunter D, Kline D, Bratton B: Histologic studies of experimental interfascicular graft repairs. J Neurosurg 51:333–340, 1979.)

## Neurotization

There are a wide variety of neural substitutive procedures that can be tried if direct neural repair is impossible for plexus proximal lesions. These include use of C3 and C4 spinal nerves or descending cervical plexus. Accessory branches and, if intact, pectoral or other branches of the plexus itself can also be used.

One of us has performed 40 intercostal neurotization procedures, with a success rate (elbow flexion only) of 46%. After the avulsion of C5 and C6 is confirmed at surgery, the musculocutaneous and axillary nerves are inspected. Sural nerves are used to bridge the gap between intercostal and recipient nerves, and this is accomplished without difficulty provided the patient has not suffered concomitant rib fractures. One of us favors cervical plexus as an outflow for loss of input to upper trunk. Rarely, the original injury has affected recipient nerves as well as avulsing the roots, and the procedure is abandoned.

## Split Repair

When a portion of the cross section of an injury site is more severely involved than the rest, the nerve can be split into fascicles or bundles of fascicles by internal neurolysis (Figure 6–19). Testing of the individual components often leads to resection of some and relative sparing of others. After clearing those to be left behind of extrinsic scar, those resected are repaired, usually by inlaying one or more grafts between

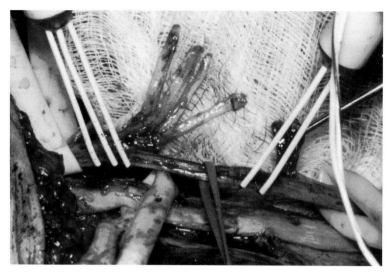

**Figure 6–19.** Stimulation (to the left) and recording (to the right) from a portion of nerve to be retained without repair because of detection of a nerve action potential (NAP) conducted across this segment. Grafts have been sewn into fascicular groups to the left and will next be sewn into those on the right of the photograph. This portion of the injury did not conduct an NAP. (From Dubuisson A, Kline D: Indications for peripheral nerve and brachial plexus surgery. Neurol Clin North Am 10:935–951, 1992.) See also color figure.

their stumps. This is termed split repair. As with end-to-end or whole nerve graft repair, it is important to resect the damaged segments back to healthy tissue and to gain as relaxed a repair as possible.

If nerve is partially transected and repaired acutely, split repair usually entails simple end-to-end suture of the transected portion. If a small gap exists, a slight undulation in the relatively uninjured portion of the nerve is acceptable with either acute or more delayed repair. On the other hand, if a good deal of undulation results, or if there is the potential for kinking to

develop, it is better to lay in grafts to fill the gap (Figure 6–20). Split repairs usually have a favorable outcome, especially if the portion spared repair is proved to be either intact, only partially injured, or regenerating by intraoperative electrophysiologic evaluation.

## Resection of Painful Neuromas

Some injuries to nerves lead to the formation of painful neuromas. If these involve relatively unimportant sensory nerves or branches of

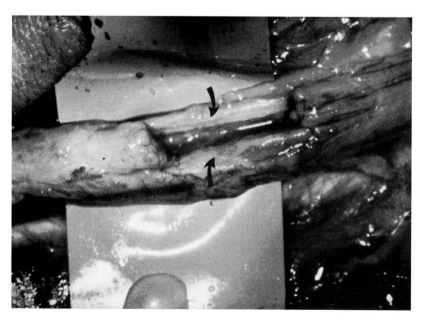

**Figure 6–20.** Preparation for split or partial repair by grafts. End to the right of the photograph has been split into bundles for receipt of grafts; the portion of the fascicular structure to the left remains to be split. Retained portions of the nerve are indicated by arrows.

mixed motor-sensory nerves, the neuroma can be resected without repair. Examples include antebrachial cutaneous nerves; lateral or forearm sensory branches of the musculocutaneous nerve; dorsal cutaneous branch of the ulnar, thenar, or palmar sensory branches of the median; superficial sensory branch of the radial (SSR); and sural and saphenous portions of the sciatic and femoral complexes. It is important under these circumstances to resect not only the neuroma but, if in continuity, portions of the nerve both distal and proximal to it. It is also necessary to remove surrounding scar and any branches from adjacent, less injured nerves. The latter can contribute to the neuroma or at least be a partial generator of painful impulses, as pointed out by Mackinnon and Dellon (Surgery of the Peripheral Nerve, New York, G. Thieme, 1988), and need resection. This is more likely to be a problem with SSR and saphenous nerve neuromas than with others.

Treatment of the freshly sectioned proximal end of nerve associated with a neuroma remains controversial. An ideal treatment to ensure against recurrence is lacking. Any injury to nerve, even fresh and sharp section of it, leads to neuroma and may eventually result in a painful neuroma. At this time, we prefer to place the freshly sectioned nerve as deep in soft tissues as possible. Preferred is placement deep to muscle. We do not suture the end to muscle, turn the nerve back on itself, curve or angulate it proximally, ligate it, or inject it with sclerosing materials. We prefer to attempt to seal shut the ends of the fascicles in the proximal stump by coagulation with the fine tips of the bipolar forceps. This is done under magnification and only in the proximal stump. The situation may be helped by resecting 6 cm or more of nerve to discourage regrowth, restoration of continuity,

and a resultant neuroma, which may again be painful.

## POSTOPERATIVE CARE

This phase of care differs somewhat from nerve to nerve, for upper and lower limbs, and for plexus and nonplexus operations (Table 6–2). Nonetheless, some common features require special emphasis.

The tensile strength of nerves, whether repaired end-to-end or by grafts, appears to be maximal by 3 weeks postoperatively. Some care in not overstretching, abducting, or extending the limb is necessary in the early weeks, but not later on. It is true that if an end-to-end repair is done under some tension, then extension of the limb even after 3 weeks postoperatively should be done gradually. A physical therapist who is aware of the implications of working out a limb after neural repair is of invaluable help. Often, a parent or other loved one can, if carefully instructed, help the patients themselves to do this.

Again, nerves do not heal by being placed at rest, nor do joints regain mobility without motion. Structured therapy is of help, but the patient and his or her family must help by moving the paralyzed or paretic limb many times a day.

Wound care is the same as that for other soft tissue operations with a few exceptions. Collections of blood or serum in and around the repair site should be minimized by careful and patient intraoperative hemostasis. If they arise postoperatively, then it is best to aspirate or surgically evacuate sizable collections; if untreated, they lead to severe scarring about the repair sites.

Although intact nerve is relatively resistant to invasion by infection, the same may not be true of injured or surgically manipulated nerve with

**TABLE 6–2**
Postoperative Care

1. Check limbs and dressings frequently for excessive swelling or bleeding and vascular insufficiency
2. Institute early and aggressive pulmonary care; chest radiograph, especially for brachial plexus dissections
3. Keep immobilization of the limb as minimal as possible
4. Institute early range of motion, especially of joints well proximal and distal to the operative site
5. Daily wound care; early mildly compressive dressings followed by noncompressive coverage by dressings
6. Removal of drain if used
7. Frank discussion with the patient and family about operative findings, repairs done, possible outcomes, expected course of rehabilitation, and pain patterns that may occur
8. Discharge instructions regarding wound care, need for physician follow-up, expected postoperative visits, and use of medications

altered blood-to-nerve barriers. A soft tissue infection in a limb after nerve has been operated on, with or without repair, requires aggressive treatment with antibiotics and sometimes incision, debridement, and drainage. All of our patients who have undergone lengthy procedures receive a perioperative intravenous antibiotic. We give the patient a week of postoperative antibiotic coverage, especially if the patient is discharged from hospital care after 1 or 2 days. This is important because a number of these patients come a distance for their operative care, and when they go home, it is difficult for them to return.

Dressings are usually changed daily postoperatively until discharge. Dressings are applied in such a fashion as to provide mild compression of the wound site and more distal limb. If the patient is discharged after a few days, he or she is usually sent home with a dressing on. The patient is urged to keep the wound dry and either to return for inspection and removal of sutures or clips in 7 to 10 days or, if from a distance, to see his or her local physician at about the same time. If the skin was closed in a subcuticular fashion, then Steri-Strips should be soaked off the wound edges 8 to 10 days after operation. Usually, patients are instructed to keep the arm or leg elevated for a portion of each day for several weeks or more postoperatively. This should not be done, however, by neglecting frequent movement of the involved limb.

In addition to receiving an antibiotic, the patient is usually sent home with one or more medications for pain. Some painful shocks and dysesthesia can occur later, even though they might not have been present immediately postoperatively while the patient was in the hospital. The patient needs to be told this. Dysesthesia or pain associated with regeneration is more painful to some patients than to others, and the nature and meaning of this should be explained to the patient. If potentially addictive drugs are prescribed for a week or two postoperatively, then it may also be necessary to provide an analgesic of lesser potency and less addictive properties so that the patient can switch over to the lesser drug after a period of time.

It is necessary to explain to the patient and to family and friends at the hospital what was done, what to expect, when the patient is to return for follow-up, and, if possible, what the realistic outlook is for recovery or improvement, especially in function. Provision of some timetable in this regard is helpful. We usually try to provide the patient with a rough drawing of the operative findings, on which we summarize special instructions for wound care, limb movement, return visit for wound check by us or another physician, and a tentative idea of future postoperative visits (i.e., 6 months, 1 year, 3 years, 5 years, etc.).

## COMPLICATIONS OR LIMITS TO OPERATIONS

Specific complications for specific nerves are discussed at the end of each appropriate chapter. Each type of operation on a particular nerve at a specific level has some limit to its ability to aid return of function. Some estimate of these limits can be given preoperatively and then refined further for the patient and family postoperatively. Failure to improve or limited improvement, as such, is not necessarily a complication. Nonetheless, it should always be pointed out as a possibility to the patient.

The second major possible negative outcome is that function of a partially injured nerve may be further decreased as a result of the operation. This is certainly the case if a lesion in continuity with partial distal retention of function is associated with severe pain and the lesion is resected or a repair of the entire cross section of the nerve is done. Further loss can also occur with external and especially with internal neurolysis of a partially injured nerve. The surgeon needs to warn the patient of these possibilities, even though their likelihood is small when the operator is experienced.

New loss in the distribution of a nearby or related nerve, branch, or element can also occur, even if the dissection seemed careful and retraction or other manipulation was not excessive. Good visualization of structures related to the injured nerve or element is paramount if new or further loss is to be avoided. Such loss may be minimized by dissecting out related structures, mobilizing them to a variable degree away from the injury site, and protecting them maximally.

Pain that was not present preoperatively can

result, or milder pain can sometimes be increased by operation. These distressing changes can also occur despite good technique and should be pointed out to the patient. If a partially injured nerve or adjacent element is stretched, bruised, compressed, or complicated by clot in a potentially tight space, or if a potential and related area of entrapment is not removed or is incompletely released, increased neuritic pain as well as further loss of function is even more possible.

Pulmonary complications can always occur, especially if general anesthesia is necessary (Figure 6–21). Complications include atelectasis, pneumonia, pulmonary embolus, and even acute respiratory distress syndrome. Careful attention must be given to good pulmonary toilet and maintenance of good pulmonary function postoperatively, especially after lengthy nerve operations with the patient under general anesthesia. Pleural effusion, pneumo- or hemothorax, and diaphragmatic paralysis are more likely with brachial plexus or thoracic outlet procedures and abdominal complications with pelvic plexus procedures.

Wound complications such as hematoma, seroma, or wound infection can occur. Exposures are often necessarily large, and wounds are exposed for a lengthy period. This can lead to infection unless care of soft tissues is as meticulous as possible and postoperative wound care is also carefully maintained. Anastomosis of the wrong proximal and distal nerve stumps or suture of nerve to tendon or vessel may complicate repair but can be avoided if the surgeon has a good understanding of the regional anatomy (Figure 6–22).

## USE OF GROSS ANATOMY DURING OPERATION

The peripheral nerve surgeon must be intimately familiar with the gross anatomic features pertaining to the site of injury and the injured nerves. Clinical examination is an exercise in applied anatomy, and it is from the clinical data that the site and completeness of nerve injury are estimated. At operation, the surgeon must be familiar with all structures in the operative field as well as those beyond the periphery of vision. Frequently, the surgeon seeks areas of normal anatomy from which to commence the dissection, because the site of peripheral nerve injury may be significantly distorted by the pathology.

### Bones or Osteology

The surgeon should first study the bones, preferably with the individual bones at hand. After knowledge of the elementary skeletal features is mastered, the soft tissues can be added until the complete anatomic picture is assembled.

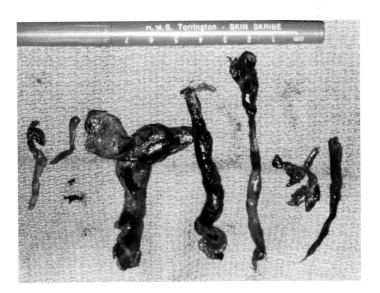

**Figure 6–21.** Clots removed from pulmonary arterial tree. Acute pulmonary embolectomy was necessary 3 days postoperatively in this patient.

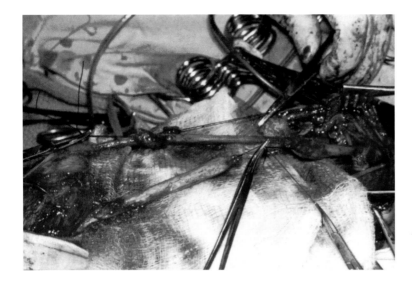

**Figure 6–22.** Proximal stump of a nerve (*to the right*) was mistakenly sewn to a severed portion of a tendon (*to the left*). Distal stump of the nerve was found at a distance from the tendon and is being drawn toward the proximal neuroma by a suture held with a hemostat.

## Upper Limb

The transverse processes of the cervical vertebrae should be studied with care. At operation, the surgeon can palpate the anterior tubercles of the transverse processes. These tubercles mark the lateral extremity of the gutters of the transverse processes, which support the spinal nerves. Scalenus anticus is attached to the anterior tubercles and scalenus medius to the posterior tubercles, so that the spinal nerves gain the posterior triangle of the neck by running between these muscles. It is appropriate also to realize the anatomy of the vertebral artery within the cervical vertebrae, because bony dissection within the foramen brings the operator close to that structure.

The bones of the pectoral girdle and shoulder joint should be examined with care. The clavicle is grooved on its undersurface by the subclavius muscle, which is always seen in brachial plexus dissections. With the clavicular bone in hand, the surgeon should review the attachment of pectoralis major and deltoid in an anatomy textbook. Division of a portion of the lateral clavicular attachment of pectoralis major is necessary to gain access to the upper medial cord and its divisions of origin. The reciprocal attachments of trapezius and deltoid to the clavicle are usually undisturbed during routine plexus surgery, but, on occasion, exposure of the suprascapular nerve proximal to the transverse scapular ligament may be improved by dividing clavicular fibers of trapezius close to the bone.

The scapular bone should be examined with care, noting the points of attachment of levator scapulae, rhomboids, serratus anterior, trapezius, deltoid, and the short scapular muscles. Careful study allows the surgeon to gain an appreciation of the combined muscle functions which result in rotation of the scapula in the later phases of shoulder abduction. An understanding of mechanisms involved in winging of the scapula, which is so characteristic of both trapezius palsy and serratus anterior palsy, is also gained by studying the exact points of attachment of these muscles to the shoulder blade. In trapezius palsy, levator scapulae has to take over the suspensory function. An appreciation of the attachment of that muscle to the scapula permits the surgeon to understand the function of the muscle in an injury to cranial nerve XI. The examiner cannot be deceived into thinking that the trapezius fibers are contracting when, in fact, levator scapulae is being examined.

The rhomboid muscle is often assessed as a clinical indicator of proximal C5 spinal nerve injury. The attachment of this muscle to the scapula should be noted in an appropriate atlas. The scapula should be examined both individually and while articulated to the clavicle so that the clinician can note the exact position of the scapular notch and transverse scapular ligament. In the articulated skeleton, the angle formed between the scapula and clavicle becomes more acute the more laterally the surgeon dissects the suprascapular nerve from its takeoff at the upper trunk, and the space becomes more and more confined. The attachment of the external rotators of the shoulder joint should be traced on the bone. Often, the surgeon hopes to regain elbow flexion in upper plexus surgery, but reinnervation of the external rotators is of the greatest importance, because failure to achieve this results in elbow flexion which is of limited use to the patient.

The very small size of the glenoid should be appreciated. The upper point of attachment of the deltoid should be delineated on the articulated scapula and clavicle. If this muscle is paralyzed from either a C5 spinal nerve, upper trunk, or axillary nerve injury, the head of the humerus slides down on the small articular surface, causing the characteristic clinical picture of subluxation of the shoulder joint. On the anterior aspect of the scapula, the coracoid process provides an extremely useful landmark and reference point during axillary dissection. Note the point of attachment of pectoralis minor and biceps. No matter how extensive the scarring is in the axilla, the coracoid can always be palpated, thus providing an anatomic landmark for the surgeon and a reference point for the neural and vascular structures contained in the axilla.

The surgeon should hold the humerus and examine the points of attachment of supraspinatus and deltoid. The C5-innervated muscles abduct the shoulder joint, and the subsequent combined action of trapezius and serratus anterior rotates the scapula to achieve the full range of scapular abduction. The exact point of attachment of pectoralis major to the humerus should also be noted. The tendon on this great muscle is usually partially and sometimes totally divided close to the humerus during the axillary exposure. While examining this region, the surgeon should note the point of attachment of latissimus dorsi. The shining tendon of this great back muscle is a constant companion during posterior axillary dissection, and the relation of this tendon to the quadrangular and triangular spaces is well appreciated by examining its point of insertion into the humerus. The surgeon should trace the humeral attachments of triceps so that the passage of the radial nerve and its relation to the spiral groove are clearly understood. Farther distally, the bony attachments of brachioradialis and extensor carpi ra-

dialis longus should be examined with care; these muscles are important in the differential diagnosis of radial nerve and posterior interosseous palsy. The point of origin of the common forearm flexors should also be observed, particularly that of pronator teres, which is frequently a feature of operations on the median nerve in the upper forearm.

The two forearm bones should be examined on an articulated skeleton. A detailed study of the insertion of the biceps tendon reveals why that muscle is a powerful supinator of the forearm. It is essential to understand the bony attachments of the two heads of flexor carpi ulnaris if the surgeon is to develop a complete understanding of the anatomy related to the ulnar nerve at the elbow joint. Similarly, the two points of origin of the supinator muscle should be carefully defined so that a subsequent understanding of the course of the posterior interosseous nerve is facilitated. One must also look carefully for the bony markings of the point of attachment of the superficial flexors of the forearm. An understanding of the anatomy of the upper portion of this muscle is essential for dissection of the median nerve distal to pronator teres. Note also the detailed points of origin of the median- and ulnar-innervated deep flexor musculature; testing of these muscles forms the basis of the clinical diagnosis of median and ulnar nerve lesions.

Next, examine an articulated hand. The four points of attachment of the transverse carpal ligament should be identified with care. Each of these four points can be palpated in the living hand. The pisiform bone is analogous to the patella in that it is a sesamoid bone. Note with care the relation of the ulnar nerve to this bone and the subsequent path of the deep motor branch around the hook of the hamate. The lateral points of attachment of the transverse carpal ligament, the scaphoid, and the trapezium should be identified, and the clinician should then understand the distal extent of the transverse carpal ligament, whose complete division in carpal tunnel surgery is so important. At this stage, it is appropriate to visualize the complex curvatures of the articular surfaces of the scaphoid and trapezium. These surfaces allow for rotation of the thumb and hence the clinical movement of opposition as opposed to pure flexion.

## Lower Limb

The bones of the lower limb should also be examined, in both the disarticulated and the articulated states. The anterior surface of the sacrum should be reviewed, drawing out the points of attachment of the pyriformis muscle. The surgeon can then get a firm appreciation of the manner in which the descending trunk formed from L4 and L5 spinal nerve crosses in front of the sacroiliac joint to join the sacral spinal nerves at the origination of the lumbosacral plexus. These neural elements escape the pelvis as the sciatic nerve and gluteal branches. The sciatic courses below or through pyriformis and is usually next observed by the surgeon in the buttock en route to the thigh. The anterior superior iliac spine should be palpated to remind the observer of its relation to the lateral femoral cutaneous nerve of the thigh. The surgeon should next examine the outer surface of the pelvic ring and trace in detail the attachments of the gluteal musculature. Note particularly the relation of the uppermost extent of the sciatic notch to the posterior iliac crest. In fashioning appropriate incisions for sciatic notch surgery, all these points are of the utmost importance if appropriate exposure is to be obtained.

Next examine the articulated hip joint. Although it is unnecessary for the peripheral nerve surgeon to master the intricate detail of the short muscles of the hip, the relation of both the sciatic nerve and the femoral nerve to the hip joint is very important. In the articulated skeleton, the bony attachments of the adductors should be examined at both the pelvic and femoral attachments. These muscles are supplied by the obturator nerve, which has the same roots of origin as the femoral nerve, a useful point of distinction between individual peripheral nerve and lumbar plexus injury. It is also important to identify and then trace the origins and insertions of the hamstring muscles, as these are frequently examined in assessing proximal sciatic nerve function. In particular, note the course of biceps femoris, because this muscle is often dissected during midthigh sciatic exposure.

The articulated knee joint should be examined from behind. The point of insertion of biceps femoris into the head of the fibula can be readily seen. This bony prominence can be pal-

pated operatively and serves as a guide to the adjacent peroneal nerve as it winds around the neck of the fibula to gain the lateral and anterior compartments of the leg. The medial and lateral malleoli should be clearly identified. The former serves as a guide to the posterior tibial nerve as it leaves the leg to gain the foot, and the latter leads to the sural nerve, which is frequently used as a source of grafts.

The peripheral nerve surgeon need not master all the details of the small bones of the foot, but several points are of importance. The bony origin of extensor digitorum brevis should be delineated, because this muscle is frequently used in electrophysiologic studies. Points of attachment of the peroneus tendons and those of the anterior and posterior tibial muscles should also be studied, because these groups are often used in assessing the nerves of the lower limb.

## Muscles

The clinician must have a complete understanding of the function of the major muscles, because weakness or paralysis is the basis of clinical diagnosis of peripheral nerve lesions. In addition, incisions to expose peripheral nerves are fashioned so that the dissection is made on the surface or edge of muscles, but occasionally muscle fibers have to be split to gain an appropriate exposure.

The posterior and somewhat lateral border of sternocleidomastoid is frequently dissected during an initial supraclavicular exposure of the brachial plexus. The clavicular origin is often divided to allow greater exposure of the lower plexus elements. The surgeon should immediately recognize the branches of the cervical plexus as they wind around the posterior border of sternocleidomastoid. These cervical plexus branches serve as a good indicator that the dissection is sufficiently extended superiorly to allow detailed dissection of the underlying C5 spinal nerve, and these nerves also serve as a preliminary guide during dissection of the accessory nerve in the posterior triangle of the neck. The omohyoid is a rapidly recognized feature in the early stages of plexus exposure, but the plexus is still obscured by the supraclavicular fat pad. Palpation of the characteristic anterior rounded surface of scalenus anticus through this fat rapidly orients the surgeon to the proximal outflow of the brachial plexus. This muscle should be studied in exquisite detail. Mastery of all the relationships of this muscle serves to elucidate the three-dimensional anatomic relationships at the root of the neck.

The function and appearance of the majority of the muscles in the upper limb can be learned by quiet periods of contemplation in the dissecting room and by studying the appropriate texts. It is well, however, to review in detail the function of the intrinsic muscles of the hand, as these structures are keys to the understanding of median, ulnar, and radial nerve injuries of the upper limb.

The appearance of the psoas muscle on retroperitoneal approach should also be reviewed. This is the guide to the dissection of the femoral nerve and its spinal nerves of origin. The anatomy of the inguinal ligament should be viewed in the dissecting room so that the surgeon clearly understands the relation of the femoral artery and the femoral nerve to that structure. On the posterior aspect of the pelvis, the peripheral attachments of gluteus maximus should be studied with care, and the relationship of the inferior border of gluteus maximus, the buttock crease, and the sciatic nerve should be reviewed. These are all points of importance during proximal exposure of the sciatic nerve. At this time, it is also appropriate to review the appearance, bony attachments, and relation of the iliotibial tract or tensor fasciae latae. In patients with femoral nerve palsies, the action of this muscle can confuse the uninitiated so that tensing of the investing fascia could be misinterpreted as evidence of quadriceps function.

It is well to become thoroughly familiar with the insertional sites and appearances of the muscles around the popliteal fossa. These structures should be viewed from the posterior aspect, because it is from this aspect that the surgeon will be operating on the posterior tibial and peroneal nerves. In the leg, the details of the relation between the peroneal nerve and the peroneus muscles should be viewed by examining a dissected specimen. The surgeon should also examine the posterior aspect of the (lower) leg so as to fully understand the plane of approach for extended exposure of the posterior tibial nerve in its course toward the ankle. The short muscles of the foot should be reviewed to the extent that the surgeon is clearly able to dissect the medial and lateral plantar nerves in their proximal portion during surgery on the distal posterior tibial nerve.

## Vessels

The peripheral nerve surgeon not only must know vascular anatomy but must also be capable of dealing with vascular pathology during nerve dissections. The anatomy of the subclavian artery should be thoroughly understood and the point of origin of the vertebral arteries mastered. These vessels must be protected during surgery on the stellate ganglion and upper thoracic sympathetic trunk. A more lateral exposure of the plexus is greatly aided by either resection or division of a portion of scalenus anticus after the phrenic nerve has been identified, mobilized, and protected. This exposure allows the surgeon to divide the thyrocervical artery and other small branches. This permits mobilization of the subclavian artery superiorly and inferiorly, offering full access to the first thoracic and eight cervical spinal nerves and the lower trunk of the brachial plexus. In supraclavicular plexus dissections, branches of the transverse cervical artery are usually secured and divided to allow detailed access to the nerve structures. In the axilla, the surgeon needs to study the course of the axillary artery. Such study pays dividends when a tedious dissection through a scarred plexus is undertaken. The origin of the median nerve embraces the artery, and following the medial motor head of the median nerve proximally leads the surgeon to the medial cord, which may be tucked out of sight behind the posteromedial border of the artery. Initial dissection of the posterior cord is usually lateral to the artery in the upper axilla and may be medial to the artery in the lower axilla. If the artery is drawn medially, the circumflex humeral vessels are revealed, and these serve as an excellent guide to the quadrangular space if the surgeon is having difficulty in locating the axillary nerve. Palpation of the brachial artery in the arm is a rapid guide to the exposure of the median nerve. In the distal forearm, the ulnar artery is very closely applied to the ulnar nerve.

In cases of combined nerve and vascular injury, it is appropriate for the surgeon to study the collateral circulation with care so that these vessels are not interrupted during subsequent peripheral nerve surgery. For example, it may be imperative to preserve the circumflex humeral vessels or to preserve the radial collateral artery running behind the humerus in the event of obstruction to the main blood supply.

In dissections at the root of the neck, the internal jugular veins are usually seen. The angle between the major draining veins of the upper limbs and the internal jugular vein should be approached with care, because numerous lymph channels, in addition to the major named lymphatic trunks, may be injured in this dissection. Previous injury may cause scarring and attachment of the internal jugular vein to the deep surface of sternocleidomastoid. This large and important draining vein in the neck should be treated with caution throughout the dissection. The cephalic or deltopectoral vein delineates the groove between deltoid and pectoralis major, and this vein is often divided during axillary exposure. As a general statement, veins that obscure the nerves under dissection are usually divided, but if the patient's venous return has previously been compromised by injury, the surgeon may have to preserve as many venous structures as possible.

Arteriovenous malformations may accompany peripheral nerve injury, and traumatic pseudoaneurysm formation is one of the causes of subsequent deterioration of peripheral nerve function after injury. When dissecting in the root of the neck or the axilla, the surgeon must always be prepared to manage such arterial or venous injuries appropriately. A particular note of caution is issued with regard to previous procedures done to repair vessels, particularly by grafts. The surgeon should ascertain before nerve surgery whether such grafts have been placed in a normal or extra-anatomic position and also have some idea of their length.

## Nerves

The clinician must be familiar enough with the course of nerves so that their surface markings at a skin level can be easily defined. Part of the clinical examination involves palpation of the nerve throughout its course. In most instances, the nerve or element of origin must also be palpated and examined for function. This type of preoperative inspection aids the placement of a proper skin incision and also helps direct the deeper portion of the dissection. Nerve masses can be moved from side to side but not axially; this point is useful in their identification by the clinician. Palpation of a mass in a peripheral nerve often results in paresthesia in the appropriate distribution.

The branches of the cervical plexus form a useful landmark during dissection for accessory nerve injury and during the dissection of the C5 spinal nerve. The phrenic nerve, attached to the front of scalenus anticus by the prevertebral fascia, is a useful guide and leads the surgeon up to the C5 spinal nerve, thus establishing the plane of outflow of the spinal nerves. The junction of C5 and C6 to form the upper trunk is usually a characteristic landmark, and the suprascapular nerve leaving the upper trunk usually indicates the point of division of that trunk into its anterior and posterior components. The position of the sixth spinal nerve having been established, it is usually fairly easy to display the seventh spinal nerve, which continues as the middle trunk. This, of course, requires a deeper dissection with removal of the overlying scalene muscles. There may on occasion be difficulty in identifying the lower trunk; it may be tucked behind the subclavian artery.

In the axilla, the median nerve is usually readily found in the distal portion of the dissection. If this nerve is followed superiorly to its lateral sensory head, the musculocutaneous nerve can be found, and if the medial head is followed, the ulnar and antebrachial cutaneous nerves of forearm are usually readily identified. The posterior cord appears as a flattened, tape-like structure in the upper axilla and is usually readily identified, but in the lower portion of the dissection, it may be easy to confuse the more rounded distal posterior cord with the distal medial cord. In the arm, the inexperienced surgeon may confuse an antebrachial cutaneous nerve of forearm with the median nerve, but the former is a much smaller nerve than the latter. In the forearm, the SSR is usually readily identified, and tracing this proximally leads the surgeon to the larger posterior interosseous nerve. The median and ulnar nerves at the wrist are usually quite characteristic in their appearance, but contusion and hemorrhage may cause confusion. We have had to reoperate on patients in whom median and ulnar nerves had been sewn to tendons at this level or more proximally in the forearm.

The appearance of the femoral nerve in the retroperitoneal space is quite characteristic, and the nerve should not be confused with a psoas tendon. In the thigh, the main trunk of the femoral nerve lies in a separate fascial compartment from the femoral artery and breaks rapidly into numerous branches in a very characteristic fashion.

In the buttock, the large sciatic nerve should be defined with ease, but care is required during that dissection with the superior and inferior gluteal nerves as well as the posterior cutaneous nerve of thigh and the proximally placed hamstring branch. The characteristic appearance of the sciatic nerve and its two divisions should guide the dissector proximally to allow identification of the other nerves mentioned. Divergence of the posterior tibial and peroneal components of the sciatic nerve in the lower thigh is quite characteristic, but the exact level of this divergence is not constant. Sural nerve usually arises from peroneal, but it may also have input from posterior tibial.

The appearance of the peroneal nerve deep to the investing fascia and just proximal to the neck of the fibula is quite characteristic. Nonetheless, the surgeon must be certain to identify the rounded tendon of insertion of biceps femoris, which on occasion may mimic the peroneal nerve in appearance. At the level of the ankle, the posterior tibial nerve must be related to vessels and surrounding tendons, and the characteristic point of branching into medial and lateral plantar nerves is another familiar landmark. In the leg, the sural nerve can be readily differentiated from its attendant lesser saphenous vein, and in similar fashion, the saphenous nerve can be distinguished from adjacent greater saphenous vein.

Inexperienced surgeons should repeatedly visit the dissection room. Review of prosected specimens helps the surgeon review the entire anatomy surrounding the proposed site of operation. In the subsequent, more limited exposure experienced in the operating room, the surgeon will be much more comfortable in establishing the relation between the structures viewed through the incision. It must be remembered, however, that dissection to display specific points in an anatomy museum in itself alters the relation among those structures. What may appear as a very straightforward pattern in a dissected anatomy specimen may be much less obvious when the surgeon deals with individual variations in anatomy as well as distortion of relations by the scar of injury.

The standard anatomy texts that should be consulted include those which display dissections in as lifelike and nondiagrammatic form as is possible. The differential coloring of tissues in these texts aids comprehension but may give a misleading impression of simplicity which is rapidly dispelled when the surgeon confronts reality in the operating room. There is, however, no substitute for gaining experience by assisting experienced surgeons who are totally familiar with the anatomy of the peripheral nerves. At the same time, the student learns technical maneuvers that enable the operator to dissect with dexterity and without causing undue damage to tissues. Finally, in this age of sophisticated imaging and electrodiagnosis, it is worth repeating that interpretation of not only the extremely important clinical findings but also the imaging and electrophysiologic studies is all based on a thorough mastery of human anatomy.

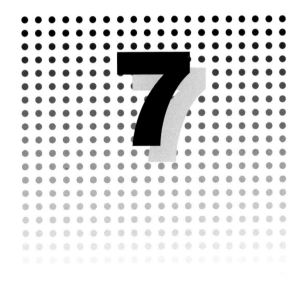

# Radial Nerve

# SUMMARY

In this and the upper extremity nerve chapters to follow, the authors have chosen to emphasize the surgical anatomy and physiology determined to be most important and applicable for the surgeon. There are many excellent anatomy texts with much more detail, and some nonanatomy texts in which the finer points of some entrapments and smaller sensory nerve injuries are described in greater detail.

The radial nerve is exceptional in many ways. Its motor input is much more important than its sensory function. These motor inputs occur at an arm and forearm level and do not include hand intrinsic muscles, as the median and ulnar distributions do. Recovery, either spontaneously or with a good repair, is excellent and is superior to that of any other major nerves except the musculocutaneous or perhaps the tibial. Nonetheless, restoration of finger and thumb extension often does not come close to the excellent function achieved in more proximal radial-innervated muscles. As a result, tendon transfers to restore finger and thumb extension remain important.

Dissection of the radial nerve at an arm level can be challenging because it is deep to triceps in the lateral arm and deep to axillary and brachial artery and other nerves in the axilla and medial arm. Results with repair of posterior interosseous (PIN) can be excellent, as can recovery after release of PIN entrapment. Both the diagnosis and the surgical dissection of PIN lesions have unique features which must be learned by both study and experience.

The tables in this and subsequent chapters provide data on treatment and outcomes according to the level of nerve involved and mechanism of injury or lesion. The data for this chapter on the radial nerve evolved from experience with 240 cases, 171 of which underwent surgery. As expected, most serious radial injuries were associated with fractures, lacerations, contusions and gunshot wounds, but a number of injection injuries and entrapments also required surgery. Some idea of the value of a neurolysis based on nerve action potential recording and of suture and graft repair can also be obtained from the Tables.

# APPLIED ANATOMY

The posterior cord of the brachial plexus is formed from divisions derived from all three trunks; consequently, there is an anatomic potential for a widespread radicular origin of the nerve fibers contained in this cord. The posterior cord of the brachial plexus is so named because of its relation to the axillary artery, but it is important to remember that the medial, lateral, and posterior cords bear that strict relation to the artery only for the short distance in which the artery is covered by pectoralis minor. Radial nerve is the major outflow of the posterior cord after the origination of the thoracodorsal and axillary nerves. The surgeon should appreciate that the point of origin of the axillary nerve is approximately at the level of the coracoid process. This bony protuberance is easily palpable and is the site of the lateral attachment of pectoralis minor.

It is useful to review some points of detail relating to branches of this complex in the axilla because these are of both clinical and surgical importance. Although the nerves to latissimus dorsi and the lower subscapular nerve are classically described as being branches of the posterior cord, we have found considerable variation in this arrangement, and it is not unusual to find the nerve to latissimus dorsi being a proximal branch of the axillary nerve and occasionally even of the radial nerve. Because the groups of fascicles are discrete within the main nerve before branching, it is possible to split both the nerve to latissimus dorsi and the axillary nerve away from the posterior cord for a matter of several centimeters.[12] This may be a useful maneuver before any nerve resection is contemplated. It may be important to stimulate all elements discussed to be certain that the surgeon knows which nerve is supplying what muscle before any decisions are made with regard to operative resection. Close to the radial nerve's origin from posterior cord, a variable number of triceps branches leave its dorsal aspect to run obliquely and to supply one or more of the three heads of the triceps muscle (Figure 7–1). At operation, the surgeon must remember to guard these triceps branches while dissecting through dense

scar and attempting to delineate the main radial nerve. Important branches to triceps which have arisen either more proximally or at that level of dissection may be encased within the scar tissue which is being removed from the radial nerve in the distal axilla.

The radial nerve can be approached from ei-

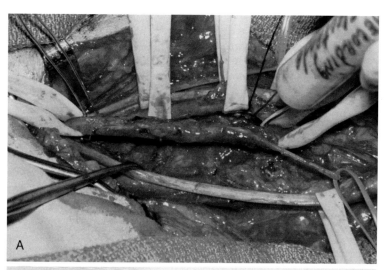

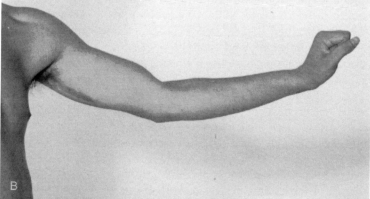

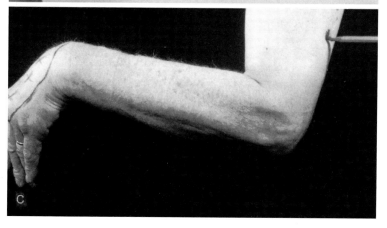

**Figure 7 – 1.** *(A)* Contusion and stretch injury caused by a gunshot wound affecting the posterior cord to radial segment. The initial triceps branch is encircled by a Vasoloop, and the more medial axillary nerve is encircled by two Penrose drains. Proximal ulnar nerve is retracted by a vein retractor inferiorly and a Penrose drain distally. Stimulation and recording over posterior cord to radial segment gave a nerve action potential at 5 months despite complete radial loss, so only a neurolysis was done. *(B)* Recovery of wrist extension after several years was substantial. *(C)* Terramycin injection injury to radial nerve at the midhumeral level. Injury spared triceps, but resulted in loss of brachioradialis, supination, and wrist and finger extension. Sensory loss on dorsum of hand is indicated. Lesion required resection and repair. *C,* from Kline D, Hudson A: Acute injuries of peripheral nerves. *In* Youmans J, Ed: Neurological Surgery, 3rd Ed. Philadelphia, W.B. Saunders Co, 1990.

ther the medial or lateral aspect of the axillary or brachial artery during the axillary dissection. Usually, there is very little difficulty in defining the radial nerve from the medial side of the artery in the inferior axilla, and dissection through the fat behind the artery rapidly reveals the characteristic tapelike nerve that is one of the largest branches of the plexus. On the other hand, if the surgeon's focus of attention is toward the axillary nerve and its relation to the radial nerve, the lateral side of the artery at the level of the coracoid process must be exposed. This is most easily accomplished by freeing up the axillary artery and displacing it and its accompanying veins medially. The vessels are tethered by the circumflex humeral vessels, which run to the level of the quadrangular space. Between the quadrangular space and the level of the coracoid process, the axillary nerve is defined behind the artery, and concomitantly, the origin of the radial nerve is noted and dissected out. At this level, the nerve itself is found just medial to the profundus branch of the axillary artery.[51] If there is a great deal of scarring superficial to subscapularis, it is usually easiest to define the radial nerve in the inferior axilla and to dissect upward, taking the precautions already described.

The circumflex humeral vessels may become crucial anastomotic branches if there has been a concomitant vascular injury. The surgeon should operate with extreme gentleness if previous vein grafts have been inserted after an axillary artery injury, and the operator must appreciate that the damaged vessels may be densely adherent to the posteriorly placed radial nerve. The profunda brachial artery, a branch of the axillary artery, accompanies the radial nerve as it leaves the axilla.

The shining, silver surface of the latissimus dorsi tendon is a welcome landmark for the surgeon as it defines the lower border of the posterior axilla. Sliding a finger upward and over teres major identifies the quadrangular space and, downward, the triangular space. In the normal situation, the dissection of the radial nerve at the lower axilla is extremely easy, but direct injury or severe scarring may require that the surgeon identify these basic anatomic landmarks before any detailed dissection of the nerve is undertaken.

In most patients, the ulnar nerve is of a smaller caliber and rounder configuration than the radial nerve. The medial cutaneous nerve of the forearm is considerably smaller than the ulnar nerve, to which it may be closely related. The ulnar nerve is initially a nerve of the flexor compartment of the arm, and it remains a close associate of the artery, whereas the radial nerve deviates progressively farther posteriorly as the artery travels distally. The motor branch of the radial nerve to the medial head of triceps may lie close to the ulnar nerve. With a little experience, the surgeon can distinguish these nerves from the much larger radial nerve, but the uninitiated may identify nerves incorrectly during dissection medially and posteriorly to the distal axillary artery through dense scar tissue. If the operator remembers that the radial nerve is destined for the extensor compartment of the arm and, in the process, enters the medial aspect to the spiral groove, he or she will be able to focus on the target by palpating the humerus and axillary and brachial arteries and demonstrating the shining surface of latissimus dorsi and the long head of triceps. It is not an easy procedure to identify the nerve deep to the fascia and posterior to the palpable brachial artery and then to trace the nerve lying on the long head of the triceps to the proximal end of the spiral groove. Once again, the individual nerve branches to triceps must be respected so that they are not injured in the process of defining the radial nerve.

## Radial Nerve in the Arm

One of the factors that may cause confusion in appreciation of the anatomy of the radial nerve in the arm relates to the peculiar nomenclature applied to the triceps muscle. Viewed from behind, the lateral head of triceps is appropriately named, and its humeral attachment is to the lateral border of the spiral groove. The head medial to the lateral head is, unfortunately, called the long head. The so-called medial head is more deeply placed but appropriately borders the medial lip of the spiral groove. The radial nerve winds around from the medial to the lateral side of the arm directly applied to the humerus and then pierces the lateral inter-muscular septum, at which point it is both rela-tively fixed and exposed. In the groove, the nerve is covered by the lateral head of triceps, and, at this point, the nerve is reduced to the least number of fascicles in its entire course (usually 4 or 5 in number). In the spiral groove, further muscular branches are given off to the medial and lateral heads of the triceps. Triceps palsy is not a feature of the usual Saturday night palsy that is caused by compression of the nerve in the spiral groove, suggesting that the more proximally placed motor branches to triceps are more important than those branches in the spiral groove.

Nerve supply to anconeus is given off in the groove. This small muscle is of little importance during the clinical examination, but an elec-trode can be placed within its substance to check for early denervation. In the presence of radial nerve palsy, denervation of anconeus signals that the injury to the radial nerve is proximal to the outflow of this branch.

The radial nerve is identified in the distal lat-eral arm by separating brachialis from brachio-radialis. The nerve lies at the bottom of this trough of muscle. The radial nerve gives a branch to the brachioradialis 2 or 3 cm proximal to the elbow and 7 or 8 cm distal to the humeral groove. Brachialis is one of the few muscles of the body that receive a twin nerve supply (mus-culocutaneous and radial), but patients suffer-ing from radial nerve injuries very seldom ex-hibit brachialis weakness. Conversely, patients suffering from musculocutaneous injuries very seldom exhibit any significant flexion power based on radial nerve supply to brachialis. These unimportant branches to brachialis arise from the medial aspect of the radial nerve. An anatomic feature of considerable clinical signifi-cance relates to the point of branching of the motor supply to brachioradialis and extensor carpi radialis longus (ECRL). Both of these mus-cles are usually supplied by the main radial nerve in the distal arm proximal to the elbow, often by several branches issuing from the lat-eral side of the main nerve. Thus, close to the elbow joint, radial branches supply a portion of brachioradialis and brachialis, sometimes ECRL, and also the radiohumeral joint and an-nular ligament of the joint.

## The Radial Nerve at the Elbow and in the Proximal Forearm

Having gained the flexor compartment of the arm by spiraling around the humerus and piercing the lateral intermuscular septum, the radial nerve enters the antecubital fossa under cover of brachioradialis and ECRL. If brachio-radialis is gently retracted laterally and the radial nerve tented up on a sling, the major divi-sion of the nerve into its direct forearm continu-ation, the superficial sensory radial (SSR) nerve, and the posteriorly inclined motor or posterior interosseous nerve (PIN) become readily appar-ent.

### Superficial Radial Nerve

This nerve is easily demonstrated in the ante-cubital fossa and equally easily identified as it courses distally in the forearm under cover of the edge of brachioradialis and lateral to the ra-dial artery. In this superficial position, it is read-ily available as a nerve graft. The fascicles des-tined for the SSR can be split off the anterior part of the distal radial nerve by dissecting from below upward under the operating microscope or loupes for approximately 4 cm proximal to the lateral epicondyle. The fascicles destined for the PIN are placed more posteriorly at this level. At the junction of the middle and distal third of the forearm, the sensory nerve once again seeks the extensor aspect of the limb and winds around the radius deep to the tendon of bra-chioradialis. The nerve pierces the deep fascia and breaks into four or five branches at this point. These branches run across the anatomic snuffbox superficial to the thumb extensor ten-dons and are thus posterior to the wrist joint and the scaphoid bone. These terminal digital branches are well described in anatomic texts, but from a functional point of view, they supply an extremely variable area of skin on the dor-sum of the hand.

### Posterior Interosseous Nerve

The remaining motor fibers of the radial nerve in the distal arm are diverted into the PIN at the level of the forearm. This nerve supplies all the extensor muscles of the back of the forearm with the exception of ECRL. Although some texts state that the point of divergence of the main sensory and main motor continuations of the nerve is at the level of the epicondyle, our operative experience is in keeping with the data reported by Sunderland. In 14 of 20 specimens, the point of divergence was between 1 and 2 cm distal to the epicondyle[58] (Figure 7–2). Having left the main radial nerve, the PIN is destined to leave the flexor compartment of the forearm and gain the extensor compartment. It achieves this by spiraling around the radius between the two heads of the supinator muscle. The surgeon must appreciate that the nerve, inclining backward and downward in its course between the radius and supinator, is surrounded by small arteries and veins. These vessels are easily seen with the naked eye, and their anatomic relation to the nerve is more exactly defined with the aid of operating loupes. An arcade of small arteries and veins usually crosses the nerve transversely and must be coagulated and sectioned to fully expose the PIN. The supinator and the important extensor carpi ulnaris are supplied by the PIN before that nerve is lost from view between the two heads of the supinator. The branches to ECRL and extensor carpi radialis brevis (ECRB) may be partially hidden by the small vessels in this area. ECRL branches may arise from proximal superficial sensory radial, distal whole radial, or, less frequently, proximal PIN. These variations are not unlike those noted at the point of origin of the radial and axillary nerves. The surgeon should define the specific anatomy with care because some of the motor branches here are of small caliber.

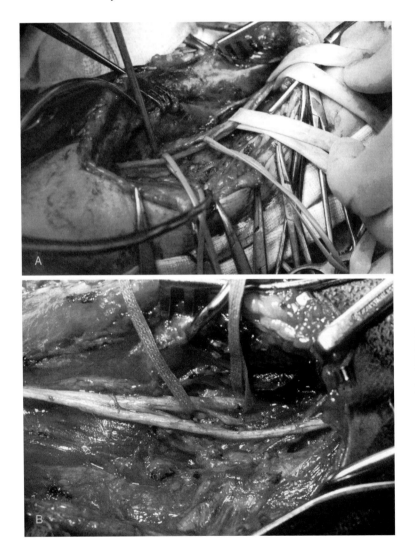

**Figure 7–2.** (A) Exposure of left superficial sensory radial nerve (SSR), encircled by two Vasoloops, and more medial posterior interosseus nerve (PIN). The instrument points to the course of the PIN beneath the volar supinator. (B) Exposure of the right PIN (encircled by tapes) and the SSR branch of radial nerve. The extensor carpi ulnaris branch can be seen arising from the proximal PIN. A portion of the volar supinator has been opened to provide this exposure.

Key to understanding the remaining course of the PIN is a clear comprehension of the anatomy of the heads of the supinator muscle. This muscle has origins from both the ulna and humeral bones. The nerve runs between the superficial and deep heads, both of which insert into the radius. The upper border of the superficial head of supinator runs at almost right angles to the course of the PIN, a feature that is quite apparent either in the anatomy dissection room or on the operating table. The PIN runs beneath the proximal edge of the volar supinator, which is sometimes fibrous and sometimes muscular. In either case, the volar supinator forms an arch or arcade around the PIN, and this is known as the arcade of Frohse. The PIN is, therefore, almost as closely related to bone as the radial nerve is to the humerus, and may be directly opposed to the radius in some cases.

## Midforearm Level

After traveling under the distal border of the supinator muscle and deep to the superficial layer of extensor muscles, the PIN immediately breaks up into short branches, which supply the extensor musculature, and two long branches, which supply extensor pollicis longus and brevis, abductor pollicis longus, and extensor indicis. Each of the three bones of the thumb receives one or more tendons on its dorsal surface: extensor pollicis longus to distal phalanx, extensor pollicis brevis and median-innervated abductor pollicis brevis to the proximal phalanx, and abductor pollicis longus to the metacarpal bone. Three of these muscles are supplied by the PIN branches and are, therefore, affected in both radial and PIN lesions. Of lesser importance is the fact that abductor pollicis longus may act as a weak wrist flexor and abductor pollicis brevis may weakly extend the distal interphalangeal joint of the thumb in the absence of function of extensor pollicis longus.

## RADIAL NERVE: CLINICAL PRESENTATIONS AND EXAMINATION

The radial nerve is the nerve of the extensor compartments of the arm and forearm. It is a mixed motor and sensory nerve, but from the clinician's viewpoint, its prime function is that of motor control. The muscles supplied are as follows: triceps, anconeus, brachioradialis, ECRL, ECRB, extensor carpi ulnaris, supinator, extensor digitorum communis, extensor digiti quinti minimi, abductor pollicis longus, extensor pollicis longus, extensor pollicis brevis, and extensor indicis. The clinical features of this major upper limb nerve are conveniently considered at axillary, arm, forearm, and hand levels.

## Upper Arm

In assessing the level of nerve injury in a patient with suspected radial nerve pathology, a key clinical point is whether that patient's latissimus dorsi and deltoid are functioning. If both of these muscles are clinically active, then the lesion is usually in the radial nerve itself and not in the posterior cord. Most surgeons are surprised to find how proximal the point is at which the medial and long heads of triceps are supplied. If a patient presents with an isolated deltoid and triceps palsy in the presence of normal wrist extension, there is only one anatomic site where the injury could have occurred, and that is in the axilla at a point where the axillary nerve and the main nerve supply to triceps are closely related to one another.

The triceps is the major extensor muscle affecting the elbow and, as such, its function is usually aided by gravity. It serves as the main antagonist of the elbow flexors, which are situated in front of the humerus. It can be readily observed and palpated as the individual attempts to extend the elbow. The triceps is best tested with the shoulder partially abducted and the elbow partially flexed to avoid the effects of gravity. If the patient is seated, ask him or her to extend the forearm parallel to the floor. If there is a question of triceps function, gravity can also be eliminated by placing the patient in a supine position and asking him or her to push up with the forearm. Outflow to triceps from the posterior cord originates primarily from the C7 root through the middle trunk and its posterior division, but also from C6 and sometimes even the C8 root. Nonetheless, its reflex is predominately a C7 one. Because the origin of the triceps branches is very proximal, few radial nerve injuries involve triceps loss (Figure 7–3). The exception is provided by distal cord-to-nerve level stretch injuries and some gunshot wounds where the cord-to-nerve level is involved. One form of Saturday night palsy of the radial nerve is caused by prolonged compression at the axillary level as a result of draping the arm over a chair back and may in some cases result in a high enough radial palsy to include triceps loss.

Occasionally, humeral fractures or operative manipulation for repair of such fractures may result in isolated injury to the triceps branches. Secondary repair of this complication is difficult owing to the branches' being torn out of muscle or injured over their entire length. Other than an occasional and unusual penetrating injury, the setting for an isolated triceps loss from nerve injury is usually a stretch injury causing combined deltoid and triceps palsies. The mechanism for such an injury is a stretch and sometimes actual avulsion, not only of the axillary nerve as it runs into the quadrilateral space, but of triceps branches, which are pulled away from the muscle itself. Effective repair of this extensive injury is difficult in our experience.

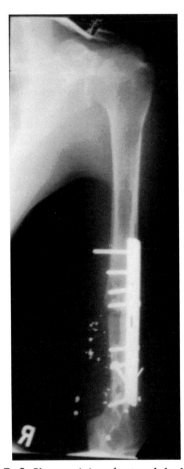

**Figure 7–3.** Shotgun injury fractured the humerus and gave a complete radial palsy. Triceps function was spared in this case. A radial lesion in continuity was resected at 4 months after injury, since there was no NAP recorded across the injury. Graft repair gave grade 3 to 4 recovery when the patient was last evaluated at 3 years postoperatively. Exploration of such a nerve injury at the time of acute fracture fixation usually shows a swollen, angry-appearing nerve. There is no way to assess the potential for recovery in such a lesion at that time.

## Midhumeral Level

Injury to the nerve at midarm level owing to humeral fracture is the most common mechanism for radial injury[21,24] (Figures 7–4 and 7–5). Approximately 20% of such fractures have associated radial palsy.[3,41] Incidence increases with oblique fractures, compound or complex fractures, and those requiring open surgical manipulation for reduction.[1,14] The nerve may be injured during subsequent removal of hardware.[18] Other mechanisms for injury at this level include gunshot wounds, contusion, simple compression or stretch without fracture, injection injury, tumor, and, on rare occasions, entrapment. The hallmarks of injury at this level are the sparing of triceps function with loss of brachioradialis and more distal radial-innervated functions.[42,47]

The patient with radial nerve injury at the midarm level retains significant triceps function because of the high origin of triceps motor branches. The brachioradialis is the first target muscle downstream, and it is this muscle that is tested on repeated clinical examination as the clinician attempts to document presence or absence of regeneration. Patients with complete radial nerve palsies at the mid-upper arm level exhibit the characteristic wrist and finger drop resulting from lack of function of all the muscles on the extensor aspect of the forearm. This includes muscles supplied by the PIN as well as a paralysis of the ECRL, which receives a branch either directly from the radial nerve or from SSR.

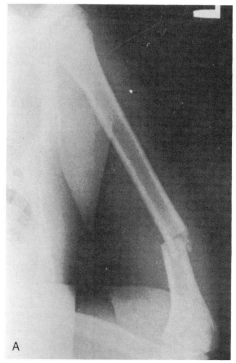

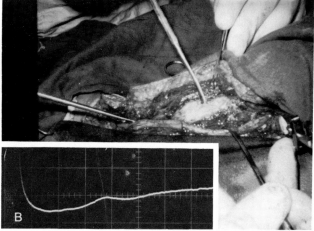

**Figure 7 – 4.** *(A)* Radiograph of a distal humeral fracture associated with radial palsy. The latter did not improve over a 4-month period, so exploration and nerve action potential (NAP) recordings were done. *(B)* The nerve was adherent to callus at the distal lateral arm level. It transmitted a small but definite NAP, so only a neurolysis was done. Subsequent recovery was excellent.

## Distal Arm

Although relatively protected because it lies somewhat beneath and between brachialis and triceps in the lower third of the arm, the radial nerve can be injured at this level by accidental drug injection, distal humeral fracture, direct contusion, or gunshot wound.[24,28] Again, the brachioradialis is the key proximal muscle involved. This muscle is best tested by asking the patient to flex the forearm with the latter placed halfway between pronation and supination. The resultant bulge of the muscle belly is felt on the radial side of the proximal and volar forearm. Biceps also contracts under these circumstances, but so does brachioradialis; inspection and palpation can separate their effects in gaining flexion of the forearm. Brachioradialis flexes the elbow joint, supplementing biceps and brachialis function, and this can be a very important substitute in a patient suffering from musculocutaneous nerve injury.

## Elbow Level

The next muscles downstream supplied by the radial nerve are the ECRL and the ECRB. Branches originate either from the whole radial nerve before it divides into PIN and SSR or from the latter itself. These muscles extend the wrist in a radial direction and are important for certain functions such as the use of a hammer. Their function is usually spared with PIN injury or entrapment but lost with elbow-level radial injury. Extension in an ulnar direction (extensor carpi ulnaris) is absent or weak with a PIN lesion. As a result, the hand deviates in a radial direction on attempted dorsiflexion of the wrist.

Elbow-level lesions to the whole radial nerve are caused by penetrating wounds in this area and, less frequently, by fracture or dislocation of the elbow, by cysts or tumors in this region, or, occasionally, by Volkmann ischemic contracture.[43] The latter is usually caused by supracondylar humeral fracture and dislocation of

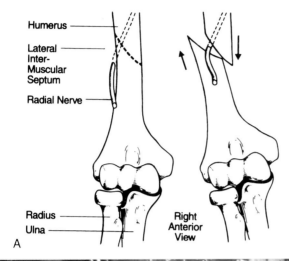

Humerus

Lateral
Inter-
Muscular
Septum

Radial Nerve

Radius
Ulna

A

Right
Anterior
View

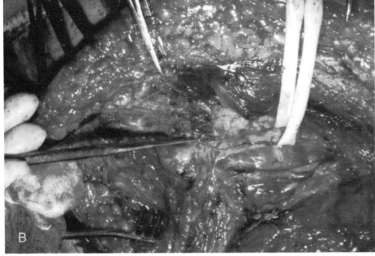

B

**Figure 7–5.** (A) Usual level and fracture mechanism for injury of the radial nerve. (B) Scar and callus involving radial nerve at the midhumeral level. Resection and repair of this lesion was necessary.

*Illustration continued on opposite page*

the elbow.[32] Brachial arterial contusion or stretch results in ischemia of forearm musculature and even of the forearm nerves themselves. Functional loss with elbow-level lesions of the radial nerve includes all muscles innervated by the radial nerve except triceps, brachioradialis, and, sometimes, extensor carpi radialis.

## Posterior Interosseous Nerve

Involvement of the PIN spares proximal muscles as well as some supination but seriously affects function of more distal muscles. PIN can be damaged or compressed by penetrating or contusive soft tissue wounds, fracture of radius or ulna, tumors originating from bone or soft tissue, or operations to repair fracture in this area.[5,9,55,57] The most common involvement of PIN is, however, by spontaneous entrapment.[23,27,33,52] The patient may present with dysfunction of all muscles innervated by PIN or, initially, with only paralysis of extension of one or more fingers at the metacarpophalangeal joints (Figure 7–6). Subsequent paralysis of other PIN-innervated muscles usually occurs. Extension of the wrist is weak, especially in an ulnar direction, and the patient cannot extend fingers or thumb at the metacarpophalangeal joints. Entrapment may be caused by a fibrous edge of the proximal portion of the superficial head of the supinator or by a scarred vascular complex or connective tissue band just before the entry of the PIN between the two heads of the supinator.[45,53] This region is complex anatomically and is known as the arcade of Frohse.

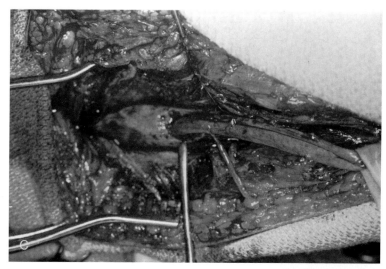

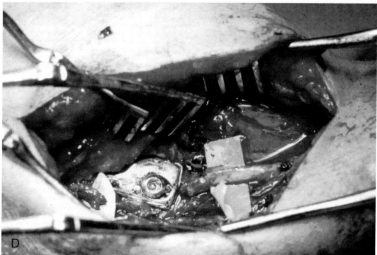

**Figure 7-5.** *Continued (C)* Radial nerve caught in the middle of a healed fracture. *(D)* Radial nerve entrapped by plate and screws used to secure a humeral fracture. See also color figure.

Spinner has described entrapment of the PIN by the edge of ECRB with pronation.[52] Chronic irritation can lead to an entrapment-like syndrome perhaps related to stressful supination and pronation; a small number of isolated cases have been reported in swimmers, frisbee and tennis players, violinists, and music conductors. These disorders should not be confused with "tennis elbow," which is related to lateral elbow pain with repetitive pronation/supination. Impingement on the PIN is not part of that problem, which instead is usually caused by epicondylitis.[13]

Some authors have characterized pain and tenderness in the region of the forearm brachioradialis, especially on deep palpation with wrist flexion or dorsiflexion, or on pronation or supination against pressure, as a "radial tunnel syndrome."[29,35] Implied is irritation of the PIN, but without any measurable clinical or electromyographic loss of function in that nerve's distribution. The exact nature of this disorder, however, remains unclear.

Branches of the supinator muscle from the PIN usually leave the nerve proximal to its entry between the two muscles' heads.[54] Supination should be tested with elbow extended to reduce the substitutive effect of biceps, which is an effective supinator if the elbow is flexed. The patient is asked to turn the hand palm up from a pronated or palm down position. The supinator muscle is a supplement to the powerful biceps

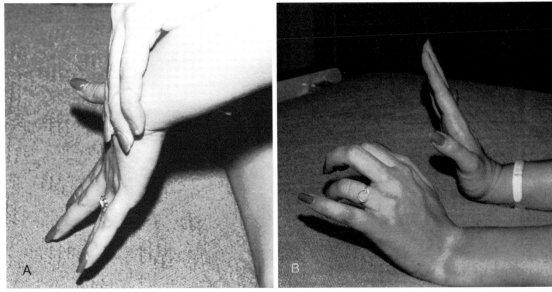

**Figure 7–6.** (A) In posterior interosseus nerve (PIN) palsy, wrist extension is poor because of weakness of the extensor carpi ulnaris, and finger and thumb extension is poor or absent altogether because of extensor communis and extensor pollicis longus weakness. (B) In early and less severe entrapment of PIN, the degree of finger extension weakness varies from digit to digit. In this case, finger extension was absent for the ring finger and the forefinger and thumb, and quite weak for the little and long fingers.

in the action of supination. The extensor carpi ulnaris branch has a variable origin but usually arises from the PIN in the region of the arcade of Frohse.[52] This muscle extends the wrist in an ulnar direction, as opposed to the extensor carpi radialis, which extends it in a radial direction and has a more proximal origin from either the SSR or whole radial nerve before it divides into PIN and SSR.

Wrist dorsiflexion can sometimes be stimulated by flexing fingers to make a fist despite the absence of extensor carpi ulnaris and extensor carpi radialis, especially if extensor communis is somewhat fibrotic and shortened because of either direct injury or chronic paralysis. Wrist extension is accomplished by the action of numerous tendons, of which ECRB is the most powerful. This movement brings the hand into the "position of function" and takes up the slack of the long flexors to the digits so that a powerful grip can be sustained by those tendons. ECRL and ECRB, however, can extend the wrist with moderate power, albeit with clear radial drift. Thus, a radial nerve palsy presents with a total wrist drop, but a patient suffering from PIN palsy exhibits wrist extension, albeit weakly and asymmetrically (Figure 7–7). After

leaving the cover of the volar supinator, the PIN reaches the dorsal expansion of the forearm and branches "pes-like" to supply the extensor communis of the forefinger, long, ring, and little fingers.

Extension of the fingers at the metacarpal phalangeal joints is by way of the long extensors of the forearm. Both radial- and PIN-palsied patients exhibit finger drop at the knuckle joint.[15] In a hand without paralysis, interphalangeal joints are extended by the function of the intrinsic musculature of the hand supplemented by long extensor tendon activity. This may give rise to some confusion in the clinician's mind, because a patient with a wrist drop may yet be able to extend the fingers. This confusion is easily removed by passively extending the patient's wrist and then asking the patient to straighten his or her fingers at the metacarpophalangeal joints. A patient with paralyzed long extensors is unable to extend the metacarpophalangeal joints, even though he or she can extend the digits reasonably well with the metacarpophalangeal joints flexed by using lumbricals. Another method for testing extensor communis and pollicis longus is to place the patient's hand palm down on a flat surface and then asking the

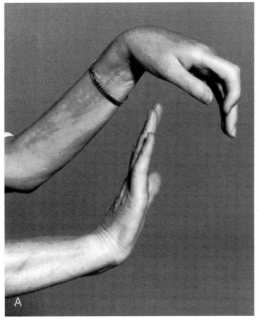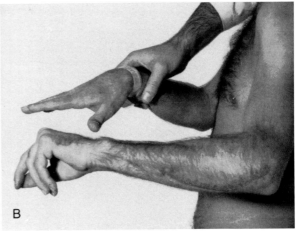

**Figure 7–7.** These figures compare the clinical presentation of a radial and a posterior interosseus nerve (PIN) palsy. *(A)* A complete radial palsy involves the patient's left arm compared with the normal function of the right arm. *(B)* A PIN palsy involves this patient's left arm. The patient can only partially extend the wrist, and finger and thumb extension is poor.

patient to lift each finger and thumb individually against resistance applied by the examiner.[17] In this fashion, the examiner can also test the extensor indicis proprius (forefinger) and the extensor digiti quinti proprius (little finger). Another test of finger extension is to have the patient make a fist and then ask him or her to extend each finger individually without holding the other fingers back with the thumb.

Most important is the method of testing extensor pollicis longus function, because abductor pollicis longus and brevis can simulate this function well. The examiner places the patient's forearm in a position halfway between pronation and the ulnar side of the hand on a flat surface.[62] The patient is then instructed to pull the thumb away from the forefinger in a parallel direction against resistance.

## Mid-Dorsal Forearm

At the level of the dorsum or extensor surface of the forearm, laceration and, less frequently, gunshot wound, fracture, and tumor provide mechanisms of injury.[2,6] Pattern of

loss in extension of fingers and thumb is quite variable according to which branches are disrupted or contused.[52] Injuries are often associated with some degree of direct muscle damage, and this makes successful repair especially difficult.

## Superficial Sensory Radial Nerve

Between elbow and wrist, the SSR may be readily injured, but with penetrating injury at the upper forearm level, the SSR is often spared, although the PIN is much more vulnerable. The sensory sphere of the radial nerve encompasses the dorsum of the hand and some of the wrist. Because of overlap from median and ulnar nerves, antebrachial cutaneous, or forearm branch of musculocutaneous nerves, the area of loss on the dorsum of the hand may be small even with complete radial nerve injury[46] (Figure 7–8). The closest the radial nerve has to an autonomous zone for sensation is the anatomic snuffbox region, which is located between the

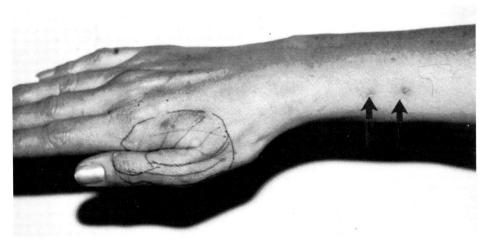

**Figure 7 – 8.** Usual sensory loss over the dorsum of the thumb and adductor space. Superficial sensory radial nerve injury was caused by the placement of transfixation pins to stabilize the forearm *(arrows)*.

abductor pollicis and extensor pollicis longus muscles.

Superficial sensory nerve damage is often associated with painful paresthesia, which may have a burning nature, making contact with the dorsum of the hand especially disagreeable. Sensory loss in the radial distribution unassociated with pain or paresthesias does not interfere with hand function.

## Substitute or Trick Movements

In testing for radial palsy, the examiner must be aware of a number of possible trick or substitute movements that can mimic radial-innervated function. Interossei can appear to extend the fingers as they are abducted, even though extensor communis is paralyzed. True extensor function can be tested by placing the hand on a flat surface and asking the patient to extend the fingers above the surface one by one. With extensor communis paralysis, the examiner may be fooled into thinking the ulnar-innervated interossei are also weak, because with finger drop or fingers in a downward flexed position at the metacarpophalangeal joints, interossei, which abduct and adduct fingers, do not perform well. This can be minimized by testing for abduction and adduction with the fingers on a flat surface such as a table or forcing the fingers into a hyperextended position, thus substituting for extensor communis function, and having the pa-

tient abduct and adduct his fingers against those of the examiner. It cannot be emphasized enough that wrist extension by radial-innervated muscles can also be mimicked by a movement in which the fingers are flexed and the wrist is forced into some degree of extension. This occurs when extensor tendons have been shortened as a result of paralysis or direct injury to muscle or tendons.

Supinator muscle function can also be mimicked by biceps/brachialis contraction, particularly if the elbow is flexed or at least not fully extended, because the partial insertion of biceps into proximal ulna tends to pull the forearm, and thus the hand, into a palm-up position. Biceps/brachialis function can be mistaken for brachioradialis function and vice-versa, particularly if the forearm is not partially pronated when brachioradialis function is tested. Gravity alone can substitute for triceps function, but palpation of triceps during extension of the forearm should confirm triceps participation.

## Electrodiagnosis of Radial Injuries

Radial nerve differs from median and ulnar nerves in that there are no radial-innervated hand intrinsic muscles, even though radial nerve function is important for a useful hand. Electrical studies therefore concentrate on the one arm muscle innervated by the nerve, the triceps, and the only forearm muscle with origin in upper arm, the brachioradialis. In addition, the proximal and midforearm muscles, the extensor carpi radialis, extensor carpi ulnaris, supinator, extensor communis, and extensor pollicis longus are evaluated. Proximal injury to upper arm is detected by denervational changes in triceps and in the more distal muscles. If posterior cord involvement has resulted in radial distribution loss, then, in addition to triceps changes, there are denervational changes in deltoid, latissimus dorsi, and, sometimes, the subscapularis muscle. Not all of triceps may show such changes, because this muscle has three parts and a number of triceps branches leave the posterior cord close to the origination of the radial nerve.[48]

Midhumeral-level injury is documented by electrical change in brachioradialis and more distally innervated muscles, but absence of the same in triceps. Of importance is the time required for reversal of denervational changes in the brachioradialis.[41] Brachioradialis receives proximal input in the distal third of the arm and other input from branches at the level of elbow and even somewhat more distally. The common axonotmetic injury associated with mid-humeral-level damage secondary to fracture may require 3 to 4 months for enough axons of sufficient caliber and myelination to reach brachioradialis and enough motor end plate reconstruction to occur so that the number of fibrillations and denervational potentials decrease in brachioradialis. Other signs of reinnervation include nascent potentials and return of evoked muscle action potentials on stimulation of more proximal radial nerve. Somewhat antedating this reversal in electromyographic denervational changes is contraction of brachioradialis in response to stimulation of the radial nerve in the lower lateral arm.[37] A stimulus site is usually found several inches above the elbow, where nerve is located usually between, although somewhat deep to, biceps/brachialis and triceps. An attempt can also be made to stimulate the radial nerve in the humeral groove as it winds around the humerus to travel from a medial to a lateral position in the mid-upper arm (Figure 7–9). After brachioradialis begins to recover, extensor carpi radialis usually shows electrical signs of recovery a few months later.[60] This recovery is then followed by recovery in

extensor carpi ulnaris. Unfortunately, electrical and clinical recovery in extensors communis, pollicis longus, indicis proprius, and digiti quinti is less certain, and if recovery does occur, it is delayed for another 6 to 9 months.[4] This is so even though more proximal muscles have recovered good function.

An interesting observation can sometimes be made by needling the anconeus, an almost vestigial muscle overlying the lateral olecranon of the ulna. Reversal of denervational changes in that muscle may antedate similar changes in extensor carpi radialis and ulnaris and, occasionally, in brachioradialis by some weeks.

With elbow-level lesions, extensor carpi radialis and ulnaris may recover electrical loss quickly. Unfortunately, with some penetrating injuries, these muscles may have sustained severe enough branch injury so that they do not recover. Return of wrist extension may under these circumstances be dependent on recovery of more distal extensor communis and pollicis longus. Electrical assessment for recovery should include these muscles, because extensor carpi radialis and especially extensor carpi ulnaris may remain deinnervated under some circumstances.

The supinator is a difficult muscle to evaluate, but fortunately the electrodiagnostic concomitants of a volar forearm PIN palsy are as striking as its clinical counterparts. Sensory conduction from superficial radial is spared or, at worst, mildly reduced in velocity. If needled by the exceptional electrodiagnostician, the supinator muscle shows only partial denervational changes, extensor carpi radialis is spared, and extensor carpi ulnaris, extensor communis, and extensor pollicis longus have changes. With supinator-level entrapment, onset of denervational changes in these muscles may be delayed beyond the usual 3 weeks, but motor conduction velocities to the same muscles are prolonged early in the course of the entrapment.[11] To stimulate PIN without surgical exposure, needle electrodes are usually necessary. Whole radial nerve can be stimulated at elbow or above with recordings from extensor indicis proprius, extensor pollicis longus, or extensor communis. Recovery of more normal conduction velocities may take many months to occur, even after a technically successful decompression of PIN.

With dorsal forearm injury to the branches of

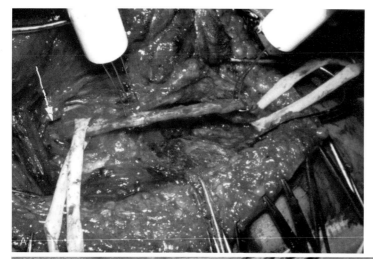

**Figure 7–9.** *(A)* Recording from the lateral arm level of radial nerve injured in association with a midhumeral-level injury. *(B)* Because no nerve action potential (NAP) was recorded, proximal radial nerve (encircled by upper Penrose drain) was exposed on the medial side of the arm and traced to the area of the humeral groove *(arrow* in *A).*

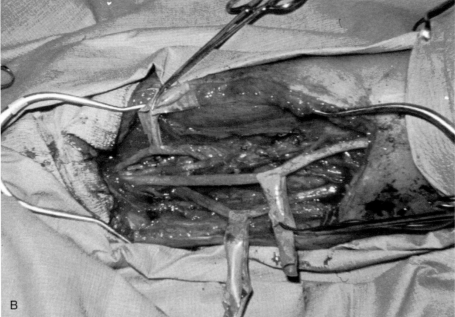

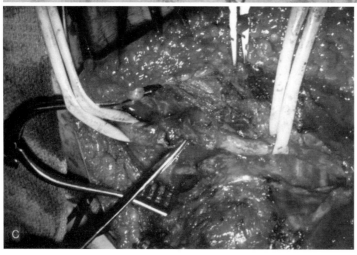

*(C)* A severe lesion in continuity was encountered. It did not transmit an NAP; therefore the lesion was resected. Nerve was repaired by transposing the distal radial stump beneath the biceps/brachialis and repairing the nerve along the medial surface of the arm.

radial nerve, the results of electrodiagnosis are variable in the sense that the distribution of loss may not be uniform: some portions of extensor pollicis longus and especially extensor communis have loss, and other portions do not. Such findings highlight the difficulties of surgical repair at this level.

## SURGICAL EXPOSURE OF THE RADIAL NERVE

### Medial Arm

Exposure of the radial nerve between its origin from the posterior cord to the medial border of the spiral groove is a straightforward matter, but the surgeon must pay particular attention to certain points of detail if injury to other peripheral nerves is to be avoided.

In the usual case, the thoracodorsal nerve is a branch of the posterior cord, and occasionally it may be a branch of the axillary nerve, but rarely is it a branch of the radial nerve. In any case, thoracodorsal fascicles are discrete, so they may be split back to the level of the posterior cord and appropriately excluded from repair. The operator must be particularly careful not to damage branches to triceps. This accident is less likely to occur if the surgical dissection proceeds in a proximal to distal direction.[22] Like the thoracodorsal nerve, the triceps branches can usually be split back and away from posterior cord and proximal radial nerve. The shining tendon and fascia of the latissimus dorsi muscle is a familiar landmark on the posterior wall of the axilla. The axillary nerve leaves the axilla by running through the quadrangular space whose lower border is the tendon of the latissimus dorsi. The axillary nerve can also be split away from posterior cord over quite a distance, but it is difficult to follow proximally through divisional and trunk levels, although the posterior division of the upper trunk is its usual origin. Although the median and ulnar nerves are nerves of the flexor compartment of the arm and the radial nerve is in the extensor compartment, these nerves are closely related through their proximal course, and prolonged retraction of median and ulnar nerve should be avoided during dissection of the radial nerve itself. The radial nerve runs across the latissimus dorsi and takes an oblique course toward the medial aspect of the arm, where it lies on the volar surface of triceps and behind the medial intramuscular septum.

As dissection nears the elbow, a number of vessels, including the radial collateral, may be encountered. The radial collateral artery may be an important component of the vascular anastomosis around the elbow joint, particularly if prior injury has resulted in occlusion of the brachial artery.[25] In this circumstance, the artery should be carefully guarded during dissection of the radial nerve.

The proximal radial nerve can also be approached from behind or posteriorly (Figure 7–10). This alternate approach to expose proximal radial nerve is the posterior approach well described by Henry.[20] The patient is positioned prone with the operative arm at the side. An incision is made curving medially beneath the lower border of the deltoid and then extended inferiorly between the long and lateral heads of the triceps. The latter are palpable because there is a slight depression between them. Fascia is then split, taking care to stay in the midline. Radial nerve, including triceps branches, is exposed and can be traced through the spiral groove to the junction of the middle and lower thirds of the forearm. This approach is excellent as long as more distal nerve does not need to be exposed to gain length or to harvest forearm-level SSR for use as a graft.

### In the Spiral Groove

The radial nerve can be exposed on both the medial and lateral aspects of the arm. By operating alternatively from lateral and medial aspects of the arm, the segment of the nerve immediately behind the humerus can be exposed without injuring triceps musculature.[25] If irreparable injury to the radial nerve immediately behind the humerus is evident grossly or by intraoperative evoked nerve action potential (NAP) studies, the radial nerve is sectioned through to areas of normal fascicular pattern both proximal and distal to the injury. As with other nerve lesions requiring resection, it is very important to section back to healthy non-neuromatous tissue before attempting repair.[31] The operator then has a proximal stump on the me-

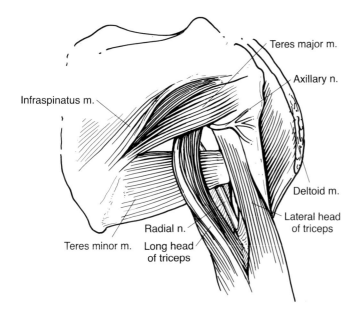

**Figure 7–10.** Anatomy concerned with a posterior approach to radial nerve at the arm level. Intermuscular septum has been sectioned, and lateral and long heads are retracted. Nerve can be seen winding around the posterior aspect of the humerus to reach the humeral groove. Superiorly, the deltoid has been sectioned and turned laterally to show the axillary nerve and its relationship to teres major and minor.

dial aspect of the humerus and a distal stump on the lateral aspect of the arm. Transposition of distal stump beneath biceps/brachialis and anterior to the humerus permits the repair to be done on the medial side of the upper arm and does regain some length, especially if the elbow is partially flexed.[36,48] Depending on the length of resection, restoration of continuity may also be accomplished by passing grafts above the humerus. The latter maneuver permits some shortening of the distance between proximal and distal stumps, but in practical terms, it is usually difficult to accomplish this maneuver with grafts of less than 5 cm in adult patients.

## Lateral Arm

On leaving the spiral groove, the radial nerve enters the lateral compartment of the arm by passing through the lateral intramuscular septum. The nerve in the lateral arm can be difficult to locate and usually requires a skin incision and deeper dissection extending from the arm, across the elbow, to the forearm (Figure 7–11). Important for this dissection is identification of the brachioradialis and brachialis muscles. The surgeon then places one thumb on the brachialis and the other thumb on the brachioradialis.[49] Pushing these two structures apart reveals the radial nerve in the depths of the valley

thus created (Figure 7–12). If this maneuver does not demonstrate the radial nerve, it can be readily located deep to the brachioradialis at the elbow and proximal forearm level and traced proximally into the arm.[25]

## Antecubital Fossa

The nerve is dissected out between brachialis and brachioradialis. At this level, it lies somewhat beneath the latter muscle, which needs to be retracted laterally in order to expose the nerve.[49] The nerve should be gently tented forward on a Penrose drain to reveal the branches to brachioradialis and ECRL, as well as its major divisions into SSR and PIN. The exact point at which the PIN leaves the SSR is variable but is easily demonstrated by gently retracting the more proximal radial nerve upward with a Penrose drain. It is essential that the surgeon have an adequate view of this region, and this is accomplished by extending the skin incision distally over brachioradialis and, if need be, onto the dorsal region of the forearm. More distal exposure of the SSR is an easy matter as overlying deep fascia is sectioned and brachioradialis is retracted. This nerve is handled with care because it may be useful as a donor graft. Fascicles of the SSR nerve can be dissected back into the main radial nerve trunk with relative

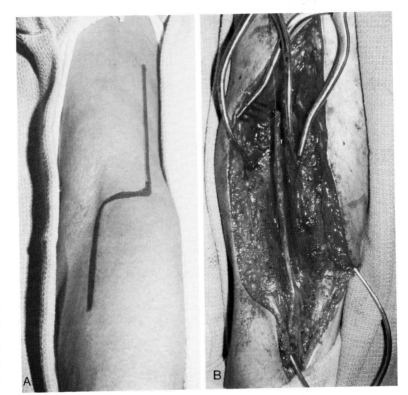

**Figure 7–11.** (A) Usual lateral arm to forearm incision used to expose radial nerve at the level of the elbow. Arm is at the top and forearm is at the bottom. The lateral side of the arm is to the right and the medial side is to the left of the photograph. (B) Exposure and neurolysis of arm and forearm-level radial nerve before transposition beneath biceps/brachialis.

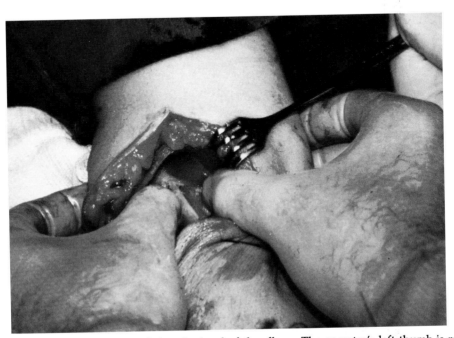

**Figure 7–12.** Method of exposing radial at the level of the elbow. The operator's left thumb is retracting against the brachioradialis and right thumb against the biceps/brachialis. At this level, nerve is found deep to the groove between these two muscles.

ease, and this may be an important maneuver to insure that subsequent regeneration of the main radial nerve is directed solely into the PIN. This is especially important if the intent of surgery is to restore the important muscles innervated by the PIN.

## Posterior Interosseous Nerve

Exposure of the radial nerve on the medial and lateral aspects of the arm and in the antecubital fossa is a relatively straightforward affair. Contrarily, dissection of the PIN is a difficult matter for the uninitiated, particularly if there is a great deal of scarring and adjacent soft tissue injury.[19] The PIN drops away from the main radial nerve to gain the interval between the superficial and deep heads of the supinator. The nerve then passes between the two heads of that muscle and winds around the lateral aspect of the proximal radius to gain the extensor aspect of the forearm. As the PIN reaches the dorsal forearm, it branches to supply most of the extensor musculature. The key to understanding this anatomy is an appreciation of the detailed structure of the supinator muscle.[63] This muscle has a humeral and ulnar head or origin and a single point of insertion onto the radius.

Numerous small vessels surround the PIN as it approaches the upper border of the superficial head of the supinator in the forearm. These vessels form leashes both volar and posterior to the

nerve and can bleed vigorously if entered without preparation. The leashes of vessels must be coagulated with the bipolar forceps in a discrete manner so as to avoid injuring the PIN itself and the branches running from that nerve to the supinator muscle. The arcade of Frohse is usually well-defined and is often of a tendinous nature (Figure 7–13). By dividing the superficial head of the supinator, the surgeon can expose the PIN as it winds around the forearm into the extensor compartment. At this point, the operator usually finds that he or she is experiencing difficulty with the exposure and should switch the approach to that placed on the dorsum of the forearm. This may be accomplished through either a separate or a single skin incision (Figure 7–14).

A surgical instrument passed from the flexor aspect of the proximal exposure along the course but superficial to distal PIN can serve as a useful landmark after the dorsal forearm approach is initiated. The surgical instrument can then be palpated and used as a guide as the operator splits the superficial extensor layer on the posterior aspect of the forearm, thus displaying the distal supinator heads. At this point, the PIN is running at right angles to the supinator fibers. Division of the superficial head of supinator is then finished so that the cut does not injure the numerous fine branches innervating the various extensor muscles. Repair of the PIN itself is usually a reasonably simple matter after the approach anatomy is mastered, but repair of the fine distal branches may be quite difficult.[38] Not

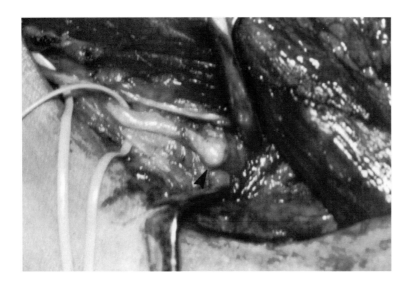

**Figure 7–13.** Neuroma of posterior interosseous nerve *(arrowhead)* located just proximal to the arcade of Frohse.

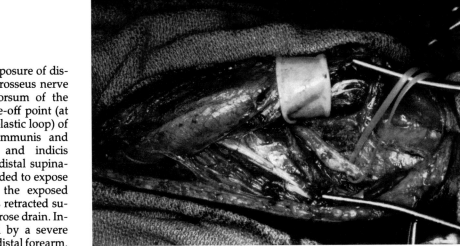

**Figure 7–14.** Exposure of distal posterior interosseus nerve (PIN) on the dorsum of the forearm and take-off point (at the level of the plastic loop) of the extensor communis and pollicis longus and indicis branches. More distal supinator has been divided to expose the distal PIN; the exposed brachioradialis is retracted superiorly by a Penrose drain. Injury was caused by a severe contusion to the distal forearm.

only are the branches small, but they are usually enmeshed in heavy scar tissue.

## Superficial Sensory Radial Nerve

Exposure of the SSR is a straightforward matter in the proximal forearm (Figure 7–15). An appropriately placed longitudinal incision defines the nerve, which may be a useful donor for graft repair of injuries of either the radial or PIN. After it arises from the main radial nerve, SSR courses beneath brachioradialis but above or superficial to ECRL. The SSR supplies skin over the radial side of the dorsum of the wrist and hand. Branches terminate on the dorsal surface of the radial three and a half digits. Particular attention should be given to the relationships between the wrist-level branches of the SSR, the brachioradialis tendon, and the three tendons destined for the proximal and distal phalanx of the thumb. In this area, there is frequent overlap with terminal branches of the lateral antebrachial cutaneous nerve of the forearm or the distal lateral branch of the musculocutaneous nerve.[33] This needs to be appreciated if the operation is intended to resolve painful neuroma problems. These branches can contribute to the neuroma, and pain can recur unless the neuroma is removed along with these involved branches.

## RESULTS: RADIAL NERVE

Outcome as a result of surgical repair of the radial nerve with or without tendon transfers is considered excellent by most workers in the field.[26,36,64] The radial nerve is felt to be the most

**Figure 7–15.** Anatomy of radial to superficial sensory radial and posterior interosseus nerve complexes viewed from a volar approach at a proximal forearm level. BR = brachioradialis nerve; ECR = extensor carpi radialis nerve; ECU = extensor carpi ulnaris nerve; SSR = superficial sensory radial nerve. (From Cravens G, Kline D: Posterior interosseous palsies. Neurosurgery 27:397–402, 1990.)

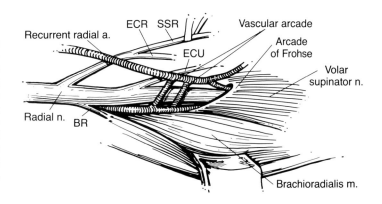

favorable major nerve in the body in terms of return of function, either spontaneously or after repair.[7,40,44] This is also reflected in our personal series.

Those patients referred for possible surgery and selected for conservative management almost invariably recovered to a grade of 4 or 5. Even those requiring operative exploration fared extremely well. This is not surprising in cases in which intraoperative NAP studies indicated significant regeneration through a lesion in continuity and, as a result, only neurolysis rather than resection and repair was done. Significant recovery also occurred with repair, however, whether by end-to-end suture or by grafts. Such good results can be related to several factors. To begin with, all muscles receiving motor input from the radial nerve receive it relatively proximal in the limb compared with the median- and especially the ulnar-innervated muscles. Thus, the terminal muscles innervated by the radial nerve are in the middle third of the forearm and not in the hand. Furthermore, although the radial nerve has a significant sensory outflow, this destination is to the dorsal aspect of the forearm and hand, sensory areas, which are relatively less important than other sensory areas. Imperfect recovery of sensation in these areas does not affect use of the limb and hand as much as it would in the median or even the ulnar distribution.

Despite favorable results with proper management of radial nerve injuries, recovery of extensor communis and especially extensor pollicis longus is difficult to obtain.[50] This is especially so with upper arm lesions, in which recovery of brachioradialis, improved supination, and some wrist extension usually provided by extensor carpi radialis is expected. In these lesions, recovery of extension of fingers and thumb and even extensor carpi ulnaris is less certain.[39] Fortunately, use of a portion of the flexor carpi ulnaris or flexor superficialis as a tendon transfer to the extensor expansion of the digits is an excellent substitute under these circumstances.[10] If it is properly done, good finger and even some degree of thumb extension can be gained.[61] Because results are good, some feel that tendon transfer rather than neural repair is the primarily indicated procedure.[16,59] We do not agree with this, preferring to reserve tendon transfer for cases in which neural regeneration

is unlikely or does not occur. On the other hand, even if transfer is done before neural regeneration is completed, we have not seen it complicate the result. Although we do not hesitate to recommend tendon transfer if appropriate, we do not advocate early transfer unless it is estimated that the chances for successful neural recovery are quite poor.

Less encouraging are those repairs attempted at the distal terminus of the PIN, where identification and reconstruction of branches on the dorsum of the forearm are difficult. Very proximal lesions involving radial outflow at posterior cord or upper radial levels and dorsal forearm injuries involving extensor communis and pollicis longus branches both share in the difficulty of obtaining recovery of digit extension and the more likely need for tendon transfer.[56]

Equally frustrating can be the treatment of SSR neuromas, which at times can resist any form of management[33] (Figure 7–16). Rather than burying nerve in bone, wrapping it in Silastic, or capping it, we prefer sharp section, bipolar coagulation of the individual fascicles under magnification, and then placement of proximal nerve in good soft tissue free of scar. If repair of the SSR is elected to try and minimize neuroma formation and recurrence of pain and paresthesias, it must be as meticulous as possible. Unfortunately, similar symptoms can occur as a result of the inevitable neuroma in continuity that occurs with either end-to-end or graft repair.

Patients likely to have prolonged wrist drop and inability to extend the fingers and thumb should be fitted with a dynamic dorsiflexion splint.[8] This splint holds the wrist in a mildly extended position and is fitted with an outrigger with rubber bands and finger pads. This permits the patient to flex against an extensor-like resistance and tends to maintain optimal length of the extensor communis and pollicis longus.

## FURTHER ANALYSIS OF RESULTS IN RADIAL SERIES

Mechanisms of injuries or lesions involving radial nerve are seen in Table 7–1. Included in the series are a relatively large number of lacerations, fractures, blunt contusions, and gunshot wounds. Although not usually injury-related,

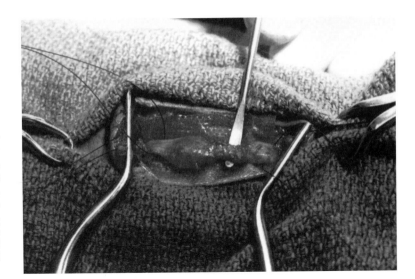

**Figure 7–16.** Superficial sensory radial nerve injury in continuity with more proximal bulbous enlargement to the left. This lesion was resected along with nerve well proximal and distal to the injury site. Proximal end was left buried beneath brachioradialis after sealing the exposed fasciculi with the bipolar coagulator.

there were also a large number of entrapments, mostly affecting PIN, and tumors, usually involving upper arm-level radial nerve. Only 69 of the 240 radial lesions evaluated did not require operation.

As can be seen in Table 7–2, lesions involving upper-arm radial nerve were the largest category, followed by those involving PIN and elbow-level radial. Radial sensory lesions and dorsal forearm radial branch lesions were less frequent, especially those requiring operation.

## Radial Results at the Arm Level

Table 7–3 shows, for operated radial nerves, the number transected and the number in conti-

nuity, operations done, and results by a whole nerve grading system. Eighteen arm-level radial nerves which were operated on were found to be transected while 53 were in continuity. Knife and glass wounds were responsible for most transections; a few were caused by fan and propeller blade injuries, gunshot wounds, and compound fracture of the humerus (Figures 7–17 and 7–18). Of the five having primary suture and end-to-end repair within 72 hours of injury, four recovered to a grade 3 or better level. Six of eight secondarily sutured nerves recovered adequately, as did three of five secondarily repaired by grafts.

A number of blunt contusive injuries to radial nerve, two injection palsies, and 4 gunshot wounds had recordable NAPs across their lesions despite total distal deficit. These lesions in continuity had neurolysis and did well. Where, despite gross continuity, there was no NAP transmitted and resection was necessary, end-to-end suture led to acceptable recovery in 11 of 14 cases and graft repair to good recovery in 13

**TABLE 7–1**
Radial Nerve — Mechanisms of Injury

| Mechanism | Operated Cases | Unoperated Cases |
|---|---|---|
| Laceration | 41 | 2 |
| Fracture | 44 | 28 |
| Gunshot wound | 14 | 5 |
| Injection | 7 | 0 |
| Entrapment | 18 | 5 |
| Blunt contusion or Volkmann | 23 | 14 |
| Dislocation | 0 | 2 |
| Sleep compression | 0 | 4 |
| Prior suture or neurolysis | 6 | 3 |
| Tumor | 18 | 6 |
| TOTALS | 171 | 69 |

**TABLE 7–2**
Radial Nerve Lesions by Level

| Level | Operated | Unoperated |
|---|---|---|
| Upper arm | 81 | 33 |
| Elbow | 31 | 14 |
| Posterior interosseus | 34 | 13 |
| Dorsal forearm | 9 | 2 |
| Radial sensory | 16 | 7 |
| TOTALS | 171 | 69 |

**TABLE 7–3**

Upper Arm Radial Nerve — Operations and Results in 71 Injuries*

| **Transected or not in continuity = 18** |
| --- |
| Primary Suture = 5/4 |
| Secondary Suture = 8/6 |
| Secondary Grafts = 5/3 |

| **Lesions in continuity = 53** |
| --- |
| (+) NAP = Neurolysis = 20/19† |
| (−) NAP =     Repair = 33 |
|          Suture = 14/11‡ |
|          Grafts = 19/13§ |

*Number of nerves operated/number of nerves reaching grade 3 or better result. Cases having poor follow-up (<1 y) were graded as less than 3.

†Excludes 10 tumors operated on.

‡Includes one split repair.

§Includes two split repairs.

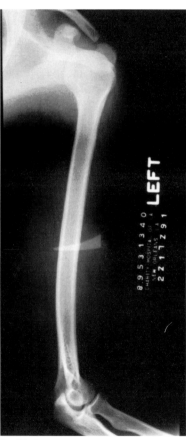

**Figure 7–17.** Penetrating glass injury at the midhumeral level transected radial nerve. This was repaired within 24 hours of the injury. Retained glass fragments can be visualized by appropriate soft tissue radiographs regardless of lead content of the glass.

**TABLE 7–4**

Upper Arm Radial Nerve — Graded Results by Mechanism in 81 Operated Cases

| **Mechanism** | | **Grade** | | | | |
| --- | --- | --- | --- | --- | --- | --- |
| | | **5** | **4** | **3** | **2** | **1** |
| Laceration | (12) | 4 | 5 | 2 | 1 | 0 |
| Fracture | (31) | 7 | 13* | 7 | 3 | 1 |
| Gunshot wound | ( 9) | 1 | 4 | 3 | 1 | 0 |
| Injection | ( 7) | 4 | 2 | 1 | 0 | 0 |
| Contusion | (10) | 1 | 4 | 3 | 1 | 1 |
| Tumor | (10) | 5 | 3 | 2 | 0 | 0 |
| Entrapment | ( 2) | 0 | 1 | 0 | 1 | 0 |
| TOTALS | (81) | 22 | 32 | 18 | 7 | 2 |

*Tendon transfers helped in 3 cases.

of 19 instances. For purposes of this table, if follow-up was not available, recovery was graded as 0.

Tables 7–4 and 7–5 show grades achieved in both the operative and nonoperative categories at this level by lesion type. Striking is the large number of grade 4 and 5 results (63%) in those selected for operation. Grade 3 or better results were achieved in 81%. These favorable figures held up even if tumors were excluded. Despite this, it was difficult to restore strong finger and thumb extension (grade 5), especially in the fracture, contusion, and gunshot wound categories (Figures 7–19 and 7–20). Here, lesions tended to be lengthier and more likely to require graft repair than the laceration and injection categories, in which, if repair was necessary, suture was more likely than graft repair. Despite inability to restore full finger extension, most patients functioned well and did not wish tendon transfers to be done. The interval be-

**TABLE 7–5**

Upper Arm Radial Nerve — Graded Results by Mechanism in 33 Unoperated Cases

| **Mechanism** | | **Grade** | | | | |
| --- | --- | --- | --- | --- | --- | --- |
| | | **5** | **4** | **3** | **2** | **1** |
| Laceration | ( 2) | 2 | 0 | 0 | 0 | 0 |
| Fracture | (17) | 7 | 4 | 4* | 1 | 1 |
| GSW | ( 4) | 3 | 0 | 1 | 0 | 0 |
| Contusion | ( 6) | 2 | 3 | 1 | 0 | 0 |
| Tumor | ( 2) | 0 | 1 | 1 | 0 | 0 |
| Dislocation | ( 2) | 1 | 1 | 0 | 0 | 0 |
| TOTALS | (33) | 15 | 9 | 7 | 1 | 1 |

*Tendon transfers helped in two cases.

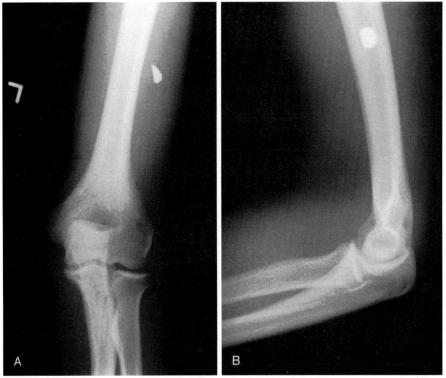

**Figure 7–18.** Anteroposterior *(A)* and lateral *(B)* radiographs of missile embedded in left arm. An ax struck metal embedded in a tree trunk. A resultant missile fragment penetrated the arm and was found embedded in the radial nerve as it lay in the humeral groove. This was repaired secondarily a few weeks after the incident. Secondary repair of a nerve injured in this fashion probably gives a better result than acute or primary repair, provided that good care is given to the soft tissue wound.

tween the injury and/or the onset of symptoms and operation is shown in Table 7–6.

The two entrapments were both spontaneous in onset and occurred at a midhumeral level in the area of the humeral groove.[30,34] In one case, a middle-aged man had overhead softball pitching as a hobby and may have had an element of chronic stretch as well as entrapment involving nerve at this level.

Five of the seven injection injuries to radial nerve required resection and repair (Figure 7–21). Results were good, although extension of fingers and thumb usually remained weak. One patient who had resection of a large neurofibroma along with nerve elsewhere required a lengthy and very proximal graft repair, with poor results.

Results in those patients selected for conserv-

**TABLE 7–6**
Upper Arm Radial Nerve — Operative Intervals (n = 81)

| Mechanism | | Months | | | | | | | | | | | |
|---|---|---|---|---|---|---|---|---|---|---|---|---|---|
| | | 0 | 1 | 2 | 3 | 4 | 5 | 6 | 7 | 8 | 9 | 12 | >12 |
| Laceration | (12) | 5 | 3 | 3 | 1 | 0 | 0 | 0 | 0 | 0 | 0 | 0 | 0 |
| Fracture | (31) | 0 | 0 | 1 | 6 | 9 | 7 | 4 | 0 | 2 | 2 | 0 | 0 |
| GSW | ( 9) | 0 | 0 | 1 | 2 | 3 | 2 | 0 | 1 | 0 | 0 | 0 | 0 |
| Injection | ( 7) | 0 | 0 | 0 | 1 | 3 | 0 | 2 | 1 | 0 | 0 | 0 | 0 |
| Contusion | (10) | 0 | 0 | 0 | 1 | 4 | 2 | 2 | 1 | 0 | 0 | 0 | 0 |
| Tumor | (10) | 0 | 1 | 2 | 0 | 1 | 1 | 2 | 1 | 0 | 0 | 0 | 2 |
| Entrapment | ( 2) | 0 | 0 | 0 | 0 | 0 | 0 | 1 | 0 | 0 | 1 | 0 | 0 |
| TOTALS | (81) | 5 | 4 | 7 | 11 | 20 | 12 | 11 | 4 | 2 | 3 | 0 | 2 |

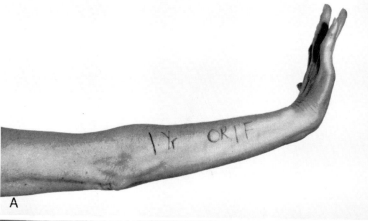

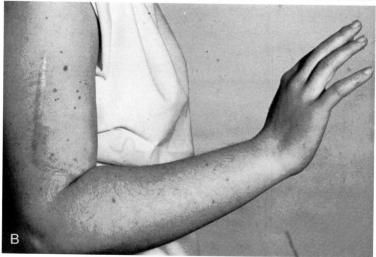

**Figure 7–19.** (A) Recovery of radial function in a patient with humeral fracture requiring open reduction and plating. Wrist extension was normal by 1 year, but finger extension, although greatly improved, had not fully recovered at that time. (B) Recovery of radial function in another patient 2.5 years after 13-cm grafts were placed at an axillary to arm level.

ative management were excellent, although functional loss was partial to begin with in almost one third of these cases. In the other cases, spontaneous improvement clinically or by electromyography was evident by 3 to 4 months after injury. Also of interest were the two tumor patients who had tumor resection elsewhere, had partial deficit, and, in both cases, improved enough spontaneously so that operative repair was not needed.

## Upper Arm Case Summaries

### Case Number 1

This 27-year-old airline stewardess noted pain radiating down her arm to the back of her hand while serving food on an air flight. If her lateral upper arm knocked against a chair back or passenger, radicular pain was reproduced. Although she had no café au lait spots or other history of tumors, subsequent examination by an

airline physician revealed a mass 3 cm in diameter below the deltoid and adjacent to the triceps. The mass could be moved side to side but not up and down. There was no neurologic deficit.

At operation, a discrete intraneural tumor was noted with fascicles spread around it like a basket (Figure 7–22). By splitting fascicles apart over the bulk of the tumor and by some interfascicular dissection proximally and distally, the tumor mass could be exposed. One fascicle entering and leaving the core of the tumor did not transmit an NAP. This feeding fascicle was sectioned, and this permitted removal of the schwannoma in toto. The capsule was then dissected from the fascicles and removed.

Postoperatively, she had only a mild sensory deficit over the dorsum of the hand and no motor dysfunction. She has done well with a 2.5-year period of follow-up.

### Comment

Nerve tumor should always be considered as a possible etiology for any mass in an extremity. Both the pa-

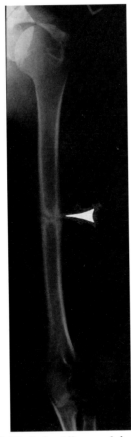

**Figure 7–20.** Healed midhumeral fracture *(arrowhead)* treated by closed reduction and associated with a radial palsy. This palsy reversed spontaneously with almost complete recovery of what must have been an axonotmetic or Sunderland grade II to III lesion by 2 years after injury.

tient's symptoms and physical findings suggested tumor involving the radial nerve. Schwannomas characteristically do not cause a neurologic deficit and usually can be removed without causing any serious loss unless there has been prior biopsy or attempted removal.

### Case Number 2

A 19-year-old male received a morphiate injection in his lateral arm below the deltoid muscle in preparation for a laminectomy. He felt an electric shock go down his arm to the back of his hand and had immediate wrist drop. Electromyography performed a week later showed absence of motor units in brachioradialis and all of the more distal radial-innervated muscles. Radial sensory responses were recorded on several occasions and seemed to show progressive decrease of sensory nerve action potential amplitudes and eventual loss. Examination a month later showed no function of brachioradialis, poor supination, and loss of wrist, finger, and thumb extension. Electromyography showed a severe denervational pattern with fibrillations as well as lack of motor units. Subsequent clinical and electrical follow-up at 2.5 months was the same, so the radial nerve was explored. Exploration began in the lateral arm between biceps and triceps. A several-centimeter segment of nerve in the spiral groove was somewhat atrophic and was also invested in some scar tissue. NAP recording on the lateral arm segment distal to the lesion gave a very small potential. As a result, radial nerve was exposed proximally by a separate incision and dissection in the high medial arm. NAP recording from nerve proximal to the spiral groove gave a response of good amplitude conducting at 80 m/sec. Recording across the spiral groove gave an NAP but of much smaller amplitude, conducting at 30 m/sec.

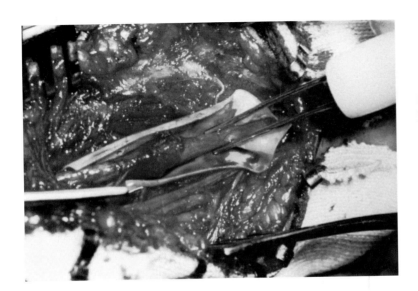

**Figure 7–21.** Radial injection site just below the two lateral heads of the triceps. There was no brachioradialis contraction in response to operative stimulation either at or above the lesion 4 months after injury, so it was resected and a repair was done. Stimulating electrodes are on the proximal stump of the nerve. (Photograph provided courtesy of Dr Glenn Meyer of Milwaukee, Wisconsin.)

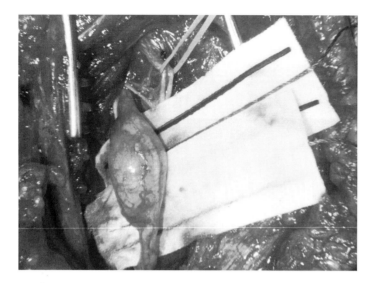

**Figure 7-22.** Typical neural sheath tumor involving radial nerve at the lateral arm level. The lateral triceps muscle has been split to expose the lesion. A plastic loop is around several triceps branches.

An internal neurolysis was done, and only a small amount of neural tissue and scar was resected. Histologic study showed myxoid material surrounding degenerated nerve fibers and forming a perineurial halo. A few of the axonal bundles had myxoid material within their confines.

He has recovered grade 4 to 5 function even in finger and thumb extension. Follow-up has extended to 3.5 years.

**Comment**

Injection injuries are preventable, and all who give injections should be thoroughly trained to avoid these painful neuropathies. In this case, the NAP recording helped make the decision against resection.

**Case Number 3**

This 20-year-old sustained a midarm humeral fracture. Radial loss was immediate and complete below the tri-

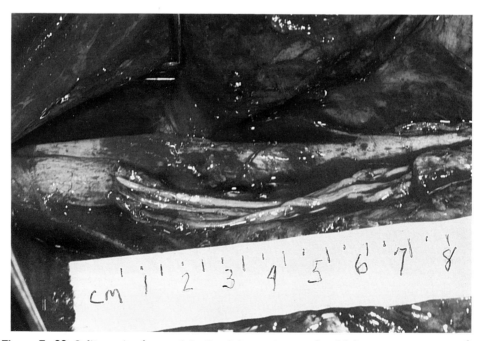

**Figure 7-23.** Split repair of nerve injection injury using antebrachial cutaneous nerve grafts.

ceps muscle. The fracture was treated in a closed fashion by cast, but clinical and electromyographic loss remained complete. As a result, radial nerve was explored at 4.5 months after injury. This was done by exposing distal arm-level nerve between triceps and biceps laterally. There was no NAP along this segment, so more proximal radial was exposed in the medial arm near the axilla. Stimulation there and recording from the lateral arm segment gave no NAP.

A lesion in continuity 3 cm in length and centered at the humeral or spiral groove was resected. Distal nerve was then mobilized to below the elbow. Branches to brachioradialis were defined and protected. Distal nerve was then transposed by placing it beneath biceps/brachialis and anterior to the distal humerus. With mild flexion of the elbow, enough length was made up to gain an end-to-end suture on the medial side of the arm.

Wrist extension returned to a grade 5, and extension of fingers to a 3, but extensor pollicis longus was only a trace. Follow-up extended to 3 years. The patient was able to use the limb quite well; therefore tendon transfer was not necessary.

### Comment

It is appropriate to wait for results because the majority of radial nerve injuries associated with fracture recover spontaneously. If no brachioradialis function is present by four months, exploration should not be delayed further.

### Case Number 4

A 42-year-old woman sustained a 38-caliber gunshot wound at midarm level. Humerus was partially splintered but not totally fractured. Loss was complete clinically and electrically and persisted for 4 months. A partially transected nerve was found at midhumeral level. Four

grafts approximately 5 cm long were sewn in place with 7-0 prolene after trimming back to healthy tissue.

Evaluation at 2 years postoperatively showed a grade 5 brachioradialis; supination graded 4, and wrist and finger extension was 3.

### Comment

Our practice is to advise radial nerve surgery where appropriate and to postpone assessment for tendon transfer until the results of nerve repair have been ascertained. Figure 7–24 shows the results in a similar case.

## Results in Elbow-Level Radial Injuries

Transections of elbow-level radial were caused by lacerations in seven cases and gunshot wound in one case. Primary repair of three sharp transections at this level was quite successful. Two gained a grade 5 result and one a grade 4 outcome. Of interest were the number of lesions in continuity having an NAP and recovery with neurolysis. This was because six of seven distal humeral fractures not only had left nerve in continuity but also were regenerating and had a recordable NAP. The one fracture-associated lesion requiring repair had lengthy grafts and only recovered to grade 2. The one case in which neurolysis did not lead to recovery was to radial nerve at the elbow level involved in a Volkmann volar compartment syndrome. The other Volkmann volar compartment syndrome case involving elbow-level radial nerve led to recovery after early fasciotomy

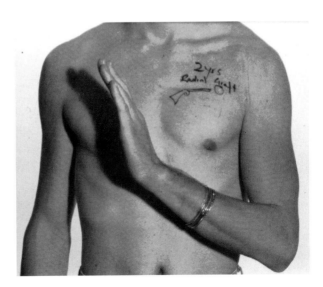

**Figure 7–24.** Radial gunshot wound in this young man was repaired by 4-cm grafts 2 years before. There was excellent return of wrist extension and some recovery of finger extension.

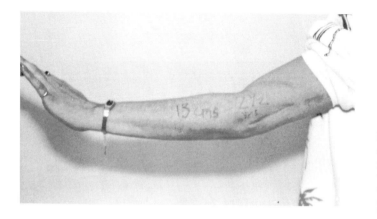

**Figure 7–25.** Recovery of most of radial function by 2.5 years after placement of lengthy grafts to repair fracture-associated injury. Note, however, that finger extension remains incomplete.

and neurolysis. Seven of the eight lesions in continuity requiring repair recovered (Figure 7–25).

Thirteen of 14 lesions treated without operation had acceptable recovery. One Volkmann-associated radial lesion remained a grade 2, and another gained a grade of 3, but only with the help of a flexor recession. See Tables 7–7, 7–8, and 7–9 for details.

## Elbow-Level Case Summaries

### Case Number 1

A 19-year-old male received a plate glass injury in which a shard of glass penetrated his lateral arm above the elbow. Acute exploration 8 hours after injury showed a transected radial nerve. Nerve was neatly but somewhat obliquely transected.

**TABLE 7–7**
Elbow-Level Radial Nerve Operations
and Results In 26 Injuries*

| Transected or not in continuity = 8 |
|---|
| Primary Suture = 3/3 |
| Secondary Suture = 2/1 |
| Secondary Grafts = 3/2† |

| Lesions in continuity = 18 |
|---|
| (+) NAP = Neurolysis = 10/9‡ |
| (−) NAP = Repair = 8 |
| Suture = 2/2 |
| Grafts = 6/5§ |

*Number of nerves operated/number of nerves reaching grade 3 or better result. Cases having poor follow-up (<1 y) were graded as less than 3.
†Includes one split repair.
‡Excludes 5 tumors operated on.
§Includes one split repair.

After minimal trimming of both stumps, an end-to-end repair was done using 6-0 nylon suture. He was fitted with a dynamic wrist and finger dorsiflexion splint with outrigger, rubber bands, and finger pads. With the help of this device and home exercises, he managed well.

At a visit 1 year postoperatively, brachioradialis graded 3, supination 2, and extensor carpi radialis 3. There was only a trace of finger and thumb extension. By 3 years after operation, brachioradialis graded 4 and wrist and finger extensors graded 3 to 4. He no longer used the dorsiflexion splint and was managing his college classes and extracurricular activities including baseball without difficulty.

**TABLE 7–8**
Elbow-Level Radial Nerve Graded
Results by Mechanism in 31 Operated Cases

| Mechanism | | Grade | | | | |
|---|---|---|---|---|---|---|
| | | 5 | 4 | 3 | 2 | 1 |
| Laceration | ( 9) | 4 | 3 | 1 | 1 | 0 |
| GSW | ( 5) | 1 | 3 | 1 | 0 | 0 |
| Fracture | ( 7) | 2 | 3 | 1 | 1 | 0 |
| Contusion | ( 3) | 0 | 1 | 1 | 1 | 0 |
| Tumor | ( 5) | 2 | 2 | 1 | 0 | 0 |
| Prior Suture | ( 2) | 0 | 1 | 0 | 1 | 0 |
| TOTALS | (31) | 9 | 13 | 5 | 4 | 0 |

### 14 Unoperated Cases

| Mechanism | | Grade | | | | |
|---|---|---|---|---|---|---|
| | | 5 | 4 | 3 | 2 | 1 |
| Fracture | ( 6) | 0 | 2 | 4 | 0 | 0 |
| GSW | ( 1) | 0 | 1 | 0 | 0 | 0 |
| Contusion | ( 2) | 2 | 0 | 0 | 0 | 0 |
| Tumor | ( 2) | 1 | 1 | 0 | 0 | 0 |
| Prior Suture | ( 1) | 0 | 0 | 1 | 0 | 0 |
| Volkmann's | ( 2) | 0 | 0 | 1* | 1 | 0 |
| TOTALS | (14) | 3 | 4 | 6 | 1 | 0 |

*Flexor recession helped in one case.

**TABLE 7-9**
Elbow-Level Radial Nerve Operative Intervals (n = 31)

| | | | | | | | Months | | | | | | |
|---|---|---|---|---|---|---|---|---|---|---|---|---|---|
| Mechanism | | 0 | 1 | 2 | 3 | 4 | 5 | 6 | 7 | 8 | 9 | 12 | >12 |
| Laceration | ( 9) | 3 | 3 | 1 | 1 | 0 | 1 | 0 | 0 | 0 | 0 | 0 | 0 |
| GSW | ( 5) | 0 | 0 | 0 | 1 | 2 | 1 | 1 | 0 | 0 | 0 | 0 | 0 |
| Fracture | ( 7) | 0 | 0 | 1 | 0 | 0 | 3 | 1 | 2 | 0 | 0 | 0 | 0 |
| Contusion | ( 3) | 0 | 0 | 1 | 1 | 1 | 0 | 0 | 0 | 0 | 0 | 0 | 0 |
| Tumor | ( 5) | 0 | 0 | 0 | 1 | 0 | 1 | 2 | 0 | 0 | 0 | 1 | 0 |
| Prior Suture | ( 2) | 0 | 0 | 0 | 0 | 0 | 0 | 0 | 0 | 1 | 1 | 0 | 0 |
| TOTALS | (31) | 3 | 3 | 3 | 3 | 3 | 6 | 4 | 2 | 1 | 1 | 1 | 0 |

## Comment

Sharp injuries due to laceration should be explored primarily before stumps have an opportunity to retract. In this case, early surgery allowed end-to-end suture.

## Case Number 2

This 8-year-old female lost her balance when she attempted to walk across the top of a swing set. While falling, she was impaled on a deer hook used to cure meat. She was rescued by her father, who found her hanging from the swing set with the hook embedded into her right elbow at the antecubital level. She required transfusions and repair of her brachial vein acutely. She had a complete radial palsy below the branches to the brachioradialis. This included supination, wrist and finger extension, and sensation on the dorsum of the hand.

A transected radial nerve at the elbow level was repaired after trimming both stumps by end-to-end suture using 6-0 nylon. This repair was done shortly after referral 4 months after the accident.

With the help of a tendon transfer a year later, a good result was gained. Wrist extensors by 3 years after neural repair graded 4 to 5, extensor communis 4, and extensor pollicis longus and supination 3.

## Comment

Complete loss of function associated with a penetrating wound of this nature could have occurred 2 to 4 weeks after injury. Tendon transfers can be tailored to specific residual defects if nerve suture is not entirely successful. Generally, we will wait several years after initial nerve repair before recommending tendon transfer, unless the likelihood of recovery is very poor.

## Results with PIN Lesions

Table 7-10 shows injured PINs which were operated on. The grading system used for eval-uating PIN lesions is found in Table 7-11. Included in Table 7-10 are six injuries caused by laceration and five caused by fracture. There were four transections caused by laceration and one associated with a fracture. Of the four lacerating injuries transecting PIN, one was repaired within 72 hours by suture and one by grafts. Despite a sharp mechanism for injury and complete preoperative loss, two nerves were in gross physical continuity. Neither transmitted an NAP, and both required a repair with eventual good results.

Each of the five fracture-associated PIN palsies had complete loss preoperatively (Figure 7-26). In three cases, prior operative manipulation and plating of the fracture may have played a role in the origin of the PIN loss. One of these had three operations in an attempt to stabilize fractures of both radius and ulna. In another case in which a fracture of the radius had been plated, there was no continuity of the PIN. Grafts were necessary because a 6.3-cm gap resulted after stumps were trimmed to healthy tissue. The other four PIN palsies associated with fracture and operated on were in continuity. Two PIN lesions transmitted NAPs and had neurolysis, but two did not and required graft repairs. One patient in each category had undergone prior neural operation. Both of these cases required graft repairs.

Excellent results were achieved by suture or grafts in both the laceration and fracture categories. Despite good neural recovery, two patients had tendon transfers to help improve their function. Both contused PINs had recordable NAPs, underwent neurolysis, and have had substantial recovery (see Table 7-10).

**TABLE 7–10**

Injured PINs — Operated

| Lacerations (Preoperative Loss Complete) (n = 6) | | | |
|---|---|---|---|
| **Operative Findings** | **Operation** | **Result** | **Follow-up** |
| Transection | Secondary Suture | 4 | 2 y |
| Transection | Secondary Suture | 4 | 1.5 y |
| Transection | Secondary Grafts | 4* | 3 y |
| Transection | Primary Suture | 5 | 3 y |
| In Continuity (−) NAP | Secondary Suture | 4 | 1.5 y |
| Prior Primary Suture (−) NAP | Secondary Grafts | 5 | 3.5 y |

*Tendon transfer helped recovery.
y = years.

| Fractures (Preoperative Loss Complete) (n = 5) | | | | |
|---|---|---|---|---|
| **Etiology** | **NAP** | **Operation** | **Result** | **Follow-up** |
| Radius F (x) plated | (−) | Grafts | 4 | 2.5 y |
| Radius F(x) plated | Transection | Grafts | 4 | 2 y 4 mo |
| Radius F (x) | (+) | Neurolysis | 4 | 2 y |
| Radius F (x) elbow disloc | (+) | Neurolysis | 4–5 | 2 y |
| Radius/ulnar F (x) 3 prior ops | (−) | Grafts | 3* | 3 y |

*Tendon transfer helped recovery.
y = years.

| Contusions (Preoperative Loss Complete) (n = 2) | | | | |
|---|---|---|---|---|
| **Means of Injury** | **NAP** | **Operation** | **Result** | **Follow-up** |
| Brick | (+) | Neurolysis | 4 | 3 y |
| Pool cue | (+) | Neurolysis | 5 | 4.5 y |

F (x) = fracture; ops = operations; PIN = posterior interosseus nerve; y = years.

**TABLE 7–11**

Grading of Posterior Interosseous Nerve Function

| Grade | Description |
|---|---|
| 0 | No extensor carpi ulnaris (ECU), extensor communis (EC), or extensor pollicis longus (EPL) |
| 1 | Trace or against gravity only of ECU but absent EC and EPL |
| 2 | Recovery of ECU but absent or trace only EC and EPL |
| 3 | Recovery of ECU and some EC but only weak or absent EPL |
| 4 | Recovery of moderate strength EC and EPL as well as full strength in ECU |
| 5 | Recovery of full strength in EPL and EC as well as in ECU |

## Forearm-Level (PIN) Case Summary

This 25-year-old motorcyclist skidded off the road and struck a barbed wire fence. He sustained multiple ragged lacerations to the forearm. These were debrided and packed open. The distal stump of a transected radial nerve was marked with a vascular clip. Several weeks later the granulated areas were covered with skin grafts. Radial deficit was total from supinator distally.

Unfortunately, repair of the radial nerve required grafts 8 cm in length. Grafts extended from main radial to the PIN just proximal to the arcade of Frohse. The latter was sectioned. No attempt was made to repair SSR, but one graft was led to a distal brachioradialis branch. Follow-up extended to 5 years. Wrist and finger extension including

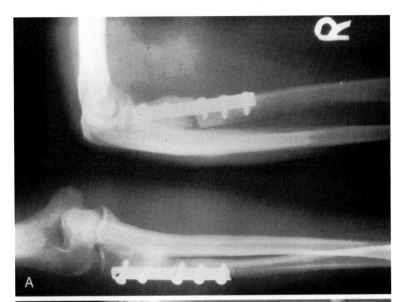

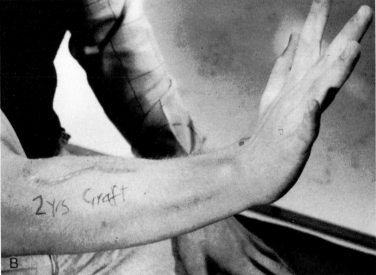

**Figure 7–26.** *(A)* Fracture of radius requiring plate and screw repair. Associated posterior interosseous nerve injury required graft repair 3 months later. *(B)* The patient recovered excellent wrist and some but not complete finger and thumb extension by 2 years after graft repair.

that to the thumb recovered to a grade 3 level; supination remained absent and there was no sensory return.

### Comment

Even in complex injury cases such as this, the radial nerve is worth repairing because of the known favorable outlook for this particular nerve.

## Posterior Interosseous Nerve (PIN) Entrapment

This entrapment syndrome is by no means rare if the examiner knows to look for it.[22] It may or may not be associated with proximal forearm pain, but it usually lacks the paresthesias and the sensory symptoms associated with most entrapments of other nerves. Instead, the patient presents with a painless decrease in extension of the fingers and thumb.[23] This may initially affect some fingers more than others. As the palsy progresses, there is weakness in extensor carpi ulnaris and extensor pollicis longus as well as extensor communis. Function of extensor carpi radialis and sensation in the distribution of the SSR branch are maintained. With dorsiflexion of the wrist, the hand drifts in a radial direction, and finger and thumb droop occur because of weakness in extension of these digits. Table 7–11 shows the LSUMC grading system used to evaluate loss and recovery in the PIN distribution. Electromyography shows denervational changes in only the more severe PIN entrapments. Conductive studies can be done but require experience if they are to be done accurately on this segment of the radial nerve.

Compression usually occurs at the arcade of Frohse, which is the proximal portion of the volar supinator, and there may or may not be a fascial edge at this level. The PIN normally travels between the volar and dorsal levels of the supinator to reach the dorsum of the forearm. After exiting between this "sandwich" of muscle, the PIN branches to supply extensors of the fingers and thumb.

In our experience and that of others, loss of function may improve spontaneously in several months, especially if the onset was related to cessation of vigorous or repetitive wrist and forearm motion. If reversal of loss does not occur or if loss progresses, operative decompression is indicated.

This is a favorable entrapment to treat surgically providing the decompression is thorough and includes division of the entire volar head of the supinator[11,63] (Figure 7–27). A vascular arcade of arteries and veins may encircle or cross over nerve proximal to the muscular or fascial edge of the true arcade of Frohse, but this is seldom responsible for the entrapment.

Results with neurolysis of PIN and division of the volar supinator for PIN entrapments are excellent in well-selected patients. In two cases in our series, entrapment was bilateral; in the re-

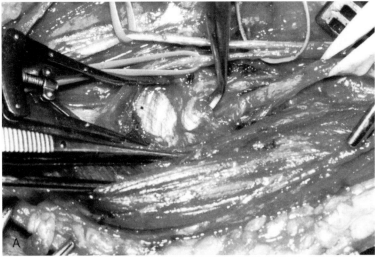

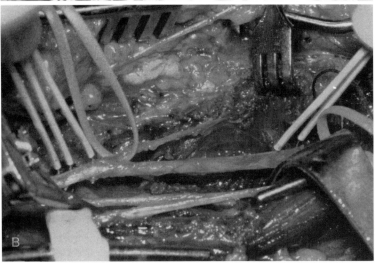

**Figure 7–27.** (A) Posterior interosseous nerve (PIN) at level of the arcade of Frohse. A double-ended dissector is beneath the somewhat fibrous edge of the volar head of the supinator. Superficial sensory radial with the extensor carpi radialis branch arising from it is seen behind or deep to the instrument. (B) The volar supinator has been incised. The recording electrode is on the more distal PIN to the right of the photograph whereas the stimulating electrode is quite proximal on the PIN and to the left.

**TABLE 7–12**

Entrapped Posterior Interosseous Nerve
Results in 16 Cases

| Preoperative Grade to Postoperative Grade = Number of Patients | | |
|---|---|---|
| 0 to 5 = 3 | 1 to 5 = 2 | 3 to 4 = 1 |
| 0 to 4 = 1 | 2 to 4 = 4 | 3 to 5 = 4 |
| 0 to 3 = 1* | | |

*Tendon transfer helped recovery in one case.

mainder it was unilateral. PIN entrapment occurred with a male to female ratio of 9 to 5, right-to-left sided ratio was also 9 to 5, average age was 30 years, and length of follow-up averaged 3.4 years.

One half of the PIN cases operated on were caused by entrapment. Table 7–12 shows the grade assigned to each case before operation and the grade achieved after operation. Despite entrapment as a mechanism, loss was complete preoperatively in five of these patients and quite severe (grade 1 or 2) in another six. In each instance, intraoperative recordings showed an NAP across the entrapment site, which was either at the arcade of Frohse or beneath the su-

pinator muscle. Conduction velocities were slowed, and NAP amplitudes were usually diminished. Fifteen of the entrapped nerves recovered to either a grade 4 (six cases) or a grade 5 (nine cases) level.

Table 7–11 shows the criteria used to grade PIN function, and Table 7–13 shows the graded results in both the operated and unoperated categories. The three tumors involving PIN that were operated on included a ganglion cyst, a lipoma, and a neurofibroma. Loss preoperatively was partial or, in the neurofibroma case, minimal. Fortunately, most neurologic function was maintained; in the ganglion cyst case, function improved from a preoperative grade 3 to a postoperative grade 4. Tumors operated on previously and having neurologic deficit included a neurofibroma in which function was graded 2 and a schwannoma in which it was 4. Both improved remarkably with time. The five entrapments not operated on were seen within 2 months of onset and had improved by 5 months after occurrence. Despite severe loss related to sleep compression in two cases and fracture in four instances, acceptable recovery occurred usually over a 6- to 7-month period.

Table 7–14 illustrates the tendency for PIN

**TABLE 7–13**

Posterior Interosseous Results Graded by Injury Mechanism

| Operated Cases | | | | | | |
|---|---|---|---|---|---|---|
| | | | | **Grade** | | |
| **Mechanism** | | **5** | **4** | **3** | **2** | **1** |
| Laceration | ( 5) | 1 | 4 | 0 | 0 | 0 |
| Fracture | ( 5) | 0 | 4 | 1 | 0 | 0 |
| Entrapment | (16) | 9 | 6 | 1 | 0 | 0 |
| Tumor | ( 3) | 2 | 1 | 0 | 0 | 0 |
| Contusion | ( 2) | 1 | 1 | 0 | 0 | 0 |
| Prior Suture | ( 1) | 1 | 0 | 0 | 0 | 0 |
| TOTALS | (32) | 14 | 16 | 2 | 0 | 0 |

| Unoperated Cases | | | | | | |
|---|---|---|---|---|---|---|
| | | | | **Grade** | | |
| **Mechanism** | | **5** | **4** | **3** | **2** | **1** |
| Sleep compression | ( 2) | 0 | 2 | 0 | 0 | 0 |
| Fracture | ( 4) | 2 | 2 | 0 | 0 | 0 |
| Entrapment | ( 5) | 4 | 1 | 0 | 0 | 0 |
| Prior Tumor Resection | ( 2) | 1 | 1 | 0 | 0 | 0 |
| TOTALS | (13) | 7 | 6 | 0 | 0 | 0 |

**TABLE 7–14**
Etiology and Handedness of Operated Posterior Interosseous Nerve (PIN) Palsy Cases

| | Female | | Male | | Total | |
|---|---|---|---|---|---|---|
| | Right | Left | Right | Left | Right | Left |
| Laceration | 1 | 0 | 3 | 2 | 4 | 2 |
| Fractures* | 2 | 1 | 3 | 0 | 5 | 1 |
| Contusion/Compression | 1 | 0 | 0 | 2 | 1 | 2 |
| Tumors† | 2 | 0 | 1 | 0 | 3 | 0 |
| Entrapment | 4 | 1 | 7 | 4 | 11 | 5 |
| TOTALS | 10 | 2 | 14 | 8 | 24 | 10 |

*PIN palsy associated with placement of plate for fracture in two cases; three prior operations in another case.
†Tumors included ganglion cyst (1), schwannoma (1), and neurofibroma (1).

palsy, whether of spontaneous or traumatic origin, to preferentially involve the right side, especially in females. The higher incidence of entrapments involving the right side versus left the left side may be related to greater use of the right arm for repetitive motions.

## Results in Dorsal Forearm Branch Injuries

As can be seen in Table 7–15, nine injuries at this level were operated on (Figure 7–28). Despite gaining some good results with the transections repaired acutely by suture and secondarily by grafts, two graft repairs failed. These dissections, especially if done secondarily, were difficult because it was a challenge to find distal branches to graft to. This was especially so in two cases in which prior operation had failed.

**TABLE 7–15**
Dorsal Forearm Branches Operative Results in 9 Cases*

| Transections or Not in Continuity = 6 |
|---|
| Primary Suture = 2/2 |
| Secondary Grafts = 4/2 |

| Lesions in Continuity = 3 |
|---|
| (+) NAP = Neurolysis = 1/1 |
| (−) NAP =     Repair = 2/1 |
| Grafts = 1/0 |
| Neurolysis/grafts = 1/1 |

*Mechanisms included lacerations (5), fracture (1), contusion (1), prior operation (2). Results show number of nerves operated/number reaching grade 3 or better result. Two contusive injuries involving forearm branches were not operated on and fortunately improved with time.

Proximal lead-out could sometimes be located only by dissecting out PIN beneath brachioradialis and tracing it through and underneath the volar head of the supinator to its transection point, either at a branch level or at the distal PIN itself. The three lesions in continuity operated on were caused by contusion in two instances and fracture of the radius in one. Two other contusive injuries at a forearm level caused by blunt objects improved with time and did not need repair. An alternative to neural repair with injury at this level is tendon transfer, and one of the failed graft repairs subsequently had this done with a good result.

## Results With Superficial Sensory Radial Nerve Lesions

Because suture of lacerated SSR nerves often results in painful hyperesthesia on the dorsum of the hand as well as a tender painful neuroma, we decided some years ago to excise such injured nerves. A similar approach has yielded even greater success with injured but painful sural and saphenous nerves. The sensory distributions of all three are not of great functional importance unless median, ulnar, or tibial sensory distributions are also absent. This approach has provided good relief in six isolated SSR lesions, but the other three have retained some symptoms. As pointed out by Mackinnon and colleagues,[33] it is important to excise the neuroma and tissues surrounding it as well as the nerve proximal to it. Fine branches from lateral musculocutaneous or antebrachial cutane-

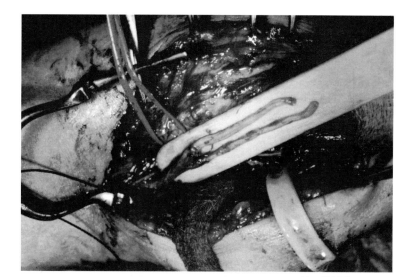

**Figure 7-28.** In this case, distal forearm-level radial branches were transected by a knife, which produced jagged transections. Grafts are attached to the distal posterior interosseous nerve and are being prepared for suture to more distal extensor branches.

ous nerves can with time contribute to or be incorporated in the SSR neuroma. This can occur whether these adjacent nerves are injured by the same forces injuring the SSR or not. Excision has also been used for the persistently painful contusion-injured SSR because earlier experience with neurolysis in two cases did not seem to work.

Seven SSR cases have been managed conservatively but not always successfully (See Table 7-16). In those with persistent symptoms, neither patient nor insurers could always be convinced of the need for operation, especially because total relief of pain could not be promised.

**TABLE 7-16**
Superficial Sensory Radial Neuroma
Results in 16 Operated Cases*

| Injury | Excision | Neurolysis |
|---|---|---|
| Laceration | 9/6 | 0/0 |
| Contusion | 3/3 | 2/0 |
| Prior Suture | 2/2 | 0/0 |

**Results in Seven Unoperated Cases**

Compression = 2/0
Prior Suture = 2/0
Contusion = 2/1
Fracture = 1/1

*Number of nerves operated/number obtaining significant relief of pain.

## Radial SSR Case Summary

This 25-year-old male sheet metal worker was carrying a pile of iron sheets when the tape holding them together broke and he sustained a laceration of the volar mid forearm area. Exploration under tourniquet showed a partial laceration of muscle including brachioradialis, flexor carpi radialis, flexor pollicis longus, superficial flexor of the long finger, and palmaris longus tendon. A partial laceration of the SSR branch of radial was noted. Muscle and tendon transections were repaired. Judging from outside notes, the partially divided area of the SSR was trimmed to healthy tissue, but it was left in continuity, and then the whole nerve in that area was placed beneath muscle.

When seen a year later, the patient was having complaints of a dull aching pain with intermittent electric shocks along the radial side of the volar aspect of the forearm. There was hypesthesia on the SSR portion of the dorsum of the hand, including the dorsum of the thumb and the anatomic snuffbox region. Motor function of the hand was quite good, but there was some sensory decrease on more volar forearm in the antebrachial cutaneous distribution. Tapping on the long volar forearm scar gave paresthesias down the radial side of the forearm. Skin-level NAP recordings showed a small amplitude SSR NAP conducting at 30 m/sec.

At exploration, neuromas in continuity were found on both the SSR and one of the lateral antebrachial cutaneous nerve branches. The former transmitted only a small, slow NAP, and the latter did not conduct at all. A proximal and distal length of both nerves, including their lesions, was resected. Proximal fascicles were sealed by use of a fine-tipped bipolar forceps and placed beneath brachioradialis muscle.

The patient did well postoperatively with good relief of pain. Unfortunately he was lost to follow-up after 1.5 years.

### Comment

Isolated SSR neuromas can present difficult management problems because the patient frequently strikes the neuroma in day-to-day tasks.

## Complications

True complications with surgery on this nerve were infrequent in our series. Failure to recover more distal radial function such as extensor communis or extensor pollicis longus is more of a recognized limitation of repair of this nerve than a true complication. If proximal nerve is involved with heavy scar, it is possible to injure otherwise uninvolved triceps branches. This can occur as the nerve is laid out on the proximal and medial aspect of the arm or sometimes even in the region of the humeral groove. This occurred twice in this series, but fortunately some of this loss reversed with time. In the region of the elbow, brachioradialis branches can be inadvertently sectioned. Of potentially even more serious import is damage to the extensor carpi radialis branch, which can be inadvertently injured because of its variable origin from whole radial nerve or SSR below the elbow.

Experience with reoperation of previously operated PIN entrapments or injuries suggests that frequently the entire volar head of the supinator has not been sectioned. This would seem to be indicated in the majority of cases at this level. Similarly, repair of an injured SSR often does not relieve the pain and paresthesias associated with such injury, and resection of a length of this nerve seems preferable if pain is the dominant problem.

### Bibliography

1. Alnot JY and Le Reun D: Les lésions traumatiques du tronc du nerf radial au bras. Rev Chir Orthop Reparatice Appar Mot 75:433–442, 1989.
2. Barton NJ: Radial nerve lesions. Hand 5:200–208, 1973.
3. Bateman JE: Trauma to Nerves in Limbs. Philadelphia, WB Saunders, 1962.
4. Bowden REM and Shell DA: The advance of functional recovery after radial nerve lesions in man. Brain 73:251–266, 1950.
5. Bowen TL and Stone KH: Posterior interossesous nerve

6. paralysis caused by a ganglion at the elbow. J Bone Joint Surg 48B:774–776, 1966.
6. Boyd HB and Boals JC: The Monteggia lesion. A review of 159 cases. Clin Orthop 66:94–100, 1969.
7. Brown PW: Factors influencing the success of the surgical repair of peripheral nerves. Surg Clinics North Am 52:1137–1155, 1972.
8. Bunnell S: Active splinting of the hand. J Bone Joint Surg 28:732–736, 1946.
9. Capener W: The vulnerability of the posterior interosseous nerve of the forearm. J Bone Joint Surg 48B:770–773, 1966.
10. Chuinard R, Boyes J, Start H, and Ashworth C: Tendon transfers for radial nerve palsy: Use of superficialis tendons for digit extension. J Hand Surg 3:560–570, 1978.
11. Cravens G and Kline D: Posterior interosseous palsies. Neurosurgery 27:397–402, 1990.
12. DiRosa F: Radial nerve: Anatomy and fascicular arrangement. *In* Brunelli G, Ed: Textbook of Microsurgery. New York, Masson, 1988.
13. Emery SE, and Gifford JF: One hundred years of tennis elbow. Contemp Orthop 12:53–58, 1986.
14. Garcia A and Maeck BH: Radial nerve injuries and fractures of the shaft of the humerus. Am J Surg 99:625–627, 1960.
15. Goldner JL: Function of the Hand Following Peripheral Nerve Injuries. Am Acad Orthop Surg Instruct, Course Lectures 10. Ann Arbor, MI, JW Edwards, 1953.
16. Griswold BA: Early tendon transfer for radial transection. Hand 8:134, 1976.
17. Guarantors of Brain: Aids to the Examination of the Peripheral Nervous System. London, Bailliere Tindall, 1989.
18. Gurdjian ES, Hardy WG, Lindner DW, and Thomas LM: Nere injuries in association with fractures and dislocations of long bones. Clin Orthop 27:147–151, 1963.
19. Hall HH, Mackinnon SE, and Gilbert RW: An approach to the posterior interosseous nerve. Plast Reconstr Surg 74:435–437, 1984.
20. Henry AK: Extensile Exposure: Applied to Limb Surgery. Baltimore, Williams & Wilkins, 1945.
21. Holstein A and Lewis GB: Fractures of the humerus with radial nerve paralysis. J Bone Joint Surg 45A:1382–1386, 1963.
22. Hudson AR and Mayfield FH: Chronic injuries of peripheral nerves by entrapment. *In* Youmans JR, Ed: Neurological Surgery, 2nd Ed., Vol. 4. Philadelphia, WB Saunders, 1982.
23. Hustead AP, Mulder DW, and MacCarty CS: Nontraumatic progressive paralysis of the deep radial (posterior interosseous) nerve. Arch Neurol Psychiatry 69:269, 1958.
24. Jayendrahumar J: Radial nerve paralysis associated with fractures of the humerus. Clin Orthop 172:171–175, 1983.
25. Kempe L, Ed: Operative Neurosurgery, Vol 2. New York, Springer-Verlag, 1970.
26. Kettlekamp DB and Alexander H: Clinical review of radial nerve injury. J Trauma 7:424–432, 1967.
27. Lichter RL: Tardy palsy of the posterior interosseous nerve with a Monteggia fracture. J Bone Joint Surg 57A:124–125, 1975.
28. Ling CM and Loong SC: Injection injury of the radial nerve. Injury 8:60–62, 1976.
29. Lister GD, Belsole RB, and Kleinert HE: The radial tunnel syndrome. J Hand Surg 4:52–59, 1979.
30. Lotem M, Fried A, Levy M, et al.: Radial palsy following muscular effort: A nerve compression syndrome possi-

bly related to a fibrous arch of the lateral head of the triceps. J Bone Joint Surg 53B:500–506, 1971.

31. Lyons WR and Woodhall B: Atlas of Peripheral Nerve Injuries. Philadelphia, WB Saunders, 1949.

32. McGraw JJ: Neurological complications resulting from supracondylar fractures of the humerus in children. J Pediatr Orthop 6:647–650, 1986.

33. Mackinnon S and Dellon A: Surgery of the Peripheral Nerve. New York, Theime Medical Publishers, 1988.

34. Manske PR: Compression of the radial nerve by the triceps muscle: A case report. J Bone Joint Surg 59A:835–836, 1977.

35. Moss SH and Switzer HE: Radial tunnel syndrome. A spectrum of clinical presentations. J Hand Surg 8:414–419, 1983.

36. Nickolson OR and Seddon HJ: Nerve repair in civil practice. Br Med J 2:1065–1071, 1957.

37. Nulsen FE: The management of peripheral nerve injury producing hand dysfunction. In Flynn JE, Ed: Hand Surgery. Baltimore, Williams & Wilkins, 1966.

38. Omer GE: Evaluation and reconstruction of forearm and hand after acute traumatic peripheral nerve injuries. J Bone Joint Surg 50A:1454–1460, 1968.

39. Omer GE: Injuries to the nerves of the upper extremities. J Bone Joint Surg 56A:1615–1624, 1974.

40. Omer GE: The results of untreated traumatic injuries. In Omer G and Spinner M, Eds: Management of Peripheral Nerve Problems. Philadelphia, WB Saunders, 1980.

41. Packer JW, Foster RR, Garcia A, and Grantham SA: The humeral fracture with radial nerve palsy. Is exploration warranted? Clin Orthop 88:34–38, 1972.

42. Pollock FH, Drake D, Bovill E, et al.: Treatment of radial neuropathy associated with fractures of the humerus. J Bone Joint Surg 63A;239–243, 1981.

43. Reid RL: Radial nerve palsy. Hand Clin 4:179–182, 1988.

44. Sakellorides H: Follow-up of 172 peripheral nerve injuries in upper extremity in civilians. J Bone Joint Surg 44A:140–148, 1962.

45. Samu M: The arcade of Frösch and its relationship to posterior interosseous nerve paralysis. J Bone Joint Surg [Br] 50:809–812, 1968.

46. Savory WS: A case in which after the removal of several inches of the musculospiral nerve, the sensibility of that part of the skin of the hand which is supplied by it was retained. Lancet 2:142, 1868.

47. Seddon H: Nerve lesions complicating certain closed bone injuries. JAMA 135:691–694, 1947.

48. Seddon H: Surgical Disorders of the Peripheral Nerve. Baltimore, Williams & Wilkins, 1972.

49. Seletz E: Surgery of Peripheral Nerves. Springfield, IL, Charles C Thomas, 1951.

50. Shaw JL and Sakellorides H: Radial nerve paralysis associated with fractures of the humerus. J Bone Joint Surg 49A:899–902, 1967.

51. Sobotta JJ: Atlas of Human Anatomy. FJ Figge, Ed. 9th English Ed., 3 Vols. Munich, Urban & Schwartzenberg, 1974.

52. Spinner M: Injuries to the Major Branches of Peripheral Nerves of the Forearm, 2nd Ed. Philadelphia, WB Saunders, 1978.

53. Spinner M: The arcade of Frösch and its relationship to posterior interosseous nerve paralysis. J Bone Joint Surg [Br], 50:809–812, 1968.

54. Spinner M, Freundlich BD, and Teicher J: Posterior interosseous nerve palsy as a complication of Monteggia fractures in children. Clin Orthop 58:141–145, 1968.

55. Stein F, Grabias S, and Deffer P: Nerve injuries complicating Monteggia lesions. J Bone Joint Surg, 53A:1432–1436, 1971.

56. Steyers CM: Radial nerve results. In Gelberman R, Ed: Operative Nerve Repair and Reconstruction. Philadelphia, JB Lippincott, 1991.

57. Strachan JC and Ellis BW: Vulnerability of the posterior interosseous nerve during radial head resection. J Bone Joint Surg 53B:320–323, 1971.

58. Sunderland S: The intraneural topography of the radial, median, and ulnar nerves. Brain 68:243–299, 1945.

59. Sunderland S: Observations on injuries of the radial nerve due to gunshot wounds and other causes. Aust N Z J Surg 17:253, 1948.

60. Trojabarg W: Rate of recovery in motor and sensory fibers of the radial nerve: Clinical and electrophysiological aspects. J Neurol Neurosurg Psychiatry 33:625–630,1978.

61. White WL: Restoration of function and balance of the wrist and hand by tendon transfers. Surg Clin North Am 40:427–459, 1960.

62. Woodhall B and Beebe WG: Peripheral Nerve Regeneration: A follow-up study of 3656 W W II injuries. VA Medical Monograph. Washington, DC, US Government Printing Office, 1956.

63. Young MC, Hudson AR, and Richards RR: Operative treatment of palsy of the posterior interosseous nerve of the forearm. J Bone Joint Surg 72A:8:1215–1219, 1990.

64. Zachary RB: Results of nerve suture. In Seddon HJ, Ed: Peripheral Nerve Injuries. Medical Research Council Special Report No. 282. London, Her Majesty's Stationery Office, 1952.

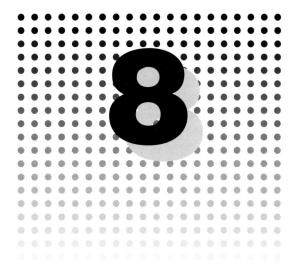

# Median Nerve

## SUMMARY

The median nerve carries important sensory as well as motor functions. Unlike the radial, the median does not innervate arm muscles, but it does provide important input to both forearm-level and thenar intrinsic muscles. Although the anatomic relations of the median are usually straightforward in the arm, they are complex at the elbow and proximal forearm, where the relations of pronator, flexor superficialis, and anterior interosseous branch to other structures are important. It is also at this level that the Martin-Gruber anastomosis can occur, or more proximally, entrapment by a Struthers ligament.

Data analyzed for this nerve indicated that for 70 patients with arm-level involvement, 76 with elbow and forearm lesions, and exclusive of carpal tunnel syndrome, there were 95 lesions at a wrist and/or hand level. Analysis of arm-level data showed surprisingly good results for not only lacerations but also gunshot wounds and even some lesions associated with fracture and contusion. Grade 5 recoveries occurred mainly with partial lesions to begin with or with complete lesions in which neurolysis was based on a positive NAP across the lesion. Major residual defects involved thenar intrinsic muscles, although lack of true opposition was usually substituted for nicely by ulnar- and radial-innervated thumb muscles. Elbow- and forearm-level median lesions also fared well with proper management, despite a diverse range in time interval between injury and operation. Twenty-six of 46 operative cases were operated on at 5 months or later. By comparison, thirty-three of the 41 operated arm-level lesions were treated surgically within 5 months of injury. Median loss due to Volkmann or electrical injury was difficult to reverse. Relief of neuritic pain was also not always possible, especially if iatrogenic injection injury was the mechanism. Wrist-level lesions involving the median nerve had similar restriction in outcome of thenar-intrinsic function to lesions more proximal in the limb, although overall grades for sensory return were higher.

The large clinical subset of carpal tunnel syndrome has been summarized with emphasis on failed carpal tunnel release, a type of case often referred to these authors for neurologic repair.

# MEDIAN NERVE ORIGIN

This nerve originates at the axillary level from large branches of the lateral and medial cords, forming the characteristic "V" that in turn overlies the axillary to brachial artery junction. The lateral cord to median nerve junction is usually easily seen on initial axillary plexus exposure, but the motor contribution from the medial cord may be posteromedial to the artery and only clearly seen when searched for and dissected away from the vessel. In a few cases, lateral or medial cord input to median nerve may pass posterior to the axillary artery. In others, the lateral cord may contribute some of its fibers destined for the median nerve by way of a proximal branch to the medial cord contribution to the median nerve. In almost a quarter of cases, lateral cord fibers destined for the median nerve can travel in more proximal musculocutaneous nerve, leaving it more distally to enter the median which has already been partially constituted by input from the medial cord and that portion of the lateral cord not contributing to the musculocutaneous nerve.[31]

Fascicles destined to form the musculocutaneous nerve may not separate from the lateral cord, but may instead travel through the lateral head of the median nerve and leave it to achieve their destination on the medial edge of biceps and brachialis. In rare cases, the median nerve in the upper arm may be bifid as far as the elbow.[74] Of surgical importance is the fact that the course of the median nerve from origin to most destinations is straight. As a result, not much length can be gained by mobilization. This makes some period of immobilization after repair of the median mandatory if there is any tension on the repair.[75]

# ARM LEVEL

Injury to this portion of the median nerve in the arm may be complicated by damage to brachial artery and vein, and even ulnar nerve damage, caused by the median nerve's close proximity to these structures. Both motor and sensory loss involve the entire distribution of the nerve and are quite characteristic (Figures 8–1 and 8–2). Radial nerve penetrates between the subscapularis muscle and the long head of the triceps, so it is deep as it descends to leave the medial upper arm to travel to the lateral side of the arm. As a result, radial nerve is more protected and is less likely to receive an injury concomitant with those involving the median and ulnar nerves and vessels, even at a proximal arm level. Exceptions are provided by stretch injuries involving the cord to nerve level of the brachial plexus and very proximal penetrating injury to the arm, in which radial nerve may also be involved.

Median nerve injuries are often associated with ulnar nerve involvement. Such injuries are devastating because, with the exception of extension of the wrist and partial extension of the fingers (radial and posterior interosseous nerve innervation), the hand is totally paralyzed.[82] Unless successful recovery is gained through regeneration, a severely clawed hand results. Such deformity involves all four fingers, resulting in a "main en griffe."[65]

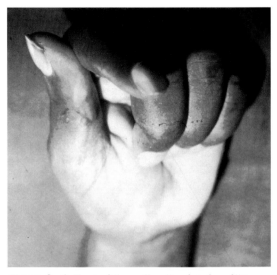

**Figure 8–1.** Typical "pope" or "prelate hand" in an individual with a complete and proximal median neuropathy. Upon making a fist, the patient is unable to flex the tip of the thumb or forefinger.

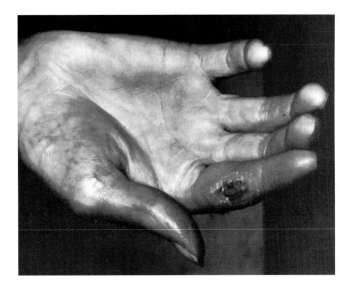

**Figure 8–2.** Burn to anesthetic zone of forefinger after proximal median nerve injury. Patients must guard and protect anesthetic skin.

Injuries to median nerve along the medial aspect of the arm can be caused by glass, knife, or gunshot wounds, or they can be iatrogenic and associated with a vascular bypass procedure or construction of an arteriovenous fistula for renal dialysis.[34] Median nerve damage at this level is rarely associated with fracture of the humerus, radial palsy being more common.[5] Mechanisms of injury to median nerve at a proximal level also include those secondary to angiography.[6] Damage results from direct penetration by a needle or catheter or in some cases, from compression secondary to pseudoaneurysm of the axillary or brachial artery or a blood clot.

High median nerve palsy, with or without radial or ulnar palsy, can be caused by compression or contusion of the nerve in the axilla or the proximal and medial arm (Figure 8–3). Such a syndrome may be seen in stuporous people who hang an arm over a chair or park bench, or after one's sleeping partner rests his or her head for a prolonged period on the medial arm. More commonly, the patient lies in a lateral recumbent position and rests his or her own head on the lateral midhumeral area of the arm; this produces radial palsy below the triceps branches. Radial palsy is also a much more common sequela of prolonged use of crutches than median palsy, but crutch palsy can, on occasion, involve

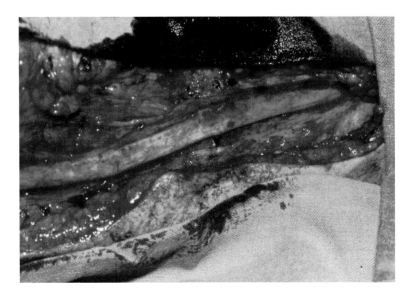

**Figure 8–3.** Contusion of median nerve at arm level, which did not transmit a nerve action potential at 6 months and required resection and repair. Note the absence of an obvious focal neuroma. You can't tell a book by its cover!

the median nerve with or without concomitant radial nerve involvement.

Loss, with proximal median involvement, is total if injury is severe enough to involve the entire cross section of the nerve. In addition to median distribution sensory loss, pronator function is markedly reduced or lost, as is palmaris longus and flexor superficialis function of all four fingers, as well as profundus function of the forefinger. In addition, it is usually obvious that more distal flexor pollicis longus is paralyzed. Pronator teres is the most proximal muscle innervated by the median nerve. Branches to the pronator, which is located in the forearm, usually arise at the level of the distal arm and innervate muscle at the level of the flexor crease of the elbow or sometimes at the proximal forearm level. Occasionally, pronator teres can be innervated by the musculocutaneous nerve, which can, even less frequently, innervate also the palmaris longus and flexor carpi radialis. The more distal pronator quadratus serves as a much weaker pronator than does the teres, receiving a branch from the median which travels along anterior interosseous membrane before branching to supply the quadratus.

## Wrist and Finger Flexion

After innervating the pronator and palmaris longus, the next important and proximal branches from the median arise 2.5 cm or so below the flexor crease of the elbow and innervate flexor superficialis.[74] In testing flexor superficialis function of the little and ring fingers, one reduces input from ulnar-innervated flexor profundi to these digits by holding the distal digits in an extended position and asking the patient to pull the straightened fingers towards the palm. Both the flexor superficialis and the flexor profundi flex the metacarpophalangeal joints towards the palm, but by isolating testing as much as possible to the metacarpophalangeal joints and the first interphalangeal joint, the superficialis is tested. Because ulnar-innervated profundi to little and ring fingers tend to pull these digits toward the palm, and because a tendon slip from the ring finger may blend in a shared fashion with that of the long finger proximal to the digits, only the tip of the forefinger cannot be flexed when the patient with median palsy attempts to make a fist. Even more commonly, long finger profundus receives dual innervation from median and ulnar nerve, sparing it from full loss of flexion in median palsy.[74] On the other hand, flexor profundus to forefinger is always median-innervated, making it a good marker muscle for the median nerve (Figure 8–4).

Wrist flexion is in an ulnar direction because flexor carpi ulnaris is no longer balanced by flexor carpi radialis longus or brevis. Distal flexion of the thumb is lost, as is pure abduction of the thumb at right angles to the palm, and true opposition movement of the thumb is also not

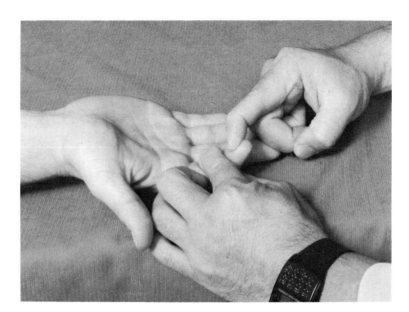

**Figure 8–4.** Testing flexor profundus to the forefinger. The first metacarpophalangeal joint is held fixed by the examiner's fingers, and the patient is asked to flex or pull the distal phalanx toward the palm. Function is graded by the examiner's applying counterpressure.

possible. With total paralysis of the flexor pollicis longus and some shortening of the tendon, the patient and examiner may yet believe that there is distal phalangeal contraction after extending the thumb and then suddenly relaxing it, because the shortened flexor tendon pulls the tip of the thumb into a partially flexed position. Lumbrical function to forefinger and long finger is weak or absent unless all lumbricals are innervated by the ulnar nerve, a circumstance occurring approximately 15% of the time.

Pronation is tested first by having the patient extend the elbow. The patient's hand is then grasped by the examiner, and the patient is asked to rotate the hand from a palm-up, or supinated, position to a palm-down, or pronated, position (Figure 8–5). Receiving innervation at a proximal forearm level is the palmaris longus, whose loss is of little functional importance because this muscle serves only as a corrugator of palmar skin. Nonetheless, the palmaris longus may be an important muscle for the electromyographer to test because it receives relatively proximal input from the median nerve.[76,84] As the median nerve passes beneath and is somewhat adherent to the under surface of the flexor superficialis, it supplies branches to this muscle. Tendons insert on the intermediate phalange of each of the four fingers and thus flex the proximal two phalanges of the fingers toward the palm.

At the level of the upper arm, and usually at its midpoint, there may be a proximal Martin-Gruber anastomosis with fibers crossing between the median and ulnar nerves. This is an unusual variation, seen in less than 3% of dissections; the true Martin-Gruber anastomosis, which is at forearm level, occurs in at least 15% of the population.[31]

## Compression by Struthers Ligament

Median nerve can be compressed beneath the Struthers ligament in the distal arm (Figure 8–6). This ligament is a rare anatomic anomaly estimated by Terry to be present in 0.7 to 2.7% of the population. Of course, not all patients with such a ligament develop compression of either the median or the ulnar nerve secondary to it. The ligament arises from a small spur or supracondylar process projecting medially from the inner surface of the distal humerus. The ligament extends to medial epicondyle, where it inserts. Ulnar as well as median nerve can be entrapped, and tenderness and a Tinel sign are often present on tapping in this region. These signs are best tested by tapping along the distal and medial groove of the arm located between biceps/brachialis and triceps and extending toward the flexor crease of the elbow.

## ELBOW LEVEL

At the elbow level, mechanisms of injury to the median are much the same as at the upper arm level, and distribution of loss may be the same, although function of pronator teres may be spared because branches supplying this muscle sometimes leave the median nerve just

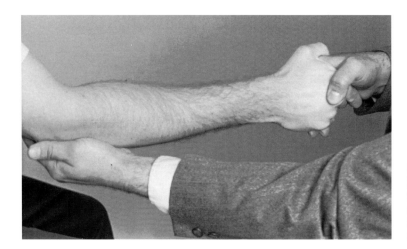

**Figure 8–5.** Pronation is readily tested with forearm relatively extended. Patient is asked to turn the palm of the hand downward against resistance.

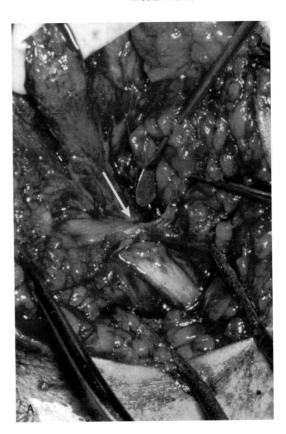

**Figure 8-6.** (*A*) Median nerve entrapped by a Struthers ligament just proximal to the elbow (*arrow*). This teenager had prior unsuccessful carpal tunnel releases bilaterally and had a contralateral Struthers ligament entrapping median at this level as well. (*B*) Drawing of usual anatomy of a Struthers ligament running volar to both brachial artery and median nerve.

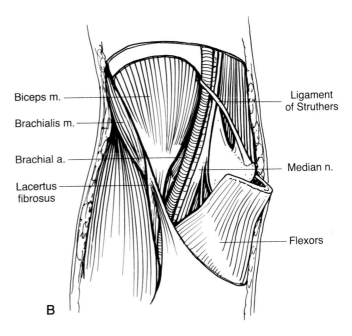

Biceps m.

Brachialis m.

Brachial a.

Lacertus fibrosus

Ligament of Struthers

Median n.

Flexors

B

proximal to this level. In addition to the usual categories of trauma, the median nerve can be injured at the level of the elbow by needles or catheter placement in the course of venipuncture or arterial catheterization.[77]

## Pronator Syndrome

The pronator syndrome consists of loss of median function distal to innervation of this muscle. Such loss is often incomplete and is usually caused by compression of the median nerve as it passes between the superficial and deep heads of the pronator teres. The nerve can be compressed by a hypertrophied pronator muscle and specifically its distal fascial edge, beneath which the main median nerve courses. Lacertus fibrosus, which is an extension of the distal biceps tendon and inserts on the flexor fascia of the forearm, can also hypertrophy and occasionally cause compression of the median nerve at this level. Testing for the pronator syndrome is described at length elsewhere; it yields variable results.[27,54,68,72] Diagnosis is sometimes provided by electrical conduction studies if they are positive, but if they are negative, it does not exclude the syndrome. Clinically, the physician looks for a history of pain and tenderness in the region of the proximal volar elbow, specifically in the area of the pronator teres, as well as symptoms of loss in the more distal median nerve distribution. Several tests have been advocated for the pronator syndrome. The patient is asked to pronate the wrist and palm and then flex the wrist. While the patient is doing this, the examiner exerts force against maintenance of this position, which reproduces the pain pattern. A simple maneuver on the part of the examiner that resists the patient's ability to pronate or rotate the palm face down without the addition of wrist flexion may sometimes reproduce the patient's complaints.

## Martin-Gruber Anastomosis

There are a number of variations of this anastomosis.[68] Fibers destined for some of the ulnar-innervated hand intrinsics may travel in an elbow-level branch from median to ulnar or through the anterior interosseous branch of the median. Loss with injury to more proximal median or to anterior interosseous may then be more serious than usual. Conversely, injury to ulnar nerve proximal to the anastomosis gives less hand-intrinsic paralysis than usual. Ulnar fibers carried by the usual Martin-Gruber anastomosis eventually innervate the first dorsal interosseous, lumbricals, adductor pollicis, and the ulnar portion of the flexor pollicis brevis.

In another variation of the anastomosis, median fibers destined for thenar eminence cross over to ulnar in proximal forearm (Figure 8-7). These fibers then return to the thenar branch of the median at a palmar level (Riche-Cannieu anastomosis). If this forearm level of crossover occurs, loss with injury to anterior interosseous gives not only paralysis of flexor profundus to forefinger and flexor pollicis longus, but also thenar intrinsic weakness.[74] Injury to median at wrist level in such a limb would spare thenar intrinsics, but injury to ulnar would involve their loss as well as the usual ulnar-innervated intrinsic paralysis.

Forearm-level connections from ulnar to me-

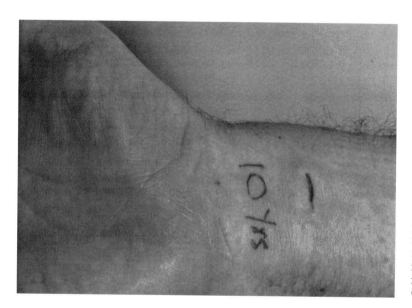

**Figure 8-7.** Thenar atrophy in patient who had an unrepaired median laceration at the lower forearm level caused by a glass injury received 10 years before in which there was no Martin-Gruber anastomosis.

dian are more unusual, but they do occur. In these cases, fibers destined for some ulnar intrinsics are carried in the median to the hand. At the palmar level, these fibers branch to trade back to the ulnar nerve branches.

## Ischemic Contracture of Volkmann

A devastating complication of supracondylar fracture or elbow dislocation caused by severe, blunt trauma is Volkmann ischemic contracture. Here, contusion or stretch of the brachial artery results in spasm of this vessel, secondary ischemia, and even frank infarction of volar flexor compartment musculature. Under these circumstances, median nerve and sometimes even radial and ulnar nerves receive not only ischemic damage but also compression secondary to ischemic infarction and swelling of the soft tissues of the volar compartment of the forearm. A less common but still observable set of circumstances occurs with acute swelling secondary to a large contusive blow to the forearm. This we have seen secondary to pool cue blows to the forearm, heavy objects falling on the forearm, and high-speed vehicular accidents in which the forearm is severely contused. Severe and prolonged compression of the forearm resulting from drug misuse and sleeping on the arm was responsible for several of our cases and has already been reported elsewhere in the literature.[60] Under these circumstances, even though there is no fracture, median nerve, and occasionally also the posterior interosseous portion of the radial nerve, can be acutely compressed by swollen tissue in the volar compartment.

In addition to a swollen, painful forearm, the patient with impending Volkmann ischemia has paresthesias, usually in the median distribution, but sometimes in the radial and ulnar distributions as well. These symptoms can progress in severity, and with time there is dampening or loss of the radial pulse and ischemic symptoms and findings in the hand, especially at the fingertips. In addition to extensive damage to volar forearm musculature, the ensuing median sensory and motor neuropathy and, at times, associated radial and ulnar losses, make

for a complex and difficult-to-reverse syndrome.[64] Early fasciotomy and neurolysis of the median and often the posterior interosseous portion of the radial nerve is necessary. Various devices and techniques have been used to measure pressure in the anterior compartment more objectively.[43] However, a good index of suspicion for the diagnosis and, as a result, early fasciotomy, are preferable in our experience.

## Anterior Interosseous Syndrome

An anterior interosseous branch leaves the main trunk of the median nerve beneath the flexor superficialis muscle to travel in a somewhat oblique and radial direction. This nerve branches to supply not only the flexor profundus to the forefinger and long finger but also the flexor pollicis longus to the thumb. Dysfunction of these two muscles results in the anterior interosseous syndrome, which consists of loss of the pinch mechanism between forefinger and thumb and difficulty on the part of the patient in making an "O" with these two digits (Figure 8–8). Function of the profundus to the long finger is seldom totally lost because of a sharing of deep flexor tendons between long and ring fingers. The latter is innervated by the ulnar nerve. Characteristically, the syndrome lacks median sensory abnormality, so that the observer may mistake anterior interosseous loss as tendon ruptures of the thumb and forefinger flexors.

The anterior interosseous syndrome can be spontaneous and related to entrapment or to penetrating or, less frequently, contusive injury of the forearm. Almost always, an individual with entrapment has onset of the syndrome heralded by spontaneous pain in the proximal forearm as well as loss of dexterity in use of the thumb and forefinger. If ulnar fibers travel in the anterior interosseous branch, then loss involves not only thumb and forefinger pinch mechanism but more distal ulnar intrinsic muscles as well.[71]

On occasion, compression of median nerve at the pronator level may selectively damage fascicles destined for anterior interosseous nerve and thus mimic a more distal lesion.

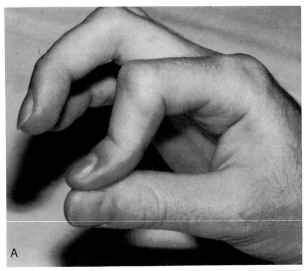

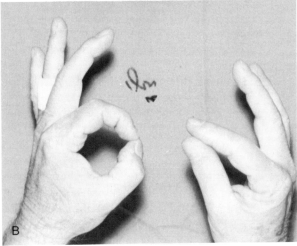

**Figure 8-8.** Anterior interosseous palsy with loss of flexor profundus to forefinger and flexor pollicis longus, poor pinch (*A*), and inability to make an "O" with forefinger and thumb (*B*).

## Anterior Interosseous Syndrome Case Summary

A 21-year-old woman had a caesarean section and postoperatively received a venipuncture injury to the volar forearm involving anterior interosseous nerve.

When seen a month after the incident, flexor profundus of the forefinger graded 3, and flexor pollicis longus was absent. Electromyography showed denervation in muscles in the anterior interosseous distribution. By comparison, there was a healthy median sensory response conducting at 55 m/sec. It was elected to follow the patient for 3 months because there was partial function of the flexor profundus.

By 3 months after injury, flexor pollicis longus had returned and graded 2 to 3. Follow-up at 3 years showed a good pinch and excellent flexor pollicis longus as well as flexor profundus.

### Comment

A similar case in an older individual was operated on at 3 months after venipuncture injury because of severe pain, although anterior interosseous deficit was partial. A neurolysis was done, and anterior interosseous function improved to a grade of 4; however, pain, although diminished, was not completely eliminated. It is difficult to relieve pain caused by needle penetration of a nerve such as the median. Sometimes external neurolysis helps even though the nerve appears, to gross inspection, to be quite normal. In other cases, neurolysis and its attendant manipulation of the nerve do not change the pain pattern.

## MIDFOREARM LEVEL

At the middle or distal forearm area, the median nerve can be injured in association with a Monteggia fracture involving the radius or ulna.[1] Loss includes flexor pollicis longus function, thenar intrinsic muscles, and lumbricals for forefinger and sometimes long finger as well. Distal forearm injuries involving median may also involve ulnar nerve, tendons, and important vessels.[11]

Other than the flexor pollicis longus branch, which usually leaves the median nerve trunk at the junction of the middle and distal third of the forearm, there are no motor branches from median nerve distal to the anterior interosseous before the nerve reaches the palmar portion of the hand. An important sensory branch originating in the distal forearm is the thenar sensory branch, which leaves the radial side of the median nerve at a variable distance proximal to the principal flexion crease of the wrist. This branch supplies sensation over the dorsoradial aspect of the thenar prominence and the intermediate and distal phalanges of the thumb.

As pointed out earlier, the Martin-Gruber anastomosis is common. Fibers destined for some of the distal median-innervated hand intrinsic muscles can leave median nerve at the forearm level as a branch anastomosing with ulnar nerve. They travel down the distal ulnar nerve to the distal third of the forearm, where a branch from the ulnar nerve may reanastomose with the distal median nerve. In many cases, fibers destined for median nerve do not leave ulnar nerve until the palmar level. Here, a branch leaving the deep ulnar nerve termed the Riche-Cannieu anastomosis provides fibers that travel back into the main median or, more commonly, to the recurrent thenar branch to innervate thenar musculature. Implications of these connections are extensive. Injury to median nerve at distal forearm level can, in some patients, result in only median distribution sensory loss with little or no thenar muscular loss. In other patients, the reverse situation may apply. Ulnar nerve fibers destined for intrinsics and lumbricals of little and ring fingers travel in median nerve for a distance down the forearm before reanastomosing with the ulnar nerve at distal forearm or palmar levels.

The thenar sensory branch can be injured during the course of median nerve dissection at the wrist level or with blind scissoring of subcutaneous and wrist-level transverse carpal ligament fibers during the course of carpal tunnel release (CTR). An occasional spontaneous laceration of the wrist with or without main median nerve transection or damage can involve this branch, as can contusive or crush injury at this level. Another mechanism producing injury to this branch is inadvertent damage or involvement during the course of tendon repair or tendon substitution and transfer procedures.

## WRIST LEVEL

At wrist level, the median nerve is in close proximity to the palmaris longus tendon, and is located somewhat laterally to it or on its radial side. It is also volar or superior to the flexor tendons, both superficial and deep.

Damage to the median nerve at the wrist level provides a common set of clinical circumstances. Because the nerve lies immediately volar to the flexor tendons, associated tendon injuries, particularly with sharp mechanisms, are common, as are injuries to the radial or ulnar arteries.[8] Loss is to all intrinsic muscles innervated by the nerve and also in the median sensory distribution, except for that of the thenar sensory branch, which again usually arises 1 cm or more proximal to wrist crease. The median sensory fascicle exclusive of the thenar motor branch provides some sensation over the volar thenar eminence of the thumb and to distal palm on the median side of the hand. It also provides sensation to the volar surface of the forefinger and usually the radial half of the long finger. Autonomous zone for the median nerve includes volar and dorsal surfaces of the distal phalanx of the forefinger and the volar surface of the distal phalanx of the thumb. Not uncommon is partial injury, with either sensory loss accompanied by partial or complete motor sparing, or vice-versa.

If injuries to the median at the wrist level are operated on acutely, the motor fascicle can be stimulated. If the patient is operated on later, while awake, the proximal face of the sensory fascicle can be stimulated.[21,81] More distally at the palmar level, median nerve gives rise to a recurrent thenar branch to the abductor pollicis brevis, opponens pollicis, and flexor pollicis brevis, the latter sharing its innervation with that of the deep branch of the ulnar nerve.

These anatomical and clinical considerations become very practical when dealing with the most common surgical neuropathy, which is entrapment of the median beneath the transverse carpal ligament.

The median nerve can, on occasion, be bifid at the wrist level and proximal palm, and this can lead to confusion at the time of carpal tunnel release (CTR). A smaller sensory branch can also leave median nerve in the distal forearm, travel parallel with it, and enter the palm along with the larger main median nerve. Some patients also have a palmar sensory branch that arises from the volar surface of the median and penetrates transverse carpal ligament to supply the palm. This branch can be inadvertently injured during carpal tunnel release, leading to a painful sensory neuroma.[44] At a variable level of the palm, the recurrent or thenar motor branch leaves the radial and somewhat dorsal side of the main nerve to supply abductor pollicis, opponens pollicis, and almost always a portion of the flexor pollicis brevis. Release of the flexor retinaculum must therefore be performed on the ulnar side of the nerve to avoid injury to the thenar motor branch. Flexor pollicis brevis flexes the proximal phalange of the thumb, and this function is aided by the flexor pollicis longus, which inserts on the more distal phalange of the thumb. The abductor pollicis pulls the thumb away from the palm at a right angle (Figure 8–9). It can be tested by placing the dorsum of the hand on a flat surface and asking the patient to raise the thumb away from the palm at a right angle. One can palpate the thenar muscle mass and, in a healthy subject, can feel and see contraction of a portion of the abductor pollicis as it is being tested. If the extensor pollicis mechanism is weak or paralyzed as a result of radial nerve injury, it is difficult to test for abductor pollicis function unless one provides some support along the dorsal aspect of the thumb. With the thumb supported in this fashion, the patient then attempts abduction against resistance.

The opponens pollicis pulls the thumb toward the palm in an oblique direction and

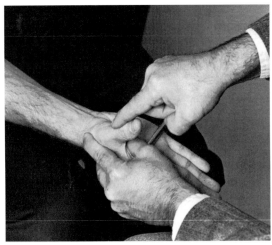

**Figure 8–9.** Abductor pollicis is tested by having the patient abduct or pull the thumb up and away from the palm and at a right angle to it.

permits the patient to touch the palmar surface of the thumb to the base of the little finger at the metacarpophalangeal joint level. The thumb rotates in opposition so that the thumb nail and small fingernail become parallel, in contrast to the position at rest, in which the nails are at right angles to one another. One can test the opponens by placing the examiner's forefinger on top of the long finger, placing both near the metacarpophalangeal junction of the patient's little finger, and asking the patient to use the thumb to press against the examiner's fingers as the examiner attempts to separate forefinger and long finger (Figure 8–10). With a healthy opponens pollicis, the examiner cannot separate the forefinger away from the long finger. It is best to ask the patient to refrain as much as possible from using the distal flexor mechanism of the thumb, which can substitute for a true opponens function. The opponens pollicis is one of the more difficult muscles in the body to test, because other thumb muscles can substitute for its function so readily.

In the presence of a distal or wrist-level median palsy, the patient may still pull the thumb away from the palm, using extensor pollicis longus and brevis (radial-innervated) and adduct the thumb across the palm with the adductor pollicis (ulnar-innervated). The patient then uses the more proximal and thus intact median-innervated flexor pollicis longus to pull the tip of the thumb and thumb phalanges down

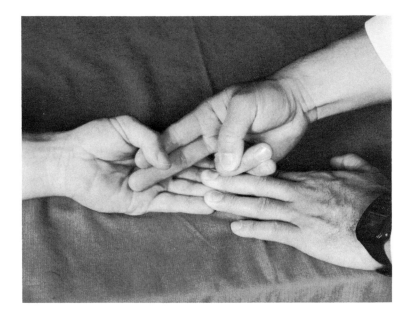

**Figure 8–10.** Opposition of the thumb is tested by having the patient press thumb down against the examiner's forefinger and long finger. When there is full strength of opponens, the examiner will have trouble separating these two fingers.

toward the palmar surface, completing a simulated opponens pollicis or opposition-like maneuver.

## PALMAR AND DIGITAL LEVELS

Median nerve injury at a palmar level can give variable findings because there is some variation of the take-off of the digital branches and even of the thenar recurrent branch. Small branches or twigs leave proximal digital nerves to supply lumbricals and interosseous muscles. The digital nerves then continue on to eventually supply sensation to the skin of the volar digits. Feeling is also provided for the volar and dorsal surfaces of the distal phalange and the volar surface of the intermediate phalange of the forefinger. Sensation is also provided to a portion of the volar surface of the long finger and sometimes to some of the ring finger along its radial aspect. Lacerations to fingers or thumb are frequent and can involve digital nerves. Crush and contusive injury can also be responsible for digital distribution sensory loss. As might be suspected under these circumstances, sensation is usually diminished or absent along the corresponding half of the palmar portion of the finger.

## COMMENTS ON ELECTRODIAGNOSTIC STUDIES

Muscles innervated by the median nerve are all distal to the level of the elbow. Therefore, for arm injuries that are severe and complete, denervational change is present in all median-innervated muscles and at loci quite distal to the injury site. This means that reversal of such electrical changes, even in proximally innervated muscles such as pronator teres, palmaris longus, and flexor superficialis, takes a number of months. Sampling of palmaris longus is difficult except for the experienced electromyographer, as is differentiating flexor superficialis from pronator teres and the median-innervated portion of the flexor profundus from that portion innervated by the ulnar nerve. Nonetheless, the profundus is a good diagnostic muscle because its ulnar half is innervated by that nerve and its radial half by the median nerve. Skillfull medial placement of the electromyographic needle can assess the ulnar-innervated profundus, whereas lateral placement assesses the median-innervated portion of the profundus.

In checking for anterior interosseous nerve syndrome, the median-innervated profundus to the forefinger is sampled along with flexor pollicis longus, the next muscle downstream from the profundus. Stimulation of the median nerve above the elbow and recording of muscle action potentials (MAPs) from the muscles provide a latency value that is increased if the anterior interosseous branch is entrapped or partially injured. With more severe injury to the proximal median nerve or its anterior interosseous branch, denervational changes are also present in the flexor pollicis longus and flexor profundus to the forefinger. With midforearm-level injury to the median nerve, the flexor pollicis longus is the key muscle to needle in addition to thenar intrinsics such as abductor pollicis brevis and opponens pollicis. These thenar intrinsic muscles should also be needled with evaluation of wrist-level injury to the median

nerve.[76] Altered latencies for MAPs can also be recorded from these muscles with entrapment of the median nerve at the wrist or with carpal tunnel syndrome (CTS).

Sensory conduction is more likely to be abnormal with early CTS than motor conduction. Sensory latencies are determined by stimulating digital nerves and recording a nerve action potential (NAP) from the wrist proximal to the flexor crease (orthodromic conduction) (Figure 8–11). The latter site can also be used for stimulation of the median nerve so that needle recordings of MAPs from thenar intrinsic muscles can be accomplished or sensory NAPs can be recorded at skin level from more distal fingers (antidromic conduction). One of the difficulties in recording digital sensory potentials in an an-

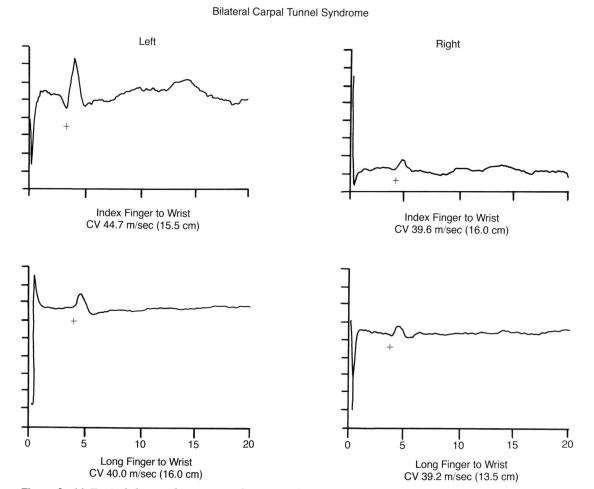

Bilateral Carpal Tunnel Syndrome

Left

Right

Index Finger to Wrist
CV 44.7 m/sec (15.5 cm)

Index Finger to Wrist
CV 39.6 m/sec (16.0 cm)

Long Finger to Wrist
CV 40.0 m/sec (16.0 cm)

Long Finger to Wrist
CV 39.2 m/sec (13.5 cm)

**Figure 8–11.** Typical abnormal sensory conduction studies in a patient with bilateral carpal tunnel syndrome. Stimulation sites were digital nerves, and recording site was the wrist. Since distance between stimulation and recording sites and latency between stimulation and onset of evoked response were known, conduction velocity could be calculated. CV = conduction velocity.

tidromic fashion is that the recordings may be contaminated by MAPs arising from thenar eminence or, more frequently, from lumbrical muscles.

Peripheral metabolic neuropathies have slowing of conduction as great as might be expected across the wrist with CTS, but conduction is also at least as slow more distally, such as from the palm to the digits. Electrical sampling of thenar eminence musculature usually does not show denervation except in severe cases of CTS syndrome. On the other hand, if a MAP is recorded from thenar intrinsics after stimulation of median at the wrist, then motor conduction across the carpal tunnel can be determined. In addition, forearm-level slowing of conduction is frequently seen in the more severe examples of CTS, indicating some retrograde degeneration of axons.

Pronator syndrome or compression of median nerve at the elbow level may be difficult to document electrically, especially in its early stages. If denervation is present, it can be found in proximal muscles as well as distal ones. Because the median nerve penetrates between deep and superficial heads of pronator in 85% of cases, a tendinous band within muscle may, in a few cases, constrict the nerve. This can result in slowing of conduction and a mild, partial median nerve syndrome distal to this level.

# SURGICAL EXPOSURE OF THE MEDIAN NERVE

## Arm Level

Exposure of the median nerve at this level can be but is not always straightforward. Incision is made superficial to the cleft between biceps/brachialis and triceps and over the course of the usually palpable brachial artery. As lateral and medial cord branches blend together to form median, they do so directly over and often somewhat attached to the volar surface of the axillary to brachial artery junction. The nerve may be somewhat adherent to the artery at this level and must be carefully dissected away. The medial antebrachial cutaneous nerve is of smaller caliber and is usually easily distinguished from the median nerve. The median nerve takes an almost straight course down the arm and toward the volar elbow but farther distally tends to lie more lateral to brachial artery, although the nerve's mesoneurium tends to adhere the nerve to vessel. By contrast, the ulnar nerve, after its origin from medial cord, begins to take a slightly oblique course as it heads for the region of the olecranon at the back of the elbow. On rare occasions, the median nerve at arm level may send a branch to biceps brachialis. Quite rare is a connection between the ulnar and median nerves at the level of the arm and comprising a proximal Martin-Gruber anastomosis. Whenever possible, these connections, if present, should be preserved during the dissection. As the median nerve approaches the elbow, it may give off an early branch to the proximal pronator.

With injury and concomitant scar, it is important to skeletonize at least a portion of the artery so it can be protected as the median nerve is manipulated away from it and repaired. In a practical sense, adequate exposure and identification usually involve some exposure of not only artery but also ulnar nerve. Venous branches running to brachial and eventually axillary vein often cross median nerve at the arm level and may have to be ligated or coagulated to adequately expose median nerve and to gain length for operative electrical studies and repair. This can be done without compromise of important venous drainage because this drainage is located medially, inferiorly, and somewhat parallel to artery and nerve rather than crossing the latter.

## Elbow and Forearm Level

Median nerve along with brachial artery runs beneath lacertus fibrosus at the level of the elbow. After giving some branches to the pronator teres, it then goes deep to this muscle. Exposure at the elbow usually begins with an incision over the distal arm's brachial groove that runs slightly transversely in the flexor crease of the elbow and then extends distally, overlying the cleft between the brachioradialis and pronator. The nerve tends to lie beneath the lateral or radial edge of the pronator as it runs deep to this muscle and the flexor superficialis. There are many branches at the elbow level, and these can be dissected out to provide some mobility for the main nerve. These take an oblique course toward the pronator, palmaris longus, and flexor superficialis and should be preserved whenever possible (Figure 8–12).

Beneath the flexor superficialis, the median divides into anterior interosseus and main median. The former supplies the median half of the profundus, primarily to the forefinger and long finger, and the latter runs beneath flexor musculature to eventually give a branch to the flexor pollicis longus at midforearm to distal forearm level. There can be some variation in take-off of the anterior interosseus, with sometimes more than one branch originating this outflow. The anterior interosseus may also penetrate through a slip of flexor superficialis muscle or fascia, and this may, on occasion, predispose it to entrapment.

### Distal Forearm and Wrist

Skin incision begins on the volar wrist and extends proximally on the forearm. It is made in an up-and-down fashion and just to the radial side of the palmaris longus. The nerve stays beneath muscle until it reaches the more distal forearm, where it nestles between multiple tendons. The wrist-level extension of the transverse carpal ligament or the antebrachial fascia covers the nerve, and this must be opened to expose the nerve at the wrist. At this level, the median nerve lies somewhat deep to the palmaris longus and yet superficial to both the flexor superficialis and profundus tendons. As the nerve

approaches the distal forearm, a branch leaves its dorsal surface to run to the pronator quadratus. Closer to the wrist, a thenar sensory branch leaves the radial side of the nerve and can usually be dissected out and spared. Most of the surrounding tendons, especially those adjacent to or somewhat overlying the median nerve, can be mobilized and encircled with a Penrose drain to retract them from nerve. Care must be taken in placing self-retaining retractors at this level because not only tendons but also nearby ulnar nerve and artery or radial artery can be easily damaged.

As the median enters the palm of the hand, it runs under the transverse carpal ligament, which should be sectioned whenever nerve is exposed and manipulated at the wrist or distal forearm levels. Soft tissue swelling can otherwise extend distally and lead to entrapment at this level.

### Palm and Hand

Incisions for exposure for injuries and CTS are usually made in the lifeline of the palm. Palmar skin is thick, but the amount of subcutaneous tissue varies from patient to patient. Underlying transverse carpal ligament usually has a grayish color and is especially thick at the heel of the palm. If there is an opportunity, we usually open the ligament first at the midpalmar level where it is not as thick, and then, with scalpel or scissors, ligament is opened more proximally and distally (Figure 8–13). Even if

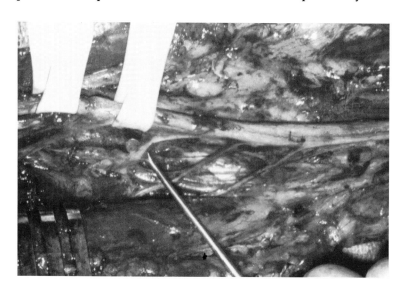

**Figure 8–12.** Anatomy of median at the level of the elbow. Arm is to the right and forearm is to the left. Lacertus fibrosus has been sectioned and pronator teres split away to expose this portion of the nerve. Pronator, flexor superficialis, and anterior interosseous branches can be seen. See also color figure.

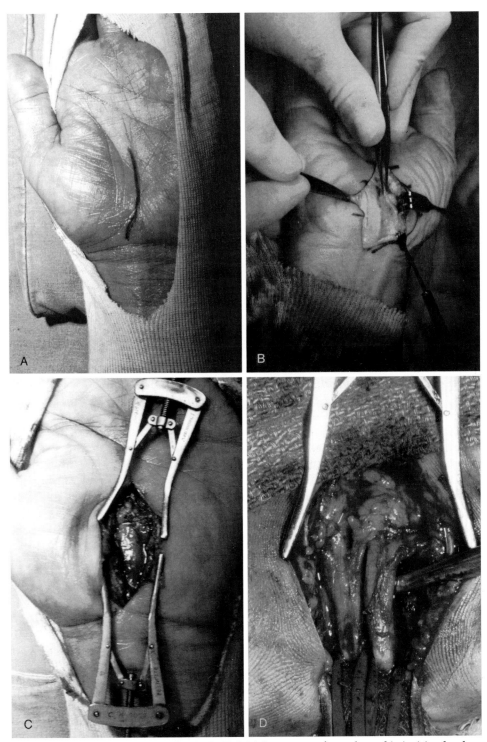

**Figure 8 – 13.** (*A*) Usual palmar incision for CTR. (*B*) Initial exposure after palmar skin incision has been made. (*C*) Median nerve, in this case somewhat scarred and thickened, is exposed by the palmar incision. (*D*) In another case, a bifid median nerve was exposed at the time of a carpal tunnel release.

the incision is not extended proximal to the wrist level, which we usually do not do for CTR, subcutaneous tissue of the wrist is undermined from the level of the palmar incision. One blade of the Metzenbaum scissors is then slid on top of the median and the other blade on top of transverse carpal ligament. Wrist-level ligament and antebrachial fascia of the forearm are then sectioned with the scissors. Usually, this is done on top of but toward the ulnar side of the median nerve to avoid cutting the thenar sensory branch. This arises usually from the radial side of the nerve 2 to 3 cm or so proximal to the distal wrist crease. In the distal palmar space, the superficial palmar arcade of vessels tends to lie superficial to the digital branches and to cross them in a transverse fashion. The deep palmar arcade is dorsal and thus deep to the digital branches. These branches head toward the base of the long finger and the forefinger. They give off small branches to underlying lumbricals and are sometimes accompanied by small arterial and venous branches from the palmar arcades of vessels.

Origin of the thenar recurrent branch is somewhat variable. This branch can run obliquely and forward from the nerve if it originates at a proximal palmar level or, as is more usual, runs transversely if it arises from the median at midpalmar level. In some instances, the thenar recurrent has a more distal origin and actually takes a backward course to go to thenar muscles. The branch can and often does divide before reaching musculature. Great care must be taken in dissecting along the radial side of the median nerve at a palmar level to preserve the recurrent thenar branch.

Serious injury involving the main median nerve before it branches at palmar level may require internal neurolysis. One way to do this and preserve as much nerve as possible is to isolate digital and recurrent thenar branches. These are then dissected proximally through the lesion in continuity. This results in an internal neurolysis of the nerve in which scar from not only epineurium but also interfascicular epineurium is removed.

Differential recording of NAPs can be done at a fascicular level or from a group of fascicles as well as from nerve as a whole. Grafts, if necessary, can extend from bundles or groups of fascicles proximally to digital and thenar recurrent branches distally.

Many lesions at this level are operated on under local anesthesia, especially CTR. A tourniquet is not used, and usually these patients are operated on and return home on the same day. In the case of CTS, the transverse carpal ligament should be inspected before incision to exclude its penetration by a palmar cutaneous sensory branch. The palmar cutaneous should be preserved to minimize palmar paresthesias and pain. Usually, we prefer to do an external neurolysis of the median, clearing or freeing the nerve at least at the palmar level 360 degrees around. Heaped up or inflamed synovia enveloping nerve is resected. We usually also resect a strip of transverse carpal ligament on either side to minimize reformation of the ligament. We do not close or imbricate the ligament, but we do close the subcutaneous tissue, with No. 3 or 4 resorbable suture, and the skin, usually but not always, with a running but buried subcuticular suture of 4-0 suture. Steri-Strips are then usually applied to the skin incision. Before closure, any oozing or bleeding points are sought out and coagulated with use of the bipolar forceps. A serious surgical complication at this level is a palmar hematoma of enough size to compress median or ulnar nerves. As a result, meticulous hemostasis is very important. A mildly compressive dressing is applied using a soft, circular wrap of dressings. A boxing glove-like dressing is fashioned, leaving the tips of the fingers and thumb exposed so the patient can be encouraged to move and use them relatively early postoperatively.

## RESULTS

### Arm-Level Lesions

Results with a number of other series of median injuries have been published and are worth careful study.[25,40,53,65,66] Some of these reports have been nicely reviewed by Cooney.[13] Most of these and other series have tended to be weighted toward more distal median injuries since they were reported by orthopedists or plastic surgeons or those interested in hand surgery.[43,46,52,83] There are a few exceptions, but most of these summarizations are based on war wounds involving this nerve[56,58,82,84] (Tables 8–1, 8–2, and 8–3). Although a variety of tendon transfers is available for median palsy, those

**TABLE 8–1**
Median Cases — Series Reported

| Series | Median Cases | Total No. of Nerve Cases |
|---|---|---|
| Alexander — Britain WW I | 179 | 876 |
| Burrow & Carter — Britain WW I | 242 | 1406 |
| Worster-Drought — Britain WW I | 323 | 1008 |
| Frazier — U.S. Army I | 269 | 2390 |
| Frazier/Silbert — U.S. Army I | 88 | 378 |
| Pollock/Davis — U.S. Army I | 172 | 985 |
| Tinel — French Army I | 67 | 408 |
| Foerester — Germany WW I | 800 | 3907 |
| Bristow — Brtain WW II | 451 | 2636 |
| Woodhall/Beebe — U.S. WW II | 707 | 2276 |
| Sunderland — Australia WW II | 66 | 365 |

done in these patients seemed much less effective than those done in other patients with radial or ulnar palsies.[59,64]

Table 8–4 lists patients seen and evaluated and those operated on by mechanism leading to loss. Lacerations and gunshot wounds were responsible for the majority of injuries. Tumors also led to operation in many cases. In our series, median nerves injured at an arm level did surprisingly well in that a very large number of those operated on had restoration of enough sensation in the median distribution to be at least protective. In addition, pronation by means of pronator teres and some degree of wrist and finger flexion was recovered. This degree of return provided a grade of 3 using the LSUMC system (Figure 8–14). In addition, 14 patients gained a grade of 4 owing to recovery of flexor pollicis longus and flexor profundus to the forefinger as well as more proximal median-innervated muscles and at least S3 sensation.

Few patients requiring proximal repair gained a grade 5, which required recovery of median-innervated thenar intrinsics as well as excellent

**TABLE 8–2**
Median Nerve Secondary Suture Repair Results (Seddon)

| | |
|---|---|
| Arm and elbow level | 36% M3 S3+ or better recovery |
| Forearm level | 25% M3 S3+ or better recovery |
| Wrist level | 43.6% M3 S3+ or better recovery |

M = motor grade; S = sensory grade.

**TABLE 8–3**
Median Repair Results (Dellon)

| | |
|---|---|
| High-level suture repair | 30% M4 or better recovery |
| | 17% S3+ or better recovery |
| Low-level suture repair | 45% M4 or better recovery |
| | 33.5% S3+ or better recovery |
| Combined high and low graft repair | 33% M4 or better recovery |
| | 26% S3+ or better recovery |

M = motor grade; S = sensory grade.

sensory return (S4 or S5). Two that did were gunshot wounds in which, at operation, a NAP could be recorded across a lesion in continuity several months after wounding. Both cases had a neurolysis and, as predicted, recovered considerable function. Other gunshot wounds had no recordable NAPs through lesions in continuity and were resected and repaired by end-to-end suture (6 cases) or graft (1 case). Despite such a proximal level for repair, function returned to a grade 4 level in six of these seven cases. Other cases recovering after operation to grade 4 or grade 4 to 5 levels included lacerations repaired either primarily or secondarily or those contused nerves needing only a neurolysis rather than resection because of the presence of a NAP (Table 8–5). In addition, one injection injury and four stretch/contusion injuries associated with fractures recovered to a grade 4 or better level. Table 8–6 provides the grades for operated arm-level lesions by mechanism of injury or lesion type.

## Laceration

Four of the 15 lesions of proximal median nerve associated with a lacerating injury left the

**TABLE 8–4**
Arm Level Median Nerve — Mechanisms of Injury — LSUMC Series

| Mechanism | No. Seen | No. Operated |
|---|---|---|
| Laceration | 18 | 15 |
| Gunshot wound | 22 | 12 |
| Fracture | 5 | 5 |
| Stretch/contusion | 5 | 4 |
| Compression | 7 | 4 |
| Injection | 1 | 1 |
| Tumor | 12 | 10 |
| TOTAL | 70 | 51 |

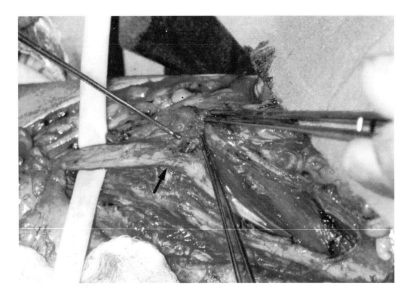

**Figure 8-14.** This median nerve was injured at a proximal level when a Swan-Ganz catheter was removed and a suture was placed in the nerve (*arrow*). Exploration was timely and was done 3.5 months later because of complete clinical and electrical loss. Resection was necessary, and, over a 3.5-year period, the patient regained a sensory grade of 3 and motor grade of 3 to 4.

nerve in continuity, had a NAP on recording across an area of contusion, and recovered to a grade of either 4 (3 cases) or 5 (1 case). Three primary suture repairs were done; of these, two gained at least a grade 4 result, and one achieved a grade 5. Three secondary grafts regained a grade 3 or better result, and three reached only a grade 2 level (Figures 8–15 and 8–16).

### Gunshot Wound

There was only one failure in this group of 12 operated patients and that was an individual who required 10-cm (4-inch) grafts to replace a segment of proximal median nerve damaged by a shotgun blast. Fortunately, most proximal median injuries caused by gunshot wound and requiring resection were focal enough to be repaired by suture or, in one case, by split repair.

### Fractures and Contusions

Eight of these nine lesions fared well with repair. The majority required placement of grafts because of their lengthy up-and-down nature. One such repair, left unrepaired until 12 months after injury, not unexpectedly failed.

### Compressive and Injection Injuries

Severe high median palsy resulting from either compression by a crutch or a sleep palsy from placing arms over the back of a chair was usually managed conservatively, although a few cases required operation. Operative results were excellent in two (grade 5), fair in one (grade 3), and poor in one (grade 2). Those treated conservatively had partial loss to begin with, and, in the early weeks after compression, showed significant improvement and had an eventual good result with spontaneous regeneration (Table 8–7).

The one injection injury was caused by an attempted needling to draw blood from the medial upper arm. Loss, although present, was minimal. Neurolysis was done for pain, and, fortunately, this improved and eventually disappeared. Damage under these circumstances is usually more extensive and may require resection and repair. Such a lengthy injection injury

**TABLE 8-5**
Arm Level Median Nerve — Operations

| | | | |
|---|---|---|---|
| Patients operated on— 51 | | | |
| Not in continuity | — 12 | | |
|    Primary repair | — 3 | Improved— | 2 |
|    Secondary repair | — 9 | Improved— | 5 |
|      Graft | — 8 | Improved— | 4 |
|      Suture | — 1 | Improved— | 1 |
| In continuity | — 29 | | |
|    Positive NAP | — 17 | Improved— | 16* |
|    Negative NAP | — 12 | Improved— | 10 |
|      Graft | — 7 | Improved— | 5 |
|      Suture | — 5 | Improved— | 5 |
| Tumors: 9 of 10 removed | | | |
|   without deficit | | | |

NAP = nerve action potential.
*Had neurolysis with improvement.

**TABLE 8-6**
Arm Level Median Nerve — Results of Operation (n = 51)

| Causes | Total Cases | Functional Grade Achieved | | | | | | Insufficient Follow-up |
|---|---|---|---|---|---|---|---|---|
| | | 5 | 4 | 3 | 2 | 1 | 0 | |
| Laceration | 15 | 1 | 6 | 4 | 4 | 0 | 0 | 0 |
| Gunshot wound | 12 | 2 | 6 | 3 | 1 | 0 | 0 | 0 |
| Fracture | 5 | 0 | 1 | 3 | 1 | 0 | 0 | 0 |
| Contusion | 4 | 0 | 1 | 3 | 0 | 0 | 0 | 0 |
| Compression | 4 | 2 | 0 | 1 | 1 | 0 | 0 | 0 |
| Injection | 1 | 0 | 1 | 0 | 0 | 0 | 0 | 0 |
| Tumor | 10 | 6 | 2 | 1 | 1 | 0 | 0 | 0 |
| TOTALS | 51 | 11 | 17 | 15 | 8 | 0 | 0 | 0 |

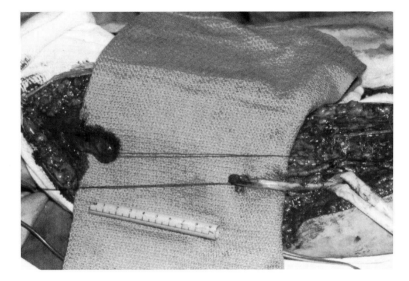

**Figure 8-15.** Long gap in median at arm level caused by a blunt transecting injury. Grafts required for repair had to be 10 cm long despite mobilization of both ends and mild flexion of the elbow.

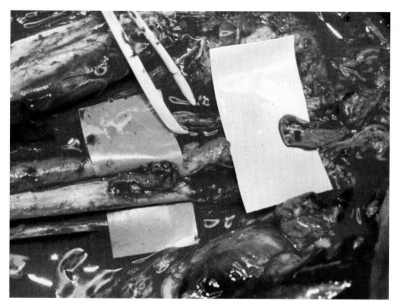

**Figure 8-16.** Preparation of bluntly lacerated median at an axillary level for repair.

**TABLE 8–7**
Arm Level Median Nerve—Results With No Operation (n = 19)

| Causes | Total Cases | Functional Grade Achieved | | | | | | Insufficient Follow-up |
|---|---|---|---|---|---|---|---|---|
| | | 5 | 4 | 3 | 2 | 1 | 0 | |
| Laceration | 3 | 0 | 2 | 1 | 0 | 0 | 0 | 0 |
| Gunshot wound | 10 | 3 | 5 | 1 | 0 | 0 | 1 | 0 |
| Fracture | 0 | 0 | 0 | 0 | 0 | 0 | 0 | 0 |
| Contusion | 1 | 1 | 0 | 0 | 0 | 0 | 0 | 0 |
| Compression | 3 | 2 | 1 | 0 | 0 | 0 | 0 | 0 |
| Injection | 0 | 0 | 0 | 0 | 0 | 0 | 0 | 0 |
| Tumor | 2 | 1 | 1 | 0 | 0 | 0 | 0 | 0 |
| TOTALS | 19 | 7 | 9 | 2 | 0 | 0 | 1 | 0 |

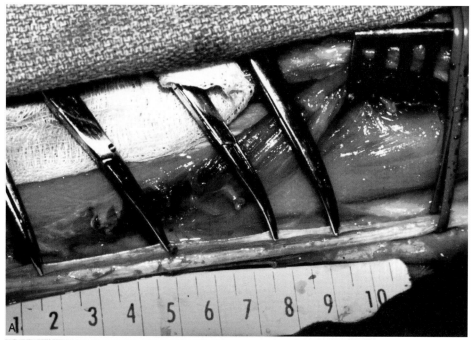

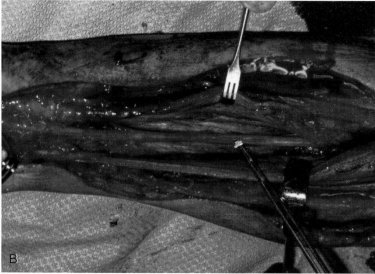

**Figure 8–17.** (*A*) Lengthy injection injury involving median nerve in a physician as the result of an axillary-level anesthetic block. (*B*) Ulnar nerve is being gently retracted to better expose injured median. This severe lesion in continuity required resection and a graft repair.

**TABLE 8–8**
Arm Level Median Nerve
Previous Operations in Operated Nerve Cases (n = 51)

| | Laceration | Gunshot Wound | Fracture | Stretch/Contusion | Injection |
|---|---|---|---|---|---|
| Vascular repair | 8 | 7 | 0 | 1 | 0 |
| Prior operation on nerve | 3 | 1 | 1 | 0 | 0 |
| Fracture operation | 0 | 2 | 1 | 1 | 0 |
| Fasciotomy | 0 | 1 | 0 | 0 | 0 |
| TOTALS | 11 | 11 | 2 | 2 | 0 |

to arm level median nerve cared for relatively recently and thus not included in Table 8–7 is seen in Figure 8–17.

## Tumors

These included a lymphoid lymphoma compressing median nerve and schwannomas and neurofibromas intrinsic to nerve. These were resected without great difficulty, although one patient with a neurofibroma had some residual hyperesthesia mixed with hypoesthesia in the thumb and forefinger following tumor resection.

Table 8–8 shows the large number of operations associated with the arm level median lesions reported in this series. This included 16 operations for vascular repair. Table 8–9 shows the array of intervals between injury and operation. Twenty-eight of the 41 injuries operated on had their procedure done within the first 3 months.

## Arm-Level Lesion Case Summaries

### Case Number 1

This 19-year-old youth was shot in the right midarm with a 22-caliber pistol. Wound of entrance was on medial arm and exit was posterolateral. There was no humeral fracture. Acutely, a repair of the brachial artery was done by use of a vein graft. Postoperatively, median loss was thought to be incomplete because of retention of some pronator and finger flexor function. Despite these findings, electromyograms done at both 1 and 2 months after injury showed a severe denervational pattern.

Median nerve was exposed along medial arm 9.5 weeks after injury. A lesion in continuity 2.6 cm in length was tested by NAP stimulation and recording. There was no distal muscle response on stimulation, and no NAP transmitted across the lesion, so it was resected. This was repaired by an end-to-end suture. Histologic studies showed the resected segment to be neurotmetic or a Sunderland grade 4 lesion.

By 3 years postoperatively, sensation in the median distribution graded 4, as did motor function. The patient was able to use his arm to work as a carpenter.

**TABLE 8–9**
Arm Level Median Nerve Operative Intervals for Injuries (n = 41)

| Mechanism | Months Between Injury and Operation | | | | | | | | | | | |
|---|---|---|---|---|---|---|---|---|---|---|---|---|
| | 0 | 1 | 2 | 3 | 4 | 5 | 6 | 7 | 8 | 9 | 12 | >12 |
| Laceration | 3 | 1 | 4 | 5 | 0 | 1 | 1 | 0 | 0 | 0 | 0 | 0 |
| Gunshot wound | 0 | 0 | 5 | 3 | 2 | 2 | 0 | 0 | 0 | 0 | 1 | 0 |
| Fracture | 0 | 0 | 0 | 1 | 2 | 0 | 0 | 1 | 0 | 0 | 0 | 0 |
| Contusion | 1 | 0 | 0 | 1 | 1 | 0 | 0 | 1 | 0 | 0 | 0 | 0 |
| Compression | 1 | 0 | 1 | 2 | 0 | 0 | 0 | 0 | 0 | 0 | 0 | 0 |
| Injection | 0 | 0 | 0 | 0 | 0 | 1 | 0 | 0 | 0 | 0 | 0 | 0 |
| TOTALS | 5 | 1 | 10 | 12 | 5 | 4 | 1 | 2 | 0 | 0 | 1 | 0 |

## Comment

Some gunshot wounds leaving nerves in continuity get better spontaneously, but if there is no substantial clinical improvement by 3 months or so, then exploration is certainly indicated.

### Case Number 2

A 24-year-old male sustained a propeller laceration just below the axilla to medial arm while water skiing. He also sustained a scapular fracture. He required acute repair of the proximal brachial artery, and then, 2 days later, he was returned to the operating room for primary suture of a divided and probably bluntly transected median nerve. Ulnar, although badly injured, was found in continuity and left alone.

The patient was then referred because of persistent complete loss of median and ulnar function clinically and electrically. When explored by us at 6 months after injury, a suture neuroma of median nerve and a lesion in continuity of ulnar nerve were found. Neither nerve transmitted a NAP beyond their lesions. Both lesions in continuity were resected to healthier tissue. Stumps were then sutured end-to-end. Length was made up by mobilization of both stumps and transposition of the distal ulnar to a submuscular position volar to the elbow.

Follow-up at 8 years showed partial median recovery with motor and sensory grades of 3. Ulnar recovery was worse and graded only a 2 overall. The patient used the arm and hand to help his dominant right upper extremity, but only as a helper limb.

## Comment

Perhaps a better initial management of this case would have been a delay of repair of the median for several weeks, because this was a blunt transection. At that time or later, the ulnar nerve could have been evaluated by NAP recordings, and a more timely repair of this nerve could have also been done.

### Case Number 3

This 36-year-old male had renal failure resulting from glomerulonephritis. A Gore-Tex shunt was placed from the brachial artery to vein for dialysis. Immediately postoperatively, he experienced arm pain radiating to the hand as well as painful paresthesias in the fingers and thumb. Both median and ulnar palsies were noted. The palsies appeared to progress in the early months after placement of the shunt. Symptoms were initially thought to be caused by a relatively ischemic limb and possible nephritic neuropathy, but when seen 8 months later, it was apparent that both the symptoms and the clinical loss related to the proximal arm-level shunt site. Electromyography showed partial deinnervation in most median- and ulnar-innervated muscles, including those proximal in the limb, such as pronator teres, flexor super-ficialis, flexor carpi ulnaris, and flexor profundi. Conduction studies showed marked slowing along more distal median and ulnar nerves.

The shunt and nerves were approached through a medial upper arm incision between the biceps and triceps and extending up to the axillary area. Both median and ulnar nerves were found entrapped and compressed beneath a limb of the shunt. There was also relatively heavy scar at this point. Nerves were cleaned by working beneath the shunt. Small but definite NAPs could be recorded across both nerves. Postoperatively, the patient had almost immediate relief of his neuritic pain. Function gradually recovered even though the shunt was still used for dialysis. Median and ulnar function each graded 4 overall when the patient was seen in follow-up 3 years later. He was using his arm for most tasks.

## Comment

Some patients who develop a peripheral neuropathy after arteriovenous shunt for dialysis have compression and entrapment as a cause rather than an ischemic or metabolic mechanism.

## Elbow- and Forearm-Level Lesions

*Lacerations* to median nerve at elbow level were fairly frequent and comprised 13 of 47 cases operated on at this level (Table 8–10). Five had prior vascular operations for repair of brachial artery or vein. Some of these cases also had primary suture repair of the nerve elsewhere, and several of these required re-repair.

**TABLE 8–10**

Median Nerve Lesions, Elbow/Forearm Level: Mechanism of Injury

| Mechanism | No. Seen | No. Operated |
|---|---|---|
| Laceration | 20 | 13 |
| Gunshot wound | 10 | 8 |
| Fracture | 7 | 4 |
| Stretch/contusion | 11 | 6 |
| Compression | 5 | 1 |
| Injection | 13 | 8 |
| Volkmann | 4 | 2 |
| Electrical | 1 | 1 |
| Arteriovenous fistula | 1 | 0 |
| Tumor | 4 | 4 |
| TOTAL | 76 | 47 |

**TABLE 8–11**

Median Nerve — Elbow/Forearm Levels —
Operations (n = 47)

| | | |
|---|---|---|
| Not in continuity | — 7 | |
| Primary Repair | — 2 | Improved — 2 |
| Secondary Repair | — 5 | Improved — 4 |
| Graft | — 3 | Improved — 3 |
| Suture | — 2 | Improved — 1 |
| In continuity | —36 | |
| Positive NAP | —23 | Improved — 22* |
| Negative NAP | —13 | Improved — 9 |
| Graft | — 9 | Improved — 6 |
| Suture | — 4 | Improved — 3 |
| Tumors: 3 of 4 removed without further deficit | | |

* 19 had an external neurolysis and improved; 2 had an internal neurolysis and improved; 1 had a split repair and improved.

The need for re-repair had no correlation with whether magnification had been used at the time of the original suture but did relate to how sharp the original transection had been.[51] Two primary repairs done by ourselves at the elbow level fared well, with recovery to grade 4 in both cases (Table 8–11). Secondary repairs of lacerations also had acceptable results. Three grafted nerves recovered, as did one of the two end-to-end sutures. The case report presented at the end of this section demonstrates the usual situation with laceration at this level.

*Gunshot wounds* all produced lesions in continuity and required operation in 8 of 10 cases. Six improved to grade 3 or better levels (Table 8–12). Not all, though, required neuroma resection and repair. Three had NAPs, indicating early and effective regeneration, were spared

resection, and recovered nicely. Three had graft repair, and two had end-to-end suture repair. Of these patients, three had acceptable results, but the other two did not.

*Fracture or contusions* to median nerve did well at this level unless they were complicated by Volkmann ischemic contracture. There were, unfortunately, four of these cases, two of which were not operated on for neural reconstruction because of late referral. The two operated on had neurolysis, one early (within 24 hours) and one late (at 4 months). Both patients had recovery of median function to grade 3 only. The other contused nerves usually had partial deficit to begin with, or they had demonstrable NAPs or muscle response to stimulation and did not have resection.

*Injection injuries* to median at the elbow provided a relatively large category with 13 cases. Deficits were usually, but not always, partial; without exception, they were associated with severe pain. Injection injuries to elbow level median were usually caused by attempted venipuncture or catheterization of the brachial artery. In eight instances, operation was felt to be indicated because of severe pain and paresthesias (see Table 8–12). Seven patients had neurolysis only, and one had a suture repair. Some amelioration of pain was gained as well as preservation of function in the cases having neurolysis. Pain was helped in the one case having resection and repair, but only a grade 3 functional result was obtained. Four cases improved spontaneously and did not require operation (Table 8–13).

**TABLE 8–12**

Median Nerve — Elbow/Forearm Levels
Results of Operated Cases (n = 47)

| Causes | Total Cases | Functional Grade Achieved | | | | | | Insufficient Follow-up |
|---|---|---|---|---|---|---|---|---|
| | | 5 | 4 | 3 | 2 | 1 | 0 | |
| Laceration | 13 | 4 | 4 | 3 | 1 | 1 | 0 | 0 |
| Gunshot wound | 8 | 0 | 4 | 2 | 2 | 0 | 0 | 0 |
| Fracture | 4 | 0 | 3 | 1 | 0 | 0 | 0 | 0 |
| Stretch/Contusion | 6 | 1 | 4 | 0 | 1 | 0 | 0 | 0 |
| Compression | 1 | 1 | 0 | 0 | 0 | 0 | 0 | 0 |
| Injection | 8 | 2 | 5 | 1 | 0 | 0 | 0 | 0 |
| Volkmann | 2 | 0 | 0 | 2 | 0 | 0 | 0 | 0 |
| Electrical | 1 | 0 | 0 | 0 | 1 | 0 | 0 | 0 |
| Tumor | 4 | 2 | 1 | 1 | 0 | 0 | 0 | 0 |
| TOTALS | 47 | 10 | 21 | 10 | 5 | 1 | 0 | 0 |

**TABLE 8–13**

Median Nerve—Elbow/Forearm Levels
Results With No Operation (n = 29)

| Causes | Total Cases | Functional Grade Achieved | | | | | | Insufficient Follow-up |
|---|---|---|---|---|---|---|---|---|
| | | 5 | 4 | 3 | 2 | 1 | 0 | |
| Laceration | 7 | 1 | 5 | 1 | 0 | 0 | 0 | 0 |
| Gunshot wound | 2 | 0 | 1 | 1 | 0 | 0 | 0 | 0 |
| Fracture | 3 | 0 | 2 | 0 | 1 | 0 | 0 | 0 |
| Stretch/contusion | 5 | 0 | 3 | 2 | 0 | 0 | 0 | 0 |
| Compression | 4 | 2 | 0 | 0 | 1 | 0 | 0 | 1 |
| Injection | 5 | 2 | 2 | 0 | 0 | 0 | 0 | 1 |
| Volkmann | 2 | 0 | 0 | 0 | 0 | 1 | 0 | 1 |
| Arteriovenous fistula | 1 | 0 | 0 | 1 | 0 | 0 | 0 | 0 |
| TOTALS | 29 | 5 | 13 | 5 | 2 | 1 | 0 | 3 |

The single *electrical injury* at this level was a late referral, required grafts over a 7.6-cm distance, and had only a grade 2 result.

Table 8–14 shows the prior operations done on the elbow-level injuries. Nine of the 19 operations were previous attempts to repair the nerve. Table 8–15 shows the interval between injury and operation by mechanism of injury.

Anterior interosseous nerve or division was injured by injection in three cases, stretch in one, and burn scar in three. The entrapments which were seen were usually helped by release and neurolysis of the nerve (Figures 8–18 and 8–19; Table 8–16).

## Elbow-Level Lesion Case Summaries

### Case Number 1

This 28-year-old female lacerated her elbow on a plate glass window. She had soft tissue repair and primary su-

ture repair of the median nerve in the antecubital fossa 4.5 hours after injury. She had a complete median palsy below the pronator teres which persisted for 6 months. Electromyography at that time showed complete denervation with no evidence of reinnervation of palmaris longus or flexor superficialis.

The median nerve was explored at 6.5 months after injury (Figure 8–20). A partially distracted suture repair was found, and it did not transmit a NAP or have muscle response on stimulation. Neuromas and intervening scar were resected and the nerve was re-repaired.

The patient has done well with recovery of acceptable median function. Median-innervated finger flexion began to occur by 6 months postoperatively. Follow-up at 5.5 years gave median sensation a grade of 3 and motor a grade of 4 to 5. Thenar intrinsics and forefinger lumbricals graded 3 to 4.

### Comment

Even with a primary repair of a sharp injury, proper mobilization of the stumps and postoperative immobilization for several weeks may be necessary to avoid distraction.

**TABLE 8–14**

Median Nerve—Elbow/Forearm Levels
Previous Operations in Operated Nerve Cases (n = 19)

| | Laceration | Gunshot wound | Fracture | Stretch/Contusion | Compression | Injection |
|---|---|---|---|---|---|---|
| Vascular repair | 5 | 1 | 0 | 0 | 0 | 0 |
| Prior operation on nerve | 5 | 1 | 1 | 2 | 0 | 0 |
| Fracture operation | 0 | 1 | 1 | 0 | 0 | 0 |
| Fasciotomy | 0 | 0 | 0 | 2 | 0 | 0 |
| TOTALS | 10 | 3 | 2 | 4 | 0 | 0 |

**TABLE 8–15**

Median Nerve—Elbow Levels
Operative Intervals for Injuries (n = 43)

| Mechanism | Months Between Injury and Operation | | | | | | | | | | | |
|---|---|---|---|---|---|---|---|---|---|---|---|---|
| | **0** | **1** | **2** | **3** | **4** | **5** | **6** | **7** | **8** | **9** | **12** | **>12** |
| Laceration | 2 | 2 | 2 | 3 | 1 | 1 | 0 | 0 | 0 | 0 | 0 | 2 |
| Gunshot wound | 0 | 0 | 0 | 2 | 2 | 2 | 1 | 0 | 0 | 0 | 0 | 1 |
| Fracture | 0 | 0 | 0 | 2 | 0 | 0 | 1 | 0 | 0 | 0 | 0 | 1 |
| Stretch/Contusion | 0 | 0 | 0 | 1 | 2 | 1 | 0 | 0 | 0 | 0 | 0 | 2 |
| Compression | 0 | 0 | 0 | 0 | 0 | 0 | 0 | 0 | 0 | 0 | 0 | 1 |
| Injection | 0 | 1 | 1 | 1 | 2 | 2 | 0 | 0 | 0 | 0 | 0 | 1 |
| Volkmann | 1 | 0 | 0 | 0 | 1 | 0 | 0 | 0 | 0 | 0 | 0 | 0 |
| Electrical | 0 | 0 | 0 | 0 | 0 | 0 | 0 | 0 | 1 | 0 | 0 | 0 |
| TOTALS | 3 | 3 | 3 | 9 | 8 | 6 | 2 | 0 | 1 | 0 | 0 | 8 |

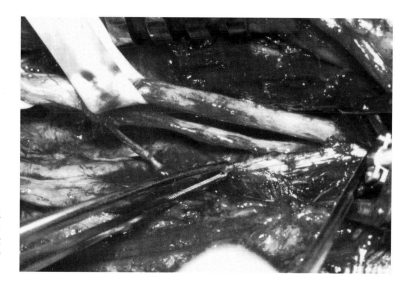

**Figure 8–18.** Fascial band compressing anterior interosseous branch of median at junction of upper and middle third of forearm.

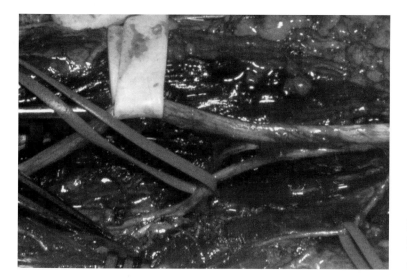

**Figure 8–19.** Anterior interosseous branch is retracted by a Vasoloop, and main median is retracted by Penrose drain.

## TABLE 8-16
## Median Nerve — Anterior Interosseous Nerve Palsies — Results*

| Mechanism | No. Cases/No. Recovered to Grade 3 or Better | |
| --- | --- | --- |
| | Operated | Unoperated |
| Compression by ligament or bone | 4/3 | 0/0 |
| Injection injury | 1/1 | 2/1 |
| Stretch | 1/1 | 0/0 |
| Burn scar | 1/1 | 2/1 |
| TOTALS | 7/6 | 4/2 |

*All lesions in continuity. Loss in distribution of anterior interosseous significant but incomplete. Neurolysis done in each case.

### Case Number 2

A 38-year-old male had open catheterization of the brachial artery for cardiac angiography. After this procedure, the patient had neuritic pain in the median distribution. He described painful dysesthesias that extended down the forearm to the hand. Sympathetic blocks were tried elsewhere but gave only partial relief. Percussion or palpation over the healed incision used for angiography gave pain and some electric shock-like stimuli radiating to the hand. Electromyography showed only mild denervational change in median-innervated muscles, but conduction across the elbow was slowed.

Exploration at 3 months after injury showed a swollen and somewhat scarred median nerve segment beneath the lacertus fibrosus. NAP conduction across the lesion was 38.5 m/sec before and after external and partial internal neurolysis. Function was maintained, and, fortunately, pain was helped a good deal. Follow-up has extended to 4 years.

### Comment

Severe, non-causalgic pain resulting from local nerve injury should usually be managed by direct operation on the nerve rather than by a more central procedure.

### Case Number 3

This 23-year-old male had a water ski flip up and strike the medial surface of the arm above the elbow. Despite direct pressure to the wound, he lost a great deal of blood and required transfusions on reaching the hospital an hour later. The wound was explored, and a short segment of brachial artery was found missing. Ends were trimmed, and an end-to-end arterial anastomosis was achieved. Lacerated and partially thrombosed veins were ligated. The distal end of the median was found beneath pronator muscle and tagged with a suture. Postop-

eratively, there was a pulse to Doppler only, but over several days, a palpable pulse returned. Two months later, the wound was re-explored, but the nerve stumps were found widely apart, and because the surgeon did not feel comfortable attempting a graft repair, the wound was closed.

The patient was subsequently referred for graft repair. He had a complete median palsy including loss of pronator both clinically and by electromyography. There was a diminished but present radial pulse and adequate vascular perfusion of the limb. At exploration 3.5 months after injury, the proximal end of the median with a neuroma was found above the elbow in the medial brachial groove and somewhat adherent to the underlying brachial artery. This was dissected off the vessel and trimmed back to healthy fascicular tissue. The tagged distal stump was found below the elbow and beneath the pronator. After trimming of this stump, a 10-cm gap existed. This was bridged with five grafts using both sural and antebrachial cutaneous nerves.

Follow-up has extended to 9 years. The patient uses the hand to turn valves in an oil refinery and has excellent wrist flexion and finger and thumb flexion. Thenar intrinsics remain quite weak, but he doesn't feel impeded by that. Sensory recovery is less complete, but grades 3 to 4. He still has some pins-and-needles feeling at the tip of the thumb and forefinger. The overall grade for median recovery is 4.

### Comment

Even though this was a complex and lengthy proximal injury, repair gave at least protective median distribution sensation despite the use of long grafts.

### Case Number 4

A 39-year-old carpenter received a stab wound at the elbow level. Entry point was superior to the medial epicondyle, and the knife had been directed laterally and superiorly. Because median loss, although severe, was felt to be partial, he was managed with physical therapy and not referred for further evaluation. On examination 1 year after injury, pronator teres graded 3 to 4, flexor superficialis was quite weak, and flexor profundus to forefinger was absent. Flexor profundus to the long finger was grade 4, probably because its tendon was shared with that to ring finger. Flexor pollicis longus function was absent. There was a trace only of abductor pollicis brevis and opponens pollicis, and forefinger and long finger lumbricals were weak. Sensory grade in the median distribution was 2 to 3. Electromyography showed a severe denervation pattern in the median distribution, with a few nascent units in flexor superficialis and pronator but not elsewhere.

At exploration, a sizable neuroma in continuity was found at the level of the elbow. There was severe scarring just distal to the neuroma. The distal median nerve

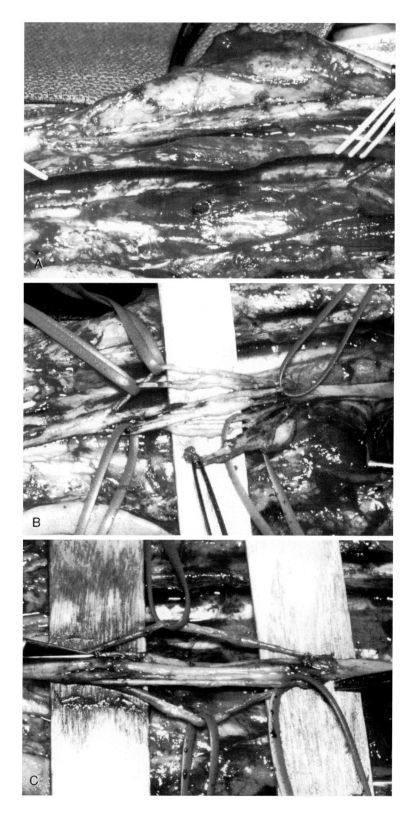

**Figure 8–20.** (*A*) Median lesion in continuity at forearm level resulting from a contusive but partial laceration. Loss before operation was partial, and neuritic pain was a major problem. A nerve action potential (NAP) could be transmitted through the lesion. (*B*) Lesion was split into groups of fascicles; some transmitted NAPs, but most did not. Others, such as the one held by forceps, were obviously neurotmetic. (*C*) A split repair was done. Three fascicular groups had a neurolysis, and four were replaced by grafts 3.175 cm (1.25 inches) in length.

appeared atrophic. Stimulation proximal to the neuroma and recording distally showed a very small NAP. Because a year had elapsed and the response was small, the lesion was resected. Conduction velocity of this small NAP across the neuroma was relatively fast at 70 m/sec. This suggested that the original laceration had spared a small portion of the nerve. This was shown to be the case on histologic examination, during which a small fascicle was found to be spared. The rest of the neuroma consisted of fine fibers mixed with scar. There were only a few moderate-sized fibers.

An end-to-end suture was done after resection of the neuroma. Follow-up was at 14 years. The patient could make a fist but still could not curl his forefinger entirely into the palm. He could, however, flex the tip of the thumb, and this function graded 3 to 4. Sensation in the median distribution graded 4. Although he had some residual stiffness and pain in the fingers, he used the hand for work as a carpenter.

## Comment

Even though a lesion may be partial or nearly complete but not complete, conservative management is not justified in the absence of appropriate improvement and

operation should not be unduly prolonged. See Figures 8–21 and 8–22 for additional examples.

Considerable judgment is required to manage cases with complete loss of function and minor degrees of recovery or cases with partial loss with little recovery. At operation a decision may have to be made even after NAP recordings to sacrifice minor function so that an adequate repair can be done to provide a better end result.

## Forearm-Level Lesion Case Summaries

### Case Number 1

A 56-year-old male sustained a 22-caliber gunshot wound to the proximal forearm. The wound was debrided acutely elsewhere and a sympathectomy was done for what was thought to be true causalgia. This gave only partial relief of his severe pain, which was primarily neuritic and not sympathetically mediated. Pronator teres and finger flexors, including flexor profundus to forefinger and flexor pollicis longus, graded 3 to 4. Thenar intrinsic and median-innervated lumbrical functions were absent. Median distribution sensation graded

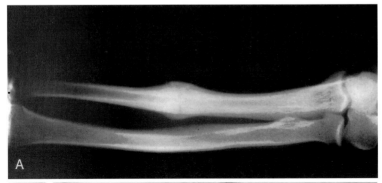

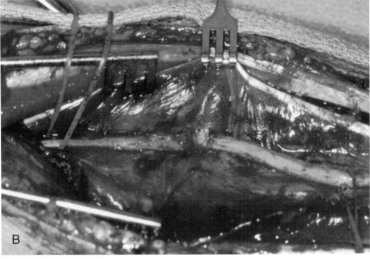

**Figure 8–21.** (*A*) Radius fracture involving median at midforearm level. Distal median loss was still complete at 5 months. Nerve was found entrapped in cicatrix at fracture site (*B*). Resection and end-to-end repair were required.

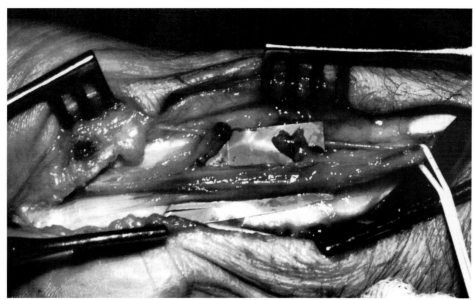

**Figure 8-22.** Distal forearm median injury from resection of "ganglion" at the wrist level. "Ganglion" was in fact a median nerve schwannoma. Preparation for split repair of damaged fascicles by graft and retention of undamaged fascicles.

3 to 4. Electromyography suggested a lesion involving median nerve but distal to the anterior interosseous branch.

Exploration at 5 months showed a lesion in continuity on the main median nerve distal to the anterior interosseous branch. A NAP could be transmitted across the lesion, but stimulation gave no distal muscle function. Only an external neurolysis was done.

The pain was helped a good deal. Follow-up at 10 years showed good use of the limb. Overall motor function graded 4 to 5; median distribution sensation was quite acceptable, but still graded 4.

**Comment**

Sometimes, even external neurolysis may help neuritic pain, but this is by no means a universal outcome. Generally, severe pain from local nerve injury is best treated at least in the early months after trauma by direct repair of the nerve rather than by more central procedures.

**Case Number 2**

This 14-year-old fell playing basketball and sustained a fracture of the radius and ulna. Weakness in finger and thumb flexion and hand intrinsics was noted, as well as sensory loss in the median distribution. Fractures were treated by closed manipulation and then casting for 6 weeks. The patient then received intensive physical therapy, but a complete median palsy involving flexor pollicis longus and more distal thenar and lumbrical function

was noted. Ulnar-innervated hand intrinsics worked but were weak, grading 3. Sensory loss was only in the median distribution.

Median and ulnar nerves were exposed at mid-forearm level 4.5 months after injury. Both nerves were bound down in cicatrix at the fracture site. Both nerves conducted a NAP before and after external neurolysis.

Follow-up after a 4.5-year period showed good recovery of motor and sensory function, not only in the ulnar but also the median distributions. He uses the arm to compete as an amateur in golf tournaments.

**Comment**

All fractures involving a limb require a thorough neurologic examination. Not all blunt injuries to nerve can be managed expectantly.

**Case Number 3**

This 33-year-old male sustained an extensive and complex plate glass laceration to the midforearm. The soft tissue wound was repaired acutely, and a large gap found in the median nerve was not repaired. Clinical examination and electromyography showed complete loss, including that to flexor pollicis longus and more distal muscles. He maintained flexor superficialis and profundus function, and ulnar and radial function were normal. Unfortunately, referral for nerve repair was quite delayed. Three interfascicular grafts 7.6 cm in length were placed at 14 months after injury.

A Tinel sign advanced down the forearm to wrist in the

early months after repair, but overall grades were only 3 for both median sensory and distal median motor evaluations at 6 years.

## Comment

Even though injury is complex to non-neural tissues and requires extensive management, any significant neural injury should not be neglected too long. Ideally, this known transection to the median nerve should have been repaired either acutely or within a few weeks of the original injury once other soft tissues had healed.

## Case Number 4

A 37-year-old female sustained a stress fracture of the right distal radius after lifting a heavy crate. This fracture was casted, but when the cast was removed at 6 weeks after injury, there was inability to flex either the tip of the thumb or that of the forefinger. There was no sensory loss. The elbow and proximal portion of the median nerve and anterior interosseous branch were surgically explored 8 weeks after injury. The median complex appeared normal, but only a very small NAP could be recorded from the anterior interosseous branch.

A neurolysis was done. Recovery began 6 months later, and function was normal by 1.5 years. At last follow-up, 3.5 years later, function of the right hand was normal. The patient had developed, in the interim and quite spontaneously, decreased pinch of the opposite left thumb and forefinger, and these muscles graded 4 on examination. The patient, however, refused further investigation and subsequently has been lost to follow-up.

## Comment

The anterior interosseous syndrome is quite characteristic, and the clinical diagnosis should be made without difficulty. The subsequent spontaneous occurrence on the contralateral side can occur with almost all entrapment syndromes.

### TABLE 8–17
Median Nerve — Wrist Level Mechanisms

| Mechanism | Operated | Unoperated |
|---|---|---|
| Laceration | 16 | 1 |
| Prior suture after laceration | 10 | 3 |
| Gunshot wound | 2 | 0 |
| Fracture | 2 | 5 |
| Prior suture after fracture | 1 | 3 |
| Contusion | 6 | 6 |
| Compression | 5 | 2 |
| Electrical | 2 | 2 |
| Injection | 0 | 1 |
| Stretch | 2 | 0 |
| Tumor | 7 | 1 |
| TOTALS | 53 | 24 |

### TABLE 8–18
Median Nerve Wrist Level Injuries*
Operations Done (n = 46)

**Cases Operated/No. Recovered to Grade 3 or Better Result**

| | |
|---|---|
| Not in Continuity | 15/13 |
|   Primary suture | 5/5 |
|   Secondary suture | 4/3 |
|   Secondary graft | 6/5 |
| In Continuity | 31/29 |
|   +NAP = Neurolysis | 14/14 |
|   −NAP = Repair | 17/15 |
|     Suture | 11/9 |
|     Graft | 6/6 |

*Seven tumors resected and not included in this table; 2 patients had mild to moderate deficit postoperatively; this table does not include carpal tunnel cases.

## Wrist-Level Lesions

*Lacerations* to nerve predominated at this level (Table 8–17). Ten of the 26 laceration cases operated on had prior suture and were thought to be failing or to have failed. Most (8 of 10) required re-repair either by suture or grafts. Despite this, only two failed to gain a grade of 3 or better. Our impression was that at this distal level, aggressive management was necessary in order to optimize results, particularly if sensory loss was significant. Some of the remaining patients had neurolysis because nerves either were recovering after suture or were left in continuity despite laceration as a mechanism of injury. Despite a sharp mechanism for injury, nerve was found to be contused rather than divided and, because of NAPs transmitted across the lesion, had only neurolysis (Table 8–18). Painful

### TABLE 8–19
Median Nerve — Wrist Level
Operative Results (n = 53)

| Causes | Total Cases | Functional Grade Achieved | | | | | | Insufficient Follow-up |
|---|---|---|---|---|---|---|---|---|
| | | 5 | 4 | 3 | 2 | 1 | 0 | |
| Laceration | 26 | 6 | 12 | 6 | 0 | 1 | 1 | 0 |
| Gunshot wound | 2 | 0 | 1 | 1 | 0 | 0 | 0 | 0 |
| Fracture | 3 | 1 | 1 | 1 | 0 | 0 | 0 | 0 |
| Contusion | 6 | 0 | 5 | 1 | 0 | 0 | 0 | 0 |
| Compression | 5 | 1 | 2 | 1 | 1 | 0 | 0 | 0 |
| Electrical | 2 | 0 | 2 | 0 | 0 | 0 | 0 | 0 |
| Stretch | 2 | 0 | 1 | 0 | 1 | 0 | 0 | 0 |
| Tumor | 7 | 3 | 2 | 1 | 1 | 0 | 0 | 0 |
| TOTALS | 53 | 11 | 26 | 11 | 3 | 1 | 1 | 0 |

**TABLE 8–20**
Median Nerve — Wrist Level
Results With No Operation (n = 24)

| Causes | Total Cases | Functional Grade Achieved | | | | | | Insufficient Follow-up |
|---|---|---|---|---|---|---|---|---|
| | | 5 | 4 | 3 | 2 | 1 | 0 | |
| Laceration | 4 | 0 | 2 | 1 | 0 | 1* | 0 | 0 |
| Fracture | 2 | 0 | 1 | 1 | 0 | 0 | 0 | 0 |
| Contusion | 6 | 0 | 5 | 1 | 0 | 0 | 0 | 0 |
| Compression† | 2 | 0 | 1 | 1 | 0 | 0 | 0 | 0 |
| Injection | 1 | 0 | 1 | 0 | 0 | 0 | 0 | 0 |
| Electrical | 2 | 0 | 1 | 1 | 0 | 0 | 0 | 0 |
| Prior Suture | 6 | 1 | 2 | 1 | 0 | 2‡ | 0 | 0 |
| Tumor | 1 | 1 | 0 | 0 | 0 | 0 | 0 | 0 |
| TOTALS | 24 | 2 | 13 | 6 | 0 | 3 | 0 | 0 |

*Refused operation
†One case was caused by tenosynovitis and one by cellulitis
‡Very late referral of both cases

paresthesias were also a problem in a few of these cases and were sometimes helped by neurolysis.

Smaller numbers of patients had nerve contused by *gunshot wound*, fracture of the wrist, direct but blunt blows, stretch, or electrical injuries (Table 8–19). Results with neurolysis if a NAP was recorded were excellent, and repair by either end-to-end suture or grafts also gave good results (see Tables 8–18 and 8–19). Even the two patients with electrical injury gained some degree of recovery (grade 3 to 4) by graft repair. Table 8–20 shows results in a group of patients with wrist-level median lesions treated without operation, at least on our part.

As can be seen in Table 8–21, there were six associated ulnar nerve lesions, mostly in the laceration category. This combination of injuries made total rehabilitation of the hand more difficult and downgraded the eventual results. The intervals between injury and operation (Table 8–22) were spread out between 0 and 12 months or more, although most wrist-level lesions were operated on during the first 6 months after injury. The three cases operated on acutely were transections caused by knives (2 cases) and glass (1 case), and each had a primary end-to-end coaptation with excellent results. Outcomes were also good with delayed repair either after blunt transection or after resection of lesions in continuity. In the entire series, only 5 of the 53 operated cases (8%) did not gain a grade 3 or better result.

The nonoperative category at this level also fared well. Failures in conservative management were mainly caused by very late referral or

**TABLE 8–21**
Median Nerve — Wrist Level — Operated Cases
Previous Operations and Associated Condition (n = 25)

| | Laceration | Gunshot Wound | Fracture | Contusion | Compression | Electrical | Stretch |
|---|---|---|---|---|---|---|---|
| Carpal tunnel release | 1 | 1 | 2 | 3 | 4 | 0 | 1 |
| Partial neuroma resection | 1 | 0 | 0 | 1 | 0 | 0 | 0 |
| Tendon/bone | 5 | 0 | 1 | 3 | 1 | 0 | 0 |
| Neurolysis | 2 | 1 | 0 | 1 | 0 | 1 | 0 |
| Prior suture | 10 | 1 | 0 | 0 | 0 | 0 | 0 |
| Arterial repair | 2 | 0 | 0 | 0 | 0 | 1 | 0 |
| Ulnar nerve injury | 4 | 0 | 1 | 0 | 0 | 1 | 0 |
| Fasciotomy | 0 | 0 | 0 | 0 | 1 | 0 | 0 |
| TOTALS | 25 | 3 | 4 | 8 | 6 | 3 | 1 |

**TABLE 8–22**
Median Nerve — Wrist Level — Operated Cases
Operative Intervals for Injuries (n = 46)

| | Months Between Injury and Operation | | | | | | | | | | | |
|---|---|---|---|---|---|---|---|---|---|---|---|---|
| **Mechanism** | **0** | **1** | **2** | **3** | **4** | **5** | **6** | **7** | **8** | **9** | **12** | **>12** |
| Laceration | 3 | 4 | 2 | 2 | 0 | 1 | 3 | 0 | 3 | 2 | 1 | 5 |
| Gunshot wound | 0 | 0 | 0 | 0 | 0 | 1 | 1 | 0 | 0 | 0 | 0 | 0 |
| Fracture | 0 | 0 | 0 | 1 | 1 | 0 | 0 | 0 | 0 | 0 | 0 | 0 |
| Contusion | 0 | 1 | 0 | 1 | 1 | 0 | 0 | 0 | 0 | 0 | 1 | 2 |
| Compression | 0 | 0 | 0 | 1 | 1 | 0 | 0 | 0 | 1 | 2 | 0 | 0 |
| Electrical | 0 | 0 | 0 | 1 | 0 | 0 | 0 | 0 | 1 | 0 | 0 | 0 |
| Stretch | 0 | 0 | 1 | 0 | 0 | 0 | 0 | 0 | 0 | 0 | 0 | 1 |
| Prior suture | 0 | 0 | 0 | 0 | 0 | 0 | 1 | 0 | 0 | 0 | 0 | 0 |
| TOTALS | 3 | 5 | 2 | 7 | 3 | 2 | 5 | 0 | 5 | 4 | 2 | 8 |

refusal of operation (see Table 8–20). Patients with prior suture were sent for follow-up care and did well in four of six cases that were seen relatively early (less than 1 year after repair). If seen late, 18 months or more after prior suture, re-repair for motor return of thenar intrinsics was not thought to be worthwhile, especially if motor rather than sensory deficit was the major remaining deficit.

## Wrist-Level Lesion Case Summaries

### Case Number 1

This 28-year-old male sustained a 22-caliber gunshot wound to the right distal forearm near the wrist. This was a through-and-through injury entering the volar forearm and wrist and exiting the dorsum of the forearm. There was no fracture, and the patient had a good radial pulse but a complete median palsy from the wrist more distally. The puncture wounds were dressed, and he received tetanus toxoid and was placed on antibiotics. The palsy did not resolve over a 3-month period. Electromyography confirmed a total median palsy with denervation in the abductor pollicis brevis and opponens pollicis. Sensory studies showed no evoked sensory NAPs after stimulation of digital nerves of the forefinger and recording from the wrist.

On exploration at 3.5 months after wounding, there was no NAP evoked across a lesion in continuity at the wrist and stimulation gave no thenar intrinsic function. The lesion was resected, and an end-to-end suture repair was done. The resected segment was neurotmetic (Sunderland grade IV injury) on histologic study.

Sensation in the median distribution at 3.5 years post-operatively graded 4, whereas thenar intrinsic motor function graded only 3. He has been able to work as an electrician's helper.

### Comment

Most of the time, gunshot wounds do not divide nerve but produce a lesion in continuity with a variable potential for recovery. Unfortunately, physical continuity does not guarantee useful recovery. Thus, in the absence of improvement in the early months after wounding, exploration and operative recordings are in order.

### Case Number 2

This 26-year-old male sustained a knife wound to the wrist and a wrist-level median palsy which was complete. At exploration 1 month later, the nerve was found to be partially transected yet still in continuity. There was no response to stimulation above or below the lesion. The partial transection was completed, and both ends were trimmed to healthy tissue. An end-to-end suture was done. Histologic examination of the resected segment showed several small but spared fascicles.

Follow-up extended to 3.5 years and indicated sensory recovery to a grade of 4; thenar and lumbricals graded 3 to 4.

### Comment

Not all penetrating, sharp injuries divide or transect nerve; some may only stretch or contuse nerve and not divide any portion of the nerve. In this case, most but not all of the nerve was divided. The remaining fascicles were, however, bruised and stretched, and this gave a complete deficit. In other cases, fascicles in continuity can be spared but on testing, those in this case were not functional and therefore they were resected. NAP recording at 1 month could not be hoped to give evidence of functional regeneration, even if it were occurring. Simple stimulation in this case did show that the fascicles had been seriously injured.

### Case Number 3

This 4-year-old child fell on a broken glass bottle and sustained a laceration of distal forearm. Initial examination showed a loss of distal thumb flexion as well as blunting of sensation on the tips of the thumb and forefinger and on some of long finger. It was impossible to test thenar intrinsics or lumbricals since the child was crying and uncooperative for most of the examination.

The wound was explored acutely, and both a divided flexor pollicis longus tendon and a transected median nerve were found. The nerve required minimal trimming of both stumps since epineurium had been neatly transected. Both the nerve and the tendon were repaired end-to-end. After closure of the forearm-to-wrist laceration, the wrist and palm were wrapped with circular gauze dressings with the fingertips and thumb tip exposed so they could be moved both voluntarily and passively.

The child did well. By 1.5 years after injury, median sensation graded 4 and thenar intrinsics almost 4. Electromyographic studies showed abundant thenar nascent changes, and sensory NAPs from forefinger to above wrist could be obtained and conducted at 30 m/sec.

### Comment

Clinical or electrical evaluation of children with nerve injury can be quite difficult. The surgeon must retain a high index of suspicion for serious injury, and examination may need to be repeated.

### Case Number 4

Another youngster, who was only 1 year of age, fell and lacerated her right wrist on a piece of metal. The soft tissue wound was cleaned out and sutured in an emergency room. The child tended to suck the fingers of this hand, and the mother brought the child back to the hospital because of ulcerated, eroded fingertips. This involved primarily the forefinger and the long finger. Further examination by another neurosurgery service showed absent median sensation, yet there was no apparent atrophy of the thenar eminence, and abduction and opposition of the thumb appeared to be done with ease.

At exploration, a neuroma in continuity involved median nerve, but it was more severe on the volar than on the dorsal surface. Nerve transmitted a NAP, so an internal neurolysis was done, splitting the nerve into bundles, half of which transmitted and half of which did not. A split repair was done, using sural grafts to replace the presumed sensory portion of the nerve.

The metal fragment must have transected the sensory portion of the nerve but spared, for the most part, the motor portion. Resolution of changes in the skin and nails and restoration of good sensory function occurred over the next 2 years.

### Comment

In this case, despite apparent retention of median motor function, exploration and eventual repair were certainly indicated because of serious sensory loss in an area of great functional importance.

## DIGITAL NERVES— PALMAR AND FINGER LEVELS

Most patients seen in consultation in this category were sent by us to a hand surgeon if repair was indicated, but 18 were managed by us.

Lacerating and contusive injuries were responsible for the majority of these lesions, but in four instances, injury was associated with carpal tunnel release (Figures 8–23 through 8–

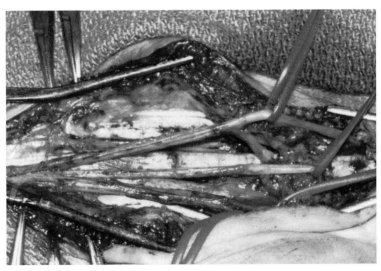

**Figure 8–23.** Internal neurolysis of median at palmar level for very painful lesion in continuity caused by contusion. A nerve action potential transmitted to recurrent thenar and each digital sensory branch, so each group of fascicles was cleared of scar tissue and none were resected.

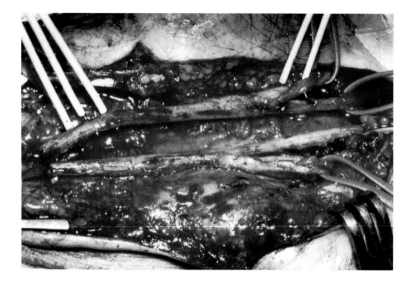

**Figure 8-24.** Direct injury to palmar median. Nerve has been split into two major bundles. One large medial bundle is being stimulated, and recording is from thenar recurrent motor branch.

25; Table 8-23). In eight instances, operation was not judged worthwhile, either because of incomplete loss predicted to improve or because the patient refused operation. Two patients with finger amputations and digital stump neuromas were helped by trimming the digital nerves back to a palmar level, coagulating the fascicles exposed with fine-tipped bipolars, and burying stumps as deeply in the palm as possi-

ble. There were three digital nerve repairs done at distal palmar or finger levels, and each had useful recovery of sensation to a grade 4 level. One of these patients had extensive tendon lacerations and a secondarily stiff hand, making for a delayed and incomplete recovery. Contusive injuries operated on usually had an extensive neurolysis without repair, but one patient with extensive palmar contusion did require a

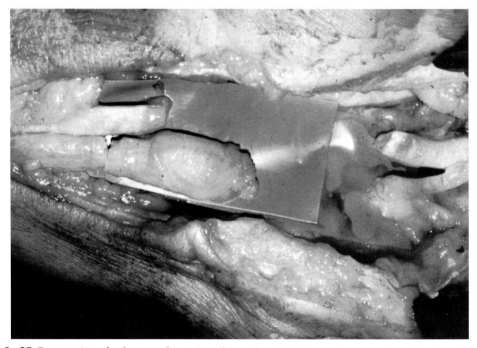

**Figure 8-25.** Preparation of palmar median injury for grafts. Digital branches are to the right. Previous suture was with catgut and no splint was used. Neuroma is undergoing resection.

**TABLE 8–23**

Median Nerve — Digital Nerve Injuries — Results (n = 18)

| Mechanism | No. Operated/No. Significantly Improved | |
|---|---|---|
| | Operated | Unoperated |
| Palmar or Finger Lacerations | 4/3 | 3/2 |
| Contusion/Finger Avulsion | 1/1 | 4/3 |
| Prior Carpal Tunnel Release | 4/3 | 0/0 |
| Electrical | 1/0 | 0/0 |
| Missile | 0/0 | 1/1 |
| TOTALS | 10/9 | 8/6 |

| Operations | | No. Operated/No. Significantly Improved |
|---|---|---|
| Neurolysis | = | 3/3 |
| Suture | = | 2/2 |
| Graft | = | 2/1 |
| Evacuation of hematoma | = | 1/1 |
| Resection of digital nerve for neuroma | = | 2/2 |

graft repair, with recovery of sensation to only grade 2 to 3.

Digital nerves inadvertently injured during CTR for CTS required neurolysis in two instances and repair in two others. Results were good for restoration of some useful sensory function (grade 3), but painful paresthesias and a tender palmar wound remained a problem in two of these patients. One patient had a hematoma of the palm caused by a duck knife wound. Sensory symptoms in the digits improved after the hematoma was evacuated. The palmar electrical injury appeared to be helped somewhat by neurolysis of the median complex in that painful paresthesias in the fingers decreased.

## Digital Nerve Case Summary

This 36-year-old gardener and handyman was injured with an electric hedge clipper, sustaining a blunt laceration to his left forefinger along its radial side at the level of the metacarpophalangeal joint. A primary end-to-end repair was attempted elsewhere. Over the next few months, he developed severe hyperesthesia and pain referred to the tip of the forefinger. There was extreme tenderness at the junction of the palm and forefinger, and tapping there gave paresthesias radiating to the tip of the forefinger.

At exploration 7 months after injury, there was a suture neuroma 2.5 cm in length, and it was apparent that there had been partial distraction of the repair site of the radial digital nerve. This was resected, and the gap was bridged by a 2.6 cm sural nerve graft. To date, the severe pain and hyperesthesia have been relieved, but sensory return on the tip of the forefinger grades only 3 after 2.5 years of follow-up.

## COMPLICATIONS

Dissection of the proximal median nerve can be associated with injury to the brachial artery, on which it lies. This occurred several times, but fortunately the vessel could be directly repaired by one or more fine vascular sutures. It helps to encircle the vessel with tapes both proximal and distal to the epicenter of the nerve injury. Then, if hemorrhage occurs during the nerve dissection, the bleed can be readily controlled and the vessel sutured. Retraction at this level can also compress proximal ulnar nerve, but we had no serious sequelae related to that.

At the elbow level and below, there is not only the risk of arterial or serious brachial venous injury, but also the risk of injury to the posterior interosseus and superficial sensory radial branches of the radial nerve. We were fortunate to be able to avoid any serious loss in those distributions, although sometimes a patient with operation on median at this level reported either a mild decrease in sensation on the dorsum of the hand or mild finger or thumb extension weakness.

Full exposure of midforearm-level median nerve includes splitting or dividing some of flexor superficialis, and some new or additional weakness in finger flexion may be present postoperatively. Thrombosis of the median artery has been reported at this level as a result of injury, or sometimes because of vasculitis or, less frequently, operation. We have not seen that occur as a result of an operation but did do a neurolysis on a patient who had thrombosis of this vessel and severe neuropathy as a result of an unspecified vasculitis.

Complications of managing injury at the wrist include injury to nearby ulnar nerve and artery and section of thenar sensory branches or, in the palm, palmar sensory or recurrent motor branches.

Each of our wrist-level median injuries operated on by ourselves had prophylactic section of the transverse carpal ligament, but despite this, one patient who regenerated through a repair appeared to develop CTS several years later and required a neurolysis at the palmar level. Wound healing or infection was seldom a problem.

## WRIST-LEVEL CARPAL TUNNEL SYNDROME

CTS is caused by compression of the median nerve at the level of the wrist or palm. The transverse carpal ligament, which is about the size of a postage stamp, extends in a somewhat quadrilateral fashion from the ulnar side of the wrist and the pisiform bone over to the base of the thumb. CTS is usually caused by hypertrophy of the ligament with secondary compressive or

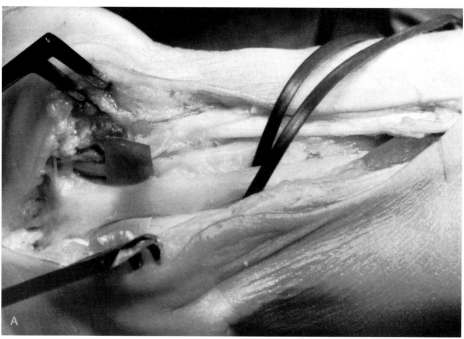

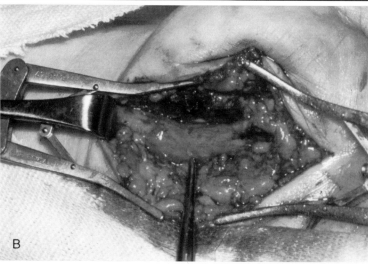

**Figure 8–26.** (A) Thinned and discolored segment of palmar-level median nerve caused by hypertrophied transverse carpal ligament. (B) Scarred and thickened segment of median nerve in patient with long-standing carpal tunnel syndrome.

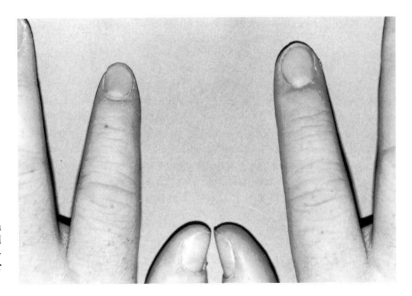

**Figure 8–27.** This child had a long-standing carpal tunnel syndrome on the left. Note tapering of the left forefinger compared with the right.

frictional injury to the median nerve.[16,50] (Figures 8–26 and 8–27). There may be a predisposition in some patients in whom the carpal canal has less volume than normal.[4] In any case, pressure within the canal and presumably on the nerve is usually elevated in the symptomatic patient.[6,23] Injury to or inflammation of soft tissues can produce swelling in this region. As a result, secondary compression of an already snug but previously uncompromised nerve in the carpal canal can also occur.

CTS has been associated with pregnancy, especially in the third trimester, rheumatoid arthritis, synovitis of the flexor tendons, prior or sometimes fresh fracture of the wrist (either a Colles fracture or a reverse Colles fracture), thyroid disorders, and a host of other less common diseases and injuries involving the wrist and wrist joints.[2,19,30,42,49] The syndrome can also occur spontaneously, and actually this is its most frequent presentation.[7,73,78]

Onset of CTS is usually associated with numbness and paresthesias in the median distribution, particularly at the tips of the fingers. Such symptoms can appear to spread to involve ulnar-innervated fingertips as well. The paresthesias frequently awaken the patient at night, and he or she gets up and attempts to "shake it off" or run cool or warm water over the hand to try and improve the symptoms. With time, the sensory symptoms become more permanent, and weakness of the hand, particularly of the thenar intrinsic muscles innervated by the me-

dian nerve, is evident. Abduction and opposition of the thumb can be weak, as can lumbricals function, especially for the forefinger and less so for the long finger. Atrophy of thenar eminence may also occur with long-standing and severe CTS. Usually, however, the patient comes to the physician complaining of only sensory symptoms and perhaps some mild clumsiness of the hand. Fine hand movements such as opening a bottle, turning a doorknob, or holding a pen or pencil between forefinger and thumb can be affected. Such symptomatology is usually evident before atrophy occurs and, in some patients, is as bothersome as the sensory symptoms.[62]

Inability to localize stimuli in the median distribution, particularly in its autonomous zones, is a late finding with CTS, whereas blunting of sensation or hyperesthesia on stroking the volar tip of the forefinger, long finger, or thumb is an earlier finding. Comparison of blunt stimuli to sharp ones may be altered relatively early as well. Often, however, there is no sensory change to testing, even to two-point discrimination, despite the fact that the patient has many sensory complaints. Tapping on the wrist and sometimes the proximal palm gives paresthesias into the hand which may not always be restricted to the median nerve distribution. A Phalen sign, in which acute flexion or sometimes extension or dorsiflexion of the wrist gives median distribution paresthesias, is occasionally present, but it is more frequently absent than one would suspect, even with an acutely symptomatic CTS.[72] Even if the Phalen sign is negative, application of pressure by the examiner's thumb over the nerve at the wrist level as the wrist is either extended or flexed sometimes reproduces the patient's median distribution paresthesias.

Although CTR for CTS is one of the most straightforward and successful operations known, it can and does fail. Of course, the leading cause for failure or partial relief is that there can be other causes for paresthesias, numbness, or pain in the fingers and hand.[28] Most of these simulators are readily differentiated from CTS. Some of these causes include cervical disc and degenerative disease of the spine, diabetic neuropathy and various arthropathies. Despite this, CTS can complicate or add to these primary diagnoses, and if so, CTR is still indicated. Less common are neural-related conditions, including cervical rib involving C7 to middle trunk, pronator or anterior interosseous syndrome, or compression of median in distal upper arm by a Struthers ligament.[32,36,37,54,57,63,70] On the other hand, patients with CTS are often subjected to repeated periods of traction, steroid therapy, myelography, scalenotomy and first rib resection, and even psychotherapy before the transverse ligament is sectioned, frequently with relief of symptoms.

The diagnosis may be missed because the numbness and pain that would be expected to be confined to the distal sensory distribution of the median can involve the whole hand and can radiate up or down the arm.[9] On rare occasions, the presentation may be confined to thenar loss and atrophy caused by compression of the recurrent motor or thenar branch,[3] and the neurologist or surgeon has difficulty conceiving of CTS as the cause of the symptoms.

Although much has been written about the workup of CTS, a few points are worth re-emphasis. Diagnosis of CTS is usually straightforward and can almost always be readily made by taking a careful history. Characteristic is a tingling pain mixed with numbness and associated paresthesias. Onset may be insidious or sudden, but discomfort is usually worse at night and often awakens the patient from an otherwise sound sleep. A Tinel sign on tapping or percussion is almost always present over the course of the nerve, particularly at the wrist and proximal

palm. There may or may not be objective sensory decrease or median-innervated motor abductor pollicis, opponens, and forefinger lumbrical weakness or thenar atrophy.

CTS can be present without electrical concomitants, but they are almost always there if searched for carefully, or there is an alternate explanation for their absence.[26,29,35] Intraoperative conduction changes are even more likely to be present than those recorded noninvasively. This is probably because the operative recordings can be made just across the involved portion of nerve and thus over a shorter segment of median than is utilized by the usual less invasive studies.[18] Even though compound MAPs recorded from thenar muscles after stimulation at the wrist or above may be normal, those sensory NAPs recorded at wrist after stimulation of digital nerves at the fingers or, better yet, in the palm, usually have a slowed conduction across the carpal tunnel.[67]

## FAILURE OF CARPAL TUNNEL RELEASE

As pointed out by Hudson and Mackinnon and others, patients with CTS can have persistent symptoms after CTR, may have temporary relief of symptoms after CTR only to have them recur, or may develop increased symptoms or even new symptoms which differ from those present before surgery.[17,27,28,45] In some clinics, this has led to attempts at conservative, nonsurgical management.[22] These methods can work but require careful, repetitive follow-up, and the patient often comes to surgery anyway.[27,48]

### Persistent Symptoms After CTR

If the initial diagnosis was correct, persistent symptoms are often caused by incomplete division of the transverse carpal ligament, either in the distal palm or at the level of the wrist[33] (Figure 8–28). There may be a proximal extension of the transverse carpal ligament or thickening of what some term the antebrachial fascia at the wrist level. A Tinel sign is usually present at the wrist or distal palm even many months after the original surgery. New sen-

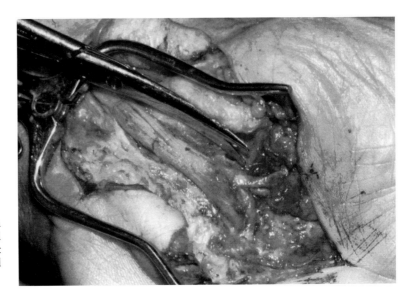

**Figure 8–28.** Median nerve in a patient with persistent carpal tunnel syndrome who did not have distal transverse carpal ligament sectioned.

sory/motor velocity studies may or may not be of help, because conductive abnormalities across the carpal tunnel may persist for many months and sometimes years even after the most successful CTR. The diagnosis of incomplete CTR may be suspected if the incision for the original CTR was placed over the wrist, suggesting the possibility of retention of distal palmar ligament. An inappropriately placed wrist or palmar incision or a very short wrist or distal palmar incision may suggest the possibility of persistent entrapment.[12] Less frequently, hypertrophic and sometimes inflamed synovium may have enveloped the nerve and may have been overlooked at surgery[38] (Figure 8–29).

Even less frequently, a ganglion cyst, lipoma, accessory lumbrical muscle, or other lesion may have intruded on the carpal tunnel and served as a precipitating or complicating feature of CTS. It is possible to overlook such a lesion, especially if the surgeon's principal focus is release of the transverse carpal ligament and not careful inspection of the median nerve and its bed. Unfortunately, incomplete resection of the ligament and injury to other structures, even the ulnar nerve, can occur if a retinaculum or arthroscope is used for the release.[10,61] Even direct exposure of the nerve at a palmar level can be complicated by direct injury to the median nerve.

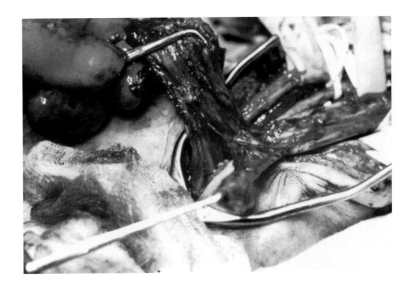

**Figure 8–29.** Tenosynovitis caused by tuberculosis and involving median nerve at the level of the distal forearm and wrist with less involvement of the ulnar nerve. The patient presented with a palpable fullness at wrist and symptoms suggestive of a carpal tunnel syndrome. An extensive synovectomy was necessary, and then the patient was begun on antitubercular drugs.

## Recurrent CTS

Although debated by some, we are convinced that the transverse ligament can reform with time. For that reason, we favor excision of a strip of ligament on either side of the transection at the time of the initial CTR. Nonetheless, reformation of the ligament is difficult to confirm without reoperation. Because such reconstitution does occur, it brings into question the efficacy of purposeful incomplete transverse ligament section or procedures to imbricate or reconstitute the ligament after section in an attempt to improve gripping power between the thumb and other fingers after CTR.[67]

Postoperative scar setting in and around the released nerve has been cited as a cause for recurrence. This is more likely to be a factor if hemostasis at the time of the original surgery was less than adequate, if a palmar or wrist hematoma complicated the original surgery, or if wound healing was incomplete or poor as a result of infection or dehiscence of the wound.

## Increased or New Symptoms After CTR

It is not unusual for numbness and paresthesias and even pain to increase after CTR (Figure 8–30). Usually such symptoms in an otherwise successful CTR are temporary. They are caused by an irritable nerve, perhaps one severely compressed but recently manipulated during CTR. If such symptoms do not resolve in a matter of weeks, or if they are very severe with or without new and significant sensory or motor loss, then there is the possibility that the nerve has been inadvertently injured during CTR. This is more obvious if there is new and significant deficit, but direct neural injury can sometimes be the source of severe pain without additional or new deficit. Sometimes this is caused by overenthusiastic manipulation of the nerve; other times, it results from inadvertent direct surgical injury to the nerve, and in other cases, it may be caused by ill-advised invasion of the nerve. At the present time, there is no indication for internal

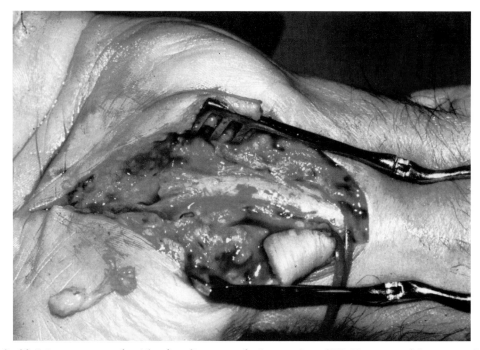

**Figure 8–30.** Injury to sensory fascicle of median nerve during previous CTR. Neuroma of the sensory fascicle has been resected and laid on palmar skin.

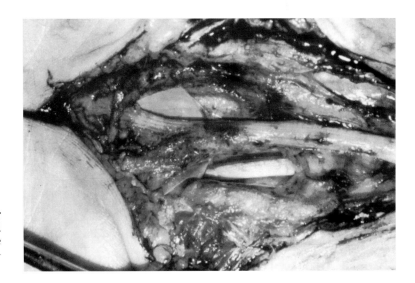

**Figure 8–31.** Injury to palmar portion of the median caused by prior carpal tunnel release attempted through a transverse wrist incision.

neurolysis on the vast majority of spontaneous and previously unoperated median nerves associated with CTS.[15,24,47] Inadvertent injury can and does occur even in the hands of surgeons who are very experienced with this operation (Figure 8–31). This is seldom related to anatomical variation of the nerve and its branches, although this is always a possibility.[39,80] The median nerve can be injured, as can the adjacent ulnar nerve during "arthroscopic" section of the ligament, but these complications can also occur when the ligament is divided under direct vision.

If the pattern of loss and pain doesn't improve in the early months after CTR, then reoperation is in order. This is especially true if a prior operative incision appears to be badly placed (Figure 8–32). Neurolysis of distal palmar branches may help but is often only the initial step in working out the extent of the direct neural injury. Internal neurolysis of the main median nerve at palmar and sometimes wrist level may be necessary. After internal neurolysis, intraoperative NAP recordings can identify or confirm the portion of the nerve that is damaged and help the surgeon decide whether to resect and repair that segment or to be content with a neurolysis. Time necessary for recovery then depends on what type of repair is necessary, time interval between injury and repair, patient age, and all the other usual factors that play a role in nerve regeneration. Restora-

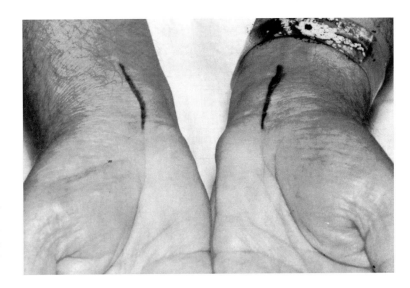

**Figure 8–32.** Failed bilateral carpal tunnel release with approach made through longitudinal wrist incisions. Some thenar eminence atrophy is evident on the right.

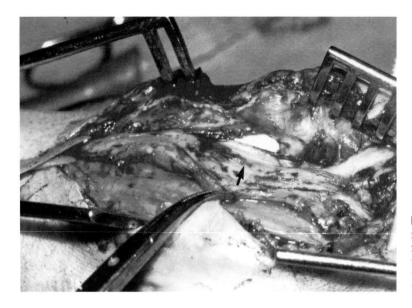

**Figure 8–33.** Severe palmar median injury (*arrow*) which required graft repair. A carpal tunnel release had been attempted through a transverse wrist incision.

tion of function once lost does not follow the usual timetable for recovery after CTR.

Sometimes, a branch of the nerve can be severed or damaged during the course of CTR (Figure 8–33). This may be the thenar, which provides median motor input to the thenar eminence and which, if damaged, produces thenar atrophy and weakness[41] (Figure 8–34). This may or may not be reparable, depending on the relation of the injury to the input of this branch to muscle. A palmar-level digital nerve can also be injured and require repair, especially if its supply is to thumb or forefinger. Digital nerves destined for long finger or, less frequently, little finger may be resected if there is

avulsion, neuroma, or severe damage over a length, because a hypesthetic long or ring finger is preferable to one with severe hyperesthesia and hyperpathia. Some surgeons, such as Mackinnon and Dellon, even purposely harvest one or more of these branches for use in repair of the median nerve at a palmar or wrist level.

Less obvious but of great diagnostic importance is damage to the palmar sensory or thenar sensory branches. These injuries can be associated not only with numbness but with painful paresthesias, especially if a neuroma forms at the injury site. The palmar sensory may penetrate the transverse carpal ligament and thus be

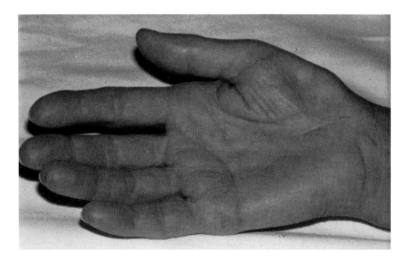

**Figure 8–34.** Thenar atrophy as a result of inadvertent section of the recurrent thenar branch during carpal tunnel release. A retinaculotome had been used through a small wrist-level incision.

damaged even with a direct exposure and section of the ligament, and especially if a less open or a closed procedure is used. Unfortunately, even direct inspection of the nerve can lead to inadvertent branch or whole nerve injury (Figure 8–35). The thenar sensory branch has a somewhat variable origin from the radial side of the distal median as it approaches wrist. This branch can be damaged if scissors are used on top of the nerve at the wrist level to divide antebrachial fascia or ligament, especially if done subcutaneously from a palmar entry site. Resection of the injured branch and any attendant neuroma is usually preferable to attempted repair, because the latter invariably leads to some degree of neuroma formation, which in itself may become painful (Figures 8–36 through 8–38).

Occasionally, a patient sustains operative injury to the ulnar nerve or its superficial or deep palmar branches. This has been seen with closed procedures for CTS but also with a direct approach to CTR.[10,41] Reoperation then depends on the severity of the loss and its attendant symptoms. Under these circumstances, it is often found that the transverse carpal ligament over median nerve has also not been released at the time of the original surgery.

Despite all of these considerations and potential complications, surgical CTR remains an extremely successful operation for a very disabling disease, provided patients to be operated on are well selected.[14,20,55,62,79]

## RESULTS WITH CARPAL TUNNEL RELEASE THROUGH A PALMAR INCISION

Outcomes in a relatively small group of patients in whom follow-up was available are summarized in Table 8–24. The procedure was relatively successful in relieving or improving pain and paresthesias. Some reversal of sensory loss or motor loss was possible but less likely, particularly if such loss was severe or had been present for some time. The majority of the patients seemed pleased with their outcomes, but as can be seen in Table 8–24, three required a repeat CTR, five had some worsening of their symptoms, and a few patients had complications which, fortunately, were usually mild.

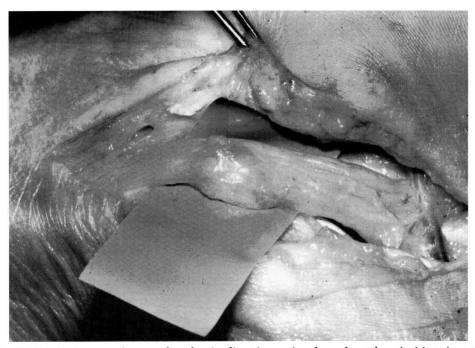

**Figure 8–35.** Direct injury to palmar median despite direct inspection through a palmar incision. A portion of this lesion required repair.

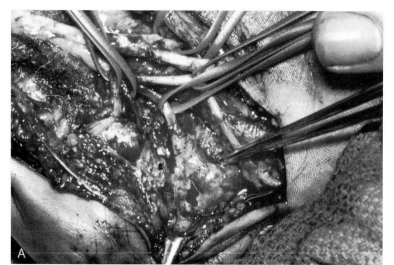

**Figure 8–36.** (*A*) Digital branch injury as a result of carpal tunnel release. Neuroma and severe scar are evident at tips of the forceps. Less involved thenar recurrent and other digital branches are encircled by Vasoloops. (*B*) Injury to sensory branch of median nerve was resected. A narrow sural nerve graft has been sewn in place with monofilament suture to replace the resected segment of sensory nerve.

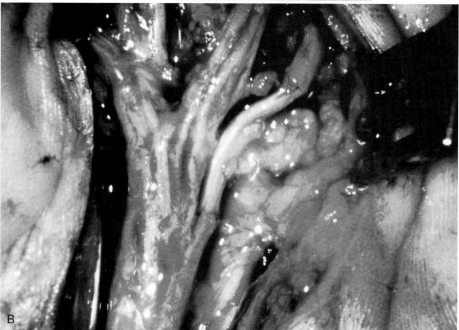

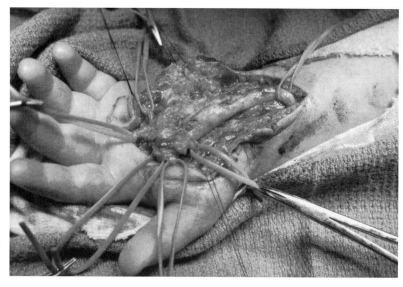

**Figure 8–37.** Contusive injury after carpal tunnel release requires dissection of all branches of median nerve.

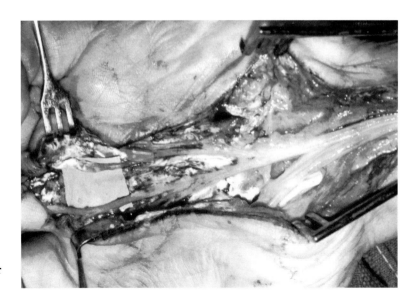

**Figure 8-38.** Distal palmar median sensory injury.

## Median Entrapment: Case Summary

This 15-year-old female had presented elsewhere with numbness and tingling in her thumbs and fingers at age 12. A bilateral CTR had been done. Symptoms quickly recurred and a repeat bilateral CTR was done 1 year later. However, after her symptoms persisted, she was seen by an orthopedist who ordered radiographs of her elbows, and bilateral medial and inferior humeral spurs were found. A presumptive diagnosis of a Struthers ligament compression of the median nerves at the level of

**TABLE 8-24**

## Results of Carpal Tunnel Release by Palmar Incision — LSUMC Series
(n = 376 CTRs in 340 patients*)

| | |
|---|---|
| Prominent pain improved | 246 of 282 (87%) |
| Prominent paresthesias improved | 230 of 249 (92%) |
| Significant numbness improved | 82 of 146 (56%) |
| Significant weakness improved | 20 of 48 (42%) |
| Patients satisfied with results | 303 of 340 (89%) |
| Major symptoms persisted | 23 cases (6%) |
| Deficit increased | 5 cases (1%) |
| Required repeat operation | 3 cases (1%) |
| Complications | |
|   Wound, hematoma | 1 case |
|   Superficial wound infection | 3 cases |
|   Addiction to narcotic | 1 case |
|   Reflex sympathetic dystrophy | 1 case |
|   Other diagnosis | 2 cases |

*Average follow-up period was 18.5 months.

the elbow was made, and the patient was then referred for further work-up and possible surgery.

Electrical work-up at LSUMC showed conductive slowing not only at the wrist but also at the elbow level for both median nerves. Both nerves were exposed at the elbow level and found to be compressed by a Struthers ligament running from the humerus to medial epicondyle (see Figure 8-6). Compression was most severe on the left. Intraoperative NAP studies showed significant slowing of conduction across both nerves at the level of the Struthers ligaments. The ligaments were resected and an external neurolysis was done on the median nerves at that level. The median nerves at wrist and palmar level were also explored. They were, as might be expected, heavily scarred. An external neurolysis was done on both nerves. Intraoperative NAP studies confirmed significant slowing at this level as well. However, it was evident from this operation that these changes were most likely secondary to the two prior CTRs and that the primary problem was at the elbow level for both limbs.

Recovery has been slow but good, and 4 years later she uses both hands and arms normally.

### Comment

Even though CTS is a common diagnosis, other disorders must be ruled out, particularly in individuals who are not middle-aged.

### Bibliography

1. Abbott L and Saunders J: Injuries of the median nerve in fractures of the lower end of the radius. Surg Gynecol Obstet 57:507–511, 1933.
2. Beard L, Kumar A, and Estep HL: Bilateral carpal tunnel syndrome caused by Grave's disease. Arch Intern Med 145:345–346, 1985.
3. Bennet JB and Crouch CC: Compression syndrome of

the recurrent motor branch of the median nerve. J Hand Surg 7:407–409, 1982.

4. Bleeker M, Bohlman M, Moreland R, and Tipton A: Carpal tunnel syndrome: Role of carpal canal size. Neurology 35:1599–1604, 1985.

5. Blom S and Dahlback L: Nerve injuries in dislocation of shoulder joint and fractures of neck of humerus. A clinical and electromyographic study. Acta Chir Scand 136:461–466, 1970

6. Boswick J and Stromberg W: Isolated injury of the median nerve above the elbow. J Bone Joint Surg Am 49A:481–487, 1967.

7. Brain WR, Wright AD, and Wilkinson M: Spontaneous compression of both median nerves in the carpal tunnel: Six cases treated surgically. Lancet 1:277–282, 1947.

8. Carroll R and Match R: Common errors in the management of wrist lacerations. J Trauma 14:553–558, 1974.

9. Cherington M: Proximal pain in carpal tunnel syndrome. Arch Surg 108:69, 1974.

10. Chow J: Endoscopic release of the carpal ligament: A new technique for carpal tunnel syndrome. Arthroscopy 5:19–24, 1989.

11. Chow J, Van Beek A, Bilos K, et al.: Anatomical basis for repair of ulnar and median nerves in the distal part of the forearm by group fascicular suture and nerve grafting. J Bone Joint Surg Am 68:273–280, 1986.

12. Connolly W: Pitfalls in carpal tunnel decompression. Aust N Z J Surg 48:421–425, 1978.

13. Cooney WP: Median nerve repairs: The results of treatment. In Gelberman R, Ed: Operative Nerve Repair and Reconstruction. Philadelphia, JB Lippincott, 1991.

14. Cseuz KA, Thomas JE, Lambert EH, et al.: Long-term results of operation for carpal tunnel syndrome. Mayo Clin Proc 41:232–241, 1966.

15. Curtis RM and Eversmann WW Jr: Internal neurolysis as an adjunct to the treatment of the carpal tunnel syndrome. J Bone Joint Surg 55:733–740, 1973.

16. Dawson D, Hallett M, and Millender L: Entrapment Neuropathies, 2nd Ed. Boston, Little Brown & Co, 1990.

17. Eason SY, Belsole RJ, and Greene TL: Carpal tunnel release: Analysis of suboptimal results. J Hand Surg 10B:365–369, 1985.

18. Eversmann WW Jr and Ritsick JA: Intraoperative changes in motor nerve conduction latency in carpal tunnel syndrome. J Hand Surg 3:77–81, 1978.

19. Freshwater F and Arons MS: The effect of various adjuncts on the surgical treatment of carpal tunnel syndrome secondary to chronic tenosynovitis. Plast Reconstr Surg 61:93–96, 1978.

20. Gainer JV and Nugent GR: Carpal tunnel syndrome: Report of 430 operations. South Med J 70:325–328, 1977.

21. Gaul J Jr: Electrical fascicle identification as an adjunct to nerve repair. J Hand Surg 8:289–296, 1983.

22. Gelberman RH, Aronson C, and Weisman MH: Carpal tunnel syndrome: Results of a perspective trial of steroid injection and splinting. J Bone Joint Surg 62A:1181–1184, 1980.

23. Gelberman RH, Hergenroeder PT, Hargens AR, et al.: The carpal tunnel syndrome: A study of carpal canal pressures. J Bone Joint Surg 63A:380–383, 1981.

24. Gelberman RH Pfeiffer G, Galbraith R, et al.: Results of treatment of severe carpal tunnel syndrome without internal neurolysis of the median nerve. J Bone Joint Surg 69:896–903, 1987.

25. Haase J, Bjerve P, and Semesen K: Median and ulnar nerve transections treated with microsurgical interfas-

cicular cable grafting with autologous sural nerve. J Neurosurg 53:73–84, 1980.

26. Harris CM, Tanner E, Goldstein MN, and Pettee DS: The surgical treatment of the carpal tunnel syndrome correlated with preoperative nerve-conduction studies. J Bone Joint Surg 61A:93–98, 1979.

27. Hudson A and Mayfield F: Chronic Injuries of Nerve by Entrapment. In Youmans J, Ed: Neurological Surgery, 2nd Ed. Philadelphia, WB Saunders, 1983.

28. Hudson A, Kline D, and Mackinnon S: Entrapment neuropathies. In Horowitz N, and Rizzoli H, Eds: Postoperative Complications of Extracranial Neurological Surgery. Baltimore, Williams & Wilkins, 1987.

29. Iyer V and Fenichel GM: Normal median nerve proximal latency in carpal tunnel syndrome: A clue to coexisting Martin-Gruber anastomosis. J Neurol Neurosurg Psychiatry 39:449–452, 1976.

30. Jain VK, Cestero RVM, and Baum J: Carpal tunnel syndrome in patients undergoing maintenance hemodialysis. JAMA 242:2868–2869, 1979.

31. Kaplan E and Spinner M: Normal and anomalous innervation patterns in the upper extremity. In Omer G and Spinner M, Eds: Management of Peripheral Nerve Problems. Philadelphia, WB Saunders, 1980.

32. Kelly MJ and Jackson M: Compression of median nerve at elbow. Br Med J 2:283, 1976.

33. Kessler F: Complications of the management of carpal tunnel syndrome. Hand Clin 2:401–406, 1986.

34. Kline DG and Hackett E: Reappraisal of timing for exploration of civilian nerve injuries. Surgery 78:54–63, 1978.

35. Kimura J: The carpal tunnel syndrome: Localization of conduction abnormalities within the distal segment of the median nerve. Brain 102:619–635, 1979.

36. Laha RK, Dujovny M, and DeCastro SC: Entrapment of median nerve by supracondylar process of the humerus: Case report. J Neurosurg 46:252–255, 1977.

37. Lake PA: Anterior interosseous nerve syndrome. J Neurosurg 41:306–309, 1974.

38. Langloh ND and Linscheid RL: Recurrent and unrelieved carpal tunnel syndrome. Clin Orthop 83:41–47, 1972.

39. Lanz U: Anatomical variations of the median nerve in the carpal tunnel. J Hand Surg 2:44–53, 1977.

40. Larsen R and Posch J: Nerve injuries in the upper extremity. Arch Surg 77:469–475, 1975.

41. Louis D, Green T, and Noellert R: Complications of carpal tunnel surgery. J Neurosurg 62:352–356, 1985.

42. Low PA, McLeod JG, Turtle JR, et al.: Peripheral neuropathy in acromegaly. Brain 97:139–152, 1974.

43. Lundborg G: Nerve Injury and Repair. New York, Churchill Livingstone, 1988.

44. MacDonald RI, Lichtman DM, Hanlon JJ, and Wilson JN: Complications of surgical release for carpal tunnel syndrome. J Hand Surg 3:70–76, 1978.

45. Mackinnon S: Secondary carpal tunnel surgery. Neurosurg Clin North Am 2:75–91, 1991.

46. Mackinnon S and Dellon A: Surgery of the Peripheral Nerve. New York, Thieme Medical Publishers, 1988.

47. Mackinnon S, McCabe S, Murray J, et al.: Internal neurolysis fails to improve the results of primary carpal tunnel decompression. J Hand Surg 16:211–218, 1991.

48. Mahoney J, Lofchy N, Chow I, and Hudson A: Carpal tunnel syndrome: A quality assurance evaluation of surgical treatment. R Coll Phys Surg Can Ann 25:20–23, 1992.

49. Massey EW: Carpal tunnel syndrome in pregnancy. Obstet Gynecol Surg 33:145, 1978.

50. McLellan DL and Swash M: Longitudinal sliding of me-

dian nerve during movements of the upper limb. J Neurol Neurosurg Psychiatry 39:566–570, 1976.

51. McManamny D: Comparison of microscope and loupe magnification: Assistance for the repair of median and ulnar nerves. Br J Plast Surg 36:367–372, 1983.

52. Michon J, Amend P, and Merle M: Microsurgical repair of peripheral nerve lesions: A study of 150 injuries of median and ulnar nerves. *In* Samii M, Ed: Peripheral Nerve Lesions. Berlin, Springer-Verlag, 1990.

53. Millesi H, Meissl G, and Berger A: The interfascicular nerve grafting of the median and ulnar nerves. J Bone Joint Surg 54A:727–730, 1972.

54. Morris HH and Peters BH: Pronator syndrome: Clinical and electrophysiological features in seven cases. J Neurol Neurosurg Psychiatry 39:461–464, 1976.

55. Mumenthaler M: Clinical aspects of entrapment neuropathies. *In* Samii M, Ed: Peripheral Nerve Lesions. Berlin, Springer-Verlag, 1990.

56. Nickolson OR and Seddon HJ: Nerve repair in civil practice. Br Med J 2:1065–1071, 1957.

57. O'Brien MD and Upton ARM: Anterior interosseous nerve syndrome. J Neurol Neurosurg Psychiatry 35:531–536, 1972.

58. Omer GE: Evaluation and reconstruction of forearm and hand after acute traumatic peripheral nerve injuries. J Bone Joint Surg 50A:1454–1460, 1968.

59. Omer GE: Tendon transfers for the reconstruction of the forearm and hand following peripheral nerve injuries. *In* Omer GE and Spinner M, Eds: Management of Peripheral Nerve Problems. Philadelphia, WB Saunders, 1980.

60. Osborne A, Dorey L, and Hardey J: Volkmann's contracture associated with prolonged external pressure on the forearm. Arch Surg 104:794–799, 1972.

61. Paine K: The carpal tunnel syndrome. Can J Surg 6:446–449, 1963.

62. Posch JL and Marcotte DR: Carpal tunnel syndrome: An analysis of 1201 cases. Orthop Rev 5:25–35, 1976.

63. Rask MR: Anterior interosseous nerve entrapment (Kiloh-Nevin syndrome). Clin Orthop 142:176–181, 1979.

64. Riordan DC: Tendon transplantations in median nerve and ulnar nerve paralysis. J Bone Joint Surg 35A:312–320, 1953.

65. Sakellorides H: Follow-up of 172 peripheral nerve injuries in upper extremity in civilians. J Bone Joint Surg 44A:140–148, 1962.

66. Samii M: Use of microtechniques in peripheral nerve surgery—experience with over 300 cases. *In* Handa H, Ed: Microneurosurgery. Tokyo, Igaku-Shoin, 1975.

67. Serodge H and Serodge E: Piso-triquetral pain syndrome after carpal tunnel release. J Hand Surg Can 14:858–873, 1989.

68. Seigel D and Gelberman R: Median nerve: Applied anatomy and operative exposure. *In* Gelberman R, Ed: Operative Nerve Repair and Reconstruction. Philadelphia, JB Lippincott, 1991.

69. Simpson JA: Electrical signs in the diagnosis of carpal tunnel and related syndromes. J Neurol Neurosurg Psychiatry 19:275–280, 1956.

70. Smith R and Fisher R: Struthers ligament: A source of median nerve compression above the elbow. Case report. J Neurosurg 38:778–781, 1973.

71. Spinner M: The anterior interosseous nerve syndrome with special attention to its variations. J Bone Joint Surg 52A:84–89, 1970.

72. Spinner M: Injuries of the Major Branches of Peripheral Nerves of the Forearm. Philadelphia, WB Saunders, 1978.

73. Sunderland S: The nerve lesion in the carpal tunnel syndrome. J Neurol Neurosurg Psychiatry 39:615–626, 1976.

74. Sunderland S and Ray L: Metrical and non-metrical features of the muscular branches of the median nerve. J Comp Neurol 85:191–200, 1946.

75. Tarlov IM: How long should an extremity be immobilized after nerve suture? Ann Surg 126:336–376, 1947.

76. Thomas CK, Stein RB, Gordon T, et al.: Patterns of reinnervation and motor unit recruitment in human hand muscles after complete ulnar and median nerve section and resuture. J Neurol Neurosurg Psychiatry 50:259–268, 1987.

77. Tindall S: Painful neuromas. *In* Williams R and Regachary S, Eds: Neurosurgery. New York, McGraw-Hill, 1985.

78. Tindall SC: Chronic injuries of peripheral nerves by entrapment. *In* J Youmans, Ed: Neurological Surgery, 3rd Ed. Philadelphia, WB Saunders, 1990, pp. 2511–2542.

79. Tuckmann W, Richter H, and Stöhr M: Compression Syndrome Peripherer Nerven. Berlin, Springer-Verlag, 1989.

80. Werschkul J: Anomalous course of the recurrent motor branch of the median nerve in a patient with carpal tunnel syndrome. J Neurosurg 47:113–114, 1977.

81. Williams H and Jabaley M: The importance of internal anatomy of the peripheral nerves to nerve repair in forearm and hand. Hand Clin 2:689–707, 1986.

82. Woodhall B and Beebe G: Peripheral Nerve Regeneration: A Review of 3,652 WW II Injuries. VA Monograph. Washington, DC, Government Printing Office, 1957.

83. Young V, Way R, and Weeks P: The results of nerve grafting in the wrist and hand. Ann Plast Surg 5:212–215, 1980.

84. Zachary R: Results of nerve suture. *In* Seddon H, Ed: Peripheral Nerve Injuries. Medical Research Council Special Report Series No. 282. London, Her Majesty's Stationery Office, 1954.

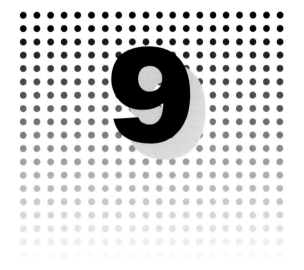

# Ulnar Nerve

## SUMMARY

The ulnar nerve takes on its greatest importance at the hand level, where it innervates most of the intrinsic muscles. Ulnar loss, when complete, is thus quite severe and is usually accompanied by clawing of the little and sometimes the ring fingers. Even though flexor carpi ulnaris receives branches from the ulnar nerve at and just below the elbow, it also receives input at the arm level, so it is frequently spared with elbow and even distal arm level lesions. On the other hand, because the flexor profundus branch supplying the little finger leaves ulnar nerve 2.5 to 5.0 cm below the elbow, flexion of the distal phalanx of the little finger is lost with complete ulnar lesions at or above the elbow. Flexion of the ring finger is not lost, however, because of the sharing of a tendinous slip with the median-innervated flexor profundus to the long finger.

Unlike the median, in which it is difficult to make up lost nerve length, the ulnar nerve can be transposed anterior to the elbow and usually deep to pronator and flexor carpi ulnaris, a maneuver that gains 2.5 to 3.8 cm of length. Despite this advantage, results with repair of this nerve at almost any level are less than those achieved with median or radial repair. Flexor profundus can usually be regained, as can ulnar sensation, some degree of hypothenar function, and even some adductor pollicis. This provides a grade 3 recovery. Harder to regain is interosseous and lumbrical function, except with lacerations or more focal injuries to nerve at the level of the wrist, at elbow level, and sometimes even at the level of the arm. Tendon transfer to substitute for lumbrical loss helps the patient extend the little and ring fingers. Despite the above, the series of 196 cases analyzed here lends strong support to the contention that ulnar repair is worthwhile and should not be abandoned in favor of reconstructive procedures only.

Intraoperative recordings on elbow-level, entrapped ulnar nerves indicated that the conductivity was most abnormal either within or just proximal to the olecranon groove and not at the level of the cubital tunnel. There were only a few exceptions to this. We favor a modified Learmouth procedure with thorough neurolysis and then the placement of nerve deep to pronator teres and flexor carpi ulnaris. This was the operation done in 296 cases in this series. We have had to redo only two such cases. A relatively large number of simple ulnar decompressions, medial epicondylectomies, and subcutaneous transpositions done elsewhere have been sent to us with severe pain, paresthesias, and sometimes progressive palsy (82 cases). Some have been helped by reoperation and submuscular placement of the nerve. These simpler procedures for entrapment work much of the time but are on the whole less effective than more formal submuscular transposition.

## SURGICAL ANATOMY

This nerve, which is so important for coordinated hand function, originates at an axillary level from the medial cord of the plexus. The medial cord, as its name implies, lies medial to the axillary artery (Figure 9–1). This cord gives a large motor branch to the median nerve and then gives rise to ulnar nerve and the medial and lateral antebrachial cutaneous nerves. The ulnar nerve travels initially posterior to artery but then takes a somewhat oblique course away from artery and down the upper arm toward the olecranon notch. At midarm level, the nerve passes either through or beneath the firm, fibrous intermuscular septum. Almost 70% of limbs have an arcade of Struthers beneath which the nerve may pass just distal to the intermuscular septum. This arcade is formed by thickening of the deep, investing fascia of the distal portion of the arm and muscle fibers from the medial head of the triceps. As one dissects proximally from the medial epicondyle, the ulnar nerve is often covered by these triceps fibers and some fascia (Figure 9–2).

In the distal arm, the nerve is usually quite

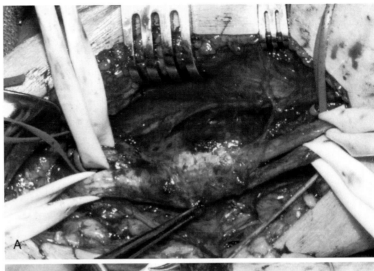

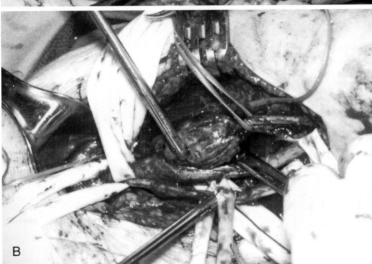

**Figure 9–1.** *(A)* Injury to medial cord to ulnar and proximal median associated with an axillary angiogram. *(B)* A pseudoaneurysm of axillary to brachial arterial junction as well as direct injury to ulnar and median nerves were present. Both ulnar and median nerves required graft repair. After proximal and distal control of the artery, the aneurysm was evacuated, but an initial repair of a large, ragged hole in the artery was unsuccessful, and a subsequent vascular graft repair by the vascular service was necessary.

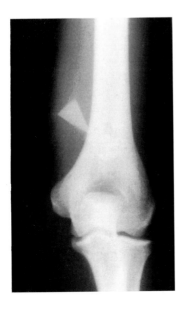

**Figure 9–2.** Radiograph showing shard of glass that transected the ulnar nerve several inches above the elbow. This glass fragment was missed on primary exploration but found when the patient was examined because of total ulnar palsy. Nerve was repaired secondarily a month later. Overlying triceps fibers, or arcade of Struthers, was divided to expose nerve at this level.

adherent to the proximal muscle belly of the flexor carpi ulnaris (FCU). Branches supplying this muscle proximal to the elbow, usually arise from the dorsal surface of the nerve and tend to tether the nerve at this level. Both arteries and veins run parallel to the ulnar nerve in this region and are usually quite adherent to it. Only 1% of the population have a Struthers ligament. In these few cases, ulnar nerve can pass beneath this structure just proximal to the notch area. The Struthers ligament arises from a small, epicondylar-like process on the medial surface of the distal humerus. The ligament usually passes over brachial artery and median nerve, and sometimes the ulnar nerve as well, on its way to insert on medial epicondyle.

As the nerve enters the olecranon notch, it tends to flatten somewhat and takes on an ovoid rather than a rounded shape. It is often adherent to the base of the notch. The nerve is covered by a raphe of connective tissue or fascia extending across the olecranon notch. Small, neural, articular branches may leave the inferior surface of the nerve and penetrate to the joint space. Small arteries and veins usually accompany the nerve into the notch and lie on the floor of the notch. In the distal portion of the olecranon notch, nerve passes into a more constricted area bounded superficially by an aponeurotic arch extending to medial epicondyle. Just distal to the notch, nerve passes beneath the two heads of FCU. Somewhat more distal to the notch, the nerve gives rise to relatively short branches that help to supply FCU. Occasion-

ally, an anomalous but radial-innervated muscle, anconeus epitrochlearis, arises from medial border of olecranon and adjacent triceps tendon and inserts into medial epicondyle. If present, this muscle forms part of the cubital tunnel, reinforcing the aponeurosis of the two heads of origin of FCU.

Branches to the medial half of the flexor profundus arise deep to FCU and about 2.5 to 5 cm distal to notch. These branches leave the radial and dorsal surface of nerve and take a relatively short course to this muscle. At this point, nerve lies on the ulnar side of the flexor profundus. If the operator places the proximal phalanx of his or her little finger into the olecranon groove and points the tip toward the ulnar surface of the wrist, the course of the nerve in the proximal forearm is outlined. In the more distal forearm, ulnar nerve remains deep to FCU and medial to flexor superficialis tendons.

Throughout the distal forearm, the nerve is closely applied to ulnar artery (Figure 9–3). This vessel usually approaches nerve at midforearm level and lies on its radial side. Its cohort, the radial artery, lies on the inner or ulnar side of the superficial sensory radial nerve. At the proximal forearm level, there may be a Martin-Gruber anastomosis. Under these circumstances, the anterior interosseous branch of the median gives rise to a branch that goes to ulnar nerve.[63] This branch can take median fibers, especially those destined for abductor pollicis brevis and opponens pollicis, from median to forearm-level ulnar nerve. These fibers then

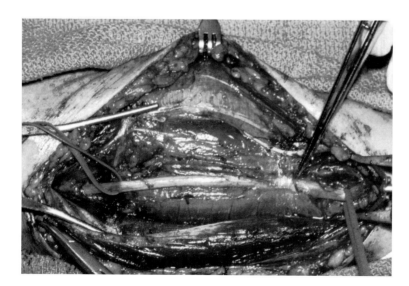

**Figure 9–3.** A relatively focal forearm-level ulnar lesion associated with fracture and contusion. At 4 months, this lesion had a recordable nerve action potential across it despite total distal loss and, as a result, had only an external neurolysis. Ulnar artery has been dissected away from injured ulnar nerve.

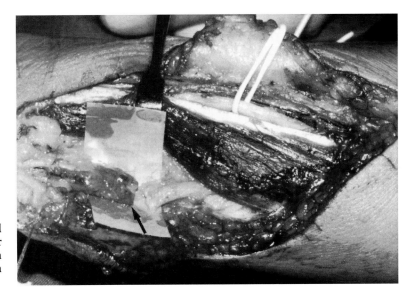

**Figure 9–4.** Transected dorsal cutaneous branch of ulnar nerve. The surgeon has made a cut on one side of the neuroma *(arrow)*.

trade back to distal median at a wrist or palmar level (Riche-Cannieu anastomosis). More commonly, ulnar motor fibers descend in proximal median nerve and then return to ulnar at a forearm level through a branch from anterior interosseous nerve.

The dorsal cutaneous nerve arises from ulnar nerve 5 to 8 cm or so proximal to wrist crease (Figure 9–4). This branch supplies sensation to the dorsum of the hand on its ulnar side. Sometimes, this branch arises separately from main ulnar nerve as far proximal as the olecranon notch. In rare cases, this branch can arise as far distally as the Guyon canal.

As the ulnar nerve passes over the wrist, it enters the Guyon canal or tunnel. The latter is formed by pisiform bone and pisohamate ligament on the ulnar side of the hand. On the radial side, it is bounded by the hook of hamate. Nerve is covered by an expansion of the FCU tendon and the antebrachial fascia. The more distal portion of the canal or tunnel is composed of pisohamate and pisometacarpal ligaments on either side, opponens digiti quinti minimi muscle deep or dorsally, and superficial or overlying hypothenar fat and the palmar fibrous arch.[75]

As the ulnar nerve passes on the radial side of the pisiform bone and superficial to the medial extension of the transverse carpal ligament, it quickly divides into superficial and deep branches (Figures 9–5). The superficial branch crosses the flexor digiti quinti brevis, gives a

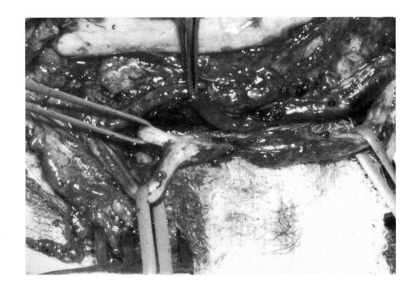

**Figure 9–5.** Ulnar injury at the palmar level in the Guyon canal and just proximal to superficial and deep ulnar branches. The injury was secondary to an attempted arthroscopic release of the transverse carpal ligament. No nerve action potential was transmitted across this lesion. After resection to healthier proximal and distal tissues, repair was done with four sural grafts 3.5 cm in length.

small branch to palmaris brevis, and then provides a variable and relatively lengthy segment composed of digital branches to the little and ring fingers. The deep branch passes backward and downward away from the operator between the heads of flexor and abductor digiti quinti minimi, winding around the hook of the hamate and running toward thumb within the concavity of the palmar arch. The deep branch divides early to supply the hypothenar muscles, which include abductor digiti quinti minimi and the opponens minimi. On occasion, a hypothenar branch may arise from the ulnar nerve proximal to the takeoff of the superficial and deep branches. The principal deep branch travels toward the thumb and through the deep palmar space to further branch and supply interossei, lumbricals for ring and little fingers, and finally the adductor pollicis.

## CLINICAL EXAMINATION

The most proximal muscle innervated by the ulnar nerve is the FCU, which is supplied by branches both above and below the elbow. It is the major wrist flexor, particularly in an ulnar direction. By grasping the patient's hand in a handshake position and asking the patient to cock the wrist in a flexed, ulnarward direction, the clinician can readily grade the strength of this muscle. Ulnar-innervated flexor profundi are another matter because that to ring finger usually shares a slip with the median-innervated profundus to the long finger. As a result,

even complete ulnar injury may cause only mild weakness of flexion of the distal phalanx of the ring finger; distal flexion of the little finger may be quite weak or its function may be absent. These subtle findings can be overlooked, especially when ulnar injury is severe, leading to extensive sensory and hand intrinsic loss with clawing of the little and ring fingers (Figure 9–6). In terms of localizing the level of injury, the profundi muscles are still extremely important to evaluate. Preservation of their function in conjunction with distal hand intrinsic loss usually indicates a more distal forearm or wrist-level lesion. An exception is ulnar entrapment at the elbow where preferentially, hand-intrinsic muscles tend to drop out with relative sparing of not only FCU but also of the profundi.

The dorsal cutaneous branch supplies sensation to dorsum of the hand and a portion of the back of the little finger (Figure 9–7). Injury distal to the origin of this branch and requiring repair may benefit by excision of this branch so that mainly motor fibers and the more important sensory fibers can be directed to distal nerve.[81] Injury proximal to this distal forearm-level branch from ulnar gives rather complete ulnar sensory loss. The latter includes loss on the dorsum of the hand and on the volar aspect of ring as well as most of little finger. Loss may at times involve the ulnar half of the long finger as well. Autonomous zone for the ulnar nerve includes the volar aspect of the distal and intermediate digits of the little finger as well as the dorsal surface of its distal phalanx.[62] Loss in that distribution can only mean injury to the ulnar

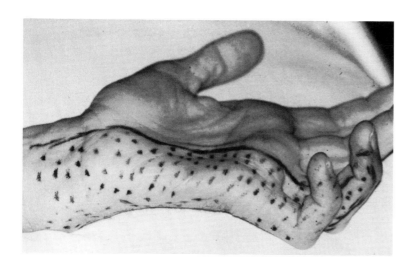

**Figure 9–6.** Ulnar sensory and motor loss with typical "clawing" of ring and little fingers caused by an arm-level ulnar injury. The denervated ulnar-intrinsic muscles fail to fix or hold the metacarpophalangeal joints, so the radial-innervated long extensors hyperextend the knuckle joints. The paralyzed intrinsics fail to extend the interphalangeal joints, so the median-innervated forearm flexors hyperflex them.

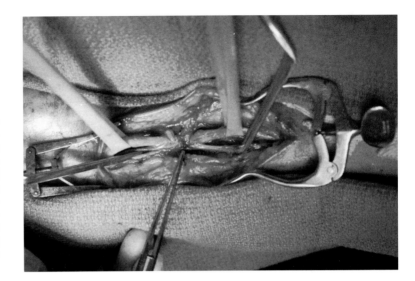

**Figure 9-7.** Distal forearm-level ulnar injury just proximal to the dorsal cutaneous branch. The latter was dissected away from proximal stump and sacrificed, so downflow to distal stump excluded the distal dorsal cutaneous branch when the nerve was repaired. Level of the wrist is to the right in this photograph.

nerve proper or its more distal superficial sensory branch. Recovery in that distribution, if loss had been present previously, can only occur as a result of ulnar nerve regeneration and is not because of sprouting from adjacent nerves[54] (Figures 9-8 and 9-9). On the other hand, injury to ulnar nerve distal to the dorsal cutaneous branch spares sensation on the dorsum of the hand and fingers.

Hypothenar function is totally ulnar-innervated. Abduction of the little finger by the abductor digiti quinti minimi is best tested by giving the patient a target to push against which is volar to the horizontal plane of the hand; otherwise, the extensor communis tendon to the little finger can mimic abduction by an ulnarward movement as the digit is extended. Opposition provided by opponens digiti quinti minimi is no

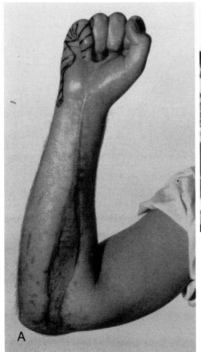

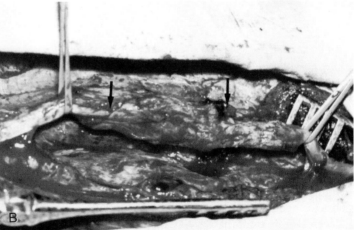

**Figure 9-8.** *(A)* Shotgun injury involving elbow and forearm-level ulnar nerve. Skin loss and defect after fasciotomy was repaired by a skin graft. Sensory loss and difficulty making a complete fist especially with little finger are evident. *(B)* At exploration, a lengthy lesion in continuity involving ulnar nerve was found *(arrows)*. This did not transmit a nerve action potential and required long grafts for repair with only partial recovery of hand function.

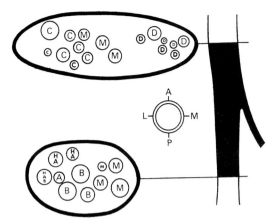

**Figure 9–9.** Ulnar fascicular pattern just proximal *(top diagram)* and then distal *(bottom diagram)* to the dorsal cutaneous branch. Repair of ulnar lesions at this level can be done by splitting away the dorsal cutaneous outflow from the more proximal nerve so that all of the proximal outflow goes to more distal downflow associated with the important hand-intrinsic muscles and sensation on the volar aspect of the little and ring fingers and hypothenar regions. (Circular diagram shows orientation of nerve cross sections: A = anterior, L = lateral, P = posterior, and M = medial.) A = cutaneous fibers from ulnar side fifth finger; B = cutaneous fibers from fourth interspace; C = combined superficial cutaneous fibers; D = dorsal cutaneous fibers; H = cutaneous fibers from hypothenar eminence; M = deep muscular fibers. (From Sunderland S: Nerves and Nerve Injuries. Baltimore, Williams & Wilkins, 1968.)

easy matter to test either, because the flexors can substitute for much of its function.[34] The examiner can cross his own forefinger and long finger and place them on the palm between palmar crease and the heel of the palm. The patient, using opponens digiti quinti minimi, should be able to reach this target and, by pressing down, be able to prevent the examiner from spreading his or her own forefinger away from long finger. The other two hypothenar muscles, flexor brevis and palmaris brevis, are more difficult to isolate and test with specificity than the abductor and opponens.[35]

Interossei are examined by having the patient place hand and fingers palm down on a flat surface and asking him to spread and then bring fingers back together. An even more reliable test of these muscles is for the examiner to place his or her fingers and thumb against the palmer surface of the patient's fingers and thumb. This is done in such a way as to place the patient's wrist and fingers in hyperextension, thus re-

moving the ability of the extensors to mimic interosseous function. Ulnar-innervated lumbricals are those of little and ring fingers. Their loss can result in an ulnar claw of one or both of these fingers. This complication of ulnar injury occurs because the function of these muscles is to set the metacarpophalangeal joint, permitting the extensor communis to extend more distal digits. If this function is absent, the flexors are not opposed by an efficient extensor mechanism, and the fingers are pulled toward the palm. Ulnar claw is more likely to occur and to be more severe with distal lesions in which flexor profundus function is intact and fingers are pulled into more flexion. Lumbricals can be tested individually by the examiner's holding the first phalanx of the finger in a somewhat extended position and asking the patient to straighten or extend the intermediate phalanx.

Adductor pollicis can be readily palpated and graded for strength by having the patient press the thumb against the side of the palm. With paralysis, a Froment sign will be present. Median-innervated flexor pollicis longus substitutes for the adductor by flexing the distal phalanx of the thumb, thus pulling the whole thumb toward and holding it against the side of the palm.

A portion of flexor pollicis brevis is also innervated by the ulnar nerve, but in the absence of median loss, it is difficult to impossible to detect any weakness in this muscle, even with complete ulnar loss.

## ELECTRICAL STUDIES

### Electromyography

Localization of the injury site is relatively straightforward for the ulnar nerve, but there are exceptions. As is the case for median-innervated pronator teres, the first discernible branches, in this case to FCU, do not reach muscle until the distal level of the arm. As a result, injury which includes FCU could be anywhere along the nerve's course in the proximal arm. Because origin of ulnar nerve is from medial cord, ulnar loss caused by severe injury at that level and mimicking ulnar injury include denervational changes not only in ulnar-innervated hand intrinsic muscles but also in those innervated by median nerve in the thenar eminence.

FCU receives neural input both above and below the elbow, but usually the two heads are sampled somewhat distal to the elbow. Denervational changes in the distribution of this muscle indicate a proximal ulnar lesion. The ulnar-innervated profundi are very important from an electrophysiologic standpoint.[44] Denervational change in these muscles but with preservation of FCU indicates injury or a lesion at the elbow or distal arm level. Needling these muscles is not easy because the median-innervated profundi are close by, and it can be difficult to be certain that the ulnar half is being sampled.

As with upper arm-level injuries, precise electrical localization of forearm-level lesions is difficult.[37] After profundi, the next muscles innervated by ulnar are the hypothenars in the hand. Sampling of the hypothenar eminence muscle mass, which is such a prominent landmark, is relatively straightforward. Nonetheless, if atrophy has occurred and the patient is unable to voluntarily contract these muscles, separation of abductor digiti quinti minimi from opponens digiti quinti minimi can be difficult to impossible. Similarly, differentiating palmar from dorsal interossei by needle examination can be difficult too. Fortunately, the two ulnar-innervated hypothenar muscles share a relatively common neural input, so their differentiation is of little practical importance in terms of localization of injury.

The first dorsal interosseous is one of the landmark muscles for ulnar electrical workup (Figure 9–10). Lumbricals, although very important for hand function, are such small, deeply-located slips of muscle that reliable sampling of their function is most difficult. Close by is adductor pollicis. With partial injuries or entrapments, this muscle is often relatively spared. Because flexor pollicis brevis has dual innervation from both ulnar and median, sampling this muscle for ulnar work-up is of limited value.

Variations in ulnar and median innervation of the hand, such as the Martin-Gruber anastomosis, are more thoroughly discussed in the chapter entitled "Median Nerve."

## Conduction Studies

Ulnar nerve injury is the classic setting for use of electrical study to assess function by conduc-

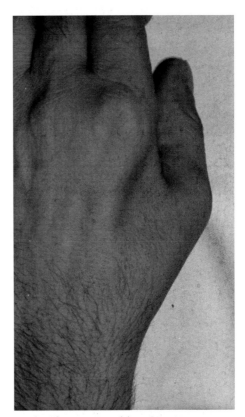

**Figure 9–10.** Atrophy of first dorsal interosseous in patient with no sensory loss in hand and normal long flexor activity to medial two digits. Electromyogram showed severe denervation in this muscle and the adductor pollicis. The deep branch of the ulnar nerve was compressed by a ganglion cyst.

tion.[3] Entrapment, whether in the olecranon notch or, as seen less frequently, beneath the more distal origins of FCU, can be readily assessed by stimulating nerve both above and below the elbow. The electrodiagnostician then records from hypothenar or first dorsal interosseous muscles and subtracts the two latencies. This gives the latency value for conduction across the elbow. An alternative is to stimulate nerve at one site well above the elbow and to record from both FCU above the elbow and ulnar-innervated flexor profundus below the elbow. Again, the latencies are subtracted to give conduction across the elbow. With entrapment at the elbow level, there is a relationship between the severity of the palsy and the amount of slowing across the notch. After transposition, conduction velocity change does not always keep pace with clinical improvement. In early or mild cases, conduction not only between the elbow and wrist, but even at the elbow, can be normal preoperatively. Distance over which latencies are recorded may play a role here, especially if conduction is normal or only slightly abnormal, not only above but below or distal to the site of compression. For some proximal, forearm-level lesions, conduction recordings from profundi instead of those from hand intrinsics can be used after stimulation of nerve at the elbow. Differentiation of Guyon canal entrapment of the deep branch can also be done by comparing conduction from proximal forearm to that across the wrist with recording from first dorsal interosseous. Wrist-level involvement of the whole nerve can also be tested by sensory nerve action potential (SNAP) studies either stimulating or recording from little finger digital nerves and vice-versa at the wrist.[32] As with the median nerve, use of sensory NAP recordings can be helpful in assessing milder lesions, especially those located at a wrist or palmar level.

# SURGICAL EXPOSURE OF ULNAR NERVE

## Arm Level

Proximal exploration of the ulnar nerve in the arm is done with a medial incision centered in the cleft between biceps/brachialis and triceps. The incision is superficial to but over the distal axillary and proximal brachial artery. Depend-

ing on the level of the lesion, exposure of medial cord, its branch to median nerve, and the antebrachial cutaneous nerves, as well as ulnar nerve, may be necessary (Figure 9–11). Although there can be variations in the anatomy at this level, the origin of ulnar from medial cord will be clearly defined after the makeup of proximal median nerve and its input from lateral and medial cords is apparent.[4,76] The ulnar nerve can then be traced distally and somewhat obliquely as it runs toward the olecranon notch, using sharp dissection and taking care to section the intermuscular septum at midarm level. There are usually no ulnar branches of concern at the arm level until the nerve approaches the elbow level, so dissection along the nerve at the midarm level is usually straightforward.

If the lesion is in more distal arm, the ulnar nerve can be most readily exposed in the olecranon notch area, or just proximal to its entry point to the notch, and traced proximally. Any dissection in this area should also include section of the intermuscular septum. In distal arm, nerve is often covered by a superior expansion of triceps muscle fibers or fascia, and these need to be sectioned for good exposure.[43] Nerve may be quite adherent to underlying muscle at this level and somewhat tethered to it by short branches to proximal FCU. It helps to dissect nerve to the epineurial level and encircle it with Penrose drains at one or more distal arm levels. The drains are then used to shift nerve as the operator clears these branches or dissects them back into main nerve to gain length. At this

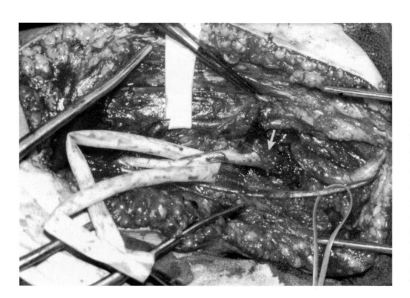

**Figure 9–11.** Ulnar nerve somewhat obliquely transected at a proximal arm level by glass (arrow). There has been only slight distraction of the stumps over a 5-week period. The Vasoloop is around an antebrachial cutaneous nerve, and the Penrose drain to the left is around the distal stump. The Penrose at the top of the photograph is around the brachial artery.

level, arteries and veins often join mesoneurium and are closely applied to nerve or epineurium itself. These vessels can usually be carefully stripped away from nerve by use of the Metzenbaum scissors for dissection and the bipolar to coagulate collateral branches. Dissection of distal arm lesions usually includes more distal elbow-level transposition of the ulnar nerve, so the lower level of the dissection usually includes clearing the nerve through the olecranon notch, opening the cubital tunnel, and splitting apart the two heads of the FCU.

## Elbow and Forearm Level

Incision begins on medial distal arm, curves over the volar elbow lateral to the medial epicondylar region, and then comes gently back down medial but proximal forearm. Dissection of the ulnar nerve through and beyond the olecranon notch region requires good lighting, some retraction, and the use of the bipolar coagulator[55] (Figure 9–12). Overlying extension of epicondylar fascia is sectioned. Nerve is carefully mobilized out of the notch using the bipolar coagulator to coagulate arteries and veins accompanying nerve through this region. Because

nerve is often somewhat snug or sometimes already entrapped at this level, technique must be especially gentle. Small articular branches are usually sacrificed; FCU branches are usually maintained but freed up over a length to aid mobilization of the ulnar nerve itself.[15,43] Nerve can then be traced below or distal to the notch by encircling it with a drain and dissecting around it while carefully sectioning overlying FCU fascia and muscle. Care must be taken to preserve the ulnar flexor profundi branch or branches which usually originate from the lateral or radial side of the nerve 2 to 4 cm distal to the olecranon notch. More superficially, originating FCU branches can be dissected back up and into the main trunk of the nerve to gain length or sectioned if necessary. It is important to split the heads of the FCU well distal to the point at which profundus branches exit the ulnar nerve so as to adequately uncover nerve. The muscle bellies of FCU can be spread and held apart with a mastoid or, in more slender patients, with an Alm retractor.

## Distal Forearm and Wrist Levels

In more distal forearm, the skin incision can parallel the superior edge of the FCU tendon.

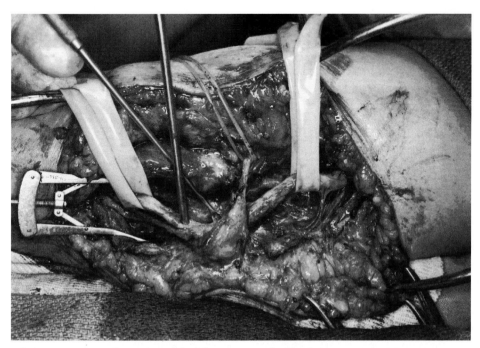

**Figure 9–12.** Ulnar injury in the region of the olecranon notch. This lesion required a split repair. Nerve was then transposed volar to the elbow and buried deep to pronator teres and flexor carpi ulnaris.

Tendon and originating muscle belly can be retracted medially after encircling them with one or more Penrose drains. The forearm portion of the nerve tends to lie beneath a line extending from medial epicondyle to the palpable portion of the pisiform bone. For midforearm-level exposure of ulnar, some of the muscle belly of FCU may have to be split as well. Nerve lies in the interval between FCU and the profundus.[76] The dorsal cutaneous branch of ulnar arises from the posteromedial or ulnar aspect of the nerve and can usually be isolated and encircled with a plastic loop. Injury to nerve at a distal forearm level often involves adjacent and parallel ulnar artery, which usually adjoins ulnar nerve at a midforearm level. This vessel may have to be isolated for subsequent repair or obliteration.[10] Most of the veins in this area can be coagulated as nerve is elevated by drains and sharply cleared of investing tissues or scar.

Exposure at the wrist and palmar level uses the distal forearm incision on radial side of FCU, curves gently on the radial side of the hypothenar eminence, and points toward the interval between the ring and little fingers. As nerve approaches wrist, it lies beneath or dorsal to the palmar carpal ligament and volar to the transverse carpal ligament and the palmar surface of the profundus tendons. The former is sectioned and the latter usually preserved as a bed for the nerve. Ulnar artery remains on the lateral or radial side of the nerve as it passes on the radial side of the pisiform bone. In the more distal tunnel, the overlying fibrous arch of the palmar fascia should be incised for adequate exposure. Artery has usually branched, as has nerve by this point, and vessels as well as superficial and deep ulnar branches are often intertwined. These relations should be worked out under magnification with the help of careful placement of one or more Alm retractors to spread adjacent tissues. The superficial palmar branch, which exits more distal tunnel along with an arterial branch, is first mobilized along with more distal sensory branches. Then, the deep palmar or terminal branch of the ulnar nerve can be exposed, usually beneath and slightly lateral to or on the ulnar side of the deep or terminal branch of the artery (Figure 9–13). As nerve and vessel exit distal ulnar tunnel, they pass around the hook of the hamate bone and deep to a fibrous arch which is the origination of the hypothenar

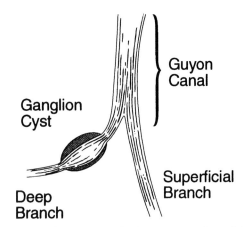

**Figure 9–13.** Drawing depicts compression of the deep branch of the ulnar nerve just distal to the Guyon canal by a ganglion cyst. Most of this patient's hand-intrinsic weakness reversed after removal of the cyst and decompression of this branch.

muscles. Dissection in the palmar area must be done in a measured and deliberate fashion, and magnification as well as use of fine instruments and the bipolar forceps are mandatory.

## RESULTS WITH ULNAR INJURIES AT ARM LEVEL

In the early literature, results reported for repair of the ulnar nerve were not encouraging.[1,65,71,72] Reports based on both world wars were especially dismal.[69,73,82,86,88] On the other hand, some more recent reports have been more optimistic.[9,38,49,59,61] Many of the more recent published series have been relatively small and, more importantly, have consisted primarily of wrist-level injuries with few injuries at an arm or elbow level.[78,79]

Associated injuries to tendons, bones, vessels, or other nerves can downgrade results, as can a fixed, clawed hand, even if successful repair returns nerve fibers to hand intrinsics.[40] Most of the ulnar nerve's input goes to fine hand intrinsic muscles, which are immensely important for a useful hand and are difficult to reinnervate in a functional fashion (Figure 9–14). On the other hand, flexor profundi to little and ring fingers and loss of sensation in the ulnar distribution are of less importance for a useful hand than hand intrinsic function.[55] Nonetheless, recovery of these functions and

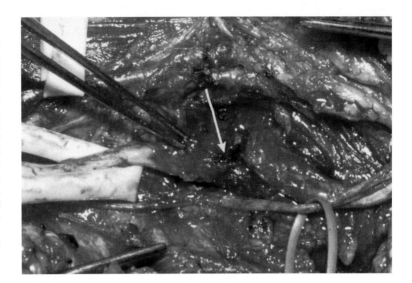

**Figure 9–14.** Old glass injury at medial cord to ulnar nerve junction *(arrow)*. Forceps is on distal stump neuroma, and the Vasoloop is around an antebrachial cutaneous nerve. Since this injury was almost a year old and involved very proximal ulnar nerve, results with repair were poor even after 3 years of follow-up. Flexor carpi ulnaris graded 4, profundus to ring finger graded 4, and profundus to little finger graded 3 to 4. Sensation in the ulnar territory graded 3. Hand-intrinsic function remained absent.

also some intrinsic function involving hypothenar and even adductor pollicis muscles is often possible, so, in our view, the nerve should be repaired whenever indicated.

As pointed out by others, we found that ulnar-injured extremities required maximal rehabilitation in terms of repetitive and sustained physical and occupational therapy and home exercises.[82,87] Pre- and postoperative grades at each level were determined by use of Table 9–1. (See also the chapter entitled "Grading Results.")

Table 9–2 shows the mechanisms of injuries or lesions involving ulnar nerve at the arm level. Thirty-five of the 46 lesions evaluated at this level were treated surgically. Twenty-six of these lesions had complete distal ulnar loss, both clinically and electrically, before operation. There were three tumors and one case of hidradenitis, and preoperative loss was mild in these cases. Despite a large number of lacerations and puncture wounds affecting high ulnar nerve, only 7 of the 17 patients operated on had complete transection of nerve; the remainder had partially transected the nerve or bruised and stretched it, giving lesions in continuity. Primary suture within 48 hours was possible in four transected cases and led to grade 3 recoveries in two (Table 9–3). Secondary suture and graft repair were less successful, with only one of three transections having good eventual re-

**TABLE 9–1**
Criteria for Grading Ulnar Nerve Injury

| | |
|---|---|
| 0 (absent) | No muscle contraction; absent sensation |
| 1 (poor) | Proximal muscles such as FCU and FP-V contract, but not against gravity; sensory grade is 1 or 0. |
| 2 (fair) | Proximal muscles (FCU and FP-V) contract against gravity, distal intrinsic muscles do not contract; sensory grade, if applicable, is usually 2 or lower. |
| 3 (moderate) | Proximal muscles (FCU and FP-V) contract against gravity and some resistance; some distal muscles, usually hypothenar muscles and occasionally lumbricals, contract against at least gravity; sensory grade is usually 3. |
| 4 (good) | All proximal and some distal hand intrinsic muscles such as interossei and lumbricals to little and ring finger muscles contract against gravity and some resistance; sensory grade is 3 or better. |
| 5 (excellent) | All muscles including hand intrinsics contract against moderate resistance; sensory grade is 4 or better. |

FCU = flexor carpi ulnaris; FP-V = flexor profundus to little finger.

**TABLE 9–2**
Arm–Level Ulnar Nerve Mechanisms (n = 46)

| Mechanism | Operated | Unoperated |
|---|---|---|
| Laceration or puncture | 17 | 5 |
| Gunshot wound | 4 | 4 |
| Stretch/Contusion | 4 | 2 |
| Fracture | 6 | 0 |
| Tumor/Infection* | 4 | 0 |
| TOTALS | 35† | 11 |

*3 tumors and 1 case of hidradenitis were operated on without significant deficit.
†26 injuries had complete clinical and electromyographic loss before operation.

**TABLE 9-3**
Arm-Level Ulnar Nerve Injuries* (n = 31)

| Operation | No. Cases/No. Recovered to Grade 3 or Better |
|---|---|
| **Transection** | |
| Primary suture | 4/2 |
| Secondary suture | 2/1 |
| Secondary graft | 1/0 |
| Secondary split repair | 2/2 |
| **In Continuity Injuries** | |
| Positive NAP | |
| Neurolysis | 10/9† |
| Split repair | 1/1 |
| Negative NAP | |
| Suture | 3/2 |
| Grafts | 5/2 |
| Neurolysis | 3/1‡ |

*There were 4 tumors at this level operated on with good results.
†4 injuries with complete preoperative loss had NAPs and neurolysis with good results.
‡3 injuries with complete loss and no NAP still had neurolysis only because of proximal level and extent of injury; one had a grade 3 recovery.

sults. Split repair was possible because of partial transection in two cases, and both of these patients experienced some degree of useful recovery.

There were 22 lesions in continuity operated upon (see Table 9-3). These included eight associated with lacerations or puncture wounds. Most of these were caused by relatively blunt objects such as fan or propeller blades or auto metal and were either partially lacerated or, more likely, contused over a length. Four lesions in continuity were associated with gunshot wounds, four with blunt soft tissue contusions, and six with fractures. In these cases, exploration was delayed for 2 to 4 months to determine whether early signs of spontaneous recovery would occur. This delay also permitted operative NAP studies to be done to prove or disprove the need for resection.[46]

Intraoperative recordings showed NAPs in 11 cases, and 10 of these had neurolysis, with 9 having recovery. One case associated with a lacerating injury had a split repair despite a NAP because one portion of the cross section of nerve was more severely involved than the rest. In the 11 cases without a NAP across their lesion in continuity, 3 had suture repair and 5 had graft repair. Despite absence of a NAP in three cases,

only neurolysis was done because of lengthy, proximal lesions. Only one of these injuries has had significant recovery, and this was only to a grade 3 level. Results with end-to-end suture and grafts were favorable for four of eight cases.

If lesions in continuity caused by gunshot wounds and stretch/contusion are grouped together regardless of presence or absence of fracture, half had neurolysis because of a NAP and half required repair. Although good intrinsic function did not recover after such proximal repair, especially if suture or graft was necessary, enough flexor profundus, hypothenar, and sensory function returned to permit many to gain a grade 3 level. The tumors fared well with resection, as did the hidradenitis case, in which ulnar nerve required extensive neurolysis.

## Arm-Level Lesion Case Summaries

### Case Number 1

This 12-year-old boy fell through a plate glass window and sustained a laceration in the axilla. The soft tissue wound was repaired, but there was an ulnar palsy. Examination 1 month later showed partial function of the FCU but a complete distal palsy. At exploration 1 week later, a lesion in continuity was found shortly after nerve left medial cord. It conducted a small NAP. Because loss was severe, it was thought that only one or two fascicles going to FCU had been spared severance. The lesion was resected, and an end-to-end suture repair was done. Histology of the resected segment showed a neurotmetic lesion save for two small, intact fascicles.

Youth served this patient well, because he recovered flexor profundi by 1 year, and by 3.5 years even hand intrinsics graded 3 to 4, and sensation had a grade of 4.

### Comment

This is a proximal ulnar nerve injury with a reasonable result, probably related to both sharp mechanism of injury and the patient's age.

### Case Number 2

This 21-year-old male lacerated distal medial surface of the arm on a piece of glass. A primary end-to-end repair without transposition was done elsewhere. He presented 10 months later with severe pain and paresthesias in the ulnar distribution. There was a tender mass 5 cm proximal to the tip of the elbow, and tapping there gave paresthesias down the ulnar side of the forearm. Motor loss was complete distal to the FCU, and this included absent flexor profundus to the little finger. Sensory loss was complete in the ulnar distribution.

The area was explored at 11 months after injury, and a suture neuroma in continuity was found. It did not transmit a NAP and was resected. The gap, which was 4 cm, was shortened by transposition of distal stump beneath FCU and pronator teres. This was done by dissecting distal ulnar nerve through the notch area and below elbow to just beyond the profundus branches. A suture was placed in the epineurium and then a large, curved hemostat was used to create a tunnel beneath FCU and pronator teres. By reaching through the tunnel from the arm to the forearm level with the long hemostat, the suture was grasped and the attached distal stump was drawn through the tunnel. Then, just proximal to the tunnel, an end-to-end repair was accomplished without tension.

Follow-up after 2 years, 11 months indicated flexor profundus to the little finger at grade 4, hypothenars 3, interossei and lumbricals to little and ring fingers 2 to 3, and adductor pollicis 3. Sensation in the ulnar distribution graded 4.

## Comment

Serious injury to ulnar nerve close to the elbow should usually include transposition as one of the surgical steps in its management.

## Case Number 3

This 11-year-old boy had an unusual story. While waiting for his father to pick him up at a boys' boarding school on the coast, he and several other boys made a small fire on the beach and placed a $CO_2$ canister, such as is used to make cocktails, into the fire in an attempt to turn it into a rocket. The cartridge exploded, and a shard of metal sharply lacerated proximal and medial arm. He was seen in a local hospital, where the wound was probed for foreign bodies; none were found. It was noted that almost all of the ulnar nerve was divided but there was a little left in continuity. He was then brought to New Orleans, where examination showed a complete ulnar palsy except for function of the FCU (Figure 9–15). Because the wound was sharp and was caused by penetrating metal rather than a gunshot wound, and because we knew the nerve was almost completely divided, we decided on a relatively acute repair. At the operating table one day after injury, a relatively clean but partial division of the nerve was found. This was converted to a complete division, ends were trimmed of a few millimeters of tissue, and an end-to-end suture was done with 6-0 nylon.

Some FCU function was still present postoperatively. By 4 months, this graded 4, and by 6 months, flexor pro-

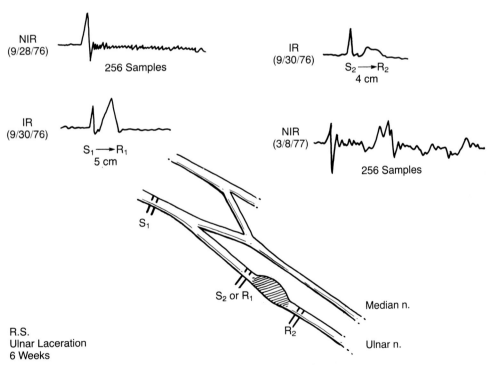

**Figure 9–15.** Partial ulnar lesion caused by an exploded fragment of a $CO_2$ canister. The flexor carpi ulnaris was spared. Although noninvasive recording (NIR) of nerve action potential (NAP) showed no ulnar conduction, a small NAP was recordable by invasive recording (IR) across the lesion *(top right recording)* and a larger one proximal to the lesion *(lower left recording)*. Lesion was resected and repaired end-to-end, and a small NAP could be recorded noninvasively from more distal ulnar nerve 5.5 months later. Because the patient was only 12 years old at the time of injury, he even regained substantial recovery of hand intrinsics (grade 3) over a 6-year period of follow-up.

fundus to the little finger had begun to return. Hypothenars began to contract by a year, and by 4 years postoperatively, intrinsics graded 3. Sensory return was a 4. Youth and the relatively sharp nature of the injury helped, and the patient now uses the limb and the hand in a normal fashion. However, some atrophy of hand intrinsics is present. His weakest muscle remains the lumbrical to the little finger.

# RESULTS WITH ULNAR INJURY AT ELBOW AND FOREARM LEVELS

Mechanisms of injury were more variable at this level than in the upper arm, but lacerations, contusions, and fracture-associated lesions still predominated (Tables 9–4 and 9–5). Complete clinical and electromyographic loss was present in 59 of the 76 cases operated on.

As with the arm-level ulnar lesions, lacerations and punctures were the largest category. Twenty of these 30 cases involved transection of the nerve (Table 9–5). Most were reparable by primary or secondary suture. Early suture was reserved for those severed by glass or knife, and secondary suture was done for those more bluntly transected and if sharply cut, those referred too late for primary repair (Figure 9–16). The patient with resection without repair had undergone several prior unsuccessful repairs and had severe pain as a result of a lengthy and large neuroma in continuity. Resection of neuroma and some proximal and some distal nerve reduced pain enough so that a nonaddictive analgesic could be used. Ten lacerating injuries either contused and stretched or partially lacer-

**TABLE 9–4**
Ulnar Nerve—Forearm and Elbow
Mechanisms for Lesions (n = 120)

| Mechanisms | Operated | Unoperated |
|---|---|---|
| Laceration/ Puncture | 30 | 14 |
| Contusion | 21 | 18 |
| Fracture/ Dislocation | 13 | 8 |
| Gunshot wound | 2 | 2 |
| Injection | 2 | 0 |
| Electrical | 1 | 0 |
| Volkmann | 1 | 1 |
| Hematoma | 0 | 1 |
| Tumor | 6 | 0 |
| TOTALS | 76 | 44 |

**TABLE 9–5**
Ulnar Nerve Injuries — Forearm/Elbow
Level* (n = 70)

| Operation | No. Cases/No. Recovered to Grade 3 or Better |
|---|---|
| **Transections** | |
| Primary suture | 6/4 |
| Secondary repair | |
| Suture | 10/7 |
| Secondary graft | 3/1 |
| Resection | 1/0 |
| **In Continuity†** | |
| Positive NAP (n = 36) | |
| Neurolysis | 36/34 |
| Negative NAP (n = 14) | |
| Split | 1/1 |
| Suture | 9/7 |
| Grafts | 4/2 |

*Six tumors also operated on without significant deficit.
†59 injuries with complete clinical and EMG loss preoperatively.

ated nerves, leaving them in continuity. One had a NAP and a split repair; five others had NAPs and only a neurolysis with adequate eventual recovery. The other four did not have a NAP and required repair, usually by suture. A few lesions had been operated on before, but repair had failed in two, and both had to be reoperated on. In both cases, acute repair of bluntly injured nerves had been attempted.[48] Almost all lesions operated on at this level had transposition and submuscular placement. In four lesions in continuity after resection, gaps were still long enough to require graft repair (Table 9–5 and Figure 9–17).

Most of the contusions and fracture-associated injuries were either partial to begin with or had a recordable NAP, and thus only had neurolysis and a transposition. One of the four gunshot wounds involving ulnar at this level required repair and subsequent transposition, whereas another had only a neurolysis and transposition (Figure 9–18).

One injected nerve required repair, but the other at 3.5 months after injection had NAPs across a lesion in continuity, had only neurolysis, and over the next 1.5 years had a very nice recovery. The Volkmann case involved median and radial as well as ulnar nerves. Neurolysis of all three nerves and transposition of the ulnar nerve as well as fasciotomy were done relatively early, but outcome was only fair.

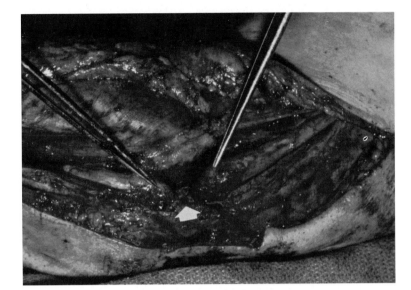

**Figure 9–16.** Ulnar nerve severed in the olecranon notch region *(arrow)* and seen several weeks later. After trimming of each stump, nerve was transposed volar to elbow. An end-to-end repair was done, and nerve was placed deep to pronator teres and flexor carpi ulnaris.

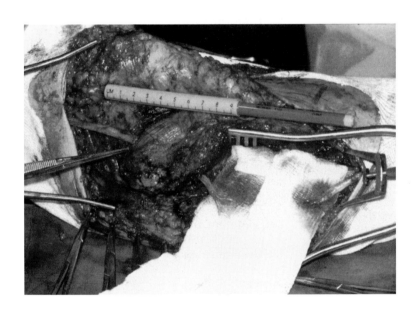

**Figure 9–17.** This lengthy gap in the ulnar nerve at a proximal forearm level was partially shortened by transposing the nerve beneath the pronator teres. The ends of the ulnar nerve have been split into fascicular groups preparatory to placement of sural grafts. The necessary grafts were 5.5 cm in length; without transposition, they would have been 10 cm in length.

**Figure 9–18.** Ulnar nerve injured by gunshot wound close to origin of the flexor profundus branch. Hand is to the left and out of the picture, and shoulder is to the right. In this case, a nerve action potential could be recorded across this lesion at 5 months after injury, so it was not resected. Stimulating electrodes are to the right and recording ones to the left. After neurolysis, the nerve was transposed and buried deep to the proximal forearm muscles.

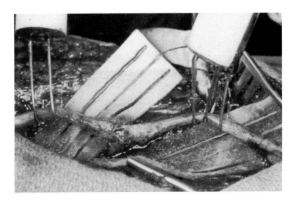

Not unexpectedly, the electrical injury required repair at 4 months after injury. Grafts were necessary, and only a grade 2 level was achieved. Burns by electricity tend to give lengthy up-and-down lesions and are often associated with other severe soft tissue damage, making these difficult lesions to treat.[21,36,52]

Recovery for most of the cases treated without operation was good; several might have benefited from surgery but were seen for the first time by us a year or more after injury. Lesions caused by mild compression, such as an operative complication, usually improved with time.[67] A few at the level of the elbow did, however, require transposition.

## Elbow- and Forearm-Level Lesion Case Summaries

### Case Number 1

This 27-year-old man sustained a gunshot wound from a 38-caliber pistol to the right elbow, resulting in an olecranon fracture which was debrided acutely with removal of bone chips and subsequent casting of the elbow. At the time, ulnar nerve looked bruised and was unroofed where it lay in the olecranon notch and more distally as it ran beneath the two heads of the FCU. After removal from the cast, it was evident that there was a complete ulnar palsy below the FCU. This was accompanied by severe pain not only at the level of the elbow but also radiating down the ulnar side of the forearm. There was an early claw deformity involving the little finger more than the ring finger. Electromyography showed complete denervation in the flexor profundus to the little finger and in the hand intrinsic muscles. These clinical and electrical findings were still present when the patient was first seen by us at 3 months after injury. As a result, the nerve was explored at 13 weeks after injury.

Nerve was found to be swollen and somewhat firm just before it entered the olecranon notch, and this change persisted through its course in the notch to the forearm level. Nerve was encased in relatively heavy scar. An external neurolysis was done. In addition, resection of some of the intermuscular septum and splitting of the two heads of the FCU were carried out. NAP recordings showed a small but definite NAP across the lesion but not beyond the point where flexor profundus branches left the nerve. Thus, there was no conducted response beyond 3.8 cm below the olecranon notch. Nonetheless, conduction velocity was 32 m/sec. As a result, a transposition was done, and nerve with its lesion in continuity was placed deep to FCU and pronator teres. Fascia and some muscle were then closed gently over the nerve.

Postoperatively, most of the patient's neuritic pain was gone, and after a 3.5-year period the functional grades achieved were sensation (ulnar), 3 to 4; flexor profundus V, 4; flexor profundus IV, 5; hypothenar muscles, 3 to 4; interossei, 4; lumbricales V, 3; lumbricales IV, 4; and adductor pollicis, 4. He has had restoration of a fair grip in the right hand, but it is still only 60% of that in the left. As a clerk in a bank, he uses the hand for both writing and some computer work.

### Comment

Despite complete distal clinical and electrical loss, intraoperative evaluation indicated neurolysis and transposition rather than resection. Fortunately, his neuritic pain improved.

### Case Number 2

This 48-year-old man was a passenger in a vehicle involved in an auto accident. His right elbow was badly contused when the door was flung open and then closed on his limb. He had bruising and swelling of the elbow and a partial ulnar palsy. The patient felt that mild, initial hand weakness had progressed with time. He was first seen 4 months after the accident. FCU and flexor profundi to the ring and little fingers worked well. Hypothenar muscles graded only 2 and interossei 1 to 2. Lumbrical to the little finger was absent and that to the ring finger graded 2 to 3. Adductor pollicis was much better at 3 to 4. Sensation was poor, but loss was partial and graded 3.

The patient underwent neurolysis, recordings, and transposition at 5 months after injury. Nerve appeared tight or snug in the region of the olecranon notch and was somewhat decreased in caliber at that level even after neurolysis. NAPs conducted across this area, but only at 20 m/sec.

He made an eventual good recovery, with hand intrinsics and sensation each reaching an overall grade of 4 by 3 years and 2 months postoperatively.

### Comment

Despite incomplete loss in the distribution of the ulnar nerve and a blunt injury, operation to provide a better environment for the nerve seemed indicated. This was especially so in this case, in which some progression of loss was suggested by the patient's history, even though there was no opportunity to document it.

## RESULTS WITH ULNAR INJURY AT WRIST LEVEL

Table 9–6 gives the mechanisms for injury at this level. In our ulnar series, injury to nerve at wrist or palm was the smallest category of injury by level. The leading mechanism of injury was

**TABLE 9–6**
Ulnar Nerve — Wrist Level Mechanisms
of Lesions (n = 42)

| Mechanisms | Operated | Unoperated |
|---|---|---|
| Laceration | 15 | 3 |
| Fracture/ Dislocation | 4 | 4 |
| Stretch/ Contusion | 2 | 3 |
| Gunshot wound | 2 | 1 |
| Tumor | 2 | 0 |
| Electrical | 2 | 1 |
| Prior surgical injury | 1 | 2 |
| TOTALS | 28 | 14 |

laceration, just as it was at the other levels. Fifteen of the 26 injuries at this level had complete loss preoperatively. There were 11 transected nerves, and 6 were sharp enough and seen acutely enough to have primary repair[47] (Table 9–7). All of those having secondary repair had at least a grade 3 recovery, with several reaching grade 4 levels. One neuroma caused by transection had been long-standing and nerve was resected rather than repaired. The other laceration-associated lesions left nerves in some degree of continuity; two had NAPs and had neurolysis with recovery, and one had a split repair based on differential fascicular recordings.[83]

**TABLE 9–7**
Ulnar Nerve Injuries — Wrist Level*
(n = 26)†

| Operation | No. Cases/No. Recovered to Grade 3 or Better |
|---|---|
| **Transections** | |
| Primary suture | 6/3 |
| Secondary repair | |
|   Suture | 2/2 |
|   Graft | 1/1 |
|   Split repair | 1/1 |
|   Resection | 1/0 |
| **In Continuity** | |
| Positive NAP (n = 9) | |
|   Neurolysis | 8/8 |
|   Split | 1/1 |
| Negative NAP (n = 6) | |
|   Suture | 3/2 |
|   Grafts | 3/1 |

*Two tumors removed without further deficit.
†15 injuries had complete clinical and electromyographic loss preoperatively.

There were eight digital nerve repairs with variable results, but usually with recovery of enough sensation to be protective. Four other patients had digital nerves with neuromas resected with improvement of pain and hypersensitivity.

Both electrical injuries operated on required graft repair, and only one regained a grade 3 functional level. A third electrical lesion was managed more conservatively because loss was partial even soon after injury. Both contusions and two of the four lesions associated with wrist fracture or dislocation had not only lesions in continuity but positive NAPs and, as a result, neurolysis with recovery.

## Wrist-Level Case Summaries

### Case Number 1

This 22-year-old male's arm went through a plate glass window, and he required immediate repair of brachial artery and biceps tendon. Nerve ends were tagged with tantalum clips, and the limb was casted. The patient had complete loss of both median and ulnar function. The only muscle partially spared was pronator teres, which graded 3. Two weeks later, we explored the wound. Median and ulnar stumps had retracted, and after trimming these, four antebrachial cutaneous nerve grafts were used to bridge the gap in the median, which was 6.4 cm in length. The gap in the ulnar was made up by transposition. As a result, an end-to-end suture repair of this nerve could be done. The immediate postoperative period was uncomplicated.

At follow-up after 6 years, the patient could make a fist and could enclose his flexed fingers with his thumb. If he extended his fingers, the little finger tended to abduct. In the median distribution, he had excellent pronation, flexor superficialis, flexor profundus, and flexor pollicis longus. Abductor pollicis brevis and opponens pollicis graded 3 to 4, and median sensation was 3. Overall median grade was 4. In the ulnar distribution, he had excellent FCU. Flexor profundus and even hypothenar muscles graded 4. Interossei and lumbricals were 3, while abductor pollicis was 3 to 4. Sensation graded 3, and overall ulnar grade was 3 to 4. He could localize stimuli, but two-point discrimination remained poor. The patient would look at his hand when he used it for fine tasks, and he still had trouble picking up fine objects and buttoning clothes, but he could use the hand to turn door knobs and could also turn the lid on a jar. As an owner of a grocery store, he stocked shelves and cut meat. He said he could use the hand to write with a pen or pencil if necessary, but his grip was somewhat different because he used more of his fingers to balance the grip of the thumb than before.

## Comment

If a decision is made not to repair a divided nerve at the time of acute operation, we recommend tacking the stump with an epineurial stitch to adjacent muscle or fascia. This prevents stump retraction. Placing a tantalum clip on a stump is of no benefit.

## Case Number 2

A 42-year-old male electronics engineer had progressive numbness and weakness in the ulnar distribution after using a hammer vigorously with the right hand. He subsequently developed a partial claw of the right little and ring fingers. There was a Tinel sign at the wrist but no palpable mass. Ulnar-innervated hand intrinsics graded 2 to 3. Sensory examination was normal. Flexor profundus to little finger was preserved. Conduction along ulnar nerves was mildly slowed at both elbows, but conduction was more markedly slowed at the level of right wrist.

At exploration several months after onset of symptoms, a ganglion cyst 1.5 cm in diameter was found compressing the deep branch of the ulnar nerve. This branch was dissected off the lateral side of the cyst. After excision, the neck of the cyst was ligated and then oversewn with fascia. He has done well postoperatively with gradual restoration of ulnar-innervated hand intrinsic function.

## Comment

Not all hand-intrinsic loss is related to the more common elbow-level lesion. In addition, a complicating mass lesion such as this patient's ganglion may play a role in entrapments. Absence of sensory loss in presence of ulnar intrinsic motor loss alerts the examiner to the wrist level as the site of pathology. An EMG report of some or slight ulnar slowing at the elbow should not outweigh the clinical findings indicating wrist as the level of involvement.

Results of repair from several other series are summarized in Tables 9–8 and 9–9.

**TABLE 9–8**

### Ulnar Nerve Secondary Suture Repair (Seddon*)

| Upper arm and elbow level | 20% M3 S3 or better recovery |
|---|---|
| Forearm level | 25% M3 S3 or better recovery |
| Wrist level | 44.5% M3 S3 or better recovery |

*British system.
M = motor grade; S = sensory grade.

**TABLE 9–9**

### Ulnar Nerve Repair Results (Dellon)

| High-level suture repair | 17% M4 or better recovery |
|---|---|
|  | 20% S3+ or better recovery |
| Low-level suture repair | 32% M4 or better recovery |
|  | 34.7% S3 or better recovery |
| Combined high and low graft repair | 43% M4 or better recovery |
|  | 21% S3 or better recovery |
| Digital Nerve |  |
|   All-level suture repair | 59% S3 or better recovery |
|   All-level graft repair | 29% S3 or better recovery |

M = motor grade; S = sensory grade.

# COMPLICATIONS

Median nerve can be injured by retraction or rough handling as ulnar nerve is approached in the proximal arm. Fortunately, we did not experience this complication.

The potential complications with various transpositions or attempts to treat ulnar entrapment at the elbow are legion. We almost always did a modified Learmouth transposition, placing nerve deep to pronator teres and FCU. Despite dividing and then reattaching a portion of these muscles, weakness in their distribution was seldom a problem. However, there were several patients who had increased weakness in flexor profundus to little finger or ring finger. In addition, a patient with partial hand-intrinsic loss before manipulation of the nerve, especially for entrapment, may have increased intrinsic loss postoperatively.

Complications at forearm level include loss of ulnar artery. This occurred in two of our patients but had no serious consequences in terms of vascular insufficiency to the hand.

Decompression of ulnar nerve through the Guyon canal can be incomplete and lead to failure to improve, with entrapment at that level. In our relatively small series of cases at this level, this complication was avoided.

A number of patients in our series of injuries, as in other authors', required tendon transfer(s) to reduce the tendency for clawing.[5,53,70] When this had not been done because stiffness in little and ring fingers had set in, progressive casting and, in a few instances, capsulotomies had to be done.[66]

# ULNAR ENTRAPMENT ELBOW LEVEL

The most common lesion to involve ulnar nerve is entrapment at the level of the elbow. Compression can occur at several levels, but the predominant involvement is within the olecranon notch. Normally, the nerve is somewhat snug as it passes over the floor of this structure. Spontaneous entrapment is usually associated with adhesions in the region of the olecranon notch. The aponeurotic arch overlying the notch and extending to medial epicondyle can also thicken and compress the nerve. Flexion of the elbow moves the nerve through this tight or snug area and may produce a frictional injury. Less frequently, the nerve is compressed more distally by the origins of the two heads of the FCU.[1,68] If this occurs, it is called the cubital tunnel syndrome.[26] Occasionally, the ulnar nerve rides up and out of the olecranon groove or notch as the arm is flexed. Rarely, the nerve is spontaneously compressed proximal to the notch by a Struthers ligament.

Entrapment is more likely to occur if there has been prior elbow fracture or dislocation, but the majority of cases seen do not give this history.[31] Soft tissue contusion to forearm and elbow without fracture can be a predisposing factor, as can diabetes mellitus, a history of alcoholism, rheumatoid arthritis, and tumors or ganglia arising at the level of the elbow. There may be a history of repetitive trauma caused by pressure. The patient may be used to resting the elbow on a hard surface such as a desk or bar top or the window ledge of a car. One patient who developed unilateral entrapment was a telephone operator who rested her right elbow on a table as she held the phone to her ear. Another patient who had bilateral entrapment worked as a fitter for wedding dresses. She would rest both elbows on a low table as she reached up to pin or sew beads or sequins on the bride-to-be or a mannequin.

## Symptoms

Patients commonly complain of paresthesias in the ulnar distribution, particularly of the little and, sometimes, the ring finger. Often, the sensory syndrome is rather specific in that symptoms are present on the ulnar but not radial side of the ring finger. Sensory fibers are usually affected before motor fibers. Paresthesias may be spontaneous or may be prompted by use of the hand. In other cases, rather than spontaneous tingling or electric shocks, the patient may notice only hyperesthesia mixed with hypoesthesia of the little and ring fingers. This is followed by numbness in a similar distribution. With time, weakness in the hand intrinsic muscles may develop. Most noticeable is interosseous and hypothenar muscle weakness. The former may be initially manifested by spontaneous abduction of the little finger or a Wartenberg sign caused by palmar interosseous weakness. With time, atrophy of these muscles is evident. Occasionally, the entrapment presents first as weakness in the hand. The patient has difficulty with fine movements. If the dominant hand is involved, holding a pen or pencil and writing is tedious. Turning a doorknob or unscrewing the lid of a jar or top of a bottle is difficult. In some cases, symptoms do not progress, and they may, on occasion, even regress if the elbow is rested or the patient avoids putting pressure on it.

## Physical Findings

Examination usually shows hypoesthesia mixed with hyperesthesia in the ulnar distribution of the hand. This is most likely on the volar surface of the little finger and the dorsum of the distal digit. Usually some degree of hand-intrinsic weakness is present, especially if the strength of the individual muscles of one hand is compared with that of the other. Intrinsics showing the earliest weakness are the lumbrical to the little finger and abductor digiti quinti minimi. Weakness of the flexor profundus of the little finger usually occurs later than weakness of the hand intrinsics. Most striking under these circumstances is the appearance of the hand. There is shrinkage of intrinsics evident by inspection of the dorsum of the hand as well as on the palmar side along hypothenar eminence. An ulnar claw may develop later in the course of the entrapment owing to lack of input of lumbricals to the little and, sometimes, the ring finger.

Tenderness is usually present at the elbow, but of even greater importance is a Tinel sign at that level. Tapping over the notch or proximal to it gives paresthesias in the distribution of the nerve, particularly into the little and, sometimes, the ring finger. The nerve may translocate out of the olecranon groove, and the examiner can feel it slip out as he or she flexes and extends the elbow. Some but not all patients with translocation of the nerve become symptomatic. Occasionally, this phenomenon is noted where there has been a prior neurolysis without transposition or a medial epicondylectomy or failed subcutaneous transposition.[13] The rate or progression of loss of function is extremely variable. At any one point in time, this progression is usually unpredictable.

## Differential Diagnosis

Differential diagnoses include those disorders or traumatic episodes that involve lower plexus elements. This includes lower cervical root radiculopathy caused by spurs or discs. Thoracic outlet syndrome with lower spinal nerve compression could in part mimic ulnar neuropathy, but in those cases there is often loss not only of hand intrinsics innervated by ulnar but also of those thenar intrinsics innervated by median. In addition, a Horner syndrome may alert the examiner to a more central or proximal pathology. Amyotrophic lateral sclerosis can begin with hand muscle loss on one side in one third of cases. With time, however, the loss involves more of the arm and also the opposite arm and hand. As with spontaneous ulnar entrapment, the peak period of presentation of amyotrophic lateral sclerosis is between 40 and 60 years of age. Another important neurologic differential diagnosis is syringomyelia (Figure 9–19). Here, truncal or contralateral hand findings may suggest the diagnosis. More distal lesions of the ulnar nerve, particularly entrapment in the Guyon canal, can mimic elbow-level entrapment, particularly if the deep branch is involved, because maximal deficit is in hand intrinsic muscles in both.

Spontaneous entrapment can be bilateral. This occurs almost 20% of the time, although the contralateral side is often not symptomatic initially, and ulnar entrapment is usually unilat-

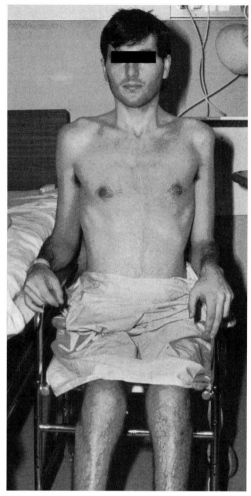

**Figure 9–19.** Paraplegic patient referred as suspected syringomyelia. Instead, compression and entrapment of both ulnar nerves at the level of the olecranon notch was found. Patient habitually rested his elbows on firm wheelchair arm rests.

eral on initial presentation. Symptoms are not always related to occupation but certainly can be. Generally, cases have been categorized as follows:

Group I    Mild symptoms without motor involvement and minimal gross abnormality found at surgery. Most will recover fully even if symptoms were present for months to years.

Group II    Various sensory symptoms and mild to moderate hand intrinsic atrophy. Almost 50% experience reversal of some

Group III  Severe sensory and motor loss with hand-intrinsic muscle wasting and not only reduced strength but loss of bulk. Surgery may relieve or help pain and may increase sensation but, at best, only gives partial return of hand-intrinsic function.

muscle loss, including intrinsic function, after careful transposition.

In the usual case, the initial symptoms include intermittent hyperesthesia and paresthesias in the ulnar distribution. These symptoms are often associated with elbow flexion. Sometimes numbness is not noticed until it is pointed out to the patient at the time of examination. The patient may or may not notice lateral instability of the fingers whereby the index finger slips sideways on gripping a knife or a pencil. There may be loss of stability of the little finger. During grasp, there may be loss of synchrony of digital flexion, and with intrinsic loss, coordination of thumb and digits may be poor.

### Electrical Studies

Electrophysiologic workup almost always confirms conductive slowing across the elbow.[8,22] Nonetheless, careful inspection and palpation of the limb and clinical testing of function remain paramount in the diagnosis of ulnar entrapment, just as with most nerve lesions.[17] This is especially so with ulnar entrapment at the elbow because most electrical conductive studies involve a segment of more normal nerve both proximal and often well distal to the area of compression in the olecranon notch. Despite this consideration, with more severe entrapment, conduction distal and for a variable length proximal to the site of compression may be slowed as well.[33] Severe and especially sustained entrapment leads to denervational changes in the hand intrinsic muscles, including hypothenars, lumbricals, and, especially, interossei.[41] Input to adductor pollicis is, on the other hand, sometimes relatively preserved. Conductive studies of wrist-level ulnar nerve can usually exclude more distal entrapment in the Guyon canal (Figure 9–20).

## WRIST LEVEL ENTRAPMENT

Three levels of entrapment can occur at the wrist level.

### Deep Branch

This is the most common ulnar entrapment at this level. Etiologies include repeated palmar trauma or pressure, ganglia, or carpal synovitis.[27,42] An unusual cause is hard labor or pressure of the palm against the handlebar in long-

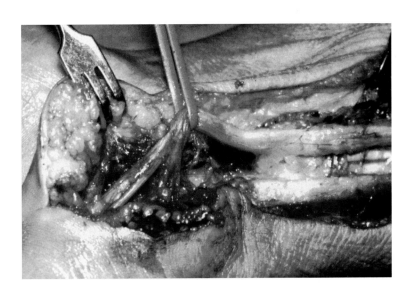

**Figure 9–20.** Ulnar nerve in the region of the Guyon canal. Both superficial and deep branches had been entrapped at this level by the ulnar expansion of the transverse carpal ligament.

distance bikers.[23,45] With trauma or pressure, the pisohamate ligament can thicken. Electrically, conduction to abductor digiti quinti minimi is usually normal but that to first dorsal interosseous is abnormal. Clinical loss and denervational changes are in interossei, little and ring finger lumbricals, and adductor pollicis.[74] Sensation is intact.

### Proximal Palmar Branch

Compression at this point gives loss in the hypothenar muscles as well as in the palmar level intrinsics. The hallmark is that despite this severe intrinsic loss, superficial sensory distribution is spared.

### Sensory and Motor Branch

This is the least frequent spontaneous distal entrapment, but can sometimes be seen with wrist fractures and ganglion cysts.[6,57] There is ulnar sensory loss that does not include the dorsal cutaneous branch distribution; loss does include distal ulnar motor loss in intrinsic muscles. Sensory conduction from the little finger and sometimes ring finger is delayed across the wrist.

## OPERATIVE TECHNIQUE FOR USUAL ULNAR ENTRAPMENT AT LEVEL OF ELBOW

The elbow is positioned in extension with a folded towel under the elbow on an arm board. The hand is placed palm up. A slightly undulating skin incision extending from the medial surface of distal arm toward the medial but volar surface of the elbow and then down along the proximal and medial side of the forearm is performed (Figure 9–21). Dissection is carried

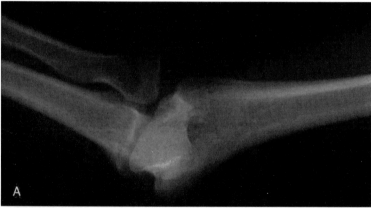

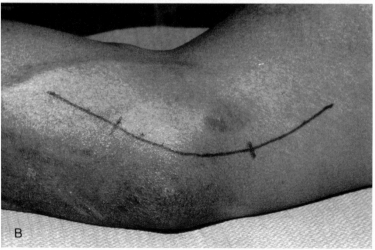

**Figure 9–21.** (A) Fracture dislocation of the elbow associated with subsequent onset of tardy ulnar palsy. (B) Usual type of incision used to expose entrapped ulnar nerve.

*Illustration continued on opposite page*

through subcutaneous tissues first, at a forearm and then at an upper arm level. Antebrachial cutaneous nerves should be preserved and, if possible, mobilized toward the radial side of the forearm. The ulnar nerve can be easily located within the olecranon notch and then traced proximally into the distal arm and distally into the proximal forearm. We have usually identified the nerve first in the arm where it lies adherent to the superior muscle fibers of the FCU and is sometimes covered by fibers from the medial head of the triceps (arcade of Struthers).[80] On its dorsal belly, nerve is also often adherent to triceps at this level and must be sharply dissected away. Major branches to proximal FCU should be preserved whenever possible. If need

be, branches can be dissected back and split away from the main trunk of the ulnar nerve so they are lengthened preparatory to transposition.

There may also be major collateral vascular input to the nerve at this level, and this should be dissected out and preserved if possible. Dissection is carried proximal enough to identify the point at which the nerve comes under intermuscular septum.[77] Septum is sectioned or a segment of septum is actually resected so that the course of the nerve in the distal upper arm is free after transposition (Figure 9–22). The nerve is then encircled with a Penrose drain. Dissection can then proceed by following the nerve distally and unroofing the olecranon

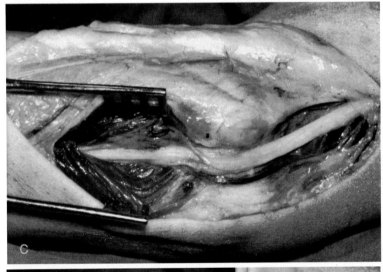

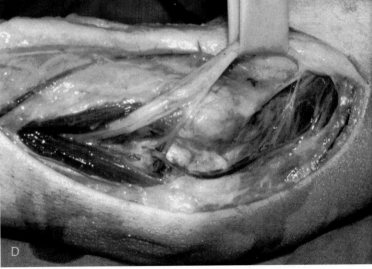

**Figure 9–21.** *Continued (C)* Ulnar nerve in olecranon notch—proximal is to the right and distal to the left where the two heads of the flexor carpi ulnaris have been split. *(D)* Nerve has been temporarily moved volar to elbow so that the line of incision in volar musculature can be ascertained.

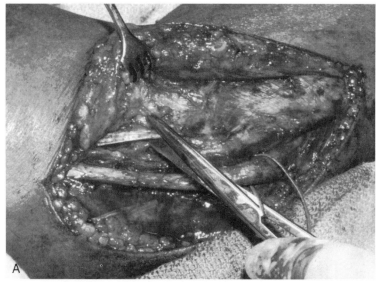

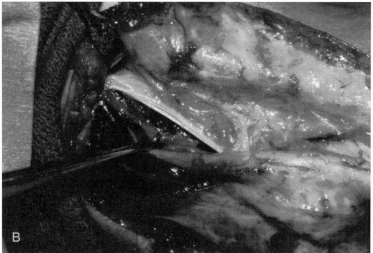

**Figure 9–22.** (A) Sectioning intermuscular septum before transposition of an ulnar nerve. An alternate step is to actually resect a segment of this fibrous tissue. (B) Repeat operation on subcutaneously transposed ulnar nerve where intermuscular septum had not been divided.

notch. The nerve is re-encircled with a Penrose drain and dissected in a circumferential fashion as it runs in proximal forearm.

An alternative for distal exposure is to place the proximal phalanx of the surgeon's little finger in the notch and to point the tip of the finger towards the ulnar side of the wrist. This gives the approximate course of the ulnar nerve in proximal forearm, where it lies deep to the two heads of the FCU but above flexor superficialis (Figure 9–23). A longitudinal incision can then be made through fascia and the fibers of the FCU muscle split to expose the deeper forearm portion of the ulnar nerve. Smaller branches to the FCU may be encountered just distal to the notch and can either be dissected

back into the main ulnar nerve to lengthen them for transposition or sacrificed by sectioning.

Some 2.5 to 5 cm distal to the notch, branches to the ulnar half of the flexor profundus arise. These take off from the radial and somewhat dorsal surface of the ulnar nerve and run a relatively short course to the profundus. It is very important to preserve this muscular input. After ulnar nerve has been cleared to 8 cm or so below the olecranon notch, it can be encircled with another Penrose drain.

Dissection is then carried into the olecranon notch alternatively from upper arm and forearm levels. Bipolar forceps should be used in the notch because both arteries and veins accompany the nerve and are deep to it, lying on the

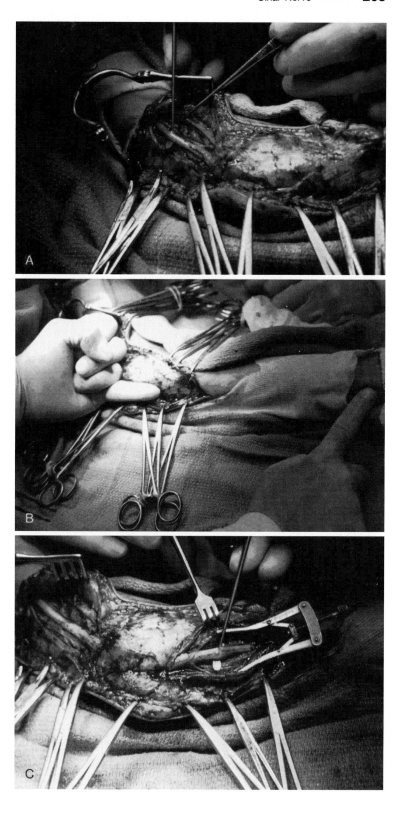

**Figure 9–23.** *(A)* Exposure of proximal-arm portion of ulnar nerve preparatory to transposition. *(B)* Method of determining forearm course of ulnar nerve. Base of surgeon's left little finger rests in the olecranon notch and points toward his right forefinger, which is placed over the wrist portion of the ulna. A line projected between the two outlines the course of the nerve. *(C)* Ulnar nerve exposed both above and below the olecranon notch. Spatula is beneath the distal or forearm level nerve.

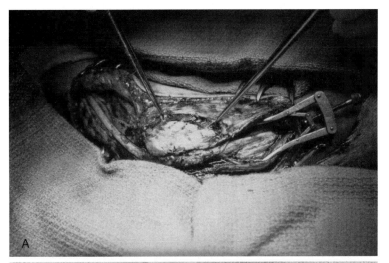

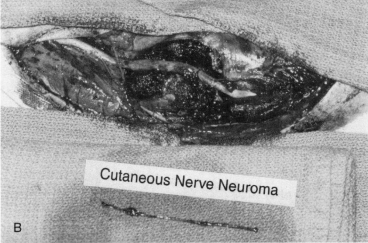

Cutaneous Nerve Neuroma

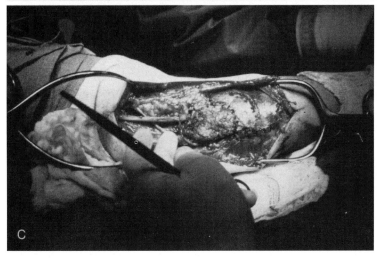

**Figure 9–24.** (A) Nerve has been cleared through the region of the olecranon notch by a complete external neurolysis. A trough has been made in the proximal forearm muscle by sectioning completely through pronator teres and the more volar portion of flexor carpi ulnaris. (B) Nerve has been placed in the muscle trough. Note that a neuroma and segment of antebrachial cutaneous nerve have been resected and are placed on the drape. This patient had prior neurolysis for olecranon notch-level entrapment and had injury to antebrachial cutaneous nerve. (C) Transposed nerve with closure of pronator teres and flexor carpi ulnaris over it. See also color figure.

floor of the notch, and these vessels bleed frequently. Neural branches to the elbow joint, which are usually small, can be cut and thus sacrificed. After nerve is free 360 degrees around, it is ready for transposition. The radial side of pronator teres is dissected distally, and some of lacertus fibrosis is sectioned to mobilize the proximal pronator muscle. Some of the pronator and FCU origins are then undermined over the medial epicondyle. A trough is made in an oblique and slightly curved fashion all the way through pronator and proximal portions of FCU. The detached distal muscle mass is then gently elevated and slightly undermined, as is that portion left attached to the medial epicondyle.

Ulnar nerve is then placed in the muscle trough, and some fascia and superficial pronator muscle is reattached to a cuff of muscle and fascia on the medial epicondyle with 1-0 suture (Figure 9–24). FCU is also reattached to the cuff of muscle along the distal portion of the medial epicondyle. Forearm FCU is then closed over the nerve, but not before gently grasping nerve proximally and distally with the gloved fingers to make sure it moves freely with a gentle tug back and forth beneath the already partially reclosed volar musculature. The longitudinal split

in more distal FCU is closed only superficially so as not to compress underlying nerve. Other soft tissues including skin are usually closed subcutaneously without a drain.

If there has been a previous operation, the older elbow incision is used but, usually, extended somewhat proximally into the arm and distally down forearm. This was especially necessary if a short elbow level incision was used for a medial epicondylectomy or a neurolysis without transposition at the elbow level. Because of prior operation and, usually, subcutaneous position of the previously transposed nerve, a good deal of scar tissue is almost always encountered. In this regard, it is helpful to extend the proximal exposure enough to find more healthy nerve and then to trace the nerve through the scar and previously placed tacking sutures using sharp dissection with a No. 15 blade on a plastic scalpel handle. In some cases, it is necessary to locate distal forearm level nerve and work this back toward and through the elbow level scar as well.

As has been reported by others, we felt that some previously operated entrapment cases were candidates for reoperation[7,56] (Figure 9–25). There were a variety of findings common to these cases.

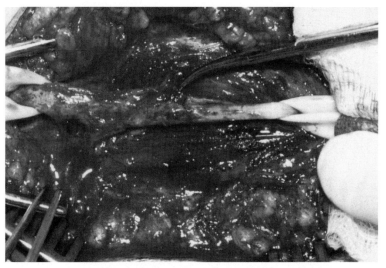

**Figure 9–25.** Appearance of ulnar nerve at the elbow after two attempts to treat it surgically for entrapment. The first operation was a simple decompression through the olecranon notch and the cubital tunnel, whereas the second was a subcutaneous transposition volar to the elbow. When seen by one of the authors, the patient had an ulnar neuropathy with motor grades averaging 3 to 4 and sensation at grade 4. The patient had painful paresthesias in the ulnar distribution and an exquisitely tender elbow with a Tinel sign over that portion of the nerve. An external neurolysis was done, and nerve was buried deep to pronator teres and flexor carpi ulnaris. Over a 1-year period, the patient's pain has improved greatly, and motor grades are 4 with a sensory grade of 4+.

1. Extraneural scar over a length of the nerve was universal.
2. Some cases had epineural thickening, intraneural scar, or even neuroma, most likely related to injury from the prior operation. Several patients had sustained damage to antebrachial cutaneous nerves or branches, and this appeared to be responsible for at least some of their persistent symptoms (see Fig. 9–24B).[19]
3. There was angulation or kinking of the nerve as it passed over volar pronator teres or, more commonly, as it left this subcutaneous site to penetrate between the two heads of the FCU. In other cases, because of slippage or initial incomplete transposition, nerve was found riding on top of the medial epi-

condyle. In some cases, the nerve was kinked or angulated at two separate levels. Usually, intraoperative NAP recording showed marked conductive delays at either or both of these sites of angulation.

4. If prior medial epicondylectomy had been tried and had failed, nerve was found to be partially volar but still riding over the medial prominence of the epicondylar region. Because of a presumed limited neurolysis, angulation or kinking either proximally or distally was sometimes found (Figure 9–26).
5. Only two transpositions with submuscular burial done elsewhere had to be redone in this series. In both of these cases, the muscle trough had been incompletely created, more medial FCU was not divided or was incom-

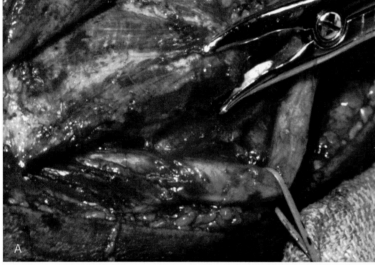

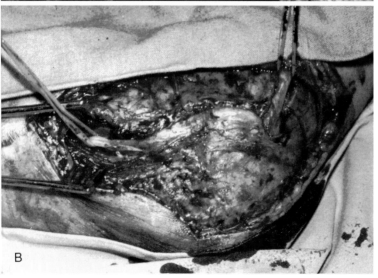

**Figure 9–26.** (A) Ehni procedure. Ulnar nerve has been mobilized, and medial epicondyle has been cleared of some of pronator and flexor carpi ulnaris origins. Leksell rongeur is used to remove some of medial epicondyle. (B) Scarred and somewhat angulated ulnar nerve which had been placed subcutaneously. Nerve was subsequently cleared of scar and placed below forearm musculature.

pletely divided, and forearm-level nerve was severely angulated. In several reoperated cases, it was apparent that nerve had been placed in pronator teres rather than below it, and this may have led to persistent symptoms, as suggested by Dellon's experimental studies.[20]

## Documentation of Ulnar Entrapment Site

For study purposes, each of the ulnar nerves in the LSUMC series of ulnar entrapments, whether previously operated or not, had intraoperative NAP recordings made from nerve both proximal to the notch and across the notch *before* nerve was released at that level. After these recordings were made and nerve was freed entirely from the notch, NAP recordings were repeated to see where abnormality in conduction velocity and NAP amplitude were first evident, and where they were maximal. Results in previously unoperated cases indicated the following.

1. The first observation was that conduction velocities were invariably much slower when intraoperative direct recording was done across the elbow than in the less invasive preoperative conductive studies. This should not be surprising, because recording distances were shorter and involved comparatively more abnormal than normal nerve with the direct intraoperative studies than with the preoperative, more classic and less invasive conductive studies.
2. Although amplitudes of NAPs across the notch sometimes increased immediately after neurolysis of the nerve, conduction velocity (CV) seldom did acutely (Figure 9–27). In a few cases, amplitude decreased, presumably because of manipulation of the nerve in the region of the notch.
3. Although CV was often slowed at the arm level in ulnar nerve involved by more distal entrapment, CV changes were usually maximal either just proximal to the notch or within the notch segment of the nerve itself.
4. Amplitude of NAPs was usually maintained in the upper arm but began to dampen as nerve approached notch or in the notch itself (Figure 9–28).

Ulnar Translocation—Nerve Action Potential Recordings

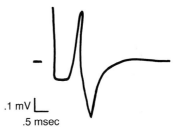

.1 mV

.5 msec

Recording proximal to notch, conduction = 78 m/sec
S→R = 5.5 cm

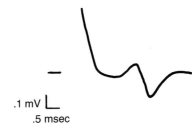

.1 mV

.5 msec

Recording in olecranon notch, conduction = 38.5 m/sec
S→R = 9.0 cm

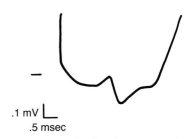

.1 mV

.5 msec

Recording distal to olecranon notch, conduction = 42 m/sec
S→R = 8.5 cm

**Figure 9–27.** Intraoperative nerve action potential (NAP) recordings on a patient with mild but significant ulnar neuropathy and translocation of the nerve over the medial epicondyle on flexion and extension. Top tracing shows recording proximal to olecranon notch. Middle tracing shows NAP recorded with electrode on the nerve in the notch (where amplitude is decreased and velocity quite slowed). Bottom tracing also shows a relatively small NAP amplitude and slowed response when recording electrode was placed about 1 cm beyond the notch area.

5. It was rare for either CV or NAP amplitude to be maintained through the notch area. In other words, the entrapment, injury, or irritative site appeared to be maximal within the olecranon notch segment of the nerve and

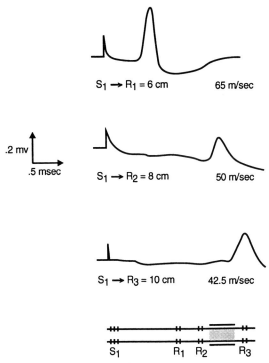

**Figure 9–28.** Typical nerve action potential recordings made operatively in a patient with ulnar-entrapment neuropathy. Top trace, $S_1$ to $R_1$, was recorded well proximal to the entrapment site; $S_1$ to $R_2$ was recorded just proximal to the olecranon notch and begins to show slowing of conduction. Recording made more distally ($S_1$ to $R_3$) is even more slowed.

not more distally beneath the two heads of the FCU or what has been termed the cubital tunnel.

These electrical observations usually correlated well with the physical appearance of that portion of the ulnar nerve in the olecranon notch or groove. Sometimes the nerve was swollen, injected, and angry in appearance in the notch area, but usually it had a compressed, narrowed, and scarred appearance.[12] In about 20% of the cases, electrical and sometimes gross pathologic abnormalities began somewhat proximal to the olecranon portion of the nerve; in most others, changes were more severe in the notch portion of the nerve. There were only four cases in which recordings were maximally abnormal just distal to the notch or in the area of so-called cubital tunnel. These observations to date support the concept that most elbow-level entrapments originate in the olecranon notch or groove and not at a more distal site.

**TABLE 9–10**
Grading for Ulnar Entrapments

| | |
|---|---|
| 0 | No hand intrinsics; sensation grades 0 to 1. |
| 1 | No hand intrinsics; sensation 1 to 3. |
| 2 | Hand intrinsics are trace (1) or to antigravity (2); sensation 2 to 4. |
| 3 | Hand intrinsics grade 3: sensation grades 3 or higher. |
| 4 | Hand intrinsics grade 4; sensation grades 4 or 5. |
| 5 | Hand intrinsics grade 5; sensation grades 4 or 5. |

The following outcomes were accumulated with the help of Dr. John Reeves.

## Results With Ulnar Entrapment at Elbow Level

The grading system used to evaluate ulnar entrapments is found in Table 9–10. The system does not match or compare proximal with distal recovery, but instead concentrates on hand-intrinsic and sensory function. These two modalities are the most seriously affected by most elbow-level ulnar entrapments. Most group I patients (see prior section on differential diagnosis) graded 5 preoperatively, whereas group II usually graded 4 preoperatively. Severe cases or group III patients graded 3 or less preoperatively. Looked at in that fashion, 27 patients in the series operated on and having some follow-up were group I, 144 group II, and 59 group III.

Table 9–11 shows the incidence of bilaterality to the 368 lesions studied and also indicates that 35 were related to prior injury, 18 to diabetes mellitus, and 3 to Hansen disease. Eighty-two patients had prior operations elsewhere in an attempt to stabilize or reverse the palsy. *Ten of the spontaneous cases presented after an unre-*

**TABLE 9–11**
Operated Ulnar Nerve Entrapments — LSUMC Series

| | |
|---|---|
| Unilateral | 308 |
| Bilateral | 60 |
| | 368 |
| Injury associated | 35 |
| Diabetic | 18 |
| Hansen disease | 3 |
| Prior operation | 82 |

*lated operation or during hospitalization.* This type of onset has been reported before.[2,24,60] In a few cases, this onset could be related to operative positioning or inadvertent compression during the course of the operation, but in most, a clear-cut cause was lacking (Figure 9–29).

The proper procedure to use for surgical management of ulnar entrapment remains most controversial, and there are advocates of each of the many different operational procedures. Operations include neurolysis without transposition, release of only the cubital tunnel, neurolysis and transposition of the nerve to a subcutaneous site, medial epicondylectomy or the Ehni procedure, transposition to an intramuscular site, and, finally, neurolysis with transposition to a submuscular site.[14,25,30,58,64,84,85] The last approach, originally described by Learmouth and refined by Leffert and Dellon and others, was used in our clinic for operative management of entrapments severe enough not to respond to conservative treatment.[16,50,51]

Table 9–12 depicts results in terms of grade stabilization or change after operation in fresh cases and in those operated previously elsewhere and requiring repeat operation. Follow-up for patients reported in this table was for at least 1 year. Grade categories are also provided for cases not operated on but seen in follow-up over a period of one or more years.

In the cases not operated on, grades tended to remain stable, and only 12 of 72 cases, or 15%, improved with time. Indeed, three cases deteriorated over time from 5 to 4, but these patients still refused operation. By comparison, in the freshly operated category, 154 of 214 cases improved their level of motor function, and usually sensory function, postoperatively. Fifty-two remained unchanged; 10 of those were at an excellent level (grade 5) to begin with, and another 28 cases were at a grade 4 level.

It was harder to improve function in those patients who had undergone prior operations. In that category, 25 of 82 cases stayed at their preoperative level, and one case deteriorated from a 3 to 0. Nonetheless, 45 patients in this category improved one grade, and 10 patients improved two grades.

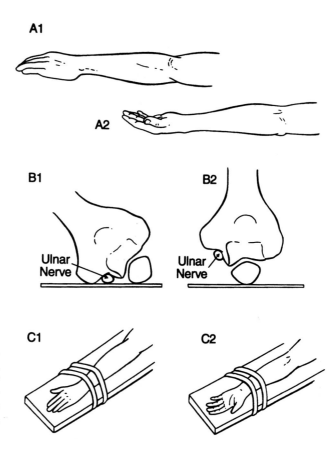

**Figure 9–29.** If arm is extended and elbow is held down on a firm surface, such as an arm board, it is better to place the hand palm up rather than palm down. The palm up position is less likely to lead to compression of the ulnar nerve in the region of the olecranon notch.

**TABLE 9–12**
Ulnar Entrapments Preoperative Grade to Postoperative Grade (n = 368 cases)*

| Grades<br>Preoperative to Postoperative | Number of<br>Operated Cases | Number of<br>Unoperated Cases |
|---|---|---|
| 2 to 2 | 3   (2) | 9 |
| 2 to 3 | 10   (4) | 1 |
| 2 to 4 | 12   (3) | 0 |
| 3 to 0 | 0   (1) | 0 |
| 3 to 3 | 11   (3) | 6 |
| 3 to 4 | 40 (16) | 3 |
| 3 to 5 | 40   (7) | 0 |
| 4 to 4 | 28 (15) | 16 |
| 4 to 5 | 52 (25) | 8 |
| 5 to 5 | 10   (4) | 20 |
| 5 to 4 | 0   (0) | 3 |
| Subtotals | 206 (80) | 66 |
| Results not known | 8   (2) | 6 |
| | 214 (82) | 72 |
| Total | 368 Cases | |

( ) = cases with prior neurolysis and/or transposition
*Patients with one or more years of follow-up

A subset of 84 patients without prior operation has been followed for 3 or more years. Table 9–13 compares preoperative with postoperative grades in this category with relatively lengthy follow-up. There were six patients who had severe preoperative loss grading 1, 14 grading 2, 27 grading 3, 28 grading 4, and 9 grading 9. With this longer period of follow-up, 51% improved one grade, 26% two grades, and 10% either three or four grades. Only 13% did not improve. Most of these latter patients were al-ready grade 5 when operated on, although one patient did drop one grade postoperatively.

Table 9–14 shows the course of 60 patients with 3 or more years of follow-up who had undergone one or more prior operations. Fifty-three percent improved one grade, but only 17% two grades and 2% three grades. Some 28% had no improvement. Only one third of these were grade 5 to begin with. Fortunately, no patient in this reoperative category had a decrease in function from the preoperative grade.

A special subset in the category of patients

**TABLE 9–13**
Ulnar Entrapment With No Prior Operation
Three or More Years of Follow-up
(n = 84)

| Postoperative<br>Grades | Preoperative Grades | | | | |
|---|---|---|---|---|---|
| | I | II | III | IV | V |
| I | — | — | — | | |
| II | 1 | — | — | — | — |
| III | 1 | 3 | — | — | — |
| IV | 1 | 7 | 13 | 2 | 1 |
| V | 3 | 4 | 14 | 26 | 8 |

**Results**
Improved 1 grade = 43 (51%)
Improved 2 grades = 22 (26%)
Improved 3 or 4 grades = 8 (10%)
No change in grade = 10 (12%)
Worse = 1 (1%)

**TABLE 9–14**
Ulnar Entrapment With Prior Operation
Three or More Years of Follow-up
(n = 60)

| Postoperative<br>Grades | Preoperative Grades | | | | |
|---|---|---|---|---|---|
| | I | II | III | IV | V |
| I | 2 | — | — | | |
| II | 1 | 1 | — | — | — |
| III | 2 | 6 | 3 | — | — |
| IV | 1 | 1 | 11 | 6 | — |
| V | 0 | 0 | 7 | 14 | 5 |

**Results**
Improved 1 grade = 32 (53%)
Improved 2 grades = 10 (17%)
Improved 3 grades = 1 (2%)
No change in grade = 17 (28%)

**TABLE 9–15**

Results With Reoperation for
Severe Pain (n = 56)

| | **No. Cases With Significant Improvement** |
|---|---|
| Patients with severe pain and severe neuropathy that improved | 4 of 11 (36%) |
| Patients with severe pain and mild or moderate neuropathy that improved | 39 of 45 (87%) |

**Conclusion:** Patients with severe pain and mild or moderate neuropathy respond well to neurolysis and deep burial of nerve.

with prior operation were those who presented with severe pain and some neuropathy. If both severe pain and severe neuropathy (grade 2 or less) were present, reoperation helped in only 36% of cases. On the other hand, if only mild or moderate neuropathy (grade 3 or better) was present along with severe pain, the response to reoperation was favorable in 87% (Table 9–15). Even though the odds of recovery with severe loss are low, reoperation is often the only treatment alternative available besides tendon transfer for clawing.[29]

These results compare favorably to those reported by some of our contemporaries.[18,28,39] Despite this, we were surprised that so much objective improvement occurred. This was not only in the previously unoperated spontaneous cases but also in those with a history of trauma to the elbow and in those patients who had had a previous operation.

## Bibliography

1. Adelaar RS, Foster WC, and McDowell C: The treatment of cubital tunnel syndrome. J Hand Surg 9A: 90–95, 1984.
2. Alvine FG and Schurrer ME: Postoperative ulnar nerve palsy. J Bone Joint Surg 62A:255–259, 1987.
3. Bauwens P: Electrodiagnostic definition of the site and nature of peripheral nerve lesions. Ann Phys Med 5: 149–152, 1960.
4. Branch C, Kelly D, and Lynch G: Surgical exposure of peripheral nerves. In Wilkins R and Rengachary S, Eds: Neurosurgery, Vol. 2. New York, McGraw-Hill, 1985.
5. Brand P: Tendon transfer in the forearm. In Flynn J, Ed: Hand Surgery. Baltimore, Williams & Wilkins, 1966.
6. Brooks D: Nerve compression by simple ganglia. J Bone Joint Surg 34B:391–400, 1952.
7. Broudy AS, Leffert RD, and Smith RJ: Technical problems with ulnar nerve transposition at the elbow: Find-

ings and results of reoperation. J Hand Surg 3:85–89, 1978.
8. Brown WF, Ferguson GG, Jones MW, et al.: The location of conduction abnormalities in human entrapment neuropathies. Can J Neurol Sci 3:111–122, 1976.
9. Buck-Gramcho D: Evaluation of perineurial repair with nerve injuries. In Jupiter J, Ed: Flynn's Hand Surgery. Baltimore, Williams & Wilkins, 1991.
10. Bunnell S: Surgery of the Hand. Philadelphia, JB Lippincott, 1964.
11. Campbell JB: Peripheral nerve repair. Clin Neurosurg 17:77–98, 1970.
12. Chang KF, Low WD, Chan SI, et al.: Enlargement of the ulnar nerve behind the medial epicondyle. Anat Rec 145:149–155, 1963.
13. Childress HM: Recurrent ulnar-nerve dislocation at the elbow. J Bone Joint Surg 38A:978–984, 1956.
14. Craven PR and Green DP: Cubital tunnel syndrome: Treatment by medial epicondylectomy. J Bone Joint Surg 62A:986–989, 1980.
15. Dellon A: Techniques for successful management of ulnar nerve entrapment at the elbow. Neurosurg Clin North Am 2:57–73, 1991.
16. Dellon AL: Operative technique for submuscular transposition of the ulnar nerve. Contemp Orthop 16: 17–24, 1988.
17. Dellon AL: Pitfalls in interpretation of electrophysiological testing. In Gelberman R, Ed: Operative Nerve Repair and Reconstruction. Philadelphia, JB Lippincott, 1991.
18. Dellon AL: Review of treatment results for ulnar nerve entrapment at the elbow. J Hand Surg 14A:688–700, 1989.
19. Dellon AL and Mackinnon SE: Injury to the medial antebrachial cutaneous nerve during cubital tunnel surgery. J Hand Surg, 19:33–36, 1985.
20. Dellon AL, Mackinnon SE, Hudson AR, et al.: Effect of submuscular versus intramuscular placement of ulnar nerve: Experimental model in the primate. J Hand Surg Br, 11:117–119, 1986.
21. DiVincenti FC, Moncrief JA, and Pruitt BA: Electrical Injuries: A review of 65 cases. J Trauma 9:497–507, 1969.
22. Ebeling P, Gilliatt RW, and Thomas PK: A clinical and electrical study of ulnar nerve lesions in the hand. J Neurol Neurosurg Psychiatry 23:1–9, 1960.
23. Eckman PB, Perlstein G, and Altrocchi PH: Ulnar neuropathy in bicycle riders. Arch Neurol 32:130–131, 1975.
24. Ekerot L: Post-anesthetic ulnar neuropathy at the elbow. Scand J Plast Reconstr Surg 11:225–229, 1977.
25. Fannin TF: Local decompression in the treatment of ulnar nerve entrapment at the elbow. J R Coll Surg Edinb 23:362–366, 1978.
26. Feindel W and Stratford J: The role of the cubital tunnel in tardy ulnar palsy. Can J Surg 1:287–300, 1958.
27. Forshell KP and Hagstrom P: Distal ulnar nerve compression caused by ganglion formation in the Loge de Guyon. Case report. Scand J Plast Reconstr Surg 9:77–79, 1975.
28. Foster RJ and Edshage S: Factors related to the outcome of surgically managed compressive ulnar neuropathy at the elbow level. J Hand Surg 6:181–192, 1981.
29. Friedman RJ and Cochran TP: Anterior transposition for advanced ulnar neuropathy at the elbow. Surg Neurol 25:446–448, 1986.
30. Froimson A and Zahrawi F: Treatment of compression neuropathy of the ulnar nerve at the elbow by epicondylectomy and neurolysis. J Hand Surg 5:391–395, 1980.

31. Gay JR and Love JG: Diagnosis and treatment of tardy paralysis of the ulnar nerve. J Bone Joint Surg 29A: 1087–1097, 1947.

32. Gilliatt R and Sears T: Sensory nerve action potentials in patients with peripheral nerve lesions. J Neurol Neurosurg Psychiatry 21:109–118, 1958.

33. Gilliatt RW and Thomas PK: Changes in nerve conduction with ulnar lesions at the elbow. J Neurol Neurosurg Psychiatry 23:312–320, 1960.

34. Goldner JL: Function of the Hand Following Peripheral Nerve Injuries. Am Acad Orthop Surg Instruct Course Lectures 10. Ann Arbor, MI, JW Edmonds, 1953.

35. Grubb W: Management of nerve injuries in forearm and hand. Orthop Clin North Am 1:419–426, 1970.

36. Grube BJ: Neurologic consequences of electrical burns. J Trauma 30:254–258, 1990.

37. Grundfest H, Oester Y, Beebe G: Electrical evidence of regeneration. In Woodhall B and Beebe G, Eds: Peripheral Nerve Regeneration. Veterans Administration Monograph. Washington, DC, US Government Printing Office, 1957.

38. Haase J, Bjerve P, and Semesen K: Median and ulnar nerve transections treated with microsurgical interfascicular cable grafting with autologous sural nerve. J Neurosurg 53:73–84, 1980.

39. Hagstrom P: Ulnar nerve compression at the elbow: Results of surgery in 85 cases. Scand J Plast Reconstr Surg 11:59–62, 1977.

40. Hubbard J: The quality of nerve regeneration. Factors independent of the most skillful repair. Surg Clin North Am 52:1099–1108, 1972.

41. Hudson AR, Berry H, and Mayfield FH: Chronic injuries of peripheral nerves by entrapment. In Youmans J, Ed: Neurological Surgery, 2nd Ed., Vol. 14, Philadelphia, WB Saunders, 1982.

42. Hunt J: Occupation neuritis of the deep palmar branch of the ulnar nerve. J Nerv Ment Dis 35:673, 1908.

43. Kempe L, Ed: Operative Neurosurgery, Vol. 2. New York, Springer-Verlag, 1970.

44. Kimura J: Electrodiagnosis in Diseases of Nerves and Muscles: Principles and Practices. Philadelphia, FA Davis, 1983.

45. Kleinert HE and Hayes JE: The ulnar tunnel syndrome. Plast Reconstr Surg 47:21–24, 1971.

46. Kline D and Hackett E: Reappraisal of timing for exploration of civilian peripheral nerve injuries. Surgery 78:54–65, 1975.

47. Kline D and Hudson A: Complications of nerve repair. In Greenberg L, Ed: Complications in Surgery. Philadelphia, JB Lippincott, 1985.

48. Kline DG and Nulsen F: Management of peripheral nerve injuries producing hand dysfunction. In Jupiter J, Ed: Flynn's Hand Surgery. Baltimore, Williams & Wilkins, 1991.

49. Kline D, Hackett E, and LeBlanc H: The value of primary repair for bluntly transected nerve injuries: Physiologic documentation. Surg Forum 25:436–437, 1974.

50. Learmouth J: A technique for transplanting the ulnar nerve. Surg Gynecol Obstet 75:792–801, 1942.

51. Leffert RD: Anterior submuscular transposition of the ulnar nerves by the Learmouth technique. J Hand Surg 7:147–155, 1982.

52. Lewis G: Trauma resulting from electricity. J Int Coll Surg 28:724–738, 1957.

53. Litter J: Tendon transfers and arthrodesis in combined median and ulnar nerve paralysis. J Bone Joint Surg 31A:225–234, 1949.

54. Livingston WK: Evidence of active invasion of denervated areas by sensory fibers from neighboring nerves in man. J Neurosurg 4:140–145, 1947.

55. Mackinnon SE and Dellon A: Surgery of the Peripheral Nerve. New York, Thieme Medical Publishers, 1988.

56. Mackinnon SE and Dellon AL: Ulnar nerve entrapment at the elbow. In Mackinnon SE and Dellon AL, Eds: Surgery of the Peripheral Nerve. New York, Thieme Medical Publishers, 1988, pp. 217–273.

57. Mallett B and Zilkha K: Compression of the ulnar nerve at the wrist by a ganglion. Lancet 1:890–891, 1955.

58. McGowan AJ: The results of transposition of the ulnar nerve for traumatic ulnar neuritis. J Bone Joint Surg 32B:293–301, 1950.

59. Michon J, Amend P, and Merle M: Microsurgical repair of peripheral nerve lesions: A study of 150 injuries of the median and ulnar nerves. In Samii, Ed: Peripheral Nerve Lesions. Berlin, Springer-Verlag, 1990.

60. Miller RG and Camp PE: Postoperative ulnar neuropathy. JAMA 242:1636–1639, 1979.

61. Millesi H, Meissl G, and Berger A: The interfascicular nerve grafting of the median and ulnar nerves. J Bone Joint Surg 54A:727–730, 1972.

62. Moberg E: Objective methods for determining the functional value of sensibility in the hand. J Bone Joint Surg 40B:454–475, 1958.

63. Murphey F, Kirklin J, and Finlaysan A: Anomalous innervation of the intrinsic muscles of hand. Surg Gynecol Obstet 83:15–23, 1946.

64. Neblett C and Ehni G: Medial epicondylectomy for ulnar palsy. J Neurosurg 32:55–62, 1970.

65. Nicholson OR and Seddon HJ: Nerve repair in civil practice. Results of treatment of median and ulnar nerve lesions. Br Med J 2:1065–1071, 1957.

66. Omer G: Tendon transfers for the reconstruction of the forearm and hand following peripheral nerve injuries. In Omer G and Spinner M, Eds: Management of Peripheral Nerve Problems. Philadelphia, WB Saunders, 1980.

67. Parks B: Postoperative peripheral neuropathies. Surgery 74:348–357, 1973.

69. Pechan J and Julis I: The pressure measurement in the ulnar nerve: A contribution to the pathophysiology of the cubital tunnel syndrome. J Biomech 8:75–79, 1975.

69. Pollock LJ and Davis L: Peripheral Nerve Injuries. New York, Paul B Hoeber, 1933.

70. Riordan D: Tendon transplantations in median nerve and ulnar nerve paralysis. J Bone Joint Surg, 35A: 312–323, 1953.

71. Sakellorides H: Follow-up of 172 peripheral nerve injuries in upper extremity in civilians. J Bone Joint Surg 44A:140–148, 1962.

72. Samii M: Use of microtechniques in peripheral neurosurgery: Experience with over 300 cases. In Handa H, Ed: Microneurosurgery. Tokyo, Igaku-Shoin, 1975.

73. Seddon HJ, Ed: Surgical Disorders of the Peripheral Nerves. Baltimore, Williams & Wilkins, 1972.

74. Shea JD and McClain EJ: Ulnar-nerve compression syndromes at and below the wrist. J Bone Joint Surg 51A:1095–1103, 1969.

75. Siegel DB and Gelberman RH: Ulnar nerve: Applied anatomy and operative exposure. In Operative Nerve Repair and Reconstruction. New York, JB Lippincott, 1991.

76. Speed JS and Knight RA, Eds: Peripheral nerve injuries. In Campbell's Operative Orthopaedics, Vol 1. St. Louis, CV Mosby, 1956.

77. Spinner M and Kaplan EB: The relationship of the ulnar nerve to the medial intermuscular septum in the arm and its clinical significance. Hand 8:239–242, 1976.

78. Strickland JW, Idler RS, and Deisignore JL: Ulnar nerve repair. In Operative Nerve Repair and Reconstruction. New York, JB Lippincott, 1991.

79. Stromberg WB, McFarlane RM, Bell JL, et al.: Injury of the median and ulnar nerves: 150 cases with an evaluation of Moberg's ninhydrin test. J Bone Joint Surg Am 43:717–730, 1961.

80. Struthers J: On some points in the abnormal anatomy of the arm. Br For Med Chir Rev 14:170–179, 1854.

81. Sunderland S: Funicular suture and funicular exclusion in the repair of severed nerves. Br J Surg 40:580–587, 1953.

82. Sunderland S: Nerve and Nerve Injuries. Baltimore, Williams & Wilkins, 1968.

83. Terzis J, Daniel R, and Williams H: Intraoperative assessment of nerve lesions with fascicular dissection and electrophysiological recordings. *In* Omer G, and Spinner M, Eds: Management of Peripheral Nerve Problems. Philadelphia, WB Saunders, 1980.

84. Tindall S: Chronic injuries of peripheral nerves by entrapment. *In* Youmans J, Ed: Neurological Surgery, 3rd Ed. Philadelphia, WB Saunders, 1990.

85. Wilson DH and Krout R: Surgery of ulnar neuropathy at the elbow: 16 cases treated by decompression without transposition. J Neurosurg 38:780–785, 1974.

86. Woodhall B, Nulsen F, White J, and Davis L: Neurosurgical implications. *In* Woodhall B and Beebe G: Peripheral Nerve Regeneration. Veterans Administration Monograph. Washington, DC, US Government Printing Office, 1957.

87. Wynn-Parry C: Rehabilitation of the Hand. London, Butterworth & Co, 1966.

88. Zachary RB: Results of nerve suture. *In* Seddon HJ, Ed: Peripheral Nerve Injuries. London, Her Majesty's Stationery Office, 1954.

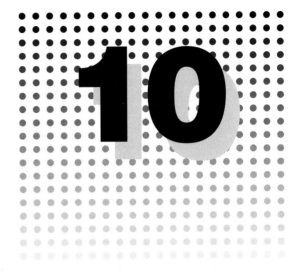

# Combined Upper Extremity Nerve Injuries

## SUMMARY

This surprisingly large category of nerve lesions is difficult to summarize because of the many combinations as well as the differing levels, injury mechanisms, and operations done. As a result, we have reported data from individual cases in the tables and have grouped these as median/ulnar (46 cases), median/ulnar/radial (4 cases), and median/radial (8 cases) injuries at various levels. Axillary and musculo-cutaneous nerve lesions seen in combination with proximal median, radial, or ulnar lesions are addressed in the chapters on the brachial plexus. Despite some impressive results, at least as judged by the LSUMC whole nerve grading system used, it was difficult for patients to regain a preinjury level of function. Exceptions were injuries in which radial was severely injured but could be repaired, damage was more partial to median or ulnar, and such partial loss reversed spontaneously. The combined median/ulnar injuries were especially devastating if loss in both distributions was complete. This resulted in "main en griffe" or clawing of all the fingers. Despite this deformity, repair of one or both nerves was worthwhile, even at proximal levels. In any combined case, it was especially important to ascertain whether any lesions in continuity could be spared complete or even partial resection by doing intraoperative nerve action potential studies. Overall recovery was, as expected, better if one or more nerves involved in a combined injury could have a neurolysis based on operative electrical evidence of either partial injury or significant regeneration. Intensive physical and occupational therapy is especially important in limbs with combined nerve injuries. Tendon transfer and other reconstructive procedures need also to be considered relatively early.

Combined nerve lesions result in greater deficit than solitary ones. Such loss is very difficult to reverse, and rehabilitation is demanding and lengthy, not only for the patient but also for those caring for the patient. Because these combined nerve lesions are so complex, they have been tabulated as individual cases in Tables 10–1 through 10–5 so that individual management and outcomes can be studied.

## COMBINED MEDIAN/ULNAR INJURIES AT ARM LEVEL

Combined median/ulnar injuries formed a relatively large category. This related to their relative juxtaposition throughout their anatomic course in the upper extremity. This was especially so in the upper arm, where muscle wounds, lacerations, fractures, contusions, and even iatrogenic causes involved both median and ulnar nerves (Table 10–1). Of the 22 patients with upper arm median/ulnar palsies studied and operated on, 12 (>50%) had undergone a prior operation. In six cases, this was a vascular repair, while in four the wounds had

prior extensive debridement. Preoperative loss was also complete in the distribution of both the median and ulnar nerves in 13 cases. Initial loss included all hand intrinsic muscles. This produced severe clawing of all fingers, or main en griffe (Figure 10–1). Unless rehabilitative exercises, nighttime splinting, or aggressive management was initiated early, the end result was a poor one. In the missile wound group of eight cases, half were caused by shotgun injury and half by single bullet and any fragments of metal or bone created by the impact. The interval between injury and operation was relatively brief and averaged 3 to 4 months. Although those elements having complete preoperative loss usually had repair, there was one exception because of a nerve action potential (NAP) across the lesion. This median nerve had a neurolysis despite complete loss preoperatively. Recovery was excellent, as it was for the ulnar nerve despite a proximal suture repair. Average grade for median in this subset of combined injuries was 4.0, and for ulnar it was 3.3.

Lacerations involving median and ulnar at the upper arm level were usually blunt and sent late for repair. Average interval between injury

**TABLE 10–1**
Combined Median/Ulnar Injuries—Upper Arm

| Age | Gender | Mechanism | Prior Operation | Loss | | Interval Between Injury and Operation | Operation | | Results (Grade) | | Follow-up (y) |
|---|---|---|---|---|---|---|---|---|---|---|---|
| | | | | Median | Ulnar | | Median | Ulnar | Median | Ulnar | |
| 50 | M | Shotgun | Vascular Repair | C | C | 3 mo | G | G | 3 | 2 | 2 |
| 32 | M | Shotgun | Vascular Repair | C | C | 4 mo | S | S | 4 | 3 | 5 |
| 30 | M | Shotgun | Debride | – | C | 3 mo | N | S | 3–4 | 2–3 | 1.5 |
| 32 | M | Shotgun | None | C | C | 5 mo | G | S | 3–4 | 3 | 5.5 |
| 23 | M | GSW | Debride | – | – | 6 mo | N | N | 5 | 3–4 | 3 |
| 44 | M | GSW | None | C | C | 3 mo | N | S | 5 | 4 | 9 |
| 6 | M | GSW | None | C | – | 4 mo | S | N | 4–5 | 5 | 17 |
| 6 | F | GSW | None | C | C | 1.5 mo | S | S | 4 | 3 | 9 |
| 42 | M | Laceration | Debride | C | – | 3 mo | G | N | 4 | 4–5 | 2.5 |
| 24 | M | Laceration/Propeller | Vascular Repair | C | C | 5.5 mo | S | S | 3 | 2 | 8 |
| 28 | M | Laceration | Vascular Repair | C | C | 7 mo | G | S | 3–4 | 2–3 | 2 |
| 45 | F | Laceration | Vascular Repair | C | C | 3 mo | N | S | 4 | 3 | 11 |
| 23 | M | Laceration/Dune Buggy | Vascular Repair | – | C | 5 mo | N | G | 4–5 | 2 | 2 |
| 22 | M | Laceration | Debride | C | C | 4 mo | G | S | 4 | 3–4 | 6.5 |
| 22 | M | Compound Fracture | Neurolysis | C | C | 7 mo | G | G | 3 | 2 | 5 |
| 48 | M | Fracture | None | C | C | 4 mo | N | N | 4 | 4 | 5.5 |
| 25 | M | Fracture | None | C | C | 11 mo | G | G | 2–3 | 2 | 5 |
| 27 | M | Contusion | None | C | C | 5 mo | S | N | 4 | 4 | 3 |
| 65 | F | Compression | None | – | – | 2 wk | N | N | 2–3 | 2–3 | 10 |
| 36 | M | A-V Fistula for Dialysis | CT Release | – | – | 8 mo | N | N | 4–5 | 4–5 | 4 |
| 60 | F | A-V Fistula for Dialysis | None | – | – | 7 mo | N | N | 4 | 3 | 3 |
| 38 | M | Venipuncture Swelling | Pain | C | C | 11 mo | G | G | 2–3 | 2 | 2 |

A–V = arteriovenous; C = complete loss of motor and sensory function; CT = carpal tunnel; F = female; G = graft; GSW = gunshot wound; I = incomplete loss of motor and sensory function distal to level of injury; M = male, N = neurolysis; S = suture; y = year(s).

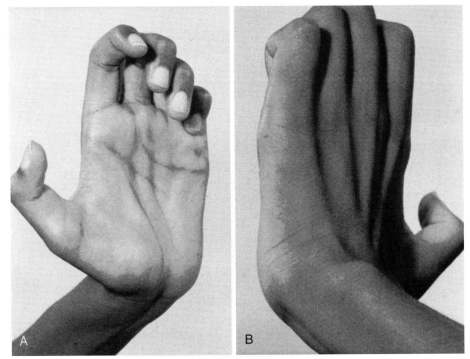

**Figure 10 – 1.** *(A)* Main en griffe hand caused by combined median and ulnar injuries. Fingers and thumb are clawed, and thenar as well as hypothenar atrophy is evident. *(B)* Interosseous atrophy is evident in the photograph of the dorsum of the same hand.

and repair was almost 5 months. Most (80%) of these combined lesions were complete preoperatively. Despite laceration as a mechanism, one ulnar and two median neuromas were in continuity, had NAPs, and required only neurolysis. Results, as with the combined missile wounds, were best for median distribution muscles and less for ulnar ones (Figure 10 – 2).

Contusion associated with fracture, blunt blows, or more sustained compression usually did not require operation. However, in five cases selected for operation involving both median and ulnar nerves, half of the injured elements required either suture or graft repair.

Two patients had iatrogenic injury resulting from an arteriovenous fistula constructed at an arm level for renal dialysis. Both had incomplete loss but also very painful paresthesias. This was caused by compression and scar enveloping proximal median and ulnar nerves. Fortunately, both patients improved with removal of the fistula and neurolysis of the nerves. In neither case was there clinical or electrical evidence of a superimposed or confusing peripheral neu-

ropathy owing to renal disease or the dialysis process itself. The combination of injury or compression by an arteriovenous fistula at the forearm level involving median and radial nerves was seen in several other cases. This more peripheral compressive neuropathy is discussed under median/radial lesions.

## Case Summary — Combined Median/ Ulnar Arm Level Injury

This 44-year-old male sustained a 38-caliber handgun wound to the medial midarm area. At admission to the hospital, he had loss of radial pulse and a complete median and ulnar palsy. Using a saphenous vein graft, a repair of the brachial artery was done by the vascular service. Median and ulnar nerves were noted to be bruised and stretched but in continuity.

There was no clinical or electromyographic evidence of reversal of loss, so the area was explored about 3 months later. A NAP could be recorded across a median neuroma in continuity. One portion of the nerve appeared to be more severely involved than the rest. As a result, the nerve was split into four bundles of fascicles. One bundle did not transmit and was replaced with two

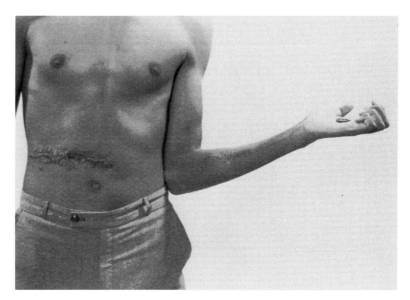

**Figure 10-2.** Combined median and ulnar injury caused by a gunshot wound that crossed the patient's abdomen and penetrated the forearm. In his hand, the patient is holding the bullet that injured both the median and ulnar nerves.

antebrachial cutaneous grafts 3.8 cm in length. The ulnar lesion did not transmit a NAP, so it was resected. Length was made up by mobilizing distal ulnar nerve to the junction of the upper and middle thirds of the forearm and then tunneling distal ulnar stump beneath flexor carpi ulnaris and pronator teres. An end-to-end suture of the ulnar nerve was thus accomplished.

Follow-up at 1 year 3 months gave an overall grade of 3 for median and 1 to 2 for ulnar. By 4 years, median function graded 4 to 5 and ulnar, surprisingly, graded 3 to 4.

### Comment

Initially and at the time of vascular repair, median and ulnar nerves were noted to be in continuity despite bruising, and therefore were not resected, and this was appropriate. Equally important is the need to explore even known lesions in continuity if there is no improvement by 3 months or so.

## COMBINED MEDIAN/ULNAR INJURIES AT THE ELBOW-FOREARM LEVEL

This was the second largest category of combined nerve injuries of the upper extremity (Table 10-2). Most of the nerves involved by laceration had complete loss and required repair. Although the average interval between injury and operative repair was relatively long, one sharp laceration by glass involving both nerves at the elbow level could be repaired

acutely. Follow-up has extended to only 1.5 years on this case, but recovery grades by that time already averaged level 3. Whether the ulnar nerve had neurolysis or repair, it was transposed and placed deep to forearm muscles.

There were six combined lesions associated with fractures of the humerus or radius-ulna (Figure 10-3). One distal humeral fracture was associated with a Volkmann ischemic contracture. A late neurolysis (at 11 months) done in conjunction with a flexor recession gave an incomplete result after 25 months of follow-up. In the other five fracture-associated cases, neurolysis of seven elements based on positive NAPs could be done. Recovery in the distribution of these nerves was, as expected, good. One other element could have a split repair, but only two of ten required suture. Results in this group of combined median and ulnar lesions associated with fractures were good. The case with a 1-year follow-up is progressing well, but further follow-up is needed. Both the laceration and fracture groups involving median and ulnar nerves at this level did surprisingly well (Figure 10-4).

Iatrogenic cases were caused by compression or were secondary to prior operation or injection injury from cardiac catheterization. Loss was incomplete, but because of pain, an operation was done. Four of six involved elements had neurolysis, one a split repair, and one a suture. Results were good. The electrical injury was an

**TABLE 10–2**
Combined Median/Ulnar Injuries — Elbow/Forearm

| Age | Gender | Mechanism | Prior Operation | Loss | | Interval Between Injury and Operation | Operation | | Results (Grade) | | Follow-up (y) |
|---|---|---|---|---|---|---|---|---|---|---|---|
| | | | | Median | Ulnar | | Median | Ulnar | Median | Ulnar | |
| 26 | M | Laceration/Glass | Vascular Repair | C | I | 5 mo | G | Split | 4 | 3–4 | 11 |
| 21 | M | Laceration/Glass | None | C | C | None | S | S | 3 | 3 | 1.5 |
| 24 | M | Laceration/MVA | 1° Repair | C | C | 7 mo | S | S | 3–4 | 2 | 2.5 |
| 28 | M | Laceration/Glass | 1° Repair | C | I | 14 mo | G | N | 3–4 | 3 | 2.5 |
| 23 | M | F(x) Humerus | F(x) Repair | I | I | 4.5 mo | G | N | 2 | 4–5 | 3 |
| 5 | F | F(x) Humerus | None | I | I | 3 mo | N | N | 4 | 4 | 6 |
| 29 | F | F(x) Humerus | Neurolysis | C | I | 4 mo | Split | N | 2–3 | 3–4 | 1 |
| 25 | M | Volkmann | F(x) Repair | C | C | 11 mo | N | N | 2–3 | 2–3 | 3 |
| 35 | M | F(x) Radius/Ulna | 1° Repair Ulnar | I | C | 8 mo | N | S | 5 | 3 | 9 |
| 10 | F | F(x) Radius/Ulna | None | C | I | 6 mo | N | N | 4 | 3–4 | 3 |
| 46 | M | Operative Compression | Neurolysis Ulnar | I (Severe loss) | (Severe loss) | 12 mo | N | S | 4 | 3 | 2.5 |
| 59 | M | Operative Compression | N/A | I | I | 13 y | N | Split | 5 | 3–4 | 2 |
| 56 | M | Cardiac | N/A | I | I | 2 mo | N | N | 5 | 4–5 | 2 |
| 34 | M | Electrical | Debride | C | I | 10 mo | G | N | 3–4 | 5 | 2.5 |

1° = primary repair or immediate repair; C = complete loss of motor and sensory function; F = female; F(x) = fracture; G = graft; I = incomplete loss of motor and sensory function distal to level of injury; M = male; MVA = motor vehicle accident; N = neurolysis and, in case of ulnar elbow/forearm, transposition as well; S = suture; Split = partial suture or graft repair with neurolysis of remainder of nerve; y = year(s).

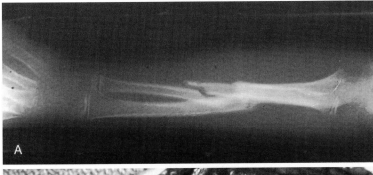

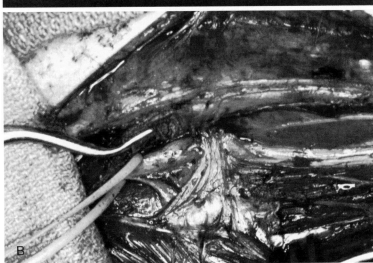

**Figure 10-3.** *(A)* Severe mid-forearm-level fractures of radius and ulna associated with midforearm-level median and ulnar palsies. *(B)* At operation 5 months after injury, median nerve was found entrapped by callus and scar. Ulnar nerve had a similar appearance. After external neurolysis, both nerves transmitted a nerve action potential beyond the injury site, so repair was not necessary. Almost full recovery occurred over the next 2.5 years.

unusual case caused by contact of an elbow with an extremely high voltage source. Debridement of extensive soft tissue damage of volar and dorsal forearm areas had been done relatively acutely. Despite a late graft repair at 10 months after injury, overall median grade was 3 to 4 by 2.5 years of follow-up. Ulnar function returned completely, but loss was incomplete in the early months after injury, grading 3, and only neurolysis and transposition of this nerve were done.

## Case Summary—Elbow-Level Lesion

### Laceration to Median and Ulnar Nerves

### Case Number 1

A 22-year-old male fell, and his arm went through a plate glass window. He required immediate repair to brachial artery and biceps tendon. The nerve ends were tagged with tantalum clips, and the limb was casted. The patient had complete loss of both median and ulnar func-

tion. The only muscle partially spared was pronator teres, which graded 3. Two weeks later, we explored the wound. Median and ulnar stumps had retracted. After trimming these, four antebrachial cutaneous nerve grafts were used to bridge the gap in the median, which was 6.5 cm in length. The gap in the ulnar was made up by mobilization and transposition volar to the elbow. As a result, an end-to-end suture repair of this nerve could be done. The immediate postoperative period was uncomplicated.

When seen for a 6-year follow-up, the patient could make a fist and could enclose his flexed fingers with his thumb. If he extended the fingers, the little finger tended to abduct. In the median distribution, he had excellent pronation, flexor superficialis, flexor profundus, and flexor pollicis longus. Abductor pollicis brevis and opponens pollicis graded 3 to 4, and median sensation was 3. Overall median grade was 4. In the ulnar distribution, he recovered excellent flexor carpi ulnaris and flexor profundus, and even hypothenar muscles graded 4. Interossei and lumbricals were 3, and adductor pollicis was 3 to 4. Sensation graded 3, and overall ulnar grade was 3 to 4. He could localize stimuli, but two-point discrimination remained poor. He would look at his hand when he used it for fine tasks, and he still had trouble picking up

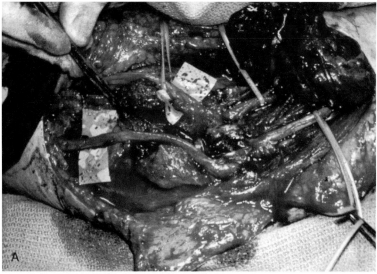

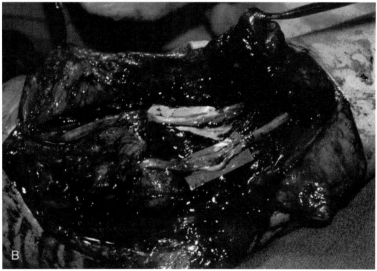

**Figure 10–4.** *(A)* Transecting injuries to median and ulnar nerves at elbow. *(B)* Ulnar nerve *(below)* required graft repair, whereas median *(top)* required split repair. This case is not included in Table 10–2 but outcome for median nerve was excellent (grade 4), whereas that for ulnar nerve was grade 3 by 3 years postoperatively.

fine objects and buttoning clothes. He could use the hand to turn door knobs and could also turn the lid on a jar. As an owner of a grocery store, he stocks shelves and cuts meat. He says he can use the hand if necessary to write with a pen or pencil, but his grip is somewhat different because he uses more fingers to balance the grip of the pen on the thumb than before.

### Comment

Even though eventual result in this case was good, the patient was a candidate for immediate, primary repair since the injury was both transecting and sharp.

## COMBINED MEDIAN/ULNAR INJURIES AT WRIST LEVEL

Most acute lacerations to these nerves at this level by attempted suicides were cared for at a primary hospital, and thus our experience with this fairly frequent injury is relatively small. However, five combined lesions that were cared for by us were caused by laceration (Figure 10–5). Three cases had primary repair and have fared well, although ulnar grades are 3 in two of these patients and 2 to 3 in the other. Two cases

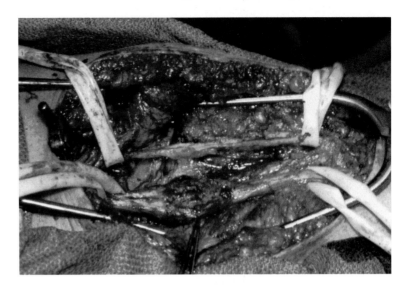

**Figure 10–5.** Combined injury involving both median and ulnar nerves at the level of the wrist.

had primary repair of both nerves and some flexor tendons done elsewhere within 24 hours of injury. Because of poor recovery, secondary exploration was done, and two of the four nerves required repeat suture (Table 10–3). Hypothenars recovered function, but interossei and lumbricals could contract only against gravity.

Two cases had pain problems associated with Colles fractures and combined median/ulnar palsies at the wrist level. Pain as well as function improved postoperatively in both of these patients. One was killed in another unrelated vehicular accident 2.5 years later.

There were two electrical injuries involving both nerves at the wrist level (Figure 10–6). One had complete loss and required graft repair; the other had incomplete loss but severe pain, had a neurolysis, and the pain subsequently improved, either because of operation or simply with the passage of time.

No patient with complete loss in the ulnar distribution gained more than a 3 as a postoperative grade. It seemed difficult to restore *strong* interosseous and lumbrical function, not only at this level, which was disappointing, but also at higher levels, which was not as surprising.

## COMBINED MEDIAN/ ULNAR/RADIAL INJURIES AT ARM LEVEL

Simultaneous injury of all three of these outflows without brachial plexus involvement was unusual, but did occur in four instances (Table 10–4). Mechanisms were diverse, but three of the four patients had required earlier vascular repair. Two patients required repair of each injured element; the third had graft repair of two elements but only neurolysis of the involved ulnar nerve; and the fourth was able to have neurolysis of all three elements (Figure 10–7). The individual case data are summarized in Table 10–4. Median and radial distribution recovery was, as might be expected, superior to that for the ulnar nerve.

## COMBINED MEDIAN/ RADIAL INJURIES AT ELBOW/FOREARM LEVEL

Although at least eight examples of this combination of injuries were seen by us, it was surprising that this did not occur more frequently

**TABLE 10−3**
Combined Median/Ulnar Injuries — Wrist Level

| Age | Gender | Mechanism | Prior Operation | Loss | | Between Injury and Operation | Operation | | Results (Grade) | | Follow-up (y) |
|---|---|---|---|---|---|---|---|---|---|---|---|
| | | | | Median | Ulnar | | Median | Ulnar | Median | Ulnar | |
| 14 | F | Laceration/Glass | None | C | C | None | S | S | 3–4 | 3 | 5.5 |
| 12 | M | Laceration/Knife | None | C | C | None | S | S | 4 | 3 | 7 |
| 28 | M | Laceration/Knife | None | C | C | None | S | S | 4 | 2–3 | 2.5 |
| 35 | F | Laceration/Glass | 1° Repair | – | – | 6 mo | S | N | 4 | 3 | 6 |
| 47 | M | Laceration/Glass | 1° Repair | – | C | 8 mo | N | S | 4–5 | 3 | 5 |
| 75 | M | Colles (Fx) | N | – | – | 19 mo | N | N | 3 (Pain Better) | 3–4 | 2.5 (Died) |
| 10 | M | Colles (Fx) | None | – | C | 4 mo | N | S | 4–5 (Pain Better) | 3 | 7 |
| 55 | F | Crush | N | – | – | 3 y | N | N | 4–5 | 4–5 | 8 |
| 46 | M | Electrical | Debride | C | C | 8.5 mo | G | G | 3–4 | 2–3 | 5 |
| 34 | M | Electrical | Debride | – | – | 5 mo | N | N | 3–4 (Pain Better) | 3 | 2 |

1° = primary repair or immediate repair; C = complete loss of motor and sensory function; F = female; F(x) = fracture; G = graft; I = incomplete loss of motor and sensory function distal to level of injury; M = male; N = neurolysis; S = suture; y = year(s).

**TABLE 10−4**
Combined Median/Ulnar/Radial Injuries — Upper Arm

| Age | Gender | Mechanism | Prior Operation | Loss | | | Interval Between Injury and Operation | Operation | | | Results (Grade) | | | Follow-up (y) |
|---|---|---|---|---|---|---|---|---|---|---|---|---|---|---|
| | | | | Median | Ulnar | Radial | | Median | Ulnar | Radial | Median | Ulnar | Radial | |
| 24 | M | GSW | Vascular Repair | C | C | C | 3 mo | S | S | G | 3 | 2 | 3 | 6 |
| 26 | M | Stab Wound | Vascular Repair | C | C | C | 4 mo | G | G | G | 3–4 | 2 | 3 | 5 |
| 26 | M | Crush | Vascular Repair | C | C | C | 3 mo | G | N | G | 3 | 3 | 3 | 14 |
| 25 | M | Contusion Swelling | None | C | C | C | 12 mo | N | N | N | 3 | 2–3 | 3 | 2 |

C = complete loss of motor and sensory function; G = graft; GSW = gunshot wound; M = male; N = neurolysis; S = suture; y = year(s).

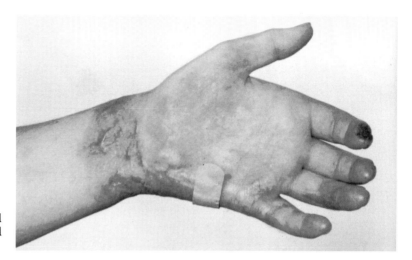

**Figure 10-6.** Severe electrical injury involving median and ulnar nerves at the wrist.

because the two nerves are in close proximity at this level. There were a variety of mechanisms responsible for injury in the cases studied, including fractures with a Volkmann contracture, shotgun wounds, laceration, venipuncture, and iatrogenic injury related to construction of an arteriovenous fistula (Table 10–5). Five prior operations had been done. Interval between injury and operation averaged 6.2 months. Eleven elements had neurolysis based on NAP recordings, four despite complete loss in their distribution preoperatively. There were five graft repairs. Average follow-up in this group at this level was 4.2 years.

Fortunately, radial grades were excellent, because median and ulnar recovery without radial function or a satisfactory substitution for such is limited in its usefulness. Median recovery had an average grade of 3.2.

## Case Summary—Laceration With Arteriovenous Malformation of Brachial Artery

A 19-year-old sustained a glass shard injury to the right antecubital fossa. He initially had a vein graft repair of his brachial artery. Median and radial nerve repair had been done 9 months previously elsewhere, and he had had a secondary procedure 8 weeks later for an arteriovenous fistula at the brachial artery repair site. For some reason, a bypass procedure was done, but the fistula was not excised. This bypass was a venous graft from upper arm brachial artery to radial artery. He presented to

us with the following functional grades: in the radial distribution, brachioradialis 2, wrist extension 2, no finger or thumb extension; in the median distribution, pronator 5 but flexor superficialis 3 to 4, no flexor profundus to forefinger, no flexor pollicis longus, no thenar intrinsics, no median-innervated lumbricals, and absent median sensation and sweating; in the ulnar distribution, hypothenar and hand intrinsics all graded 3.

Intraoperative angiography showed continued fill from a varix arising from the brachial artery repair which still had flow through it despite the prior attempt to bypass this. A single varix arising from the artery was coagulated, then ligated and excised, and the vascular problem subsided. The original injury site was encased in a heavy vascular scar. The median nerve, on exposure, had a large neuroma in continuity. NAP recording showed a good NAP proximal to the neuroma, a smaller one to the midpoint of the neuroma, but no NAP beyond. Despite some proximal and distal mobilization, a gap of 2.8 cm remained after the resection of the neuroma. This was closed with eight pieces of sural nerve 3.2 cm in length. Histology confirmed an arteriovenous malformation and a neurotmetic Sunderland grade IV lesion in continuity to the median nerve. Scar was removed from around radial nerve at the elbow level and from ulnar nerve proximal to the olecranon notch.

Postoperative angiography showed resolution of the malformation and flow through both the original repair and the bypass. At clinical and electromyographic follow-up 4 years postoperatively, he presented with recovery of full wrist and finger function in the radial distribution; full hand intrinsic function in the ulnar distribution; and full flexor superficialis, flexor profundus, and flexor pollicis longus function, plus partial recovery (2 to 3) of abductor pollicis longus, opponens pollicis, and median lumbrical function in the median distribution. Median sensation graded 4.

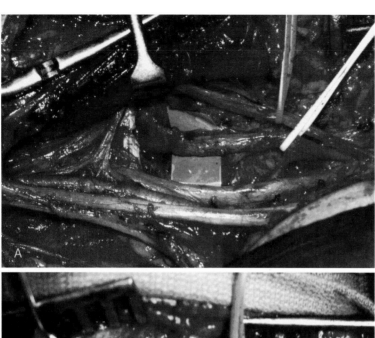

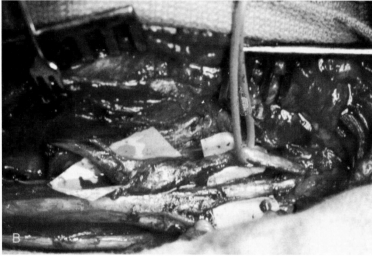

**Figure 10–7.** Sorting out injuries involving radial as well as median and ulnar nerves along the proximal and medial aspect of the arm requires careful dissection and a lot of patience.

## Comment

Arteriovenous fistulae or pseudoaneurysms involving nerve usually require resection and occlusion so that adequate decompression is obtained.

The results recorded in this chapter for combined or multiple lesions involving median, ulnar, and radial nerves should be compared with results collected over a similar 15-year period but affecting solitary nerves in the arm (Table 10–6).

**TABLE 10–5**
Combined Median/Radial Injuries—Elbow/Forearm

| Age | Gender | Mechanism | Prior Operation | Loss | | Interval Between Injury and Operation | Operation | | Results (Grade) | | Follow-up (y) |
|---|---|---|---|---|---|---|---|---|---|---|---|
| | | | | Median | Radial | | Median | Radial | Median | Radial | |
| 27 | M | Shotgun | Vascular Repair | C | C | 3 mo | G | G | 3 | 3–4 | 3 |
| 19 | M | Laceration A-V Fistula | 1° Repair Artery, Median Nv, Radial Nv | C | I | 8 mo | G | N | 5 | 5 | 10 |
| 23 | M | F(x)-Radius/Ulna | F(x) Repair | C | I | 4.5 mo | G | N | 2 | 4–5 | 1 |
| 20 | F | Volkmann | None | C | C | 6 mo | N | N | 2–3 | 3–4 | 7 |
| 28 | M | Volkmann | Fasciotomy | C | I | 8 mo | G | N | 3 | 4 | 5 |
| 58 | F | A-V Fistula for Dialysis | None | C | C | 6 mo | N | N | 3 | 4 | 2.5 |
| 49 | M | A-V Fistula for Dialysis | CT Release | I | C | 8 mo | N | N | 2–3 | 3 | 3 |
| 46 | M | Venipuncture | None | (Severe Loss) I | (Severe Loss) I | 6 mo | N | N | 4–5 | 5 | 2.5 |

1° = primary repair or immediate repair; A-V = arteriovenous; C = complete loss of motor and sensory function; CT = carpal tunnel; F = female; F(x) = fracture; G = graft; I = incomplete loss of motor and sensory function distal to level of injury; M = male; N = neurolysis; Nv = nerve; y = year(s).

287

**TABLE 10-6**

Results Radial, Median, and Ulnar Nerves by Procedure Done and Level of Lesion*
(Collected over a 15-year period ending in 1985)

| | Partial or Complete Transection | | | | | In Continuity | | | | |
| | Suture | | Secondary Graft | Split Repair | Resection | Positive Nerve Action Potential | | Negative Nerve Action Potential | | |
| Level | PRIMARY | SECONDARY | | | | NEUROLYSIS | SPLIT REPAIR | NEUROLYSIS | SUTURE | GRAFT |
|---|---|---|---|---|---|---|---|---|---|---|
| **Upper Arm** | | | | | | | | | | |
| Radial | 5/4 | 8/6 | 5/3 | 0/0 | 0/0 | 9/19 | 0/0 | 0/0 | 10/8 | 11/7 |
| Median | 3/2 | 1/1 | 8/4 | 0/0 | 0/0 | 21/19 | 1/1 | 0/0 | 5/5 | 6/4 |
| Ulnar | 4/2 | 2/1 | 1/0 | 2/2 | 0/0 | 10/9 | 1/1 | 3/1 | 3/2 | 5/2 |
| **Elbow Level** | | | | | | | | | | |
| Radial | 3/3 | 2/1 | 3/2 | 0/0 | 0/0 | 10/9 | 0/0 | 0/0 | 2/2 | 6/5 |
| Median | 2/2 | 2/1 | 3/3 | 0/0 | 0/0 | 30/28 | 0/0 | 0/0 | 4/3 | 9/6 |
| Ulnar | 6/4 | 10/7 | 3/1 | 0/0 | 1/0 | 36/24 | 1/1 | 0/0 | 9/7 | 4/2 |
| **Forearm or Wrist** | | | | | | | | | | |
| Posterior Interosseus Nerve Radial | 3/3 | 2/2 | 7/5 | 0/0 | 0/0 | 19/18 | 0/0 | 0/0 | 2/1 | 5/4 |
| Wrist Median | 13/11 | 2/1 | 2/2 | 0/0 | 0/0 | 15/14 | 0/0 | 0/0 | 11/9 | 6/5 |
| Wrist Ulnar | 6/3 | 2/2 | 1/1 | 1/1 | 1/0 | 8/8 | 1/1 | 0/0 | 3/2 | 3/1 |
| TOTALS | 45/34 | 31/22 | 33/21 | 3/3 | 2/0 | 158/148 | 3/3 | 3/1 | 49/39 | 55/36 |

*Number of lesions operated/Number of lesions gaining grade 3 or better results.

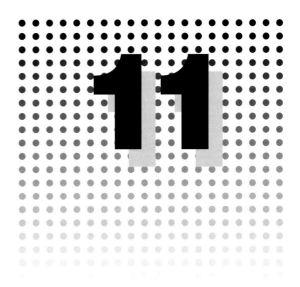

# Lower Extremity
# Nerves

## SUMMARY

A relatively large number of lesions involving the sciatic complex were cared for and operated on (324 cases). Many injuries occurred at a fairly proximal level, including the area of the sciatic notch and buttocks as well as that of the thigh. Most fracture and contusion-associated lesions and gunshot wounds involving sciatic nerve were followed and evaluated periodically for 2 to 5 months before exploration, intraoperative nerve action potential (NAP) recordings, and repair. Usually a surgical split of the nerve into its peroneal and tibial divisions was done to allow for separate evaluation and repair. This was important for most sciatic lesions in continuity, whether at a buttock or thigh level. By comparison, an attempt was made to repair sharp transections of the sciatic as acutely as possible; when this could be achieved, results were excellent.

Results with management of the tibial division were excellent, even if graft repair was necessary, and were universally good if neurolysis based on positive NAP recording across the lesion was done. Exceptions were provided by lesions that must have had their origin at a pelvic level and then extended through the sciatic notch to buttock level, and by a few very lengthy lesions in continuity at the buttock or thigh levels. Tibial repair done in the popliteal fossa behind the knee also fared quite well, but peroneal nerve repairs at this level did not do as well. In part, this was related to the nature of the usual peroneal injury, a stretch/contusion injury involving a long length of nerve. As expected, lacerations, gunshot wounds, and local iatrogenic injury involving peroneal nerve fared much better than the stretches, even if repair was necessary. Neurolysis based on a positive NAP also gave good results. Repair did lead to enough recovery in about 30% of cases so that use of a kick-up foot brace was no longer necessary. Loss from peroneal nerve entrapment was sometimes, but not always, helped by decompressive neurolysis.

Less frequent than proximal injury was involvement of tibial at the leg and ankle levels. Operation was usually worthwhile but the leg dissection is a deep one, and exposure of posterior tibial nerve at the level of the ankle is technically much more difficult than that for median nerve at the wrist and palmar levels. Electrical sensory studies showing conductive delay should be positive before entertaining the diagnosis of tarsal tunnel syndrome.

Femoral nerves can be injured at the pelvic or thigh levels, or both. Seventy-eight cases were evaluated and 54 operated on. Iliacus and quadriceps loss is especially disabling because there are not any good ways to substitute for these functions. Fortunately, proper management can lead to functional although incomplete recovery in most cases even though the femoral nerve is a mixed sensory-motor nerve. Perhaps this is because the muscles innervated by femoral nerve are large and are relatively close to both injury and potential repair sites. In this series, failures occurred in cases in which grafts had to be long and extended from pelvic to thigh levels, and in elderly individuals requiring repair rather than neurolysis. Loss from iatrogenic causes was the largest category of injury; herniorrhaphy, hip repair, femoral popliteal bypass, appendectomy, and even gynecologic procedures can lead to femoral palsy.

The pelvic plexus group of femoral injuries was a challenge to manage (49 cases evaluated). In general, surgery for injury to the lumbar plexus, which provides femoral outflow, gave better results than that for the sacral plexus, which provides sciatic including peroneal division outflow. Nonetheless, several lacerations involving sacral plexus were managed with some recovery. Most of these operations were done with the help of a general or gynecologic surgeon.

We favor resection of lateral femoral cutaneous nerve rather than decompression. In part, this prejudice has formed because we have had to resect a number of such nerves after prior unsuccessful decompression elsewhere.

The two major motor and sensory inputs to the lower extremity, the sciatic complex and the femoral complex, have separate anatomic courses. Because the patient is unlikely to have injured both concomitantly, except at a pelvic level, the overall functional result is better than might be expected, for despite some degree of paralysis, the patient is often able to use the extremity to bear at least some weight. For example, if the sciatic is out below the hamstring branches but the femoral complex is working, the patient can extend, lock, and flex the leg on the thigh and, with a kick-up foot brace to substitute for loss of foot dorsiflexion, can bear weight and walk with a surprisingly normal gait. Most patients with an intact sciatic outflow are able to compensate a great deal for a complete femoral palsy. The patient learns to throw out the lower leg or thigh, although it cannot be locked at the level of the knee. The hamstrings provides knee flexion, and the foot gives good stability because of intact plantar flexion and dorsiflexion. Another favorable factor for lower extremity nerve injuries is the fact that two of the three major territories are served by nerves, the tibial and the femoral, that can regenerate very well with proper management.

Despite these favorable considerations, the distances required for regeneration from injury site to significant motor inputs are some of the greatest in the body. As a result, the time required for regrowth is lengthy. By the time fibers reach innervational input sites, irreversible atrophy or replacement by fibrosis or fat may have occurred. In addition, although the peroneal nerve, like the radial nerve, supplies extensors, and its sensory inputs, like the radial's, are relatively unimportant, results gained by spontaneous regeneration after injury or from repair can be relatively poor. Another set

of factors frequently limiting recovery is the high association between sciatic injury and serious bony or vascular damage in the leg.[21,61] Sciatic complex cases evaluated and those operated on are summarized in Table 11–1.

## CLINICAL EXAMINATION OF SCIATIC COMPLEX

Injury to the sciatic nerve at a buttock level can give a variable pattern of loss. The components of loss may include those in the distribution of the peroneal and tibial divisions of the sciatic nerve with or without hamstring branch loss. It is rare for lesions at this level to involve the gluteal branches that supply gluteus maximus and medius. Exceptions are occasionally provided by a penetrating injury close to the sciatic notch. If glutei are not paretic, the proximal level of the lesion may be evident because of lateral (short head) hamstring paresis. The peroneal division at a buttock level carries fibers destined for a more distal portion of this hamstring complex.[26] It is also rare for a buttock level sciatic injury to totally paralyze the hamstrings. The major hamstring branch arises from proximal sciatic at the level of the notch and travels separate from it but parallel and medial to it on the underside of the glutei. More certain loss with complete sciatic injury at a buttock level gives lack of plantar flexion, foot inversion, and toe flexion as well as toe spread (tibial or posterior division). There is also a lack of eversion and dorsiflexion of the foot and extension of the toes (peroneal or anterior division).

The peroneal division is often preferentially injured at this high proximal level. Reasons for this are not clear, but it could be related to the peroneal division's more lateral position rela-

**TABLE 11–1**
Lower Extremity Nerves — Sciatic Complex

|  | No. Evaluated | No. Operated | % Operated |
|---|---|---|---|
| Sciatic — Buttock | 110 | 56 | 51 |
| Sciatic — Thigh | 136 | 93 | 68 |
| Peroneal — Knee & Leg | 217 | 145 | 67 |
| Tibial — Knee & Leg | 45 | 30 | 67 |
| Tibial — Ankle | 33 | 26 | 79 |
| Sural | 22 | 16 | 73 |
| TOTALS | 498 | 324 | 65 |

tive to the tibial division and thus more exposure to stretch/contusion during blunt trauma such as fractures or dislocations of the hip.[62] It also, however, seems to be preferentially involved if sciatic nerve is injured by injection at the buttock level. Sunderland has listed the possible reasons for the peroneal division's frequent involvement as well as difficulty in obtaining recovery.[68] Factors include a relatively poor blood supply, course of the nerve, particularly its relative lateral position close to the hip joint, amount of connective tissue between fascicles, and relative tethering, especially at head of fibula. Recovery also requires coordinated reinnervation up and down the course of the long extensor muscles of the anterior compartment of the lower leg.

Examination for sciatic palsy is relatively straightforward. With the patient in a sitting position, the patient is asked to flex the knee. The examiner can palpate and see contraction of both the lateral and medial hamstrings. With the leg extended and gentle pressure against the sole of the foot, the examiner can check plantar flexion. The examiner's other hand can be used to palpate the gastrocnemius-soleus in the calf. Inversion of the foot and flexion and spread of toes are readily checked, as is response to touch and pinprick on the sole of the foot. The saphenous branch of the femoral nerve may supply skin distal to the medial malleolus, and this should not be misinterpreted as sciatic innervation. Dorsiflexion or extension of the foot can be seen and the muscles palpated. Eversion of the foot by peronei is looked for, as is extension of the toes, particularly of the big toe by way of the extensor hallucis longus.

## CLINICAL EXAMINATION OF TIBIAL NERVE

The important sensory supply to the foot is through the posterior tibial nerve, which gives rise to calcaneal (heel) and lateral and medial plantar nerves. The sural nerve supplies the lateral side and the saphenous nerve a patch below the medial malleolus. Thus, with complete tibial division or nerve injury, sensory loss on the sole and heel of the foot is severe. An insensitive foot is a problem until enough sensation returns to

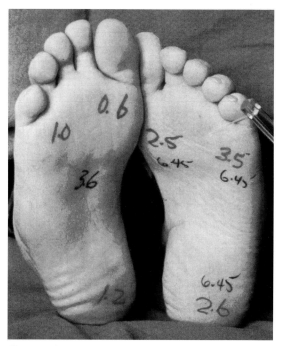

**Figure 11–1.** Comparative sensory tests on soles of feet. Left foot *(to the viewer's right)* is in a limb that had lengthy (30-cm) allografts for multiple-level propeller-blade injuries to the sciatic nerve from buttock to knee. (From Mackinnon S, Hudson A: Clinical application of peripheral nerve transplantation, Plast. Reconstr. Surg. 90:695–699, 1992.)

be protective (Figure 11–1).[10] Blisters, ulcers, and even osteomyelitis can occur unless the patient is instructed to inspect the foot daily and to wear footgear that prevents undue pressure on the heel and ball of the foot. Partial injury to the tibial complex is often very painful. Causalgia can be a major complication of injury to the tibial, but even if this does not occur, the mixture of hyperesthesia, hypoesthesia, and neuritic pain that results can be most disabling.[39,46]

Although foot intrinsic muscle loss is not a serious sequela of tibial dysfunction, it can result in a clawing of the toes, much as occurs in the hand with some distal ulnar and, especially, combined ulnar/median injuries. Some patients can abduct the big toe on the healthy side. If this is the case, the good side can be compared with the injured side. Inversion of the foot, which is a tibial function, can sometimes be partially mimicked by co-contraction of the peroneal-innervated anterior tibialis and the usually stronger gastrocnemius-soleus.

Unlike the peroneal-innervated muscles, the gastrocnemius-soleus contracts effectively after a relatively small aliquot of fibers regenerate back to it and connections are re-formed between the axons and motor end plates. Input sites for effective contraction are relatively proximal in this muscle complex. As a result, with effective regeneration of a knee-level injury to the tibial nerve, gastrocnemius-soleus contraction may begin recovery by 3 to 4 months, and with a midthigh-level lesion, by 5 to 9 months. The examiner must extend the leg when asking the patient to push down with the foot to make sure the foot is not being passively thrust down by hip and knee muscles. Early contraction of gastrocnemius-soleus can also be palpated in the proximal posterior compartment of the leg.

Recovery of plantar flexion with buttock-level sciatic lesions may require a year or more to begin. Speed of recovery depends on severity of the injury, the capacity for spontaneous recovery, and whether end-to-end repair of grafts is required. Inversion is more difficult to obtain, especially with proximal division injury and toe flexion, and other intrinsic foot function may not occur at all, even with a thigh-level tibial lesion. Tibial repair at any level, however, is always worthwhile provided the potential for poor spontaneous regeneration is proven. This is not only because there is great opportunity for recovery of plantar function, which is so important for push-off in walking, but also because at least protective sensation to the sole of the foot can be regained.

# CLINICAL EXAMINATION OF PERONEAL NERVE

With complete peroneal injury, sensory loss, which is of a variable extent on the dorsum of the foot, is of less functional consequence than with tibial injury. Of great importance is the loss not only of eversion of the foot but of dorsiflexion or extension. Toe extension loss is of less consequence because use of shoes mitigates the importance of this function for most humans. Fortunately, use of a plastic shoe insert dorsiflexion splint or, for heavier and more active individuals, a spring-loaded kick-up foot brace

built into a good shoe, substitutes for foot extensor loss magnificently. These devices are so effective that many patients, after they get used to them, are unwilling to accept the uncertainties of results from repair of the peroneal nerve, especially if the lesion is severe.

Other than lateral hamstring (short head of biceps femoris) loss with high peroneal division injuries, important muscles innervated by this nerve are, as with the tibial, all below the knee. Eversion of the foot is provided by peroneus longus and brevis and is innervated by the superficial branch of the nerve, which usually arises just distal to the fibular head. Peroneus contraction can be palpated and observed. With knee-level injury and subsequent successful regeneration, peroneus contraction can begin by 3 to 5 months. Muscle lateral to proximal fibula can be seen to quiver on attempted eversion. Tendon tightening behind and above the lateral malleolus can be seen. Recovery of anterior tibialis does not usually occur until 9 to 12 months, and return of extensor hallucis longus takes even longer. With early recovery of anterior tibialis, its tendon may be seen to tighten as it passes over the dorsum of the foot. The remainder of the toes may not recover extension after severe peroneal nerve injuries, even those at the level of the knee.

Recovery of peroneal-innervated muscular function is difficult to obtain with thigh-level repair. Return of some peroneus function may not take place for 6 months or more, and early contraction of anterior tibialis may not occur until after a year or more. Unfortunately, repair of the peroneal division at a buttock level seldom results in significant peroneal motor recovery. On the other hand, if the lesion at this level, even though complete, is one that permits spontaneous regeneration, then recovery of both eversion and dorsiflexion can occur.

Sural origin can be predominantly from either peroneal or tibial nerve, but it can also receive input from both. Thus, proximal involvement of the sciatic nerve may affect the sural sensory distribution. At a midthigh level, complete sciatic injury involves total distal tibial and peroneal loss and often sural sensory loss as well. Hamstring function is totally spared unless this function is compromised by direct injury to the muscle. Examples in our series of cases include several patients who sustained guillotine injuries not only to nerve but to all hamstring muscles as well.

The level of bifurcation of the sciatic nerve in the thigh is variable. It usually occurs at junction of the middle and distal thirds of the thigh but, in our experience, can occur at a higher level in a third of the cases. Thus, injury at a thigh level can involve either tibial or peroneal nerve. It can appear as an incomplete injury to the whole sciatic nerve but in reality be a complete injury to one nerve with sparing of function of the other.

At the level of the knee, injury usually results in either a tibial or peroneal palsy. If loss is complete, the clinical presentation is straightforward. There is complete loss of inversion, plantar flexion, and hypoesthesia on the sole of the foot with tibial involvement, and lack of eversion and extension of the foot and toes with peroneal involvement.

Injury, particularly penetrating injury near the head of the fibula, can damage either the superficial or deep branch of the peroneal nerve and spare the other. The superficial branch innervates the peronei that evert the foot, and the deep branch innervates the extensors of the foot and toes.

Because of overlap from saphenous and sural nerves, sensory loss over the dorsum of the foot may be variable with a peroneal palsy. There is not an autonomous sensory zone in which loss can be counted on, even with a complete injury. If there is sensory loss, it is over the dorsum of the foot, particularly just proximal to the web space between the large or first toe and the second toe.

Anterior compartment injury can involve a variable portion of the deep peroneal branches, depending on the level of injury. By comparison, posterior compartment injury of tibial nerve in the leg can affect sensation on the sole of the foot and toe flexion and spread, but usually spares gastrocnemius-soleus function, because branches to this large muscle complex enter it at the proximal calf level.

Ankle-level injuries may involve distal tibial nerve. As nerve approaches the ankle it gives off a calcaneal branch supplying the area of the heel of the foot. Just distal to the medial malleolus, nerve divides into medial and lateral plantar branches. These branches supply sensation to the sole of the foot and intrinsic motor function of the toes and foot.

# ELECTRICAL STUDIES OF SCIATIC COMPLEX

## Electromyography

Careful electromyographic (EMG) study of the lower limb can help differentiate pelvic plexus injury from proximal sciatic injury. Denervational changes in quadriceps, obturator, or glutei suggest a pelvic level for the lesion. Occasionally, a penetrating wound of the buttock affects gluteal nerves or muscles as well as sciatic nerve, in which case an EMG taken without the clinical history and examination could suggest a pelvic lesion. Noninvasive sampling of muscles such as the piriformis, the quadratus femoris, and, sometimes, the glutei is not always practical. Branches to these muscles can, in any case, originate at a pelvic level and leave with the sciatic nerve through the notch. A related electrodiagnostic challenge centers on the hamstring muscles. It is true that most of the hamstring input derives from proximal sciatic nerve. Nonetheless, the course of these fibers is mainly through a large hamstring branch that travels parallel to the sciatic nerve at buttock to proximal thigh level. Despite serious injury to the sciatic nerve at that level, this branch is often spared. As a result, only a few of our buttock-level sciatic lesions had hamstring loss, either by clinical or electrical examination. On the other hand, if loss was in the peroneal distribution, search for denervational changes in the lateral hamstring muscle suggested a proximal sciatic lesion. The occasional painless foot drop associated with a lateral disc herniation was sometimes differentiated from peroneal division injury not only by magnetic resonance imaging or computed tomography scan findings of the spine but also by finding paraspinal as well as dorsiflexor muscles denervated.[65] An inappropriate lumbar laminectomy can be all too easily performed if the peroneal nerve is not appreciated as the true site of pathology.

The most valuable muscle to study electrically for early recovery of sciatic function was the gastrocnemius-soleus. Even though eventual recovery may prove useful in the peroneal and other tibial-innervated portions of the sciatic complex, electrical and clinical recovery is much delayed in the peronei compared with the gastrocnemius-soleus. The other important electrical corollary is that nascent or reinnervational changes in tibial-innervated muscles are more likely to presage useful recovery than such changes in peroneal-innervated muscles. Enough fibers may return to the peroneal-innervated muscles in the anterior compartment to reverse some denervational change. There may not, however, be enough fibers of sufficient maturity in terms of size, myelination, and, perhaps most importantly, reinnervational complexity to restore peroneal function.

Besides gastrocnemius-soleus, the usual muscles sampled for tibial division injuries include tibialis posterior, which provides foot inversion, and the flexor hallucis longus, which extends the large toe. Muscles sampled for the peroneal division or nerve are usually the peroneus longus and brevis, which together provide foot eversion, the anterior tibialis, the extensor digitorum longus, and the extensor hallucis longus. Reinnervation and the electrical changes accompanying it do not always proceed in an orderly fashion down these two cascades of muscles, especially with injury to the peroneal nerve. For example, peronei may recover, anterior tibialis and extensor hallucis may not, and yet extensor digitorum longus may. Even the tibial division displays some electrical and clinical peculiarities as far as reinnervation is concerned: tibialis posterior recovery may not approach that seen with gastrocnemius-soleus, and flexor digitorum longus recovery may, if it occurs at all, be superior to flexor hallucis longus recovery.

Partial lesions to the sciatic complex, whether caused by compression or more direct injury, tend to affect maximally more distal muscles, just as with similar radial, median, and ulnar lesions.[23] As a result, the electromyographer may have to sample toe flexors and extensors or, on occasion, foot intrinsic muscles to document milder sciatic lesions, particularly those caused by compression.

## Conduction Studies

These tests are of greatest value for entrapment or compression of peroneal nerve over the head or neck of the fibula and for posterior tibial entrapment in the foot (tarsal tunnel syndrome). It is important, however, whenever possible, to compare conduction in the symptomatic limb with that in the contralateral limb.

Effective study for peroneal entrapment usually includes stimulation of the nerve well proximal to the head of the fibula.[7] Latencies are then determined for conduction to the peronei and to a more distal muscle such as extensor hallucis longus. Conduction velocities are slowed for both, but usually more so to the peronei than to more distal muscles. Even after successful neurolysis and relief of compressive bands or tissues, latencies remain prolonged, often for years. As a result, clinical evaluation, including careful grading of anterior compartment muscles, is of greater value as an index of recovery than postoperative conductive studies. The latter, however, should not be neglected if there is failure of improvement or a plateau to the clinical recovery.

Conduction velocity studies are also of great value for suspected tarsal tunnel syndrome.[19,32] This is especially so if values from the involved foot are compared with those in the contralateral limb.[8] The extreme values and the normal limits are far less precisely defined than they are for carpal tunnel studies.[52] Surgeons should concentrate on an accurate and thorough clinical examination, and use electrical studies to supplement these findings.[20] This is important because true tarsal tunnel syndrome is an infrequent diagnosis.[37] Of course, other causes for foot pain must be eliminated.[38] Sensory NAPs can be evoked by toe stimulation and recorded at a lower shin level from posterior tibial nerve proximal to the ankle. Muscle action potentials can also be recorded from foot intrinsic muscles after more proximal stimulation of the nerve. This is despite the fact that well-done sensory studies reflect earlier and more severe conductive changes in tarsal tunnel syndrome than do motor studies.[53] Needle sampling of foot intrinsic muscles can be painful for some patients but may be a necessity if loss is severe or sensory potentials are not recordable.

## SELECTED SCIATIC NERVE ANATOMY

The sciatic nerve is formed from the anterior and posterior divisions of the L4, L5, S1, and S2 spinal roots, as well as the anterior division of S3. In general, the anterior divisions make up the tibial nerve and the large nerve to the hamstring musculature, and the posterior divisions make up the peroneal nerve. Divisions combine to form the sciatic nerve. At the buttock level, the divisions may pass through or between the two heads of the piriformis or combine into the whole sciatic nerve, which may lie beneath or anterior to it. Sciatic then passes posterior to quadriceps femoris, internal obturator, and both gemelli.

The major hamstring branch arises proximal to or in the notch region after the posterior elements give rise to the superior and inferior gluteal nerves in the pelvis. The gluteal branches emerge from the pelvis through the sciatic notch, where they lie beneath the gluteus maximus. Branches to muscles such as the piriformis, along with the gluteal branches, the major hamstring nerve, and the gluteal vessels, leave the notch in conjunction with the sciatic nerve. The contiguous nature of these structures, as well as the vasculature to the nerves and the gluteal vessels themselves, make dissection at this level of the notch difficult although not impossible. The posterior femoral cutaneous nerve of the thigh usually has a separate but contiguous course to the sciatic, lying somewhat posterior to it but deep to gluteus maximus. The nerve becomes more superficial at the gluteal crease. At the level of the thigh, it innervates skin posteriorly. It also innervates posterior leg skin for a variable distance toward the ankle. At this level, the major nerve to the hamstrings is medial to the sciatic and the nerve to the short head of the biceps is lateral.

The major branch to the hamstring muscles travels close to the medial or tibial division of the nerve through the buttocks. On reaching the upper thigh, it branches to supply the long head of the biceps, the semitendinosus, the semimembranosus, and the ischial portion of the abductor magnus. One or more branches to hamstrings also arise from the sciatic nerve itself, usually at the level of the proximal thigh. A proximal peroneal division injury is likely if lateral hamstring weakness or paralysis accompanies foot drop.

The sciatic divisions lie on top of or dorsal to the obturator internus, gemelli, and quadratus femoris in the midportion of the buttocks and

enter the thigh somewhat deep and between medial and lateral masses of the hamstring muscles. As the sciatic nerve proceeds distally and deep to the hamstrings, it bifurcates into tibial and peroneal nerves. The level at which this bifurcation occurs is somewhat variable, but it is usually at the junction of the middle and lower thirds of the thigh. Injury at or close to these levels can involve tibial or peroneal nerve, or both, rather than sciatic nerve as a whole.

## SURGICAL APPROACH TO SCIATIC NERVE AT THE BUTTOCK LEVEL

Approach is with patient in the prone position with padding around the knee and some flexion of leg on the thigh. A folded sheet placed under the anterior iliac crest on the side of the dissection tends to rotate buttock up and somewhat medially.

The skin incision for the buttock-level exposure is curvilinear and is placed around the lateral aspect of the buttock mass. The incision must be sufficiently high so that after the gluteal lid is retracted medially, the notch is displayed without difficulty.[64] If the sciatic nerve in the proximal thigh and beneath the buttock needs to be exposed, the incision is swung into the buttocks crease and then down the posterior midline of the thigh. The sciatic nerve can always be identified at this point, and it can then be followed up to the notch area (Figure 11–2).

The incision extends deep between the hamstring muscles for thigh-level exposure of the sciatic nerve, whereas the gluteus maximus and a portion of the medius are separated close to the lateral pelvic brim and mobilized medially to expose the nerve up to the sciatic notch. This musculature is retracted medially with rakes or Richardson retractors. Enough of a rim of gluteal muscular attachment should be left laterally to facilitate later closure. This retained rim of musculature is usually marked by heavy sutures left attached to their needles for subsequent repair. There is a somewhat avascular plane beneath the gluteal musculature and posterior to the neural structures. This plane can be followed medially to the sciatic nerve. Care must be taken with the dissection to preserve the hamstring branch, which lies somewhat medial and superior to the main sciatic nerve.

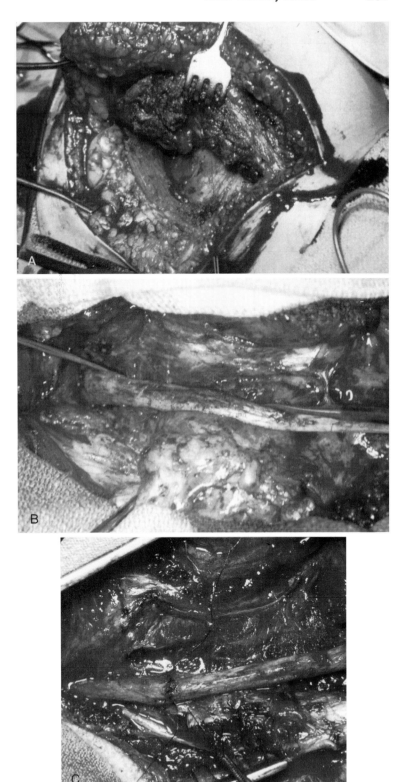

**Figure 11–2.** (A) Exposure of sciatic nerve at the level of the buttock includes transection of lateral gluteus maximus and medius muscle, leaving a cuff of muscle laterally to sew back to. Here a rake is being used to retract left buttock muscula-ture medially. Patient is prone; back is to the left and thigh to the right. (B) Contusion of scia-tic nerve close to sciatic notch area. Notch is to the left, and thigh level is to the right. (C) Suture of sciatic nerve at a but-tock level after resection of neuroma in continuity. Injury to this nerve was caused by contusion associated with hip fracture. See also color figure.

As one approaches the area of the notch, gluteal nerves and vessels need to be preserved. Innervation of the gluteus medius is critical to stability of the hip joint. It is the "deltoid" of the hip and maintains the pelvis whenever the patient takes his weight solely on that limb.

Division of gluteal vessels high in the region of the notch without their ligation or coagulation may be disastrous because the open vessels can retract into pelvis and bleed unchecked. This requires an emergent transabdominal approach and a difficult pelvic dissection for correction.

Because the usual operation on the sciatic nerve is done with the patient prone, positioning for harvesting one or both sural nerves is ideal.[45]

## RESULTS—SCIATIC COMPLEX AT THE BUTTOCK LEVEL

Results are reported by injury or lesion category, divisions operated on, and type of operation done (Table 11–2). Although most injuries required operation on both divisions, the specific operation varied. Some cases had neurolysis of both divisions, others had repair of both divisions, and still others had neurolysis of one division and repair of the other. In a few cases, only one division required an operation. Tumors are not included in the results cited in the tables but are sometimes referred to in the text. There are only a few series of sciatic injuries of any size previously reported[15,16,35,41] although a number of articles have attempted to summarize management.[2,5,36,44,55,75] Most series have concentrated on gunshot wounds involving sciatic nerve.[11,42,54,57,59]

## Results With Injection Injuries

One-fifth of sciatic lesions were at the buttock level. The largest category was those caused by injection injury (see Table 11–2). Patients with injection injuries are often, but not always, either constitutionally thin or chronically ill and thus debilitated.[14] Poor gluteal covering predisposes to this type of injury, particularly if the injection is given with a long needle in other than the upper outer quadrant of the buttocks (Figure 11–3). There appear to be two patterns of onset of pain and disability after such injury to the sciatic nerve. The first and by far the more frequent is radicular pain and paresthesias with some degree of distal deficit of almost immediate onset. The second and much less frequent pattern, occurring in 10% of patients, is delayed onset of pain, paresthesias, and deficit appearing minutes to several hours after the injection, which may or may not have produced severe local pain shortly after administration.[29] These two patterns suggest the possibility that, on occasion, noxious drugs do not need to be injected directly into the nerve to damage it but rather may be deposited within epineurium or perhaps even adjacent to the nerve, and with time, may diffuse into or penetrate the intrafascicular structure.

To date, only 37% of the sciatic injection injuries seen have warranted operation. Partial injuries sparing some function in both the tibial and peroneal divisions can usually be treated with vigorous physical therapy, pain medications, and time. Because of persistent symptoms, similar injuries may occasionally require exploration and external or internal neurolysis, which may or may not relieve the pain. More

**TABLE 11–2**
Operative Results — Sciatic Nerve — Buttock Level*

| | Neurolysis | | Suture | | Graft | | No Operation |
|---|---|---|---|---|---|---|---|
| | T | P | T | P | T | P | |
| Injection | 13/11 | 13/10 | 2/2 | 1/0 | 5/4 | 4/1 | 30/20 |
| Fracture/Dislocation | 4/4 | 4/3 | 0/0 | 0/0 | 5/3 | 4/1 | 12/7 |
| Contusion | 6/6 | 5/5 | 0/0 | 0/0 | 0/0 | 0/0 | 8/6 |
| Gunshot wound | 4/4 | 4/3 | 2/2 | 2/1 | 4/4 | 3/1 | 2/1 |
| Laceration/Stab | 1/1 | 1/1 | 2/2 | 2/1 | 3/3 | 3/1 | 1/0 |
| Compression | 2/2 | 2/1 | 0/0 | 0/0 | 0/0 | 0/0 | 1/1 |
| TOTALS | 30/28 | 29/23 | 6/6 | 5/2 | 17/14 | 14/4 | 54/35 |

P = peroneal division; T = tibial division.
*Number of divisions operated/number reaching a grade 3 or better result. Tumor cases not included.

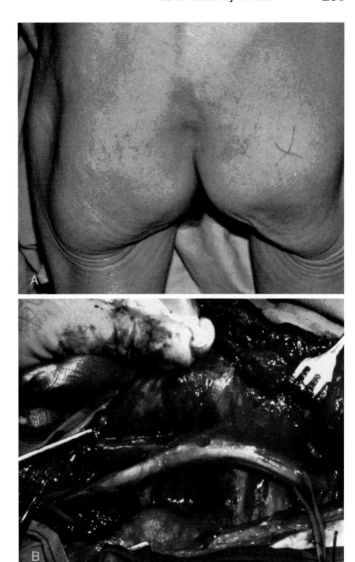

**Figure 11 – 3.** *(A)* Presumed injection site in the right buttock of a thin and cachectic individual resulted in a sciatic palsy. *(B)* Sciatic nerve is adherent to underside of gluteus musculature at injection site.

complete lesions to the sciatic as a whole or to all of one division may benefit from relatively early exploration. Intraoperative recording of nerve action potentials (NAPs) is used. Differential neurolysis of each division is done if NAPs are present, or resection and suture is performed if they are absent. Time for such exploration is best 3 to 5 months after the injection injury occurs. Results are poor if resection and suture are indicated for the peroneal division, but better with tibial repair (Figure 11 – 4). Even resection of a division, if it is thought to be nonreparable, may not help the pain associated with some injection injuries. One of our patients who had resection of a segment of the peroneal divi-

sion at the buttock level eventually had a sympathectomy with some relief, even though the pain was not of a classic, sympathetically mediated nature.

In this series of injections, two thirds (20) of those cases treated conservatively improved. These cases usually had incomplete or partial loss in the distribution of one or both divisions. Pain was a problem in most of these cases, but fortunately it usually responded to conservative management. Twenty patients were operated on. Five of nine divisions that required grafts had substantial recovery, as did two divisions that required sutures. If neurolysis was indicated based on NAP recordings, 21 of 26 divi-

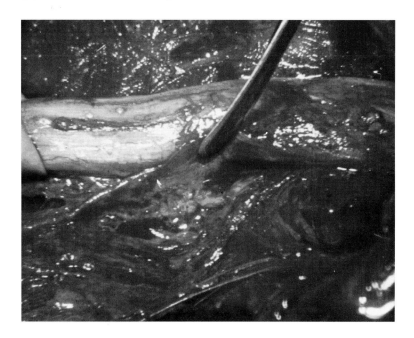

**Figure 11-4.** This individual required resection and repair of one division of the nerve at a buttock level because of an injection injury by morphine. Note the appearance of the tissue adjacent to the injected segment of nerve.

sions improved. Three of these patients had complete loss clinically and by EMG, but because they had NAPs across their lesions, neurolysis was performed, and they improved.

## Case Summary — Injection Injury

A 52-year-old woman received an injection of a morphiate drug in the right buttock. She had pain radiate down posterior thigh to calf and foot and onset of immediate sciatic palsy. Within a few days, some degree of foot dorsiflexion returned, but no plantar flexion. EMG at 4 weeks after injection injury showed severe denervational change in tibial muscles and partial denervational change in the peroneal distribution. At examination 4 months later, peroneal-innervated muscles graded 3, tibial-innervated motor and sensory function was absent, and hamstring function was normal. EMG was similar to that done at 1 month after injury and showed no nascent activity.

Exploration of the sciatic nerve at a buttock level revealed a swollen nerve, especially along its medial aspect. A NAP was recorded across the sciatic lesion, so it was split into its tibial and peroneal divisions. Both divisions appeared to transmit a NAP. However, the main hamstring branch was adherent to the side of the tibial division, and after this was dissected free, there was no NAP conducted through the tibial division. As a result, the tibial division was resected, and three 5.8-cm grafts were placed. Only an external neurolysis of the peroneal division was done. The resected segment showed de-

generated axons with marked epineurial and interfascicular fibrosis. Endoneurium was thickened. Only fine axons were present, and they were mixed in with a moderately heavy proliferation of scar tissue.

Follow-up at 2 years and 2 months showed considerable restoration of calf girth. Circumferential measurements 12 cm below the patella were equal bilaterally. Plantar flexion graded 3, and inversion was also 3. There was no toe flexion. Sensation on the sole was protective only. She had maintained excellent peroneal-innervated function.

### Comment

Some injection injuries, even to sciatic nerve at a buttock level, may be operative candidates. In this case, tibial loss predominated, and repair of this division was helpful. Pain may also sometimes be helped, especially if tibial division is involved. Lesions due to injection are not always focal. If resection is indicated by operative electrical studies, it must be lengthy enough to encompass the entire injected segment.

## Results With Fracture-Dislocations of the Hip

Injury to the sciatic nerve at a buttock level was frequently caused by fracture-dislocation of the hip or attempts to repair the same (Figure 11-5). This mechanism for proximal injury to the sciatic complex has been reported fairly fre-

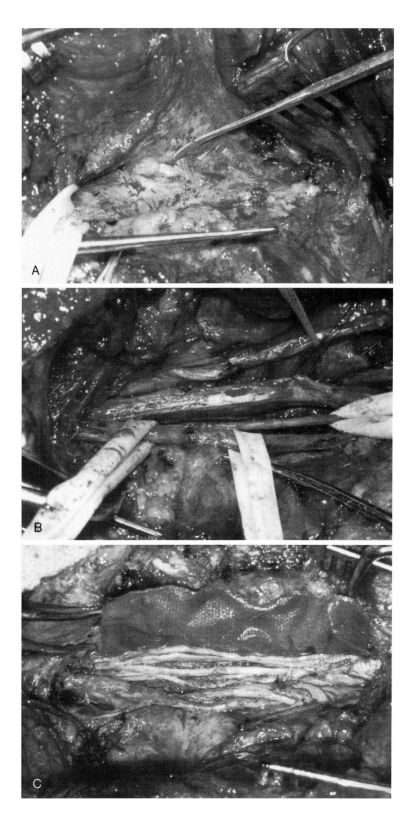

**Figure 11–5.** (A) Usual scar involving sciatic nerve in the notch area and associated with hip dislocation with proximal fracture of femoral head. (B) After neurolysis on another buttock-level lesion associated with fracture, nerve action potential (NAP) recording was positive, so nerve has been split into its two divisions. Penrose drains are on the peroneal division, which had a high or proximal bifurcation. A plastic loop is on the hamstring branch; tibial division is between it and the peroneal division. (C) The tibial division had transmitted a NAP, and an internal neurolysis was done. The peroneal division was repaired by sural grafts.

quently.[1,31,43,71] The patient presenting with a complete sciatic palsy caused by fracture or dislocation sometimes has resolution of the tibial division loss but seldom of the peroneal division loss. Unfortunately, peroneal division loss usually predominated in this series. Such loss, if complete to begin with, seldom was reversed either in the nonoperative or operative cases. One of four patients with grafts to the peroneal division at the buttock level had enough recovery so that continued use of a kick-up foot brace was no longer necessary. Three of the four patients whose peroneal divisions had neurolysis at that level improved, but that was because they had NAPs across their lesions and were thus shown at the operating table to be regenerating adequately. Significant peroneal return, including some eversion and dorsiflexion, gave these cases a grade of 3 or more. Toe extension was seldom regained, except in a few cases in which early spontaneous regeneration was evident.

Either conservative management or operation, if correctly chosen, led to some significant degree of tibial division recovery in the majority of cases. Three of five grafts succeeded, and each of the four tibial divisions having neurolysis based on presence of intraoperative NAPs across their lesions had some useful degree of recovery. Adequate recovery at this level consisted of plantar flexion of grade 3 or more, and usually, but not always, some degree of inversion and some protective sensation on the sole of the foot. It was unusual for any patient to regain toe flexion or foot intrinsic function.

## Case Summary — Fracture-Dislocation of Hip

A 23-year-old male was injured in an oil rig accident when his left leg was caught by a drill and wrapped around it. The right leg was drawn in and twisted as well. The patient sustained a dislocation of the left hip and a right midshaft fracture of the femur. The left hip was relocated a few hours later, and the right femur was pinned after several weeks of balanced skeletal traction. The accident resulted in an initially complete sciatic palsy involving the left leg. After a few weeks, a little plantar flexion returned. When seen by our service 4 months later, medial hamstrings graded 3 to 4 but lateral was trace only. Plantar flexion was 3, but there was no foot inversion or toe flexion. Sensation was absent on the sole of the foot. Peroneal-innervated muscles were completely paralyzed. EMG showed a complete denervational pattern in the sciatic distribution, except for gastrocnemius-soleus, which was only partially denervated. There were no nascent units, even in tibial-innervated muscles.

Sciatic nerve at the buttock level was surgically exposed at 4.5 months after injury. A lesion in continuity measuring 3.6 cm long began close to the sciatic notch portion of the nerve and extended inferiorly. A NAP could be recorded across this lesion and several centimeters distal to it. The nerve was split into its two divisions. Re-recording showed a NAP across the tibial half of the nerve but not across the peroneal half. Nonetheless, the tibial portion was firm and swollen. An internal neurolysis was done on this division, and the peroneal division lesion was resected. A 3.2-cm gap was replaced by six sural grafts 3.8 cm (1.5 inches) in length (Figure 11–6). Buttock glutei were reattached laterally, and other soft tissues were closed. The limb was not casted or placed in a splint. Ambulation was begun 24 hours postoperatively with the help of a shoe insert kick-up orthosis.

Follow-up at 4 years showed excellent tibial division return. Plantar flexion graded 5 and inversion 4, but toe flexion remained absent. Sensation on the sole of the foot graded 3 to 4. Both lateral and medial hamstrings graded 5. In the peroneal distribution, eversion was 2 to 3, but there was no dorsiflexion of the foot or toe extension. The patient uses his kick-up foot brace, but only for the portion of the day when he is most active. Follow-up at 6 years showed improved eversion, but anterior tibialis graded only 2, and there was no toe extension.

### Comment

This case shows the usual clinical course and results of a severe proximal sciatic injury complicating hip injury. Toe flexion seldom is regained, and practical dorsiflexion of the foot is extremely difficult to obtain.

## Results — Contusive Injuries and Gunshot Wounds

The contusive injuries operated on were caused by falls on the buttocks and vehicular accidents; they were characterized by incomplete loss and pain not responsive to medications, physical therapy, or time. An occasional painful sciatica was caused by an embedded gunshot shell fragment or a piece of bone from a fracture secondary to the gunshot wound. Operative manipulation sometimes helped the pain, and, in each case, whether pain was helped or not, eventual function was excellent (Figure 11–7).

By comparison, most of the gunshot wounds involving sciatic nerve at this level caused severe loss of function that usually did not im-

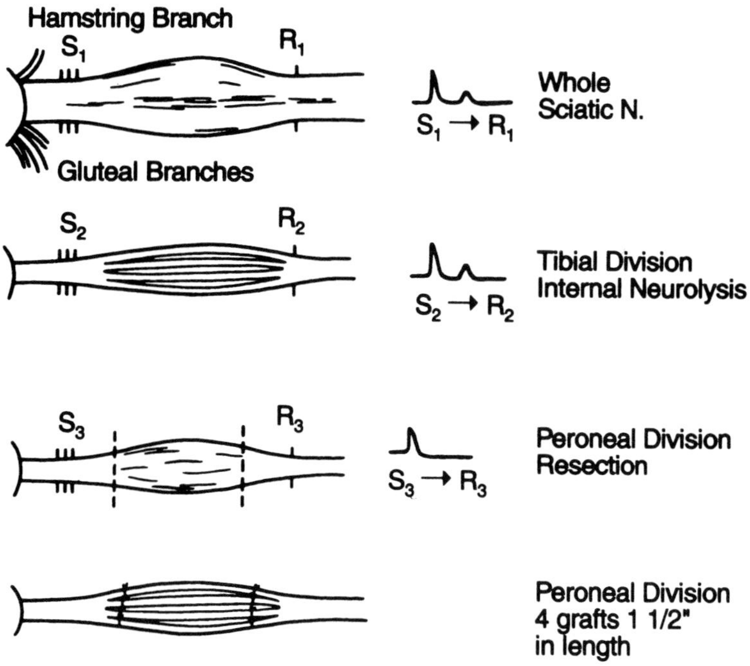

Hamstring Branch

$S_1$  $R_1$

Gluteal Branches

$S_1 \rightarrow R_1$

Whole
Sciatic N.

$S_2$  $R_2$

$S_2 \rightarrow R_2$

Tibial Division
Internal Neurolysis

$S_3$  $R_3$

$S_3 \rightarrow R_3$

Peroneal Division
Resection

Peroneal Division
4 grafts 1 1/2"
in length

**Figure 11–6.** Sciatic lesion in continuity resulting from contusion at the buttock level. Top diagram shows nerve action potential (NAP) recorded across the lesion. Tibial division that conducted a NAP had a neurolysis, in this case an internal one, since pain was also a severe problem in this patient *(second diagram)*. The peroneal division did not transmit and, as can be seen by the *third diagram*, was resected and repaired by four sural grafts 3.8 cm (1.5 in) in length *(bottom diagram)*.

prove over a 2- to 5-month period. Neurolysis based on positive NAPs led to the expected good result in seven of eight divisions managed in this fashion. Repair was necessary on 11 divisions. Significant recovery occurred in each of six repaired tibial divisions but in only two of five repaired peroneal divisions (Figure 11–8).

## Case Summary—Gunshot Wound

This 10-year-old male sustained a shotgun blast to the right buttock with severe soft tissue loss and extensive,

lengthy injury to sciatic nerve. He required shortening of femur to remove necrotic nonhealing bone several months after wounding. At that time, he had an end-to-end secondary repair of the tibial and peroneal divisions of the sciatic nerve. He was placed in a hip spica postoperatively. Follow-up 8 years later showed recovery of tibial function with an overall grade for that nerve of 3 to 4. As expected, there was very little peroneal recovery. The patient wears a kick-up foot brace and is now in college.

### Comment

If possible, bony fixation should be achieved prior to nerve repair even though both are done at the same operation.

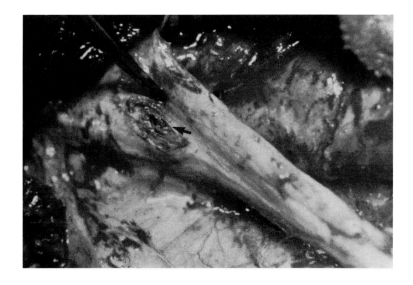

**Figure 11–7.** Shell fragment *(arrow)* imbedded in tibial division of sciatic nerve close to region of the notch. This patient had excellent peroneal function and partial tibial function grading 3 to 4, but had severe neuritic pain with some autonomic component. The latter was helped by removal of the fragment, but the patient subsequently required a sympathectomy for more complete relief of pain.

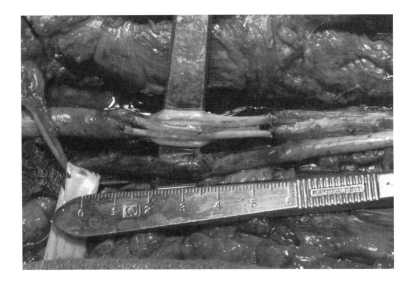

**Figure 11–8.** Split repair of the sciatic nerve close to the buttock crease in nerve injured by a gunshot wound. In this case, the peroneal division *(bottom)* transmitted a nerve action potential, but the tibial division *(top)* did not. Five grafts 4.5 cm in length were sewn in place using a grouped interfascicular repair.

## Results With Lacerations/ Stab Wounds

This was a favorable category of injury even at such a proximal level (see Table 11–2). Because of the nature of the injury, relatively early operation was always indicated. One patient refused operation and has not recovered function. Results with operation, whether by suture or by graft repair, were usually favorable. Unlike contusion or stretch involving sciatic at this level, grafts, when necessary, were relatively short, seldom exceeding 3.8 to 5.0 cm in length. Tibial division repairs, whether by suture or by graft, recovered to a grade 3 or better, whereas only two peroneal division repairs at this level recovered to a grade 3 or better score.

Despite a relatively sharp mechanism for transection in most of these cases, retraction of nerve ends occurred, and grafts were sometimes necessary because of a delay in repair. In addition, despite complete loss in the distribution of the sciatic nerve preoperatively, contusion and thus a lesion in continuity was found in one instance. NAPs were recorded across both divisions of this lesion, and this led to neurolysis with eventual satisfactory recovery.

### Case Summary—Laceration/ Stab Wound

This 4-year-old female had learned to climb her family's refrigerator shelves to get to the top shelf for milk and juice. One day, she fell backward, landing on her buttocks shortly after a glass jar had fallen and shattered. A shard of glass was driven into her left buttock, and she sustained an immediate and complete sciatic palsy. She was referred several weeks later for surgical exploration. At that time, the nerve was found transected 2.5 cm distal to the sciatic notch. Stumps had retracted, and after trimming of proximal and distal neuromas, a 3.8-cm gap resulted. Both stumps were split into tibial and peroneal divisions, and each of these into several groups of fascicles. The gap was bridged with grouped interfascicular grafts using sural nerve. Seven grafts 4 cm in length were placed. Follow-up at age 8 gave an overall grade of 4 for tibial nerve and a grade of 2 for peroneal nerve.

### Comment

Although done secondarily, buttock-level repair was especially rewarding in this youngster with a very sharp injury. Had facilities and experienced personnel been available locally, this would have also been a good case for primary (early) repair.

## Sciatic Entrapment

Entrapment resulting from piriformis syndrome has been reported.[3,22,70] This was rare in our experience; we saw only two examples over a 25-year period (Figure 11–9). One was helped by operation and removal of piriformis, and the other was not. Other than those cases associated with hip repair, operative iatrogenic causes of injury to the sciatic nerve at a buttock level are unusual. Compression can occur as a result of proximal placement of stimulators, and scarring associated with such a device may require a sec-

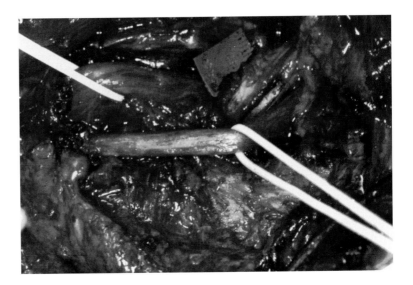

**Figure 11-9.** Exposure of left sciatic nerve in the region of the notch. Origin of tibial *(upper loop)* and peroneal *(lower loop)* divisions has been split by piriformis muscle under the short ruler at the top right of the photograph. This child had presented with progressive peroneal palsy associated with gluteal wasting and was thought to have piriformis syndrome.

ondary operation.[51] One patient in this series had a neurolysis for such scarring after removal of a stimulator at a buttock level.

## SURGICAL APPROACH TO SCIATIC NERVE AT THE THIGH LEVEL

Approach to the portion of the sciatic nerve located in the thigh is relatively straightforward. Preferred is a curvilinear posterior thigh skin incision. This incision may be taken in a lateral and curved direction around the edge of the buttocks for more proximal exposure or extended into popliteal fossa for more distal exposure of the sciatic complex. At the thigh level, hamstring muscles are readily split in the midline and retracted with Weitlaner self-retaining retractors or by use of Army-Navy or Richardson retractors. The long head of biceps lies between the operator and the sciatic nerve. This muscle is easily mobilized, displaying the sciatic nerve in the posterior thigh (Figure 11-10).

Whenever possible, more distal hamstring branches and major collateral vessels to sciatic nerve are spared, although, if need be, the latter can be sacrificed. Sharp dissection is done with a No. 15 scalpel blade mounted on a long-handled plastic knife supplemented by use of Metzenbaum scissors. Such dissection is used to expose nerve proximal and distal to the injury site in a circumferential fashion. Dissection is

then carried from either end of the exposure toward the injury. After intraoperative stimulation and recording on those lesions in continuity, whole sciatic can be split into its two divisions and each evaluated independently. The natural plane between the two divisions can be visualized with the aid of eye loupes or a low-power setting of the microscope. If there is difficulty in developing this plane, then tibial and peroneal nerves are isolated in the popliteal fossa. Penrose drains are placed around them, and they are gently spread apart as more proximal whole sciatic is split into its two divisions by working from a caudal to cephalad direction. After the sciatic nerve bifurcates at a mid-thigh or higher level, this portion of the dissection becomes easier.

## RESULTS—SCIATIC NERVE AT THE THIGH LEVEL

More than 25% of those lower extremity nerve lesions evaluated occurred at the level of the thigh. Of those 208 divisions of sciatic nerve evaluated at the thigh level, 152 (73%) were operated on (Table 11-3). Those evaluated included 38 patients with gunshot wounds, 39 with fractures, usually of the femur, 21 with laceration or stab wounds, 14 with tumors of the sciatic nerve, and 13 with contusive lesions.

At the thigh level, injuries to the sciatic nerve can produce a complete lesion that is total to both divisions, complete to one division and in-

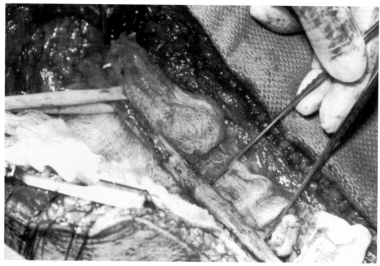

**Figure 11–10.** The long head of the biceps has been displaced to expose a severe compressive lesion of sciatic nerve at the midthigh level. This unusual circumstance occurred in a female accountant who habitually sat forward on an unpadded wooden chair without using the back rest. As a result, a good deal of her weight compressed the posterior right thigh, and she developed a severe and progressive sciatic palsy involving both divisions. There was local tenderness and a Tinel sign at a midthigh level. Nerve action potential (NAP) amplitude and velocity, although somewhat reduced and slowed, were easily measured down to the top forceps tip. There was a marked drop in NAP amplitude and slowing of velocity to 20 m/sec beyond this point, with these reductions being most prominent between the two forceps tips. An external neurolysis was done.

complete to the other, complete to one division and nonexistent to the other, incomplete to both divisions, or incomplete to one division and nonexistent to the other. This observation made it important to split the nerve into its two divisions whenever there was a lesion in continuity. Each division could then be evaluated individually by stimulation as well as by stimulation and recording techniques.[34] If relative sparing or regeneration was proved by NAP recording, then external neurolysis sufficed: 36 of 38 tibial divi-

sions at the thigh level receiving neurolysis based on intraoperative recordings recovered to grade 3 or better (see Table 11–3). This was also the case with the peroneal divisions, because 31 of 34 having physiologic evidence of early regeneration or relative sparing recovered.

If the injury was lengthy or if transection with retraction of stumps was present, graft placement was the predominant method of repair, so that distraction could be avoided[72] (Figure 11–11). Nonetheless, a number of more focal

**TABLE 11–3**
Operative Results — Sciatic Nerve — Thigh Level*

| | Neurolysis | | Suture | | Graft | | No Operation | |
|---|---|---|---|---|---|---|---|---|
| | T | P | T | P | T | P | T | P |
| Gunshot wound | 17/17 | 16/15 | 8/8 | 9/5 | 8/5 | 8/2 | 4/4 | 5/4 |
| Fracture | 11/10 | 9/9 | 1/1 | 1/0 | 4/4 | 8/2 | 9/7 | 10/2 |
| Contusion | 3/3 | 2/2 | 0/0 | 1/1 | 0/0 | 1/1 | 8/7 | 8/6 |
| Laceration/Stab | 1/1 | 2/1 | 5/5 | 6/4 | 11/10 | 9/4 | 2/1 | 2/0 |
| Compression | 4/4 | 4/3 | 0/0 | 0/0 | 0/0 | 0/0 | 1/0 | 1/0 |
| Iatrogenic | 2/1 | 1/1 | 0/0 | 0/0 | 0/0 | 0/0 | 3/2 | 3/2 |
| TOTALS | 38/36 | 34/31 | 14/14 | 17/10 | 23/19 | 26/9 | 27/21 | 29/14 |

P = peroneal division; T = tibial division.
  *Number of divisions operated/number reaching a grade 3 or better result. Not included in this table: 3 sympathectomies, 14 tumors which were resected, and one sciatic nerve repair for a recluse spider bite.

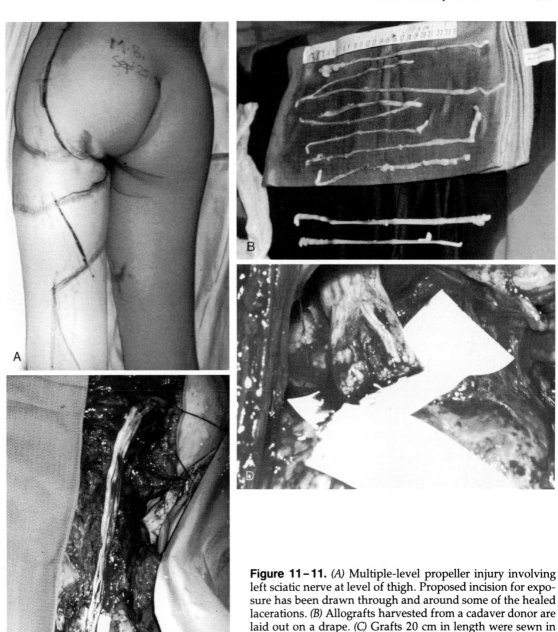

**Figure 11–11.** *(A)* Multiple-level propeller injury involving left sciatic nerve at level of thigh. Proposed incision for exposure has been drawn through and around some of the healed lacerations. *(B)* Allografts harvested from a cadaver donor are laid out on a drape. *(C)* Grafts 20 cm in length were sewn in place. *(D)* The proximal stump neuroma had been resected back to an excellent fascicular pattern. The patient was kept on immunosuppression therapy for 2 years and has regained some sensory return to the sole of the foot at 3 years. (From Mackinnon S, Hudson A: Clinical application of peripheral nerve transplantation, Plast. Reconstr. Surg. 90:4:695–699, 1992.)

lesions could be resected and repaired by end-to-end suture with relative immobilization of the limb for 3 to 4 weeks postoperatively. All 14 end-to-end sutures to the tibial division at this level worked or at least had a functional level of plantar flexion and return of protective sensa-tion on the sole of the foot. Even grafts to this division at this level fared exceptionally well, with grade 3 or better recovery in 19 of 23. As might be expected, peroneal division repairs did not fare as well, and only 10 of 17 sutures recovered enough function to not require use of a kick-up foot brace. The success rate was even less with grafts: only 9 of 26 patients could escape use of the brace. These figures make it important to protect the peroneal division as much as possible in operating on incomplete lesions involving the sciatic nerve, especially if there is partial injury or relative sparing of the peroneal division to begin with.

## Results With Gunshot Wounds

This frequent injury to the thigh level of the sciatic nerve had a surprisingly good outcome. A relatively aggressive approach was taken by exploring those patients without significant spontaneous recovery within the first 3 to 5 months post injury[73] (Figure 11–12). As can be seen by Table 11–3, all but one peroneal division selected for neurolysis based on NAP recordings recovered to grade 3 or better levels. Eight of eight tibial and five of nine peroneal divisions having suture recovered. Results with grafts were less favorable: five of eight tibial and two of eight peroneal divisions recovered adequately. In the five cases selected for nonsurgical management and having follow-up, recovery was adequate in eight of nine divisions.

## Results With Fracture

Results in this category were quite comparable to those seen with gunshot wounds at this level (see Table 11–3). All but one element having neurolysis based on presence of a NAP recovered acceptably. Sutures and grafts succeeded frequently, except for the peroneal division, in which six of eight grafts and the one end-to-end suture repair failed to produce a good result. Those patients not having surgery recovered tibial function better than peroneal function.

## Results With Lacerations/ Stab Wounds

Sharp injuries responded well, especially if repaired acutely, just as they did at the buttock level. Incidence of such lesions was surprisingly high in part because of falls or pushes through plate glass windows. For example, four limbs in three patients had guillotine-like injuries in which the limb was sectioned posteriorly through all soft tissue, including hamstring muscles and sciatic nerve, right down to the femur. Whenever it was possible, primary repair (within 72 hours) was favored for these as well as other sharp injuries in which transection was suspected. Because of referral patterns, such acute repair was not always possible, but if it could be done, suture rather than grafts could be used, and results were some of the best seen for completely injured sciatic nerves. Repair of blunt transections was delayed for several weeks or done later if referral had been late (Figure 11–13).

## SURGICAL ANATOMY AND APPROACH TO TIBIAL NERVE

Tibial nerve arises from the medial half of the sciatic nerve, usually at the level of the middle to distal third of the thigh. Nerve is deep to hamstring muscles on either side of the leg, and in the popliteal fossa it lies posterior to the popliteal artery and vein. Occasionally, a medial hamstring branch may leave tibial nerve at this level. More commonly, sensory branches to proximal calf may arise before the nerve reaches its first major innervational site, particularly as it courses through popliteal fossa. On reaching gastrocnemius-soleus muscle, the tibial nerve tends to run beneath this muscle, giving a "pes-like" profusion of branches to it. These branches provide input to plantaris, popliteus, and tibialis posterior as well as to the gastrocnemius-soleus. Such branches usually begin to define themselves as separate tibial branches proximal to the superior edge of this muscle complex.

A deep or posterior tibial branch or nerve accompanies tibial artery and vein to run through the leg medial and posterior to tibia and to the intermuscular septum separating anterior from posterior compartments. The posterior tibial nerve carries fibers destined for the foot, but it gives off branches in the more proximal leg to supply flexor digitorum and hallucis longus. As posterior tibial nerve approaches the ankle, it courses inferior to the medial malleolus. At this

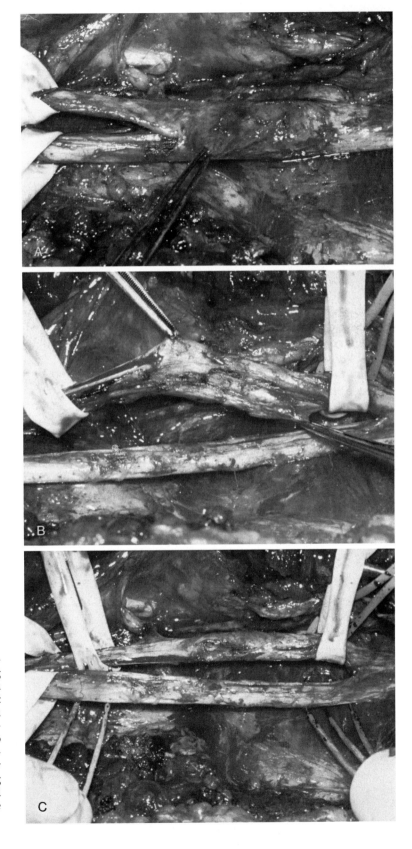

**Figure 11-12.** (A) Typical lesion in continuity involving sciatic nerve at a midthigh level caused by a gunshot wound. (B) Because the lesion transmitted a nerve action potential (NAP), it was split into its two divisions. (C) Each division was then evaluated by NAP recordings. Stimulating electrodes are to the right and recording ones to the left. See also color figure.

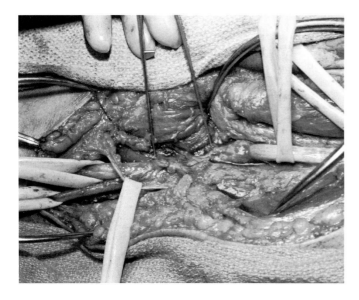

**Figure 11 – 13.** Blunt transection of the sciatic nerve at the level of the thigh explored several months after injury. Stumps were not only neuromatous but had retracted several centimeters, as shown by the spread tips of the forceps. A sural graft repair was necessary.

level, it passes beneath the medial collateral ligaments and branches into medial and lateral plantar nerves. These nerves can also arise and be well-defined before posterior tibial nerve reaches the malleolus. The lateral plantar nerve runs deep in the instep and supplies foot intrinsic muscles and sensation on a portion of the sole of the foot. A calcaneal branch can usually be found either proximal to these nerves or arising from the medial one. Thus, injury to the medial and lateral plantar nerves may spare sensation on the heel of the foot.

Surgical exposure of the proximal portion of the tibial nerve is straightforward. An incision is made in popliteal fossa by beginning in the midline between hamstrings. Incision is then extended distally to run laterally behind the knee or popliteal crease (Figure 11 – 14). Dissection must be careful enough to isolate tibial nerve from popliteal artery and vein without injury to these important vascular structures. The surgeon can usually dissect out the nerve without the necessity of skeletonizing the artery unless there has been or is a need for a concomitant vascular repair. Branches running to gastrocnemius-soleus muscles and the deeper posterior tibial nerve destined for ankle and foot can be readily isolated with Penrose drains or plastic loops.

Dissection of the nerve in the lower leg is not

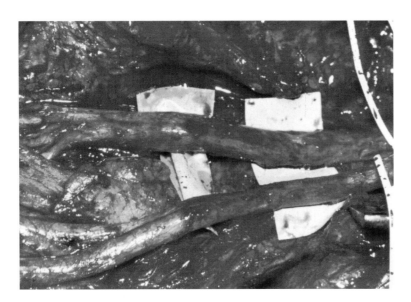

**Figure 11 – 14.** Contusive injuries to tibial and peroneal nerves behind the knee. This was caused by a blown-out hydraulic door. Acutely, the patient required a vascular repair. Both nerves subsequently required a graft repair.

as readily accomplished, but if only a short distance is needed, some of the gastrocnemius-soleus mass can be partially elevated at its superior and medial border to expose the deeper and more distal few centimeters of posterior tibial nerve. Most leg level lesions that require surgery, however, need to be approached by a medial leg incision posterior to the tibia and anterior to the bulk of the gastrocnemius-soleus. This requires an up-and-down incision paralleling the posterior edge of the tibia. This is a deep dissection, and, if injury has involved deep popliteal artery or vein as well as nerve, it is not an easy one. Proximal and distal vascular control by plastic loops or small vascular clamps may be necessary before neuromatous nerve or transected nerve stumps can be dissected free.

Exposure of posterior tibial nerve at the ankle is more straightforward than at the leg level (Figure 11–15). It can be found medial to Achilles tendon just proximal to the medial malleolus and traced beneath this structure by dividing overlying flexor retinaculum. Exposure of posterior tibial nerve at this level, though often compared with that for median nerve in the carpal tunnel, is much more complex, and thus the dissection is more tedious. The artery has a serpiginous course, and arterial and venous branches intertwine with the nerve as it, at the same locus, forms medial and lateral plantar and calcaneal nerves. Magnification, use of the bipolar forceps, and plenty of drains

or vascular loops for retraction help, as does a good deal of patience in dissection. For entrapments at this level, the job is to clean nerve and branches 360 degrees around and to provide a bed free of scar or compressive tissues for them. This includes sectioning overlying muscle and its fascial edge in the instep portion of the foot.

## RESULTS—TIBIAL NERVE AT THE KNEE AND LEG LEVELS

This was one of the more favorable nerve injuries or lesions to manage. Similar experiences have been reported by others, even for war wounds (Table 11–4). Results in this series were also good providing a proper decision was made for or against surgery (Figure 11–16). If the lesion was partial or shown to be regenerating by intraoperative electrical studies, results with neurolysis were excellent, with 12 (92%) of 13 patients achieving a grade 3 or better recovery. Results with repair, whether by suture or grafts, were equally good (Table 11–5). Ten of 11 patients with repairs reached a grade 3 or better level.

Lacerations or penetrating injuries not related to gunshot wounds were usually caused by knife or glass. In one case, however, a lawn mower struck a wire and a piece was driven into the popliteal space, partially lacerating and

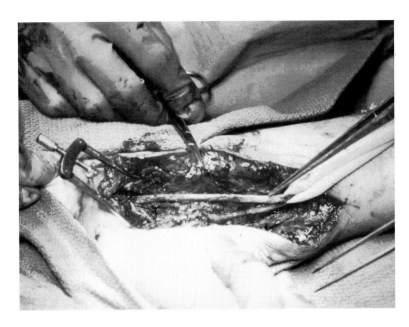

**Figure 11–15.** Posterior tibial nerve exposed at the level of the ankle. Dissection has extended to the level of the instep *(to the left of the photograph).*

**TABLE 11–4**

Tibial Nerve Primary and Secondary
Suture Repair (Seddon)

| All Levels | 78.7% plantar flexion recovery |
|---|---|
| | 61.7% sole sensation recovery |

contusing the tibial nerve. Loss was partial, but pain was the main feature in this case. Fortunately, internal neurolysis and a split repair helped the pain, and function 2 years later graded 4 in both the motor and sensory spheres.

The other relatively large categories of poste-

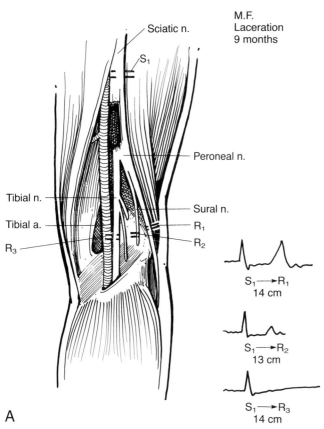

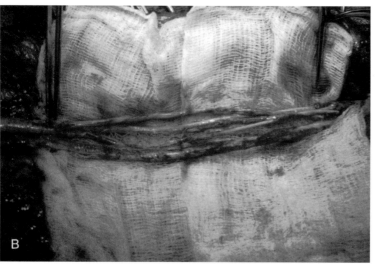

**Figure 11–16.** *(A)* Drawing of 9-month-old blunt laceration to the popliteal area involving the tibial division of the sciatic and extending to tibial nerve. Peroneal was partially injured, but overall function in that distribution graded 3 to 4. Not unexpectedly, there were good nerve action potentials from whole sciatic ($S_1$) to more distal peroneal ($R_1$ and $R_2$) but not to tibial ($R_3$). Tibial division was repaired with four sural grafts 5.0 cm long. *(B)* Tibial grafts are shown going from the tibial division of the sciatic to more distal tibial nerve.

**TABLE 11–5**
Tibial Nerve — Incidence/Results*

| | Total Cases | Neurolysis | Suture | Graft | No Operation |
|---|---|---|---|---|---|
| Laceration | 12 | 3/3 | 2/2 | 5/4 | 2/1 |
| Contusion/Crush | 10 | 3/2† | 0/0 | 1/1 | 6/4 |
| Fracture | 7 | 3/3 | 0/0 | 1/1 | 3/3 |
| Gunshot wound | 5 | 2/2 | 0/0 | 0/0 | 3/2 |
| Iatrogenic | 4 | 2/2 | 0/0 | 1/1 | 1/1 |
| Unknown | 1 | 0/0 | 0/0 | 1/1 | 0/0 |
| TOTALS | 39 | 13/12 | 2/2 | 9/8 | 15/11 |

*Number of nerves operated/number reaching a grade 3 or better result. Six tumors were removed and not included in the table. (No repair was necessary.)

†Lengthy tibial neuroma extending from leg to branches in the foot, resected for severe pain in one case. This patient had undergone several prior operations on the nerve. No repair was possible so there was no functional recovery.

rior tibial injuries were contusion or crush without fracture and fracture-associated contusion and stretch. Slightly less than half of these lesions required operation, because either the tibial lesion was partial to begin with, or there was substantial recovery in the early months following injury. Five of the eight operated contusions, although having lesions of some length, transmitted NAPs and underwent only neurolysis.

Iatrogenic causes of injury were associated with vascular repairs and both open and closed operations on the knee joint. Unless transection was observed by the original operating surgeon or suspected by us, such lesions were managed for 3 to 4 months with physical therapy and outpatient follow-up visits plus EMG. If improvement did not occur, as it did not in three of four lesions, then exploration and intraoperative electrical recordings were done. Fortunately, recovery occurred in these three operative cases and in the single nonoperative case.

If denervation is severe in the tibial distribution, great care must be taken of the sole of the foot. Proper shoes with a good fit are mandatory, and sometimes special shoes and support are necessary to prevent ulceration.[10]

## Case Summary — Tibial Nerve at Leg Level

A 17-year-old male sustained a chain saw injury to his medial leg at its midpoint. This was debrided acutely, and pieces of wood, dirt, and some tibial bone chips were removed. Tibial nerve was found to be transected. The ends were marked by suture, and the tibial artery was repaired by a vein graft. When seen by our service 5 days later, his wound was healing well. Plantar flexion graded 5 and inversion 3, but there was no toe flexion or foot intrinsic function. Sensation on the sole of the foot was absent. At exploration, a good deal of care had to be taken to protect the repaired artery. Neuromas were trimmed and the gap bridged with four grafts 7.6 cm in length. No cast or splint was used.

The patient was begun on ambulation several days later. Follow-up at 5 years showed improved but still diminished sensation on the sole of the foot, fully restored inversion, and some but still poor (grade 2 to 3) toe flexion.

### Comment

Repair of this nerve at this level is worthwhile provided that enough sensation returns to the sole of the foot so that it is not hyperesthetic to touch, weight bearing, or both.

## RESULTS — TIBIAL NERVE AT THE ANKLE LEVEL

Ankle-level injuries involving posterior tibial nerve, plantar nerves, or both were often associated with fracture, but occasionally were caused by blunt contusion or by gunshot wound without fracture (Figure 11–17). Twenty-six of 33 such injuries seen were operated on because of severe pain with or without sensory disturbance on the sole of the foot. Three patients sustained blunt transections and required delayed repair by grafts. Twelve patients had an external neurolysis only, and eight of these had improvement in pain. Seven patients with significant sensory deficit preoperatively eventually had improvement in this category. Three patients with especially severe neuritic pain had

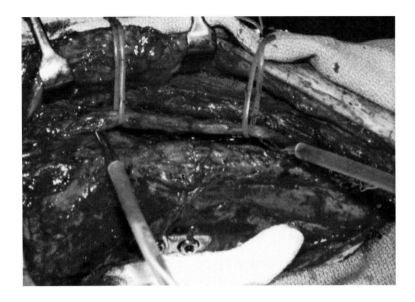

**Figure 11–17.** Posterior tibial nerve near the ankle. This nerve was contused in association with a tibial fracture (see screw at bottom of photograph) but conducted a nerve action potential (see electrodes placed on either side of the lesion). After neurolysis, the patient eventually had a nearly full recovery.

internal neurolysis, and two were helped; the third patient had to have resection of the posterior tibial nerve and gained partial improvement in pain despite an insensate sole of the foot. Including the blunt transection and the contusive injuries, 11 patients had graft repairs varying from 4 to 9.2 cm in length (Figure 11–18). Seven patients regained a sensory level of 3 or better on the sole of the foot, but only three regained any degree of foot intrinsic muscle function.

Table 11–6 summarizes the results with operations on injured posterior tibial nerves at the ankle level. If neurolysis was done based on

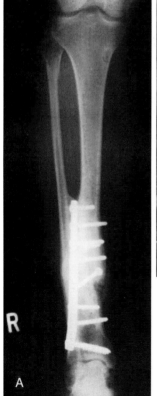

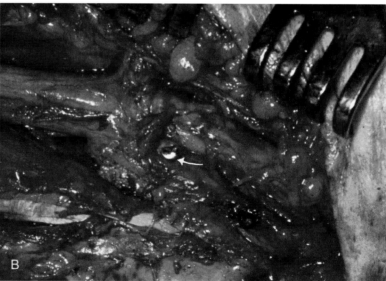

**Figure 11–18.** (A) Radiograph shows severe distal tibial fracture in a patient with complete posterior tibial palsy. (B) In addition to the severe stretch and contusive injury to the nerve, one of the screw tips was found in the nerve (arrow) when it was explored. A graft repair was necessary. Compare this lesion with that in Figure 11–17.

**TABLE 11–6**
Operated Ankle-Level Tibial Nerve Injuries

| | No. of Cases | (+) NAP External Neurolysis | (+) NAP Internal Neurolysis | Grafts* | Resection |
|---|---|---|---|---|---|
| Contusion with fracture | 14 | 7/5† | 2/1‡ | 5/3 | 1/1 |
| Contusion without fracture | 6 | 4/2† | 1/1 | 1/1 | — |
| Blunt transection | 3 | — | — | 3/2 | — |
| Gunshot wound | 2 | 1/1 | — | 1/1 | — |
| Iatrogenic | 1 | — | — | 1/0 | — |
| TOTALS | 26 | 12/8 | 3/2 | 11/7 | 1/1 |

*Number cases done/number with significant sensory recovery as well as relief of pain if significant preoperatively; if resected, those with improved pain.

†Improvement in these cases where neurolysis was done included at least partial relief of pain.

‡One patient with internal neurolysis which failed had excision with partial relief of pain.

a positive NAP across the lesion, pain was not always helped, even though in most cases further improvement in sensory and sometimes foot intrinsic muscle function occurred.

## DIAGNOSIS AND RESULTS — TARSAL TUNNEL SYNDROME

Thirty-five patients with the diagnosis of tarsal tunnel syndrome were operated on (Figure 11–19). Those patients selected for an initial operation to release the tarsal tunnel had a history of painful paresthesias on the sole and sometimes the heel of the foot. A Tinel sign producing paresthesias on the bottom of the foot was usually present inferior to the medial malleolus and sometimes proximally or distally in the region of the instep. Sometimes, there was either a mild hypoesthesia or hypoesthesia mixed with hyperesthesia on the sole or heel of the foot. Toe flexion and foot intrinsic function were spared in the majority of cases unless there had been a prior operation or injury to the ankle or foot as a precipitating factor, or if symptoms had been long-standing. Sensory conduction studies from toes or instep to tibial nerve proximal to malleolus were abnormal.

Operation included exposure of the nerve and its branches well above and below the ankle. A complete external neurolysis was always done, along with sectioning of medial collateral ligaments and splitting of the muscles of the instep. In 22 patients without prior operation, outcome was excellent in 10, good in 6, fair in 2, and poor in 4.

Thirteen patients had undergone prior neurolysis and attempted decompression of the posterior tibial nerve elsewhere and yet had recurrent or worsening symptoms. Repeat neurolysis by the LSUMC service sometimes helped and sometimes did not help pain, paresthesias, and dysfunction. Six of ten reoperated patients

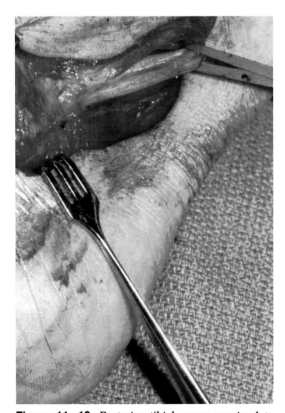

**Figure 11–19.** Posterior tibial nerve proximal to malleolus. Unusually high division into medial and lateral plantar nerves is shown. Tarsal tunnel had not yet been divided.

were helped, but four were not. Three patients had resection of the posterior tibial nerves because of severe intraneural and extraneural scar after multiple previous operations in an attempt to relieve severe neuritic pain and paresthesias associated with a hypersensitive foot. Pain was helped dramatically in two cases and less so in one. Hypoesthesia was substituted for hyperesthesia on the sole of the foot and, surprisingly, each patient not only maintained plantar flexion and inversion of the foot as expected but also some amount of toe flexion and foot intrinsic muscles. Ulceration of the sole has not occurred over an average of 3.2 years of follow-up in these three cases.

## Case Summary — Tarsal Tunnel Syndrome

This 79-year-old woman developed tingling and burning sensations in the soles of both feet. This progressed, and it became very difficult for her to bear weight, so she took to a wheelchair. There was no background of diabetes and no history of alcohol misuse. Posterior tibial conduction across the tarsal tunnel was 31 m/sec on the left and 36 m/sec on the right. At operation, nerves were flattened and grayish in color from just distal to the medial calcaneus down into the insteps of both feet. A complete external neurolysis of both nerves was done. Operative NAP conduction across these segments was in the mid-twenties and was slower than the preoperative studies, probably because it was done over a shorter segment of pathologic nerve.

Fortunately, she did well with this procedure. Although toe intrinsics remained weak, toe flexion was better, and she had good sensation on the soles of the feet. By 3 weeks postoperatively, she was able to bear weight and walk without difficulty. Follow-up was over a 2-year period, and she continued to do well.

### Comment

Tarsal tunnel syndrome is neither as easy a diagnosis to make or condition to treat as carpal tunnel syndrome. If both the clinical and electrical findings fit, then a thorough neurolysis of the nerve and its plantar branches will help. It is important to exclude diabetic and alcoholic neuropathy and to make certain that the foot has an adequate blood supply before operating on this condition.

## SURGICAL ANATOMY AND APPROACH — PERONEAL NERVE

The peroneal nerve originates at the bifurcation of the sciatic nerve and includes nerve above, at, and below the head of the fibula and the nerve's superficial and deep branches in the lower leg. The level of take-off of peroneal from sciatic nerve varies somewhat according to level of sciatic bifurcation. Close to its origin, or sometimes somewhat proximal to it, one or more branches leave to form sural nerve, either complemented or not by a branch from the tibial nerve. The peroneal nerve then takes an oblique course laterally to lie over the head and neck of the fibula.

As the nerve approaches the fibular head, it sometimes lies beneath the medial edge of the lateral hamstring. The nerve tends to curve over the posterior rim of the fibular head to travel toward the anterior compartment of the lower leg. The superficial branch takes a relatively straight course, lying beneath the fascia and some of the muscle of the peronei. It is eventually nestled between the two heads of these muscles. The superficial branch descends the lower leg, becoming somewhat more superficial at its midpoint where peronei muscles blend into their tendons. It lies between these tendons and the lateral edge of the gastrocnemius-soleus. As the nerve approaches the ankle, it is located anterolaterally and branches to supply sensation on the dorsum of the foot. This sensory territory includes anterolateral ankle and most of the dorsum of the foot.

The deep branch of the peroneal nerve quickly divides after passing over and around the head and neck of the fibula. The initial deep branch usually supplies anterior tibialis, and subsequent branches go to extensor digitorum longus and extensor hallucis longus. In some persons, the deep branch may supply peroneal tertius, a muscle that is usually not present. The anterior tibial nerve branch also supplies extensor digitorum hallucis brevis and a small area of sensation over the first dorsal web space of the foot.

For exposure, the patient is placed prone with cushioning beneath knee and ankle. For the more common lesions at the level of the fibula, a curvilinear incision is made extending from lateral lower thigh to a position posterior to the head of the fibula and curving toward the anterior compartment of the leg. An alternative is a midline posterior distal thigh incision combined with a transverse incision in the popliteal space that runs laterally and then over the head of the fibula onto the leg. On occasion, the lateral tendon of the biceps inserting onto the head of the fibula may resemble the peroneal nerve as it courses down to cross the neck of the fibula.

A key portion of the deep dissection occurs just below the head of the fibula, where the superficial and deep branches are exposed. The posterior edge of the peroneus fascia and muscle is cleared by sharp dissection, retracted, and partially split inferiorly to expose the superficial branch. With the help of a narrow Penrose drain placed around peroneal nerve at the level of the neck of the fibula, the deep branch is traced around the fibula. Of help is dissection onto the underside or anterior side of this branch. Use of plastic loops around the branches also helps, as does magnification. Small vessels are coagulated by the bipolar forceps. Fine neural branches going to the knee joint can be sacrificed if necessary to gain length along the course of the deep branch.

There is no reason for a small or focal exposure of the nerve and its branches. Short incisions and exposures are generally to be avoided in nerve surgery. This is certainly the case for peroneal nerve operations. Even with adequate exposure, it may be difficult to define a viable distal stump or branch to tibialis anticus. NAP recording is paramount to avoid needless resection, which is an especial disservice with this nerve because functional regeneration after repair is limited. On the other hand, if, despite gross continuity, the lesion is severe and does not conduct, the possibility of significant spontaneous recovery is nonexistent. As a result, a correct decision about resection is paramount.

## RESULTS— PERONEAL NERVE

Unfortunately, the largest peroneal injury category was caused by stretch/contusion. Traction injuries involving the peroneal nerve remain very difficult to manage successfully.[27,52] Most in this series were caused by vehicular accidents or sports such as football and usually occurred in relatively young individuals. Many peroneal palsies were associated with serious injury to the knee joint or surrounding structures (Figure 11–20). Some (35%) of these traction injuries were not operated on because of late referral (≥1 year after in-

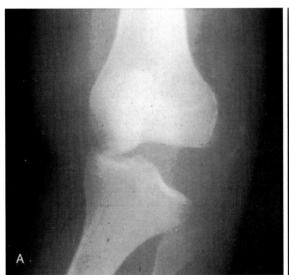

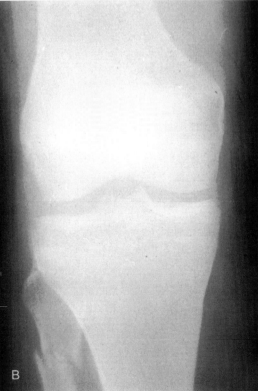

**Figure 11–20.** Common bony injuries associated with stretch injuries to the peroneal nerve: severe dislocation of the knee joint *(A)* and fracture of the neck of the fibula *(B)*. These patients had equally devastating, lengthy stretch injuries of the peroneal nerve.

jury) or, in eight cases, because of spontaneous and relatively early recovery. Of those operated, 16 had a neurolysis either because of a partial but significant injury to begin with or because, despite more complete clinical and EMG loss, there was early evidence of significant regeneration by intraoperative NAP recording (Table 11–7). Twelve of these patients recovered to a grade 3 or better level. Seven of these 12 patients even reached a grade 4 level. In 41 cases, interfascicular graft repair was necessary, either because of total distraction of the nerve (11 cases) or because of lengthy severe lesions in continuity that did not transmit a NAP (30 cases). Average graft length was 10 cm, but lengths varied between 4 and 20 cm. Sixteen (40%) of 41 patients recovered to a grade 3 level and only 9 (22%) to a grade 4 level. Only ten cases with graft repair had enough function over a 5-year period not to require continued use of a kick-up foot brace. Graft lengths for successful cases were usually less than 6 cm in length and shorter on the whole than in those cases in which sufficient recovery did not occur (Figure 11–21). The interval between injury and operation was 4 to 9 months.

Those nerves injured by stretch in association with fracture or dislocation and requiring operation had a similar fate, although two had lesions that were shorter in length and could be sutured. Both of these patients recovered significant dorsiflexion of the foot. Fractures associated with stretch injury usually involved the head of the fibula and tibial plateau. Such lesions tended to be a bit more focal than those associated with knee dislocation with or without ligamentous tears. As a result, even if grafts were necessary, recovery was better (50% to a grade 3 or better level) with fracture-related injuries than in those patients with stretch associated with dislocation of the knee or severe ligamentous injury.

## Results With Lacerations/Stab Wounds

Six of 31 lacerations to soft tissues involving peroneal were assumed to have left the nerve in continuity. In the four cases operated on, a NAP was recorded across the lesion, and significant recovery occurred with neurolysis (Figure 11–22). End-to-end or epineurial suture was possible in transections, and recovery to a grade 3 or better level was achieved (see Table 11–7). Most of these patients had primary repair within 72 hours of sustaining a sharp injury. Grafts were necessary in ten others, with five (50%) recovering to grade 3 level or better. Most of these patients had blunt transecting injuries caused by propellers, fan blades, or shards of metal (Figure 11–23). In six cases, loss was either partial and not severe or reversed, so these patients were not operated on (see Table 11–7).

## Results With Gunshot Wounds

This was another relatively favorable category compared with stretch injuries, because

**TABLE 11–7**
Injuries and Operations—Peroneal Nerve*

| | Neurolysis | Suture | Graft | No Operation | Other | Total Cases |
|---|---|---|---|---|---|---|
| Stretch/Contusion | 16/12 | 0/0 | 41/16 | 30/8 | 0 | 87 |
| Stretch/Fracture | 8/6 | 2/2 | 7/3 | 8/4 | 0 | 25 |
| Laceration/Stab | 4/4 | 11/7 | 10/5 | 6/5 | 0 | 31 |
| Gunshot wound | 4/4 | 2/2 | 4/2 | 6/4 | 1† | 16 |
| Entrapment | 14/11 | 0/0 | 4/2 | 4/1 | 0 | 22 |
| Iatrogenic | 2/2 | 0/0 | 4/2 | 7/3 | 0 | 13 |
| Injection | 0/0 | 0/0 | 0/0 | 2/2 | 0 | 2 |
| Compression | 9/8 | 0/0 | 3/2 | 9/6 | 0 | 21 |
| TOTALS | 57/47 | 15/11 | 73/32 | 72/33 | 1 | 217 |

*Number of nerves operated or evaluated/number recovering to grade 3 or better function. Twenty tumors seen were operated on; ten were ganglion cysts. Eight were neural sheath tumors and two were associated with onion whorl disease. Four tumor patients required graft repair; one of these recovered to grade 3 and one to grade 4 level.

†One lumbar sympathectomy was done in a patient with a gunshot wound involving peroneal nerve in whom direct operation on the nerve was not necessary. Patient had acute causalgia which reversed with a sympathectomy.

Compression category did *not* include peroneal entrapments.

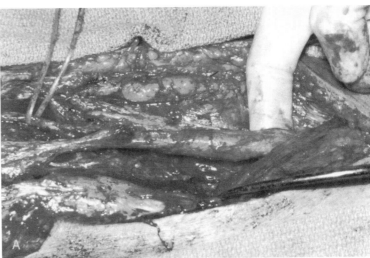
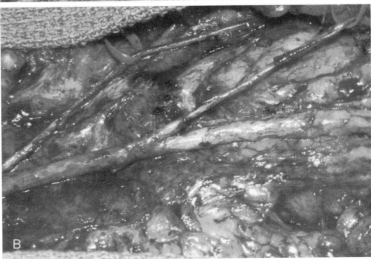

**Figure 11–21.** *(A)* A segment of a stretch/contusion injury involving peroneal nerve caused by a motorcycle accident. The lesion extended from the surgeon's gloved finger to the superficial and deep branches seen exposed to the left. In this case, the nerve was both swollen and firm. *(B)* The nerve in the lower inset had a stretch injury resulting from a ski accident. The nerve was thinned out and narrowed over an 11-cm segment. Neither lesion transmitted a nerve action potential at 5 months after injury, and both were resected and repaired by lengthy sural grafts.

some of the lesions were more focal. Even so, only three of six requiring repair gained enough function not to use a kick-up foot brace any more. Five cases had mild peroneal loss, and four of these recovered full function with conservative management. One other patient had incomplete loss that went on to recovery without operation on the nerve. Severe causalgia complicated this case and was helped by a lumbar sympathectomy.

## Results With Entrapment

The differential diagnosis of spontaneous peroneal nerve entrapment at the neck of the fibula includes L5 spinal radiculopathy. This distinction must be carefully made because mistakes in diagnosis of these widely separated sites of pathology are not infrequent.

A past history of trauma involving the knee or, occasionally, a postural habit such as frequently sitting with crossed legs, can serve as contributing factors, but most of the patients we operated on for peroneal entrapment had no such antecedent history[49,74] (Figure 11–24). Eleven of the 14 patients having a neurolysis of the nerve and a partial fibulectomy went on to recover significant function.

Loss resulting from entrapment was not always readily reversed by operation. Failure of operation to improve function was more likely if loss was severe on presentation. Functional status was usually stabilized by operation, but in two cases this was not so, and loss even progressed despite neurolysis and partial fibulec-

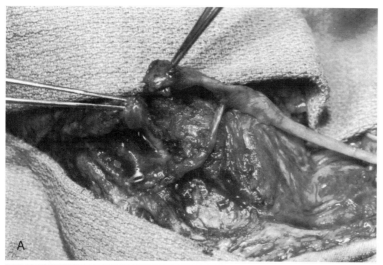

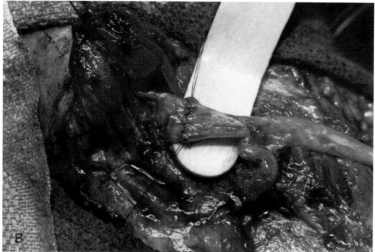

**Figure 11–22.** *(A)* A laceration of the peroneal nerve just distal to the head of the fibula caused by a knife wound. *(B)* End-to-end repair with a 6-0 prolene suture done within 72 hours of injury. The head of the fibula was then leveled off and waxed before closing the soft tissues.

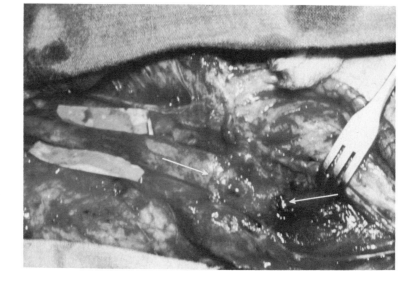

**Figure 11–23.** A propeller injury *(arrows)* at the point where the peroneal nerve passes over the head of the fibula. Injury site is bracketed by white arrows. This was repaired with sural grafts 5 weeks after injury.

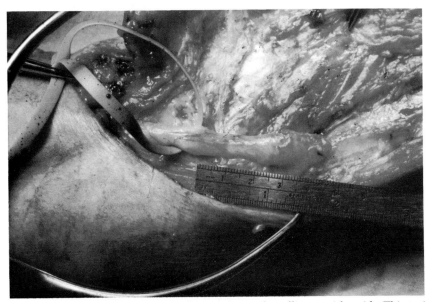

**Figure 11–24.** Left peroneal nerve with an area of narrowing and swelling on either side. This patient received a contusive blow behind the knee and over a period of several years developed a progressive peroneal palsy. The palsy was considered to be the result of a trauma-induced entrapment. The lesion conducted, and thus a neurolysis was done. (Courtesy of Dr. Jack Hurst, Lafayette, LA.) See also color figure.

tomy. In four other cases, graft repair was necessary after one to three operations done elsewhere had failed to halt progression.

## Results With Compression and Tumors

Peroneal nerve was compressed by poor positioning during anesthesia or malposition due to alcohol- or drug-induced stupor. In addition, exostosis or tumor sometimes involves this nerve (Figure 11–25).

Most of the patients in the tumor categories had ganglion cysts involving peroneal nerve. Further data is reported in the chapter entitled "Tumors Involving Nerve." Four of these patients had extensions of synovia from the knee joint into a cystic mass in the nerve, but six did not. In two of the latter cases, ganglion cyst ex-

**Figure 11–25.** A peroneal nerve entrapped by a bony exostosis near the head of the fibula (arrow). The posterior tibial nerve is at the top of the picture and the peroneal is at the bottom.

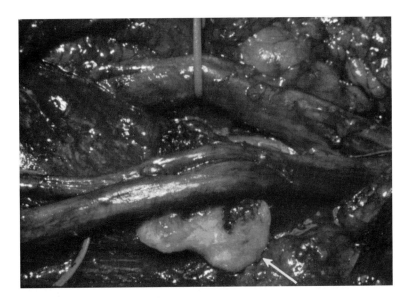

tended very proximally in the peroneal division of the sciatic complex and reached as far as the buttock level. Subtotal resection was attempted in both of those cases because of progressive, severe loss and pain. Functional loss in the peroneal distribution remained severe. A sizable number of patients had benign neural sheath tumors, which were removed in most cases without the need for repair. Two patients had localized hypertrophic neuropathy or "onion whorl" disease involving the peroneal nerve at the knee level. One of these patients recovered some function after resection of the lesion and graft repair, and one did not. One malignant schwannoma was treated with a wide local resection followed by irradiation. Other compressive causes included arteriovenous malformation (two cases) and compartment syndromes involving leg caused by soft tissue swelling or a tight cast, or both (Figure 11–26).

## Results With Iatrogenic and Injection Injuries

Two patients had somehow received injection injuries to the peroneal nerve at the level of the knee. Both lesions were relatively mild and did not require operation. Iatrogenic injury was usually associated with open operation on the knee, but in two instances it was secondary to arthroscopic examination of the joint. Two thirds of those iatrogenic cases operated on had recovery. By comparison, only three had recovery out of seven who were either referred a year or more after injury and thus did not have a secondary operation or who refused surgery.

## Summary of Peroneal Results

If the various peroneal injury categories are summarized, it can be seen that 57 nerves underwent external neurolysis based on a positive NAP (Figure 11–27; see Table 11–7). Recovery to a grade 3 or better level occurred in 84% of these patients, and 62% reached at least a grade 4 level. Return of function began earlier than in the group of patients with repairs; contraction of peronei was usually evident by 6 months and anterior tibialis by 12 to 14 months.

If the injury had transected or pulled apart and thus distracted nerve, end-to-end repair was often not possible. However, if such repair could be done, recovery was good. Seventy-three percent of the patients having end-to-end suture recovered function to a grade 3 level, and 55% recovered to at least a grade 4 level.

Seventy-three patients with a variety of peroneal injuries required graft repair. Thirty-two (44%) recovered to a grade 3 level, but only 21% obtained a grade 4 level. Many patients continued to need a kick-up foot brace to provide optimal ambulation. This was even true of patients reaching a grade 3 level in cases in which patients felt more comfortable in a brace, often despite eversion and dorsiflexion against some resistance.

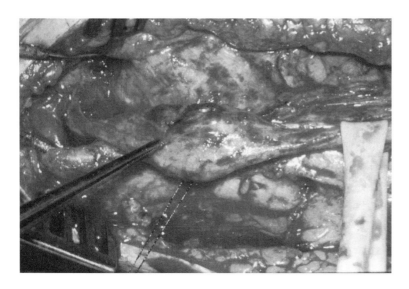

**Figure 11–26.** Large neuroma in continuity caused by a hemangioma involving peroneal nerve and after a prior operation for resection. This lesion was located behind the knee of a 17-year-old girl. The neuroma transmitted a nerve action potential (NAP) but required a split graft repair. The inferior or lower portion of the nerve transmitted a NAP, but the superior or upper portion did not and was replaced by sural grafts. Over a 3.5-year period, the patient gained peroneal function to a grade 4 level.

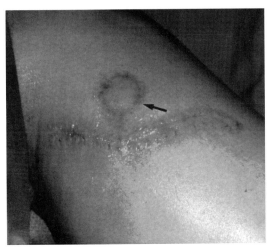

**Figure 11–27.** Lateral view of the leg of a patient struck by a pool cue over the head of the fibula *(arrow)*. He developed a partial peroneal palsy. Several weeks later, the nerve was decompressed as it crossed over the head of the fibula through the incision seen below the pool cue mark.

In our series, functional recovery after graft repair was very dependent on the length of the grafts necessary to close a gap. More than 70% of those with grafts 5 cm (2 inches) or less in length reached a grade 3 recovery. Only 35% of those with grafts 6 to 12 cm (2.4 to 4.5 inches) in length reached a grade 3 level. Those with grafts longer than 13 cm (5 inches) in length reached a grade 3 level only 18% of the time.

These results can be compared with an earlier series reported by Seddon in which repair by suture or grafts had been done.[63] Recovery of dorsiflexion averaged only 34.7% but included lesions at all levels of the peroneal nerve.

The peroneal nerve innervates slender antigravity muscles such as anterior tibialis, extensor communis, and extensor hallucis longus. These muscles require multiple-site input for effective antigravity function. This input is analogous to the input required by a pianist's fingers while playing a chord of music: coordinated firing must be regained. It is difficult for regeneration to reconstruct this patterning of innervation.

Tendon transfer or partial fusion of the ankle can sometimes ameliorate the foot drop seen with peroneal palsy.[9,18] This approach has been combined with graft repair of the nerve by Millesi with good results.[45] Those patients having

such an operation and seen by us did best if they were young, slender individuals in whom there was less of a load on the foot.[15] On the other hand, if peroneal injury is lengthy, such a substitutive approach can be more efficacious than a lengthy graft repair.

## SURAL NERVE ANATOMY

This nerve takes its origin from variable portions of peroneal and tibial nerves in the popliteal fossa. Sometimes, its entire origin is from one nerve, and that usually is the peroneal. Sural nerve enters the leg beneath the gastrocnemius fascia on medial posterior leg. After traveling beneath this fascia to the junction of the upper and middle thirds of the leg, it lies subcutaneously in the posterior calf. Nerve tends to angle towards medial calf, giving it a somewhat oblique course, at least in the lower half of the leg. As sural approaches the ankle region, it lies somewhat lateral to the gastrocnemius-Achilles tendon. The nerve is most readily located at this level, where it lies deep to and somewhat adherent to the lesser saphenous vein (Figure 11–28). As it approaches lateral malleolus, it branches, and these nerves supply sensation to the non–weight-bearing surfaces of the lateral foot. Sural nerve can branch and take separate courses anatomically, not only in distal lower leg but also in its course in proximal leg. Sometimes these branches rejoin in more distal leg, and sometimes they do not. Section of the sural nerve or its removal, which is commonly done for graft repair, leads to a fairly reproducible sensory deficit on the dorsolateral surface of the foot. This is a non–weight-bearing area, so its loss does not lead to a significant functional deficit. With time, this sensory deficit decreases in size, presumably because of overlap innervation from both the tibial and peroneal nerve distal branches.

## SURAL INJURY

Those injuries not of iatrogenic origin and involving sural nerve were most frequently caused by laceration. Most (6) were caused by glass, in several cases glass fragments exploding from soda pop bottles that had been dropped.

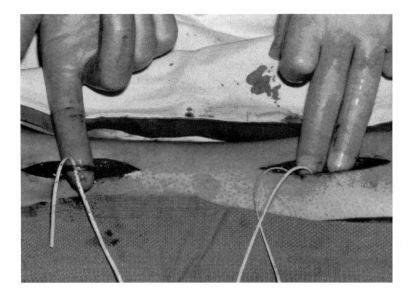

**Figure 11–28.** One method of harvesting sural nerves is by using multiple incisions on the posterolateral leg.

Two nerves were injured by knife wounds and one by a lawn mower accident in which a piece of metal was driven into the popliteal area, injuring the sural close to its take off from the peroneal nerve (Table 11–8). Sural injuries usually came to attention because of painful neuromas (Figure 11–29). Sometimes these neuromas were palpable, and sometimes not. Percussion or tapping over them usually gave paresthesias in the distal sural distribution, especially in the foot. Treatment was by relatively lengthy excision of nerve above and below neuroma rather than by repair, because sensory loss in this distribution is of little functional consequence and repair could lead to a painful neuroma in continuity. Nerve was sharply sectioned well above the injury site, and the neuroma and some of the more distal nerve were removed as well. Then, the proximal stump was visualized under loupes. The individual fascicles were then grasped by fine bipolar forceps and coagulated in an attempt to seal them shut. To date, to our knowledge, although neuromas have recurred in a few cases, they were not unduly painful and were managed conservatively without reoperation.

Several patients with gunshot wounds to the lower leg developed painful sural neuromas requiring surgical excision. These were managed in the same fashion as the lacerated sural nerves, by wide up-and-down resection. Iatrogenic injuries have been associated with sural nerve biopsy, venous stripping and ligation, and, occasionally, with orthopedic operation on ankle or lower leg. Excision was less effective in relieving pain in this category than in those related to laceration or gunshot wound. This was especially so if excision was delayed for many months after the onset of the painful syndrome.

## Case Summary — Sural Injury

This 30-year-old physician had congenital venous varicosities with venous insufficiency of the leg. He had had three venous strippings and ligations. Several months after the last venous operation, he had onset of pain radiating down the lateral lower leg to the ankle. Resection of a sural neuroma and repair of the nerve was done elsewhere. However, within a year, he had recurrence of pain, discrete tenderness, and a painful Tinel sign when-

**TABLE 11–8**
Sural Injuries — Operated

|  | Operated* | Unoperated |
|---|---|---|
| Glass laceration | 5 | 1 |
| Knife wound | 2 | 0 |
| Lawn mower/metal wire | 1 | 0 |
| Gunshot wound | 3 | 1 |
| Contusion caused by fracture | 0 | 2 |
| Sural nerve biopsy | 1 | 1 |
| Venous stripping/ligation | 2 | 0 |
| Orthopedic operations | 2 | 1 |
| TOTALS | 16 | 6 |

*Neuroma, surrounding scar, and nerve well proximal and distal to injury site were resected. Recurrence of some symptoms in two cases has been mild enough not to require reoperation.

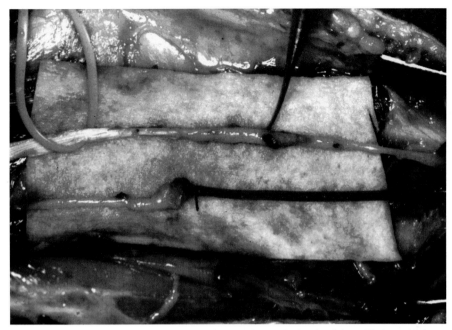

**Figure 11–29.** A sural nerve is found sewn to a tendinous slip at the back of the calf. A painful proximal sural neuroma *(to the left)* is seen attached to a plastic loop at the bottom *(to the right)* and a distal sural neuroma *(to the right)* is attached to a tendinous slip at the top *(to the left)*.

ever the repair site was bumped. There was hyperesthesia and hyperpathia distally but also somewhat proximal to the repair site. If clothing or even a breeze touched these areas, the patient experienced painful tingling and electric shocks. Tapping there seemed to produce a Tinel sign, but so did tapping or deep palpation just below the knee and just inferior to the popliteal fossa. There were a number of transverse healed incision sites up and down the leg.

At exploration, we found a sural suture neuroma in continuity in the distal leg. We could record no NAP across this, nor could we record a NAP proximal to the lesion. As a result, we followed the sural nerve proximally to where the nerve lay beneath the gastrocnemius-soleus fascia. A second neuroma was found on the sural nerve just below the knee. There was no NAP recordable across this lesion either. Both neuromas and intervening sural nerve were resected and a long segment of nerve was removed.

The patient has had excellent relief of his symptoms despite hypoesthesia along the lateral foot. The hyperesthesia is not at all bothersome to him. Histologic examination of resected tissues showed a distal suture neuroma, a smaller but still quite disorganized proximal neuroma, and intervening nerve with axons that were less than 5 μm in diameter.

**Comment**

Many transections of the sural nerve do not lead to neuromas that are exquisitely tender and painful. For ex-

ample, harvest of the sural nerve for use as a graft seldom results in a painful neuroma. What makes a given neuroma painful is not well understood. Nonetheless, in well-selected cases in which pain is a problem, resection of neuroma and a length of nerve can be effective.

# PELVIC PLEXUS

## Lumbar Plexus Anatomy and Clinical Correlations

The lumbar portion of the plexus originates from the anterior primary rami, which are formed in turn by the spinal nerves or roots of L1 through L4. The lumbar plexus spinal nerves are located in the posterior portion of the psoas major and in front of the transverse processes of the vertebrae. L1 may receive a communication from T12, the subcostal nerve. The anterior primary ramus of L4 also contributes to the sacral plexus by way of the lumbosacral trunk. Because the spinal cord usually terminates at the L1 level of the spine, both anterior (motor) and posterior (sensory) divisions of the various roots have a variable length within the spinal canal. The sensory divisions or roots are the central extensions of the dorsal root ganglia and do not regenerate after injury, whereas the motor are peripheral nerves even though they are in the spinal canal and do have the potential for regeneration. The two divisions combine within the intervertebral portion of the nerve root canal and exit the foramen as a single motor-sensory spinal nerve, just as brachial plexus roots do in the neck. As with the brachial plexus, the sensory division or root goes to a dorsal root ganglion, and a peripheral extension of this then goes to join the motor root and form the spinal nerve. Spinal nerves are then located within the psoas muscle, which is innervated by branches from the anterior primary rami; proximal femoral outflow gives short branches to the iliacus muscle. The L1 root of the lumbar plexus also gives rise to the iliohypogastric, ilioinguinal, and genitofemoral nerves, the latter also receiving input in most cases from L2. L2 also contributes to the obturator nerve, as do L3 and sometimes L4; the femoral nerve is formed by contributions from L2, L3, and L4. The lateral femoral cutaneous nerve is formed by L2 and L3. Thus, not unexpectedly, lumbar plexus injuries result in variable patterns of loss related to the sensory dermatomes and muscle myotomes corresponding to the above roots.

The *iliohypogastric nerve* passes through the psoas muscle and anterior to the quadratus lumborum to reach the area superior to the iliac crest. There it lies between the transverse and internal oblique muscles, which it supplies in part. The nerve penetrates the internal and external obliques as it extends anteriorly. Its sensory distribution is through a lateral cutaneous branch to the skin of the superior gluteal region and through an anterior branch to the lower abdominal skin above the pubis. Injury to this nerve is usually iatrogenic, from abdominal procedures, and can result, unfortunately, in painful paresthesias or a sensory deficit in these distributions.

The *ilioinguinal nerve* circles the trunk just below the iliohypogastric, and laterally is located between the transverse and internal oblique muscles. Part of its more medial course is along but superior to the inguinal ligament and then through the superficial inguinal ring and external spermatic fascia. This nerve also supplies the internal oblique and transversalis muscles, but, more importantly, it supplies cutaneous sensation to the skin over the symphysis pubis, the dorsum of the penis, the upper scrotum, and the upper thigh medial to the fem-

oral triangle. In the female, sensory distribution includes the mons and labia major. This nerve can also be inadvertently injured or entrapped by scar after pelvic or lower abdominal procedures, especially operations for hernias.

The *genitofemoral nerve*, unlike the iliohypogastric and ilioinguinal nerves, takes a straight inferior and somewhat caudal course along with iliac vessels and forms two branches: the genital branch, which innervates the cremaster muscle and a portion of scrotal skin in the male and the round ligament in the female, and the femoral branch, which penetrates the fascia of the thigh to supply sensation to the skin in the region of the femoral triangle.

The *femoral nerve* is one of the major outflows of the lumbar plexus. After its formation by the anterior divisions of L2, L3, and L4 spinal nerves, it courses for 8 to 10 cm within the pelvis in a retroperitoneal position, but superior and somewhat lateral to the psoas and medial to the iliacus muscles before passing beneath the inguinal ligament. At this level, it is lateral to the femoral artery and vein. Several centimeters distal to the ligament, it divides pes-like into a number of branches supplying the quadriceps muscle, which is composed of the rectus femoris and the three vasti. Sensory contributions from the femoral nerve go to the anteromedial thigh but also form the saphenous nerve, which courses obliquely along the medial thigh and knee, and then branches to supply the medial surface of the lower leg and the medial aspect or instep region of the foot.

In the pelvis, branches of the femoral nerve supply the iliacus, which is a major flexor muscle of the thigh on the abdomen. This muscle is best tested with the patient supine. The examiner then holds the leg beneath the knee with the lower leg flexed on the upper, and asks the patient to pull the thigh up or flex the hip against resistance and toward the abdomen. Less important are branches to the sartorius ("tailor") muscle which aides flexion at the hip and knee and assists lateral rotation of the hip. The function of the sartorius can be inferred from the fact that it arises from the anterior superior iliac spine above and inserts on the medial and proximal tibia below.

Injury to lumbar plexus or the femoral nerve within the pelvis may thus produce loss of hip flexion (iliacus) as well as an inability to extend the knee. The latter loss interferes with a normal gait, the knee usually being hyperextended by the tensor fascia lata and gracilis muscles. Classically, going up stairs or climbing is very difficult or impossible under these circumstances. Pelvic-level femoral nerve palsies related to penetrating lower abdominal injuries caused by gunshot wounds, motorcycle handlebars, and stab wounds have been seen in our clinic. Iatrogenic causes included packing of the pelvis or manipulation of pelvic contents in association with bleeding during lower abdominal operations and pelvic hematomas related to anticoagulation or femoral artery manipulation for angiography. A not infrequent cause is surgical section of a portion of the plexus for tumor removal. These tumors are often either benign neurofibromas or schwannomas. The femoral nerve can be mistaken for the lateral femoral cutaneous nerve and can be inadvertently resected in the treatment of meralgia paresthetica, or it can be injured by investment with methyl methacrylate during hip repair. Sensory loss in the anteromedial thigh is variable, as is the degree of hip flexion weakness, but the absence of quadriceps function with loss of the knee jerk is unmistakable.

Radiation plexopathy is less frequent than that involving the brachial plexus, but it does occur.[69] The three patients seen by us have been managed conservatively but have required intensive pain management and have had progressive loss of leg function.

The *lateral femoral cutaneous nerve* (lateral cutaneous nerve of the thigh) penetrates the psoas, crosses the iliacus, and, at the level of the anterior superior spine of the ilium, courses downward between the attachments of the inguinal ligament. It supplies sensation to the lateral thigh but, if stretched, entrapped, or injured during removal of bone grafts from the ilium, can give rise to the characteristic syndrome of meralgia paresthetica, with a tingling, burning pain in the lateral thigh and often hyperesthesia so severe that the lateral thigh is easily irritated by clothing or touch.[67] Patients often report normal sensibility to pinprick but an increased and painful sensibility to testing by touch.

The *obturator nerve* also originates from the anterior divisions of L2, L3, and L4. It reaches the medial border of the psoas, travels below or deep to the iliac vessels, and takes a rather vertical course toward the obturator foramen. There, it divides into an anterior or superficial branch, which supplies primarily the adductor longus and gracilis muscles, and a posterior or deep branch, which supplies the obturator externus and adductor magnus muscles. Because the adductor magnus is also innervated by the sciatic nerve and the adductor longus sometimes by the femoral nerve, complete loss of adduction and complete atrophy are seldom seen with obturator nerve injury. However, gait is mildly disturbed, because the leg is externally rotated or tends to swing outward. Damage to this nerve can occur as a portion of a lumbosacral plexus injury; less commonly, as an isolated palsy associated with a pelvic fracture; or, even less frequently, secondary to surgical injury. Sensory loss is quite variable and unreliable, in our experience, as an index of involvement of this nerve. Relative loss is sometimes present in a patchy distribution in the lower medial thigh, but at other times, there is no sensory loss at all.

## Sacral Plexus Anatomy and Clinical Correlations

The L4 spinal nerve of the lumbosacral plexus contributes to the sacral plexus through the lumbosacral trunk, as do all of L5 and the individual primary rami of S1, S2, S3, and a portion of S4, which also contributes to the coccygeal plexus. Each ramus receives postganglionic sympathetic fibers destined for blood vessels and sweat glands of the limb; S2, S3, and S4 include parasympathetic fibers destined for the bladder and anal sphincter. As with the lumbar portion of the pelvic plexus, loss with sacral plexus injuries is variable, but one can identify the contributions involved if one knows the sensory dermatomes and myotomes innervated by the various lumbar and sacral roots, especially in the lower extremity. The posterior divisions form the gluteal nerves and the peroneal division of the sciatic; the anterior divisions form the tibial, hamstring, pudendal, and posterior cutaneous nerves of the thigh. The sacral plexus lies deep and medial in the pelvis, overlying the sacroiliac and sacrococcygeal junctions. Plexus nerves exit the pelvis, for the most part, by the greater sciatic foramen (sciatic, hamstring, gluteal, and posterior cutaneous nerves), whereas the pudendal reaches the perineum through the lesser sciatic foramen.

As the *gluteal nerves* leave the sciatic notch, the superior travels lateral to the sciatic nerve and upward to supply the gluteus medius and minimus. These muscles aid in abduction and medial rotation of the thigh at the hip joint. With injury, the leg tends to rest in an outwardly rotated position in the recumbent patient, but during walking, the trunk is bent toward the side of the palsy. On standing, the contralateral pelvis drops down, causing a discrepancy in the height of the two anterior superior iliac spines. The inferior gluteal nerve exits the sciatic foramen somewhat medial to the sciatic nerve and supplies the gluteus maximus. An injury to this nerve results in weak extension of the hip, making it difficult for the patient to climb steps or to rise from a sitting position. With sagging of the muscle belly, the infragluteal fold is decreased or lost, and atrophy of the buttock is obvious with time.

The *pudendal* or *pubic nerve* is seldom injured in an isolated fashion, but loss can occur in its distribution if the sacral plexus is injured, or sometimes secondary to gynecologic operations. Nerve exits pelvis through greater sciatic foramen between piriformis and coccygeus muscles and lies on sacrospinous ligament. Branches include inferior rectal and perineal nerve and dorsal nerve of the penis or clitoris. It supplies sensation to the perineum and portions of the scrotum and penis in the male and labia in the female, including the mucous membranes of the urethra and the perianal region. Motor fibers go to the external sphincter of the anus, and both the bulb and the corpus spongiosis of the penis. Because of its input to the external sphincter of the bladder, it is concerned with voluntary control of urination.

## PELVIC PLEXUS INJURY

Pelvic plexus injuries are unusual, and most appear in the literature as a small series of case reports or solitary cases. In addition to gunshot wounds and other penetrating injuries to the pelvic region, fractures of the pelvis and of the sacrum and rare primary tumors of the pelvic plexus provide the usual cause.[12,30,58] However, the pelvic plexus has been reported to be in-

volved secondary to hematomas caused by anticoagulation, usually heparinization for thrombosis, phlebitis, or pulmonary embolus, and even in patients with disseminated intravascular coagulation[24,76] (Figure 11–30).

Our experience has included a number of gunshot and iatrogenic wounds (Table 11–9). Patients with fractures and incomplete pelvic plexus loss have been treated expectantly and have had acceptable results. We have followed patients who had pelvic, usually sacral, plexus involvement secondary to pelvic fractures, and most of these have improved at least partially without operation (Figure 11–31). There have been exceptions, because some gunshot wounds and pelvic fracture–associated lesions have required surgery. See Table 11–10 and also pelvic-level femoral lesions in Table 11–11. Results have been variable, but if a repair was necessary, results were generally acceptable for lumbar plexus outflows and poor for those of the sacral plexus.

The hallmark of panpelvic plexus involvement is combined femoral or obturator and sciatic involvement. Branches leading to ilioinguinal, genitofemoral, saphenous, and lateral femoral cutaneous nerves can be involved but usually are not. Injury and entrapment are more likely to occur with distortion of the lower abdominal, inguinal, or upper thigh anatomy (Figure 11–32). One of our patients had a large, recurrent intraspinal neurofibroma at the L3 to L4 level with tumor in the pelvis as well as in a greatly dilated intervertebral foramen at that level. Origin was thought to be from a root in the pelvis with extension into the spinal canal. Because of extensive intraspinal recurrence, an attempt at total excision was elected. After subtotal removal of the intraspinal portion of the tumor to the level of the intervertebral foramen, the pelvic portion was resected using a transabdominal approach in conjunction with the general surgery service. The psoas muscle was split to locate the tumor, which was enucleated, sparing most, but unfortunately not all, of the root input to the femoral nerve.

A number of sacral plexus neurofibromas and schwannomas have been operated on and successfully removed. One patient, a female, presented with dyspareunia, and a mass was not palpable by vaginal or rectal examination. However, digital percussion of the lateral vagi-

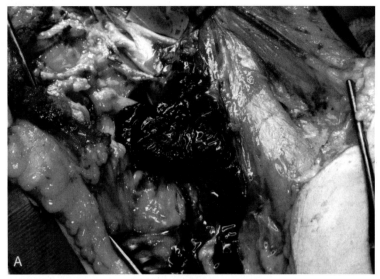

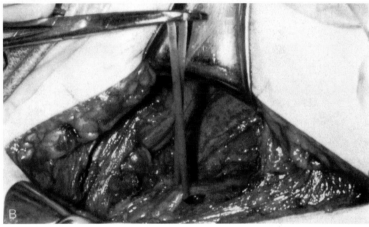

**Figure 11–30.** *(A)* A retroperitoneal clot due to anticoagulation that resulted in a femoral palsy. Clot was approached by a muscle-splitting incision in the lower quadrant of the abdomen and the right flank. *(B)* Retroperitoneal exposure of the pelvic portion of a femoral nerve that had been badly compressed by a retroperitoneal clot.

nal wall gave paresthesias into the medial thigh and vagina. This finding, combined with a history of the patient's having had a mediastinal neurofibroma removed some years earlier, led to exploration of the sacral portion of the plexus,

**TABLE 11–9**

Pelvic Plexus Injuries* (n = 47)

|  | **Operated** | **Unoperated** |
|---|---|---|
| Pelvic ± lumbar fracture | 3 | 15 |
| Gunshot wound | 4 | 6 |
| Stab/Laceration | 3 | 1 |
| Irradiation change | 0 | 3 |
| Stretch avulsion | 1 | 5† |
| Iatrogenic injury | 3 | 5 |
| TOTALS | 14 | 35 |

*Tumors operated on, including 11 neurofibromas, five schwannomas, one ganglioneuroma, and one sarcoma, are not included in the table.

†Includes one birth palsy.

where a solitary neurofibroma was found and successfully excised. Several other unsuspected neurofibromas were found attached to the intestinal mesentery and omentum, presumably arising from autonomic fibers.

Some other tumors of neural sheath origin in the pelvis have been exceptionally large and required extensive exposure of pelvic contents, including mobilization of bowel, identification of ureters, and as much protection of aortoiliac vessels and plexus nerves as possible. For these cases, we have enlisted the input of a general surgeon or sometimes a gynecologic surgeon to provide the initial exposure and to mobilize abdominal contents. If the sacral plexus or deep pelvis is to be explored, a transabdominal approach is favored by us, even though a lateral muscle splitting approach similar to that used for lumbar sympathectomy is also available if

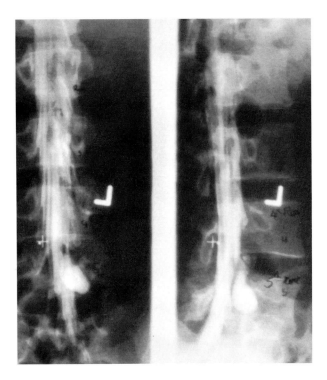

**Figure 11–31.** Two radiographic views show a large meningocele involving the fifth lumbar root and a smaller abnormality involving the fourth lumbar root. This patient had a severe pelvic plexus stretch injury associated with multiple fractures of the pelvis.

the lesion involves lumbar rather than sacral plexus.

Secondary attempts at repair of plexus element injury after resection of intrapelvic tumors, often unsuspected neurofibromas in the subrenal region, have usually met with frustration brought about by inability to find a proximal end for repair.[28]

Pelvic plexus palsies associated with lumbar, sacral, or pelvic fractures should be evaluated by myelography because the presence of a meningocele usually impedes successful repair, at least at that level, just as in brachial plexus injury.[4,25,47]

**TABLE 11–10**
Lower Extremity Nerves — Femoral and Pelvic Plexus

| | Evaluated | No. Operated | % Operated |
|---|---|---|---|
| Femoral | 78 | 54 | 69 |
| Lateral femoral cutaneous | 19 | 17 | 89 |
| Saphenous | 7 | 5 | 71 |
| Pelvic plexus | 49 | 14 | 29 |
| Obturator | 3 | 1 | 33 |
| TOTALS | 156 | 91 | 58 |

# FEMORAL, LATERAL FEMORAL CUTANEOUS, AND SAPHENOUS NERVES

*Femoral nerve* has its origin from the anterior divisions of L2, L3, and L4 roots or spinal nerves. The nerve has a relatively lengthy retroperitoneal course, lying initially on top of the large psoas muscle, which has its origins from lumbar transverse processes. By the pelvic level, the femoral nerve lies along the medial edge of this muscle. The iliacus muscle is supplied by relatively short branches arising from the posterior aspect of the femoral nerve. Iliopsoas muscles serve as the major flexor of the thigh. Femoral nerve also supplies branches to the sartorius or tailor muscle. The origin of the sartorius innervational branch is somewhat variable, but it usually arises from the more distal intrapelvic portion of the nerve. This muscle provides some upward and rotary lift of the thigh as the heel is raised to the opposite knee.[33]

As femoral nerve leaves the pelvis, it travels under the inguinal ligament along with more medially located femoral artery and vein. The nerve is in a separate fascial compartment and is more easily identified by dissection proximal in the thigh (Figure 11–33). Dissection a few cen-

**TABLE 11–11**
Femoral Nerve Injury Mechanisms and Results*

| Mechanism | Average Interval Between Injury and Operation (mo) | Neurolysis | | Suture | | Grafts | | Average Follow-up (mo) Operative | No Operation | Average Follow-up (mo) Nonoperative |
|---|---|---|---|---|---|---|---|---|---|---|
| | | Thigh | Pelvis | Thigh | Pelvis | Thigh | Pelvis | | | |
| Laceration (6) | 6 | 1/1 | 0/0 | 1/1 | 0/0 | 1/1 | 2/2 | 30 | 1/1 | 32 |
| Gunshot wound (7) | 5 | 0/0 | 2/2 | 0/0 | 0/0 | 2/1 | 1/1 | 20 | 2/1 | 26 |
| Hip or pelvic fracture (18) | 11 | 2/2† | 1/1 | 2/1 | 0/0 | 2/1 | 5/2 | 26 | 6/3 | 24 |
| Iatrogenic | | | | | | | | | | |
| Angiographic (6) | 5 | 3/3 | 0/0 | 0/0 | 0/0 | 0/0 | 0/0 | 18 | 3/2 | 9 |
| Arterial bypass (9) | 4 | 1/1 | 1/1 | 0/0 | 0/0 | 2/2 | 2/1 | 16 | 3/1 | 18 |
| Gynecologic surgery (5) | 7 | 0/0 | 2/2 | 0/0 | 0/0 | 0/0 | 1/0 | 23 | 2/1 | 12 |
| Lumbar sympathectomy (2) | 6 | 0/0 | 0/0 | 0/0 | 0/0 | 0/0 | 1/1 | 29 | 1/1 | 8 |
| Appendectomy (1) | 8 | 0/0 | 0/0 | 0/0 | 0/0 | 0/0 | 1/1 | 27 | 0/0 | — |
| Hernia repair (9) | 11 | 5/5‡ | 0/0 | 1/1 | 0/0 | 1/1 | 0/0 | 22 | 2/0 | 16 |
| Hip surgery (12) | 7 | 1/1 | 2/2 | 1/1 | 0/0 | 2/1 | 3/1 | 32 | 3/1 | 19 |
| Injection (1) | 6 | 0/0 | 0/0 | 0/0 | 0/0 | 0/0 | 0/0 | — | 1/1 | 23 |
| L.F.C. (2) | 7 | 1/1 | 0/0 | 0/0 | 0/0 | 0/0 | 1/0 | 25 | 0/0 | — |
| TOTALS (78) | 7.6 (averaged) | 14/14 | 8/8 | 5/4 | 0/0 | 10/7 | 17/9 | 26.1 (averaged) | 24/12 | 20.3 (averaged) |

L.F.C. = lateral femoral cutaneous nerve operation resulting in damage to femoral nerve.

*Number of operations/number reaching grade 3 or better level.

†Both patients had incomplete loss and severe pain. Loss as well as pain improved.

‡Includes two cases with preoperative function of one in whom internal neurolysis was done with function and pain improved. The other three patients had no function preoperatively but transmitted a nerve action potential and function returned.

(Adapted from Kim D, Kline D: Surgical outcome for intra- and extrapelvic femoral nerve lesions, J Neurosurg 1995, in press.)

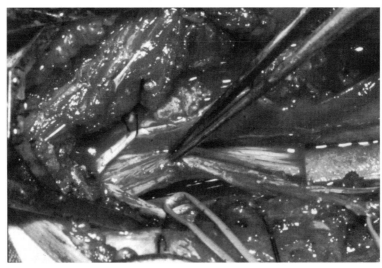

**Figure 11–32.** Exposure of the cauda equina in a child with pelvic plexus stretch injury. Several nerve roots were extended by grafts through the intervertebral foramina to the iliofemoral outflow. This required a two-stage procedure. Laminectomy exposed the cauda equina. Grafts were attached to proximal cauda equina. Sutures at the distal ends of the grafts were then placed through the intervertebral foramina at several levels, using Keith needles. The iliofemoral outflow at a pelvic level was then exposed by a flank and retroperitoneal approach. The Keith needles, sutures, and grafts were pulled into the pelvis, and the grafts were then sewn to the pelvic portion of the femoral nerve.

Femoral Nerve in Inguinal Region

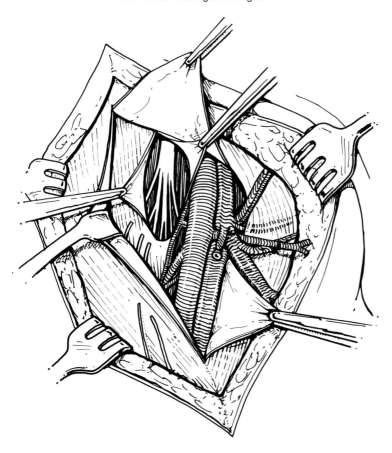

**Figure 11–33.** Drawing of the left femoral nerve, demonstrating the need to open iliacus fascia for exposure of the nerve in its position lateral to the femoral artery and vein at the level of the inguinal ligament and below.

timeters distally may be more difficult because the larger main nerve divides into numerous smaller branches destined for quadriceps. Lymph tissue, including nodes, also lie close to nerve at this level. During its relatively short course in the thigh, femoral nerve lies beneath a rather thick layer of fascia which is an extension of the iliacus fascia. Approximately 3.8 cm distal to inguinal ligament, nerve divides pes-like into a variable number of motor, sensory, and mixed motor-sensory branches supplying quadriceps musculature and anterior thigh sensation down to and including that to skin on the medial surface of the knee (Figure 11–34). A large sensory branch, the *saphenous nerve*, arises from anteromedial femoral nerve close to inguinal ligament. This nerve descends the thigh, running in the subcutaneous level to supply sensory fibers to skin around the medial knee. Usually, by means of several branches, saphenous then descends

the leg, supplying sensation to the medial leg and to the instep region of the foot. Saphenous nerve is usually accompanied by saphenous vein and, at times, small arterioles.

*Lateral femoral cutaneous nerve* arises from L1 and L2 spinal nerves and courses obliquely through the pelvis lateral to femoral nerve, but not as lateral as ilioinguinal and genitofemoral nerves. Nerve then courses anteriorly at the level of the lateral pelvic brim to exit pelvis medial to the anterior superior spine of the iliac crest. In doing so, it runs beneath and sometimes through the more lateral fascial fibers of the inguinal ligament. Sometimes nerve is branched as it runs over pelvic brim, but in other cases, it branches distal to this level.[50] The course of this nerve approaching and below or distal to pelvic brim can be variable. The surgeon must be prepared to look further if nerve is not found at its usual locus just medial to the anterior superior spine of the ilium. It supplies sensation to the skin of the lateral thigh, and with loss, an ovoid area of hypoesthesia over the lateral thigh is quite distinctive as the "trouser pocket" area. If lateral femoral is entrapped, this region is quite hyperesthetic.

The number of femoral, lateral femoral, saphenous nerve, and obturator cases evaluated or operated on is shown in Table 11–10.

## Clinical and Electrical Examination of Femoral Nerve

Examination for femoral nerve injury or neuropathy is straightforward. The grading characteristics used for pelvic- and thigh-level femoral nerve are found in Tables 11–12 and 11–13.

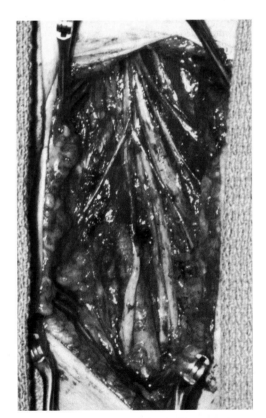

**Figure 11–34.** Thigh-level femoral nerve showing the complexity of branches just distal to the inguinal ligament. This nerve was contused, and the patient had partial dysfunction and severe pain and paresthesias.

**TABLE 11–12**
Grading Characteristics—Pelvic
Femoral Nerve

| Grade | Description |
|-------|-------------|
| 0 | No iliopsoas or quadriceps contraction |
| 1 | Trace iliopsoas, usually no quadriceps |
| 2 | Iliopsoas against gravity, trace quadriceps |
| 3 | Iliopsoas against gravity and some pressure, quadriceps against at least gravity |
| 4 | Iliopsoas against moderate pressure and quadriceps the same |
| 5 | Both iliopsoas and quadriceps contract against considerable pressure |

**TABLE 11–13**
Grading Characteristics — Thigh
Femoral Nerve

| Grade | Description |
|-------|-------------|
| 0 | No quadriceps contraction |
| 1 | Trace quadriceps but not against gravity |
| 2 | Contraction against gravity |
| 3 | Contraction against gravity and some pressure |
| 4 | Quadriceps contraction against moderate pressure |
| 5 | Quadriceps contraction of full strength |

Iliopsoas can be readily seen in the groin and palpated as the patient attempts to flex the hip. These large muscles can also be readily graded for strength of contraction. Sartorius is more difficult to assess with certainty. As the tailor muscle, it helps the individual to attain a sitting cross-legged position. However, by placing the heel of the limb to be tested on top of contralateral knee and then asking the patient to rotate thigh up and medially, one can sometimes see and palpate the tendon of this muscle. Quadriceps is best tested with the patient seated, and anterior thigh can be easily palpated as the patient extends the knee. As with the psoas muscle, fairly accurate grading of quadriceps can be achieved. The examiner does have to be careful that tensor fascia lata (supplied by the superior gluteal nerve) is not providing some extension of the leg when quadriceps is absent or very weak. If this is occurring, the examiner can usually see the patient tensing lateral thigh skin and underlying soft tissues rather than anterior thigh mass. Thigh adduction is provided by the three adductor muscles, which are innervated by obturator nerve, and not by the femoral-innervated quadriceps; abduction and some extension is also provided by more posteriorly located gluteus maximus and medius, innervated by gluteal nerves.

EMG studies of femoral nerve may include attempts to sample iliacus function and that of three portions of the quadriceps — lateral, intermediate, and medial muscle groups.[13] Nerve can also, if partially injured or regrowing, be stimulated at the level of inguinal ligament, and an attempt can be made to measure latencies of any evoked muscle action potentials recorded from quadriceps. Lateral femoral cutaneous has no motor component, and it can be difficult to measure conduction along this sensory nerve with certainty.[6] Assessment of the saphenous,

another sensory nerve, is more straightforward. Sensory NAPs can be evoked at a skin level by stimulating over the instep of the foot and recording over medial knee or sometimes even more proximally over anteromedial thigh.

## Surgical Exposure of the Femoral Nerve

Femoral nerve exposure is helped by flexing the knee to 30 to 45 degrees. Usually, posterior knee can be supported by a pillow or rolled sheets. If pelvic exposure of the nerve is anticipated, it may be best to place a few folded sheets beneath ipsilateral buttock as well. Initial incision has usually been placed in the femoral triangle in an up-and-down direction extending from inguinal ligament to the junction of the upper and middle thirds of thigh. More medial femoral artery requires isolation, as does some of femoral vein and its branches. Such branches may require ligation or bipolarization to expose femoral nerve branches down the thigh. The latter are encircled with plastic loops, and main femoral nerve is encircled by a Penrose drain.

If the injury involves intrapelvic femoral nerve, pelvic exposure is usually gained by a retroperitoneal approach combined with dissection of nerve in the femoral triangle (Figure 11–35). After exposure of the nerve in the triangle, it is traced retroperitoneally by sectioning the inguinal ligament and then curving the soft tissue incision laterally. Lower abdominal and flank musculature is split as much as possible in the direction of its fibers to expose the peritoneum. Peritoneum is then dissected away from the lateral and posterior false pelvis in an extraperitoneal fashion. Retroperitoneal space can usually be swept medially with the gloved hand, and then intraperitoneal abdominal contents and the abdominal wall can be retracted superiorly and somewhat medially by a Deaver or a large Richardson retractor. During this portion of the dissection, care is taken to spare lateral femoral cutaneous nerve as it runs medial to the anterior superior spine of the ileum and beneath the lateral portion of the inguinal ligament. Care should also be taken with ilioinguinal and genitofemoral nerves. Because the incision is initially kept close to the inguinal lig-

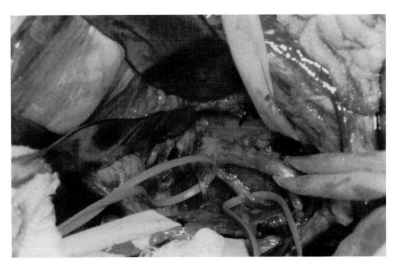

**Figure 11–35.** Retroperitoneal exposure of the pelvic portion of a femoral nerve (encircled by a Penrose drain). The plastic loop on the right is around the lateral femoral cutaneous nerve, and that on the left is around the ilioinguinal-genitofemoral origin. This exposure can be combined with that of thigh level femoral nerve for lesions extending from pelvis to thigh.

ament and then curved laterally and the dissection is kept retroperitoneally, these nerves should not be encountered until higher in the flank.

In the pelvis, the relations of femoral nerve as it is formed by the anterior divisions of the spinal nerves have already been discussed. Care must be taken to dissect nerve along the course of the iliopsoas. Iliac vessels and ureter lie more medially and must be excluded from the dissection. Smaller vessels coursing with the pelvic portion of the femoral outflow can usually be isolated from it and spared.

If exposure of the spinal nerves and divisions making up femoral nerve is necessary, a more direct approach though a lateral flank and muscle splitting incision is advisable. This approach is identical to that used for lumbar sympathectomy. The patient is placed in a partial lateral decubitus position with a roll or support under the flank to be opened. Skin and subcutaneous tissues are opened in the lateral flank with a somewhat oblique incision beginning beneath the lateral rib cage and extending inferiorly towards the anterior iliac crest or midportion of the inguinal ligament. External and internal oblique and transversalis muscles are split in the direction of their fibers and retracted by Gelpi, mastoid, or other self-restraining retractors. Then, the peritoneum is dissected away from the retroperitoneal fat, and the retroperitoneal space is dissected by the gloved fingers or a sponge stick until the iliopsoas is located. The anterior surface of the vertebral column lies midline and medial to the iliopsoas as the latter originates from transverse processes. Spinal

nerves usually penetrate through some of the psoas to form the upper pelvic plexus and, further distally, the femoral nerve. Sympathetic chain lies over the anterolateral vertebral column between the medial edge of the psoas and the midline of the anterior surface of the lumbosacral vertebral bodies.

## RESULTS— FEMORAL NERVE

The results provided in previously published series have been limited in their size or number and their lack of detail. However, it is apparent from such a review that this is a relatively favorable nerve for management.[56,60,62,63,68] Table 11–11 summarizes injury mechanisms and results in 78 femoral injuries in that series of patients.

### Results With Lacerations

Five of six lacerations involving femoral nerve were operated on, three at a thigh level and two at a pelvic level. Two of the five lacerations to femoral nerve were associated with vascular injury. One injury at a pelvic level was the result of an accidental lower abdominal stab wound inflicted by a pair of scissors. Other thigh- or pelvic-level injuries were caused by falls on broken glass or, in one instance, a stab wound from a kitchen knife. In retrospect, some of these femoral nerve injuries might have been repaired acutely or primarily because it seemed that the transections were sharp and relatively neat. Because of delay in referral, most were repaired secondarily. In one of these cases, repair had been attempted acutely, but distal femoral nerve stump had been sewn into the side of femoral artery at the level of the inguinal ligament. At the time of a secondary repair some 7 months later, it was found that the proximal stump had retracted into pelvis, was displaced medially, and had formed a large neuroma. After taking down the distal stump from the artery and trimming neuroma on the proximal stump, a gap of 10 cm (4 in) remained, and this was closed with interfascicular grafts. Acceptable recovery of quadriceps to a grade 4 level occurred, but 4 years was required for this degree of recovery.

## Results With Gunshot Wounds

The seven gunshot wounds involving femoral nerve were of low caliber, and this permitted survival because there was no major vascular injury (Figures 11–36 and 11–37). Five of the seven lesions were operated on. Three patients had repairs, and two of those recovered significant function. Two patients had a neurolysis with subsequent recovery. In one case with complete clinical and EMG loss, a NAP was transmitted across the lesion in continuity at 7 months after wounding. Only a neurolysis was done, and recovery was satisfactory. In another patient, an extensive shotgun wound to the abdomen involved bladder and bowel. This led to acute exploration and repair of these injuries. Secondary graft repair of the femoral nerve after resection of a lengthy intrapelvic lesion in continuity gave only grade 3 quadriceps recovery.

## Results With Iatrogenic Causes — Vascular Repair and Angiographic Complications

The most frequent etiology of injury to femoral nerve was iatrogenic and related to femoral artery repair or angiography, hip surgery, or herniorrhaphy (Figure 11–38). Vascular repairs in which nerve was secondarily involved were usually aortofemoral bypasses. Exposure of the injured femoral nerve at the time of repair was difficult because the bypass had to be protected. In most of these cases, more normal femoral nerve had to be located proximal to the inguinal ligament at a pelvic level and then traced by sharp dissection through the scar associated with the vascular repair. In some of the vascular cases, neural damage began at a pelvic level because nerve there had been directly injured by a needle or catheter or a hematoma had dissected beneath the inguinal ligament to involve the pelvic portion of the nerve. Identification of distal femoral branches, particularly if repair by grafts was necessary, was especially difficult. This was usually accomplished by carefully splitting the atrophied muscle fibers of the midportion of the quadriceps in a segmental, longitudinal fashion.

Despite resection of a large femoral artery pseudoaneurysm in an elderly lady, lengthy neural graft repair was still required, and only grade 1 to 2 quadriceps function was obtained by 1.5 years postoperatively. The aneurysm was not discovered until 7 months after angiography despite persisting complete femoral palsy. The extent of her vascular injury was so great that an arterial bypass had to be routed from the opposite femoral artery across the lower abdomen to the distal femoral artery on the injured

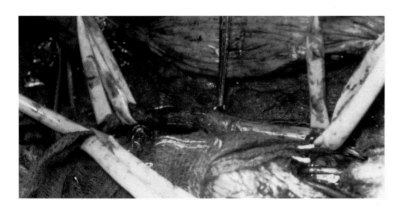

**Figure 11–36.** Gunshot wound involving a segment of a femoral nerve at the level of the inguinal ligament. The pelvic segment is to the left and the thigh segment is to the right. When operated on 6 months after injury, a graft repair was necessary.

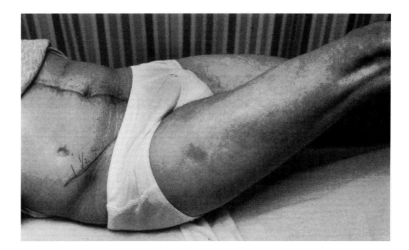

**Figure 11–37.** Recovery of the iliopsoas and some quadriceps function after an intraperitoneal graft repair of a gunshot wound injury to femoral nerve that was repaired 1.5 years earlier.

side. Another patient, who was a child, had a large pseudoaneurysm of the femoral artery because of catheterization for cardiac study. After resection of the aneurysm, she required a graft repair extending from the pelvic portion of the nerve to that in the thigh. Function was regained in this patient. In other cases associated with angiography, loss was incomplete, but pain and paresthesias were a problem despite vigorous physical therapy and pharmacologic management. Neurolysis seemed to help the pain syndrome in most of these cases.

## Other Operations With Iatrogenic Damage to Femoral Nerve

Involvement of femoral nerve by direct injury, scar, or suture as a result of hernia repair usually occurred at the level of the inguinal ligament. Neurolysis helped pain in two cases with incomplete loss. There was, as expected, a recordable NAP across these lesions. Three other patients with more severe loss before operation had a neurolysis because of a NAP and recovered (Figure 11–39). In one case, suture was found not only around but in nerve. Grafts 5 cm in length were required for repair, and quadriceps graded 3 at follow-up 3 years later.

Femoral nerve injury also occurred during the course of lateral femoral cutaneous nerve resection for meralgia paresthetica. In one case, a segment of femoral nerve was resected instead of lateral femoral cutaneous nerve. This required repair of femoral nerve by grafts from an intrapelvic to femoral triangle level.

Femoral palsy has been previously reported as a complication of total hip replacement.[66,71] A

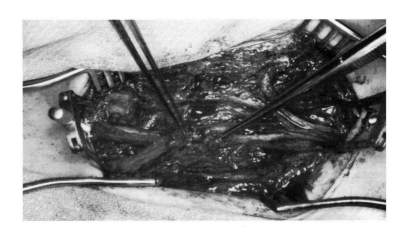

**Figure 11–38.** A femoral nerve injury secondary to an iliofemoral arterial bypass. Resection and graft repair were necessary.

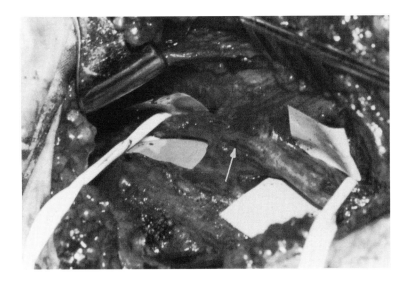

**Figure 11–39.** Femoral nerve at a pelvic level injured by a retractor during the course of an abdominal operation *(arrow)*. This lesion transmitted a nerve action potential. As a result, a neurolysis was done. Recovery to a grade 4 level occurred over a 2-year period.

number of cases of contusion and stretch associated with hip operations required operation. After a NAP recording most required a repair, although three could have had a neurolysis (Figure 11–40). Two cases of femoral palsy associated with hip repair were caused by neural encasement with methyl methacrylate. In each case, a lengthy segment of nerve had to be replaced by sural grafts, and results were poor.

## Results With Stretch/ Contusion in Hip or Pelvic Fracture

This was a relatively large category of injury and included evaluation of 18 patients (Table 11–11). Nonetheless, stretch involving femoral nerve alone and unassociated with a more widespread pelvic plexus lesion is less frequent than plexus injury. Compared with brachial plexus stretch injuries, those to pelvic plexus are infrequent. Six patients were managed without operation, and three recovered sufficient function to straighten and lock the knee on walking. Three patients had a neurolysis based on a NAP and recovered, but one had incomplete loss initially. Nonetheless, this patient's pain also improved, and this was evident immediately on recovery from anesthesia. One of two patients having suture repairs recovered substantial function. The other patient was grateful for the reversal of pain after resection of a lesion in continuity, but recovery of quadriceps was only to

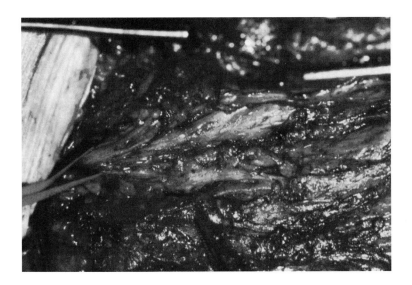

**Figure 11–40.** A severely contused femoral nerve just distal to the inguinal ligament. This patient had a hip replacement operation. A graft repair was necessary.

grade level 1 to 2. Seven patients had graft repairs, five at a pelvic level and two at a thigh level. Three of the seven patients recovered femoral function to a grade 3 or higher level. One patient required 9-cm sural grafts, and although some recovery was gained (grade 3), individual muscle grades were better for iliopsoas than for quadriceps.

## Results With Tumors

It was rather interesting that tumors primary to nerve were found, even in the femoral nerve (Table 11–14). There were three neurofibromas and one schwannoma involving proximal femoral nerve. One neurofibroma had been resected elsewhere and, as a result, had complete loss of function. Grafts 6 cm in length were necessary for repair, but acceptable recovery occurred. A second neurofibroma was successfully resected without loss of function. A third tumor associated with von Recklinghausen disease was resected but femoral nerve required almost complete replacement by grafts 8 cm in length. Recovery has been partial over a 3-year period of follow-up and grades 2 to 3. A moderately large schwannoma was removed successfully from the femoral nerve just distal to the inguinal ligament in another patient who was 47 years old. A malignant schwannoma involving a femoral sensory branch at midthigh level was treated by wide local resection and local irradiation. The patient has remained free of recurrence over a 4-year period.

Four benign neural sheath tumors involved spinal nerves leading to femoral nerve at a pelvic level, and three were totally resected without subsequent femoral deficit. A ganglion cyst of the thigh was removed elsewhere with partial, incomplete femoral deficit. This patient has been followed without further surgery and has improved. One patient had a large leiomyosarcoma involving femoral nerve, which was resected with graft repair of pelvic femoral nerve; he has had extensive intra-abdominal recurrence 1.5 years after a gross total resection of tumor and the involved nerve.

Spontaneous pelvic hematomas associated with anticoagulation or hemophilia can cause femoral neuropathy (see Figure 11–30).[13] Fortunately, most of these neuropathies are usually reversible without surgery. One case that presented recently with rather acute and extremely severe neuropathy and a very large hematoma required hematoma evacuation and neurolysis of a severely stretched pelvic to thigh level femoral nerve. This patient, who had been given anticoagulant for cardiac disease, had early grade 2 recovery of quadriceps after hematoma evacuation, but follow-up is too short for inclusion in this series.

## Results — Saphenous Nerve

This sensory nerve was sometimes inadvertently injured during the course of venous stripping and ligation or occasionally during operative procedures around the knee (Figure 11–41). This type of iatrogenic involvement has been reported previously.[17] The nerve,

**TABLE 11–14**
Tumors Involving Femoral Nerve

| Number of Cases | Description of Treatment and Results |
| --- | --- |
| **Pelvic Level** | |
| 5 | Neurofibromas (one bilateral). Retroperitoneal approach. Result: 3 patients without deficit including the one with bilateral lesions. |
| 1 | Leiomyosarcoma. Wide resection and graft repair of pelvic femoral nerve. Recurrence at 1.5 years. |
| **Thigh Level** | |
| 3 | Neurofibromas and schwannoma. One, resected elsewhere, required graft repair and recovered. One solitary schwannoma was successfully resected. One tumor with VRD was resected and required graft repair. Limited recovery so far. |
| 1 | Malignant nerve tumor on femoral sensory branch. Wide local resection. No recurrence in 4 years. |
| 1 | Ganglion cyst resected elsewhere. Partial loss improved without further operation. |

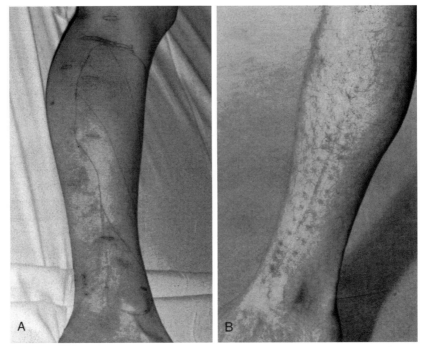

**Figure 11–41.** *(A)* Saphenous nerve injuries at several levels associated with a venous stripping and ligation. Sensory loss is outlined. The nerve was resected from the knee to the ankle level because of painful paresthesias. *(B)* Another mechanism for saphenous injury is harvesting of a saphenous vein for arterial repair.

which is entirely sensory, originates from femoral in the proximal anterolateral thigh and descends the medial thigh and leg as one or more branches. Injury at any point along its course can lead to a painful neuroma. We have favored wide excision of the neuroma and attached scar and removal of nerve well proximal and distal to the injury site rather than repair. This nerve serves a functionally less important sensory territory than tibial or even peroneal, and attempts to resect the neuroma and repair the nerve can lead to another painful neuroma as the suture or graft site matures. To date, five saphenous nerves associated with neuroma have been resected with satisfactory relief of pain and paresthesias. Two other patients with saphenous branch injuries associated with arthroscopic procedures of the knee have been managed conservatively without further operation. Occasionally, a mass such as a lipoma, cyst, or, in one patient, a venous aneurysm, involves this nerve, but we have not seen a spontaneous entrapment unassociated with injury.[40,48]

## Results — Lateral Femoral Cutaneous Nerve

This nerve originates high in the pelvis, usually from the L2 and sometimes L1 spinal nerve. It travels over proximal psoas muscle in an oblique fashion and remains retroperitoneal as it approaches ilium of the pelvis. It exits the pelvis at the level of the anterior superior spine of the ilium. It passes medial to this process and is covered by a portion of the inguinal ligament. Nerve enters the anterolateral thigh deep to the iliacus fascia (Figure 11–42). It soon branches to supply lateral thigh skin. This nerve can be difficult to find if dissection is confined to the thigh alone. On the other hand, if the spine of the ilium is exposed, so will be the nerve. If the nerve is entrapped, contused, or stretched, excision of the nerve may be indicated. Preferred is an approach to the nerve close to the anterior superior spine of the ilium and the removal of enough of the nerve on the side of the peritoneal cavity so that proximal stump lies retroperito-

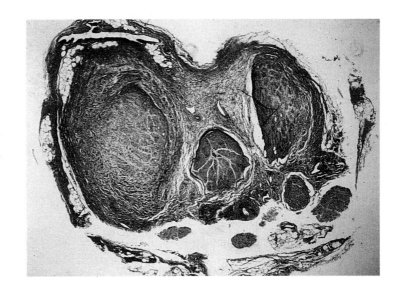

**Figure 1–7.** Cross section of an injured nerve showing intrafascicular as well as extrafascicular scar. Masson stain.

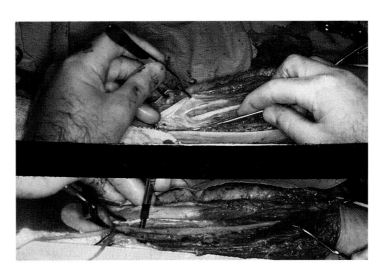

**Figure 2–16.** Long-standing Volkmann contracture caused by intra-arterial morphine injection. Top shows fatty replacement of muscle grasped by forceps. Lengthy ischemic as well as acutely compressed segment of median is shown at bottom. Area to the right looks like a finger but is caused by a bloodied stockinette.

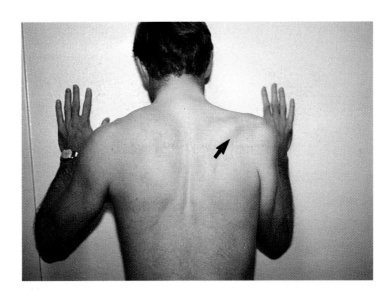

**Figure 4–4.** In this patient, there was loss not only of deltoid but of supraspinatus and infraspinatus function. Note the muscular atrophy on either side of the scapula's spinous process *(arrow)*. Supraspinatus function was trace only, as was that of deltoid; infraspinatus function was absent (0). This gave an overall grade for C5 function of 1.

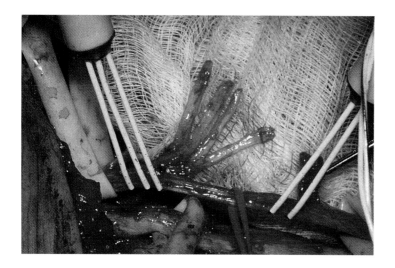

**Figure 6 – 19.** Stimulation (to the left) and recording (to the right) from a portion of nerve to be retained without repair because of detection of a nerve action potential (NAP) conducted across this segment. Grafts have been sewn into fascicular groups to the left and will next be sewn into those on the right. This portion of the injured nerve did not conduct an NAP. (From Dubuisson A, Kline D: Indications for peripheral nerve and brachial plexus surgery. Neurol Clin North Am 10:935–951, 1992.)

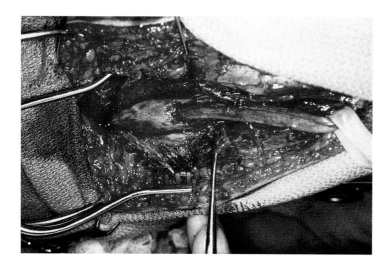

**Figure 7 – 5.** Radial nerve caught or entrapped in the middle of a healed humeral fracture.

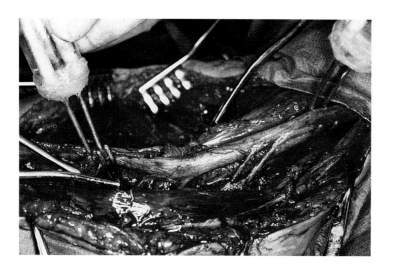

**Figure 8 – 12.** Anatomy of median at the level of the elbow. Arm is to the right and forearm is to the left. Lacertus fibrosus has been sectioned and pronator teres split away to expose this portion of the nerve. Pronator, flexor superficialis, and anterior interosseous branches can be seen. This figure is similar but not identical to the one in the text.

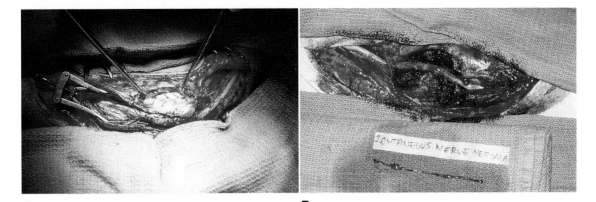

A                                    B

**Figure 9-24.** (A) Nerve has been cleared through the region of the olecranon notch by a complete external neurolysis. A trough has been made in the proximal forearm muscle by sectioning completely through pronator teres and the more volar portion of flexor carpi ulnaris. (B) Nerve has been placed in the muscle trough. Note that a neuroma and segment of antebrachial cutaneous nerve have been resected and are placed on the drape. This patient had prior neurolysis for olecranon notch-level entrapment and had injury to antebrachial cutaneous nerve.

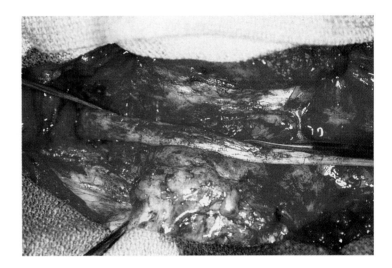

**Figure 11-2.** Contusion of sciatic nerve close to sciatic notch area. Notch is to the left, and thigh level is to the right.

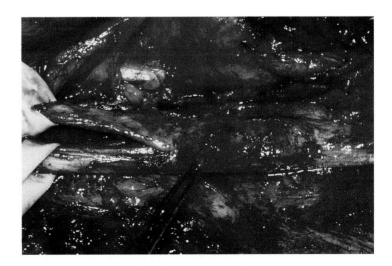

**Figure 11-12.** Typical lesion in continuity involving sciatic nerve at a midthigh level caused by a gunshot wound. Proximal sciatic nerve is to the right, and origin of tibial and peroneal nerves is to the left.

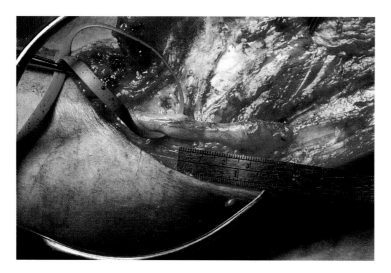

**Figure 11-24.** Left peroneal nerve with an area of narrowing and swelling on either side. This patient received a contusive blow behind the knee and over a period of several years developed a progressive peroneal palsy. The palsy was considered to be the result of a trauma-induced entrapment. The lesion conducted, and thus a neurolysis was done. (Courtesy of Dr. Jack Hurst, Lafayette, LA.)

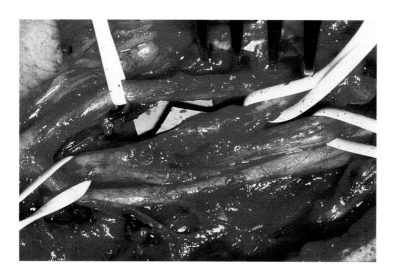

**Figure 13-3.** Stab wound involving middle trunk of the plexus (encircled by plastic loop at left bottom) and explored at 1 month. This lesion was resected and an end-to-end repair was done. This lesion could have been repaired acutely had there been the opportunity.

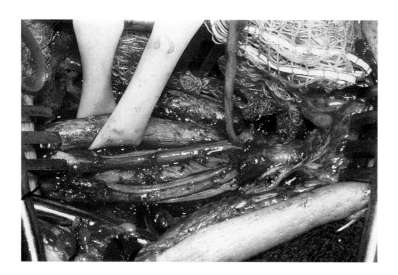

**Figure 14-4.** Missile wound injury to C5, C6, and upper trunk. Function had not improved clinically or electrically by 5 months after wounding. Operative stimulation and recording showed only a small nerve action potential from a portion of the C6 outflow to upper trunk. This was split off and spared resection; the rest of C6 and all of C5 outflow to the upper trunk were replaced by grafts. One graft, which is elevated at the upper right of the picture, remains to be attached distally.

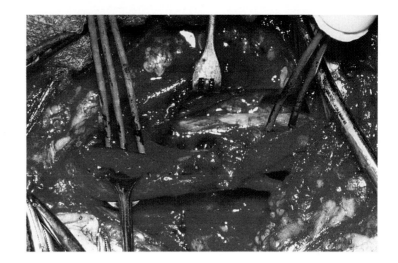

**Figure 14–7.** Gunshot wound involving upper trunk. C6 is being stimulated to the left, and recording electrodes are placed on the anterior division of the upper trunk to the right. This truncal lesion, which was exposed 3.5 months after injury, required resection and repair. Outcome was good. At 3.5 years, biceps graded 4 to 5, brachioradialis 3, deltoid 3, and supraspinatus 3.

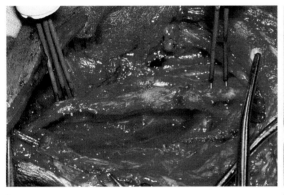

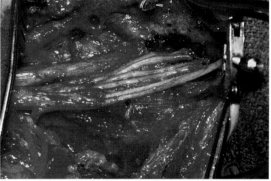

A            B

**Figure 15–16.** (A) Right C5 and C6 stretch injury extending into upper trunk. Clavicle is to the right. After exposing spinal nerves and more distal elements, nerve action potential recordings were done. Here C5 is being stimulated (to the *left*), and recording electrodes are on one of the upper trunk divisions (to the *right*). (B) Graft repair of another but left-sided C5-C6 stretch injury. Sural grafts run from an intraforaminal level of both C5 and C6 to distal upper trunk (to the *left*). Less injured or involved C7 to middle trunk is seen in the background.

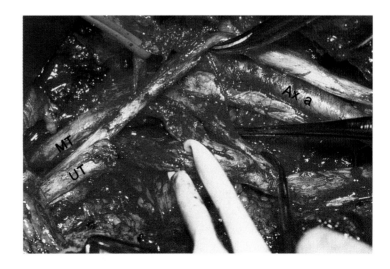

**Figure 15–40.** This unusual stretch injury involved only the posterior divisions of all three trunks. These elements did not transmit nerve action potentials, were resected, and were then replaced by grafts. Loss was to the deltoid and to all of the muscles in the radial distribution. Ax a = axillary artery; MT = middle trunk; UT = upper trunk.

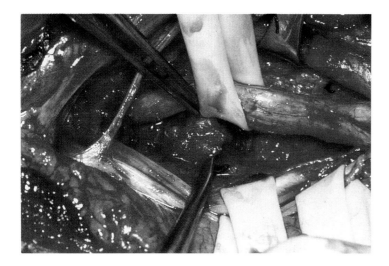

**Figure 17-5.** Elongated process of C7 vertebra exposed beneath C7 nerve to the middle trunk area in a patient with TOS. Lower trunk is retracted slightly by vein retractor at the top of the picture.

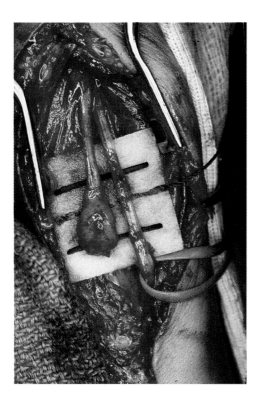

**Figure 20-3.** Neuroma on dorsal cutaneous nerve at the forearm level caused by a lacerating injury. Remainder of ulnar nerve is to the right and is headed toward Guyon canal. After resection, proximal nerve was trimmed sharply and fasciculi were grasped with fine-tipped bipolar forceps and bovied in an attempt to seal them shut.

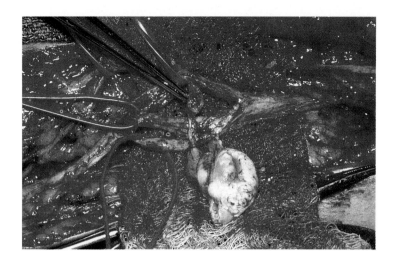

**Figure 21–14.** Relatively small neurofibroma of ulnar nerve at the elbow level which has been worked free of most of the fascicular structure.

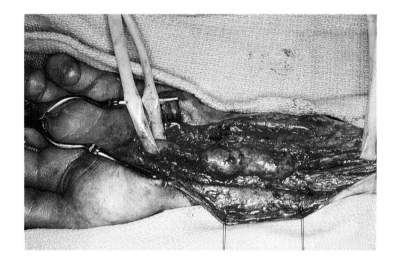

**Figure 21–46.** Venous angioma or aneurysm involving distal forearm-level median nerve. Patient worked stocking shelves in a store. While stocking lower shelves, he experienced painful paresthesias in the median distribution that dissipated when he worked on higher shelves. The lesion was resected by clearing individual fascicles of vessels and scar. Five years later, however, this angioma recurred and required resection and sural graft repair of the median nerve.

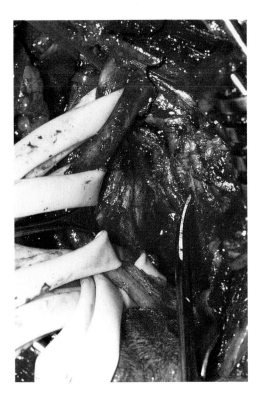

**Figure 21–49.** Metastatic pulmonary carcinoma (at tip of scissors) attached to proximal humerus and compressing plexus (retracted to the left) at a cord level. Plexus elements have been dissected away from the tumor and are retracted medially by Penrose drains.

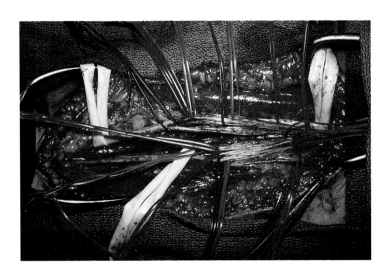

**Figure 21–57.** Internal neurolysis on sciatic complex; both divisions were involved by hypertrophic neuropathy.

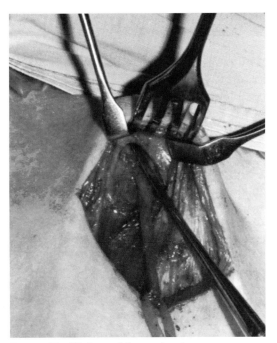

**Figure 11–42.** Lateral femoral cutaneous nerve exposed in the region of the anterior superior spine of the ileum and more distally in the thigh. Dissector points to the region of the ligament overlying the nerve. Note the relative size of the nerve.

neally. This is because of experience with nerves previously sectioned just distal to the anterior superior spine. Neuroma intermixed with scar resulted at this level, and because it was located on the pelvic brim, it was usually painful or more painful than the original problem. In several cases, this nerve was inadvertently injured during the course of bone removal from the ilium for use as graft material (Figure 11–43). Procedures to harvest bone from iliac crest for grafts should be kept well lateral to this site. Table 11–15 categorizes results as good, fair, or poor and includes experience with 12 entrapments, two injuries associated with operations on the iliac crest, one injection palsy, and two lacerations, both from knife wounds.

## COMPLICATIONS

Operations on the sciatic nerve at an extrapelvic level are amazingly free of most complications. At the level of the sciatic notch, gluteal vessels can be transected and retract into the pelvis, producing a large retroperitoneal hema-

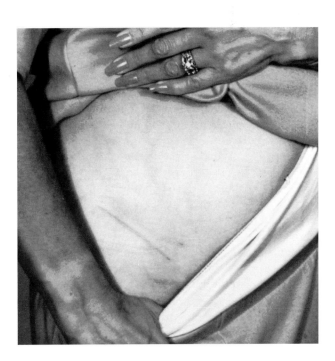

**Figure 11–43.** Incision used for harvesting an iliac crest bone graft where the lateral femoral cutaneous nerve was injured.

**TABLE 11–15**

Results From Resection of Lateral
Femoral Cutaneous Nerves

| Mechanism | Results | | |
|---|---|---|---|
| | Good | Fair | Poor |
| Entrapment | 8 | 3 | 1 |
| Iliac crest resection | 1 | 1 | 0 |
| Injection | 1 | 0 | 0 |
| Laceration | 2 | 0 | 0 |
| TOTALS | 12 | 4 | 1 |

toma. This complication was not seen in our series but has been reported by John McGillicuddy. Because gluteal muscles must be transected laterally and then reopposed after the sciatic operation, some loss of gluteal bulk and contraction strength can occur. More serious at this level is inadvertent injury to a less involved sciatic division, and this can occur as the injured division is split away from the less involved one. This occurred several times in our series, but loss in the newly injured distribution was partial and usually reversed with time.

One end-to-end sciatic repair for blunt transection at the thigh level distracted by several months postoperatively and required re-repair by grafts. Neurolysis of the peroneal nerve for entrapment in the region of the head and neck of the fibula either failed to reverse loss or helped only temporarily with return of loss over a period of months. This occurred despite neurolysis, splitting the peroneus fascia and muscle over the peroneal branches, and partial fibulectomy. One potential complication of the latter procedure is incorporation of the peroneal nerve by a bony callus. To our knowledge, that has not occurred in this series, at least not in a symptomatic fashion. However, we have not done postoperative radiography on all of those patients in whom a partial fibulectomy was done.

As might be predicted, we found dissections very difficult for branch level injury of either peroneal nerve in the anterior compartment of the leg or posterior tibial nerve deep to gastrocnemius in the posterior compartment of the leg. In the latter cases, injury to the posterior tibial artery, if not already present, can readily occur, and in one case, required ligation of this vessel at the time of posterior tibial repair. Fortunately,

there was sufficient blood supply to the foot maintained by other vessels.

Surgical wounds around the distal leg and foot were slow to heal and had about a 1% incidence of wound infection, which was higher than that at other sites in the leg or elsewhere in the body.

The list of potential complications is great if the pelvis has to be entered for nerve repair or neural tumor removal. Ileus, urinary retention, and urinary urgency and incontinence with or without urinary tract infection were the most frequent. Intraperitoneal or retroperitoneal bleeding can also result in significant hematoma. Although not experienced in this series, ureteral injury, aortic or iliac arterial injury, significant venous injury, and colonic or even small intestine injury, are potential complications.

### Case Summary — Stab Wound With Postoperative Complications

A case too recent for the analysis of this reported series illustrates some of these points. This individual received an abdominal stab wound resulting acutely in a large retroperitoneal hematoma and injury to mesenteric vessels as well as a lumbar plexus injury. At the time of a retroperitoneal approach for graft repair of the plexus 2.5 months later, a greatly scarred retroperitoneal space was found. Sural grafts were placed to fill an 8-cm gap from lumbar roots to iliofemoral outflow. Some of this gap was made up by mobilization of distal femoral outflow to the level of the thigh, but grafts still had to be 6 cm in length. It was noted that most of the posterior peritoneum had been torn by the original injury and necessary surgery, and the large bowel was scarred and thickened. The patient had to be returned to surgery on the third postoperative day to evacuate a large retroperitoneal hematoma. He then developed pneumonia and acute respiratory distress syndrome and required intubation and ventilatory support under anesthesia for 4 days. He recovered well from this pulmonary problem but then developed a small bowel obstruction and a retroperitoneal collection thought to be an abscess. A transperitoneal exposure by general surgery revealed torsion of the mid-portion of the small bowel beneath a scarred and perforated portion of the transverse colon. A portion of the small intestine was not viable and required resection and reanastomosis, and a temporary colostomy was necessary. A recurrent collection of retroperitoneal blood grew out gram-positive and gram-negative organisms. He finally recovered well enough to be sent home. In each of the reoperations, the graft repair site was exposed and protected. Outcome in terms of femoral recovery remains to be seen.

## Bibliography

1. Adams JC: Vulnerability of the sciatic nerve in closed ischiofemoral arthrodesis by nail and graft. J Bone Joint Surg Br 46:748–753, 1964.
2. Aldea PA and Shaw WA: Lower extremity nerve injuries. Clin Plast Surg 14:691–699, 1986.
3. Banerjee T and Hall CD: Sciatic entrapment neuropathy. J Neurosurg 45:216–217, 1976.
4. Barnett HG and Connolly EJ: Lumbosacral nerve root avulsion. J Trauma 15:532–535, 1975.
5. Bateman JE: Trauma to Nerves and Limbs. Philadelphia, WB Saunders, 1962.
6. Behse F and Buchthal F: Normal sensory conduction in the nerves of the leg in man. J Neurol Neurosurg Psychiatry 34:404–414, 1971.
7. Berry H and Richardson PM: Common peroneal nerve palsy: A clinical and electrophysiological review. J Neurol Neurosurg Psychiatry 39:1162–1171, 1976.
8. Borges LF, Hallett M, Selkoe DJ, and Welch K: The anterior tarsal tunnel syndrome. J Neurosurg 54:89–92, 1981.
9. Bourrel P: Transfer of the tibialis posterior to tibialis anterior, and of flexor hallucis longus to the extensor digitorum longus in peroneal palsy. Ann Chir 21:1451–1456, 1967.
10. Brand P and Ebner JD: Pressure sensitive devices for denervated hands and feet. J Bone Joint Surg 51A:109–116, 1969.
11. Bristow WR: Injuries of peripheral nerves in two World Wars. Br J Surg 34:333, 1947.
12. Byrnes O, Russo GL, Ducker TB, and Cowley RA: Sacrum fractures and neurological damage. J Neurosurg 47:459–462, 1977.
13. Calvery JR and Mulder DW: Femoral neuropathy. Neurology 10:963–967, 1960.
14. Clark K, Williams P, Willis W, and McGavran WL: Injection injuries of sciatic nerve. In Ojemann RG, Ed: Clinical Neurosurgery 17:111–125, 1970.
15. Clawson DK and Seddon HJ: The late consequences of sciatic nerve injury. J Bone Joint Surg Br 42B:213–225, 1960.
16. Clawson DK and Seddon HJ: The results of repair of the sciatic nerve. J Bone Joint Surg Br 42B:205–213, 1960.
17. Cox SJ: Saphenous nerve injury caused by stripping of long saphenous vein. Br Med J 1:415–417, 1974.
18. Cozen L: Management of foot drop in adults after peroneal nerve loss. Clin Orthop 67:151–158, 1969.
19. DeSeze S: Electromyography of the tarsal tunnel syndrome. Rev Rheum 37:189–195, 1970.
20. Edwards WG, Lincoln CR, Bassett FH, and Goldner JL: The tarsal tunnel syndrome. JAMA 207:716–720, 1969.
21. Fried G, Salerno T, Brown HC, et al.: Management of the extremity with combined neurovascular and musculoskeletal trauma. J Trauma 18:481–486, 1978.
22. Gelmers H: Entrapment of the sciatic nerve. Acta Neurochir (Wien) 33:103–106, 1976.
23. Gentilli F and Hudson AR: Peripheral nerve injuries: Types, causes, grading. In Wilkins RH and Rengachary SS, Eds: Neurosurgery, Vol. 2. New York, McGraw-Hill, 1985.
24. Gilden DH and Eisner J: Lumbar plexopathy caused by disseminated intravascular coagulation. JAMA 237:2846–2847, 1977.
25. Harris WR: Avulsion of lumbar roots complicating fracture of the pelvis. J Bone Joint Surg 55A:1436–1442, 1974.
26. Haymaker W and Woodhall B: Peripheral Nerve Injuries. Principles of Diagnosis, 2nd Ed. Philadelphia, WB Saunders, 1953.
27. Highet WB and Holmes W: Traction injuries to the lateral popliteal and traction injuries to peripheral nerves after suture. Br J Surg 30:212, 1943.
28. Hudson AR, Hunter GA, and Waddell JP: Iatrogenic femoral nerve injuries. Can J Surg 22:62–66, 1979.
29. Hudson AR, Kline DG, and Gentilli F: Peripheral nerve injection injury. In Management of Peripheral Nerve Problems. Philadelphia, WB Saunders, 1980.
30. Huttinen V: Lumbosacral nerve injury in fracture of the pelvis. A postmortem radiographic and pathoanatomical study. Acta Chir Scand Suppl 429, 1972.
31. Johnson EW: Nerve injuries in fractures of the lower extremity. Minn Med 52:627–633, 1969.
32. Johnson EW and Ortiz PR: Electrodiagnosis of tarsal tunnel syndrome. Arch Phys Med 47:776–778, 1966.
33. Kline DG: Diagnostic approach to individual nerve injuries. In Wilkins RH and Rengachary SS, Eds: Neurosurgery, Vol. 2. New York, McGraw-Hill, 1985.
34. Kline DG: Operative experience with a major lower extremity nerve lesion. In Omer G Jr and Spinner M, Eds: Management of Peripheral Nerve Problems. Philadelphia, WB Saunders, 1980, pp. 607–625.
35. Kline DG: Operative management of major nerve lesions of the lower extremity. Surg Clin North Am 52:1247–1265, 1972.
36. Kopell HP: Lower extremity lesions. In Omer G Jr and Spinner M, Eds: Management of Peripheral Nerve Problems. Philadelphia, WB Saunders, 1980, pp. 626–638.
37. Lam SJ: Tarsal tunnel syndrome. J Bone Joint Surg 49B:87–92, 1967.
38. Lassmann G, Lassmann H, and Stockinger L: Morton's metatarsalgia: Light and electron microscopic observations and their relation to entrapment neuropathies. Virchows Arch A Pathol Anat Histopathol 370:307–321, 1976.
39. Long DL: Electrical stimulation for relief of pain from chronic nerve injury. J Neurosurg 39:718–722, 1973.
40. Luerssen TG, Campbell RL, Defalque RJ, and Worth RM: Spontaneous saphenous neuralgia. Neurosurgery 13:238–241, 1983.
41. MacCarty CS: Two-stage autograft for repair of extensive damage to the sciatic nerve. J Neurosurg 8:319–322, 1951.
42. Marcus NA, Blair WF, Shuck JM, et al.: Low-velocity gunshot wounds to extremities. J Trauma 20:1061–1064, 1980.
43. McLean M: Total hip replacement and sciatic nerve trauma. Orthopedics 9:1121–1127, 1986.
44. Millesi H: Lower extremity nerve lesions. In Terzis J, Ed: Microreconstruction of Nerve Injuries. Philadelphia, WB Saunders, 1987.
45. Millesi H: Nerve grafts: Indications, techniques and prognosis. In Omer G Jr and Spinner M, Eds: Management of Peripheral Nerve Problems. Philadelphia, WB Saunders, 1980, pp. 410–430.
46. Mitchell SW, Morehouse GR, and Keen WW: Gunshot Wounds and Other Injuries of Nerves. Philadelphia, JB Lippincott, 1864.
47. Moosey JJ, Nashold BJ, and Osborne D: Conus medullaris nerve root avulsions. J Neurosurgery 66:835–841, 1987.
48. Mozes M, Ouaknine G, and Nathan H: Saphenous

nerve entrapment simulating vascular disorder. Surgery 77:299–303, 1975.

49. Nagler S and Rangell L: Peroneal palsy caused by crossing the legs. JAMA 133:755–761, 1947.

50. Nathan H: Ganglioform enlargement of the lateral cutaneous nerve of thigh. J Neurosurg 17:843–850, 1960.

51. Nielson KD, Watts C, and Clark WK: Peripheral nerve injury from implantation of chronic stimulating electrodes for pain control. Surg Neurol 5:51–53, 1976.

52. Nobel W: Peroneal palsy due to hematoma in the common peroneal nerve sheath after distal torsional fractures and inversion ankle sprains. J Bone Joint Surg 48A:1484–1495, 1966.

53. Oh SJ, Kim HS, and Ahmad BK: The near-nerve sensory nerve conduction in tarsal tunnel syndrome. J Neurol Neurosurg Psychiatry 48:999–1003, 1985.

54. Omer G Jr: Nerve injuries associated with gunshot wounds of the extremities. In Gelberman R, Ed: Operative Repair and Reconstruction. Philadelphia, JB Lippincott, 1991.

55. Omer GE Jr: Results of untreated peripheral nerve injuries. Clin Orthop 163:15–19, 1982.

56. Osgaard O and Husby J: Femoral nerve repair with nerve autografts. Report of two cases. J Neurosurg 47:751–754, 1977.

57. Paradies LH and Gregory CF: The early treatment of close-range shotgun wounds to the extremities. J Bone Joint Surg 48A:425–429, 1966.

58. Patterson FP: Neurological complications of fractures and dislocations of the pelvis. J Trauma 12:1013–1023, 1972.

59. Pollack LJ and Davis L: Peripheral nerve injuries, the sciatic nerve, the tibial nerve, the peroneal nerve. Amer J Surg 18:176–193, 1932.

60. Rakolta GG and Omer GE: Combat-sustained femoral nerve injuries. Surg Gynecol Obstet 128:813–817, 1969.

61. Rich NM and Spencer FC: Vascular Trauma. Philadelphia, WB Saunders, 1978.

62. Rizzoli HV: Treatment of peripheral nerve injuries. In

Coates JB and Meirowsky AM, Eds: Neurological Surgery of Trauma. Washington, DC, Office of the Surgeon General, Department of the Army, 1965.

63. Seddon HJ, Ed: Surgical Disorders of the Peripheral Nerves. Baltimore, Williams & Wilkins, 1972.

64. Seletz E: Surgery of Peripheral Nerves. Springfield, IL, Charles C Thomas, 1951.

65. Singh N, Behse F, and Buchthal F: Electrophysiological study of peroneal palsy. J Neurol Neurosurg Psychiatry 37:1202–1213, 1974.

66. Solheim LF and Hagen R: Femoral and sciatic neuropathies after total hip arthroplasty. Acta Orthop Scand, 51:531–534, 1980.

67. Stevens H: Meralgia paresthetica. Arch Neurol Psychiatry 77:557–574, 1957.

68. Sunderland S: Nerves and Nerve Lesions. Edinburgh, Churchill Livingstone, 1978.

69. Thomas J, Cascino T, and Earl J: Differential diagnosis between radiation and tumor plexopathy of the pelvis. Neurology 35:1–7, 1985.

70. Wagner FC: Compression of the lumbosacral plexus and the sciatic nerve. In Szabo R, Ed: Nerve Compression Syndromes: Diagnosis and Treatment. Thorofare, NJ, Slack, 1989.

71. Weber ER, Daube JR, and Coventry MB: Peripheral neuropathies associated with total hip arthroplasty. J Bone Joint Surg 58A:66–69, 1976.

72. Whitcomb BB: Separation at the suture site as a cause of failure in regeneration of peripheral nerves. J Neurosurg 3:399–406, 1946.

73. White JC: Timing of nerve suture after gunshot wound. Surgery 48:946–951, 1960.

74. Woltman HL: Crossing the legs as a factor in the production of peroneal palsy. JAMA 93:670–672, 1929.

75. Wood MB: Peripheral nerve injuries to the lower extremity. In Operative Nerve Repair and Reconstruction. Philadelphia, JB Lippincott, 1991.

76. Young MR and Norris JW: Femoral neuropathy during anticoagulant therapy. Neurology (Minneap) 26:1173–1175, 1976.

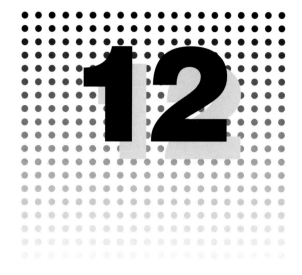

# Brachial Plexus Anatomy and Physiology

## SUMMARY

The elements or portions of the nervous system that usually comprise the brachial plexus are the C5, C6, C7, C8, and T1 nerves. These elements begin as roots until they penetrate dura and lie in their intervertebral foramina; then, they are known as spinal nerves. Fixation of the spinal nerves in their bony canals and their relative intraforaminal length and obliquity become important as the mechanisms involved in stretch and avulsive injuries are studied and operations are designed to attempt correction of proximal injury. The patterns with truncal, cord, and cord-to-nerve level injuries are relatively constant. An exception is the wrist and finger function remaining after combined middle and lower truncal damage. In addition, lower trunk loss sometimes involves more than hand intrinsic muscle and ulnar distribution sensory loss. The pattern of loss for a single spinal nerve can also vary, especially for C6, C7, and C8. Divisional-level injury can also give variable patterns of loss, depending on which truncal outflows are involved and the proportion of anterior and posterior division loss.

The differentiation of trapezius, serratus anterior, and rhomboid loss by a thorough clinical examination of the upper back and shoulders is very important, as is testing for supraspinatus, infraspinatus, and latissimus dorsi loss. The clinician's understanding of plexus anatomy, its variations and response to injury, is tested by the necessity of ordering the appropriate diagnostic tests and placing them in context with the clinical examination. Electromyographic sampling of proximal muscles such as paraspinals, rhomboids, serratus anterior, and spinati is of help, as are carefully done sensory conduction studies if preganglionic injury is suspected. Denervational changes may persist for months after clinical contraction of a muscle is evident in recovery. By comparison, a muscle such as the deltoid or biceps may show some nascent or early reinnervational activity in the early months after injury and yet never gain enough new input to restore useful contraction. Plain film radiographic studies may show humeral, clavicular, scapular, rib, or spine fractures, which sometimes helps the clinician weigh the severity and level of the injury. Of even greater potential importance is the use of myelography for evaluation of plexus stretch injuries (including anterior-posterior, lateral, and oblique views), in spite of possible false-positive or false-negative studies. Computed axial tomographic scan myelography may miss meningoceles or other root abnormalities because it is based on transverse cuts. The magnetic resonance imaging scan has difficulty displaying all of each root and spinal nerve at all of the levels necessary for adequate evaluation of brachial plexus injuries. This deficit will most likely be corrected in the future.

## SURGICAL ANATOMY

The brachial plexus originates at the level of the spine and usually includes the C5, C6, C7, C8, and T1 spinal nerves, the three trunks of the plexus, and their anterior and posterior divisions. Spinal nerves and trunks are supraclavicular, whereas divisions tend to lie beneath the clavicle. Lateral, posterior, and medial cords are infraclavicular, as are their origins for the major nerves of the upper extremity (Figure 12–1).

## Spinal Nerves

Several texts have thoroughly summarized the anatomy of the roots or spinal nerves as well as their variations.[4,17,21,22,26,34,45] A thorough exposition of anatomy and physiology was provided by Wilbourn.[44] Summarized as well was the literature available on some of the nonsurgical conditions responsible for brachial plexopathy, such as neuralgic amyotrophy, athletic "burners or stingers" affecting the plexus, and rucksack paralysis. We have selected the most

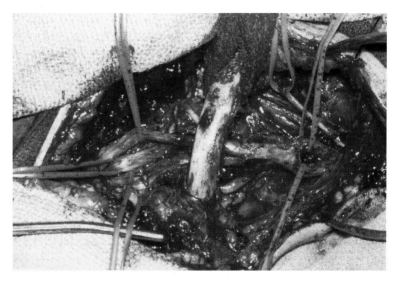

**Figure 12-1.** View of left plexus from the side of the neck and shoulder. Supraclavicular plexus is to the right of the clavicle and infraclavicular plexus is to the left. Right lower two loops are on C5 and C6 spinal nerves, and upper right loop is on the phrenic nerve. Left loops are on, from top to bottom, lateral, medial, and posterior cords. Sponges are around the clavicle so it can be moved up or down during the dissection.

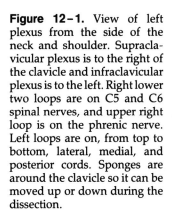

useful surgical information from these sources as well as from our own experience.

Each individual spinal nerve or root of the plexus originates as multiple sensory rootlets from the dorsal root entry zone of the posterolateral sector of the spinal cord and usually as one ventral or motor rootlet from the ventrolateral portion of the cord. The dorsal rootlets combine, usually at the entrance of the intervertebral foramen, to form one dorsal root per spinal segment. At the same time, the anterior or motor root enters the foramen. The foraminal course of the rootlets varies between 10 and 16

mm (Figure 12-2). The dorsal root ganglion is located at an intraforaminal level and usually at its midpoint. Shortly distal to this, the anterior and posterior roots blend together to form the spinal nerve. Then, posterior primary branches go to the paraspinal muscles and a larger anterior branch contributes to the brachial plexus.

Spinal nerve is not tethered within the intervertebral foramen but is bound by attachments to the cervical transverse processes.[40] Dura changes to epineurium and is continuous with it within the foramen, and the arachnoid usually ends close to or on the posterior root ganglia.

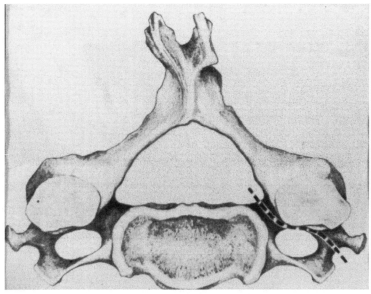

**Figure 12-2.** Intraforaminal course of spinal nerve *(dotted line)*. Nerve lies posterior to foramen transversarium, which contains vertebral artery. Note that intraforaminal course of the spinal nerve is considerable. (Adapted from Sunderland S: Nerve and Nerve Injuries, 2nd Ed. Edinburgh, E. Livingstone, 1984.)

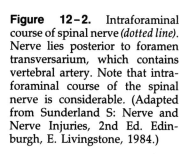

Vertebral artery originates from subclavian artery and travels superiorly to enter the foramen transversarium of C6 and to run through those of C5, C4, C3, and C2. The artery lies anterior to the spinal nerves at these levels. Small branches from this vessel supply the spinal nerves and anastomose with spinal cord vasculature. Vertebral branches also anastomose with branches from ascending cervical, deep cervical, and superior intercostal arteries.[1,18]

Within the foramen, the C5 spinal nerve gives rise to a dorsal scapular nerve branch, which supplies the rhomboids. In addition, a branch to form long thoracic nerve, along with C6, C7, and even occasionally C8 exits the foramen posterior to the spinal nerve. The caliber of C5 is usually smaller than that of the other spinal nerves. Exposure requires soft tissue dissection high in the neck. Descending cervical plexus must be mobilized and moved away, as must phrenic nerve. Small arteries and veins cross the root or travel with it as it exits the foramen and they must be coagulated. Dissection into the foramen requires resection of origins of the anterior scalene and resection of some of the transverse process of the fifth cervical vertebra (Figure 12–3). The extraforaminal course of C5 is along the lateral edge of the anterior scalene, and sometimes the nerve may be partially embedded in it. C4 may make a small contribution to the plexus. Rarely, this may be substantial and thus represent a prefixed plexus.

C6 has a slightly longer intraforaminal course than C5 but a shorter extraforaminal course before blending with C5 to form the upper trunk[26] (Figure 12–4). The extraforaminal course of C6 is somewhat oblique posterior to the anterior scalene. It joins C5 at the lateral edge of the anterior scalene to form the upper trunk of the plexus. Most frequently, long thoracic nerve arises from the dorsal surface of the distal portion of C6. Branches contribute to this nerve also from C5 and C7 and sometimes C8 as well as C4. Nerve is usually posterior to the junction of C6 to upper trunk and dives downward to penetrate and course through the middle scalene.

The intraforaminal portion of the C7 spinal nerve is 12 to 15 mm in length. Extraforaminal C7 spinal nerve has the straightest course of any of the spinal nerves of the plexus, and it blends imperceptibly into the middle trunk with little to differentiate the two (Figure 12–5). C7 lies posterior to the medial edge of the anterior scalene and may be adherent to it. C8 has an intraforaminal course of 10 to 15 mm; after exiting its foramen, C8 combines with T1 to form lower trunk.

The course of C8 is slightly oblique, and this root is usually larger in caliber than either T1 or C7. Its extraforaminal extent is relatively short, for it blends with T1 to form the lower trunk. It lies on top of the middle and posterior scalene muscles, and in some cases is covered by Sibson fascia, which extends from the transverse processes of the seventh cervical and sometimes the sixth cervical vertebra to the apical pleura. C8 root is closely covered by or accompanied by

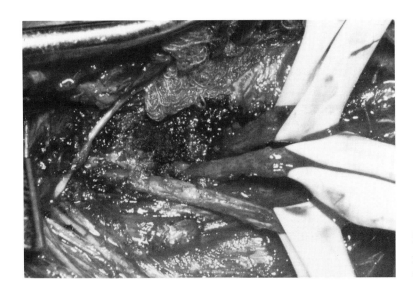

**Figure 12–3.** Dissection of spinal nerves into foramina. The bipolar coagulator and Oxycel cotton is used to control bleeding at these levels. Penrose drains are around distal spinal nerves. Foramina of spinal nerves are to the left. The descending cervical plexus is seen at lower lefthand corner.

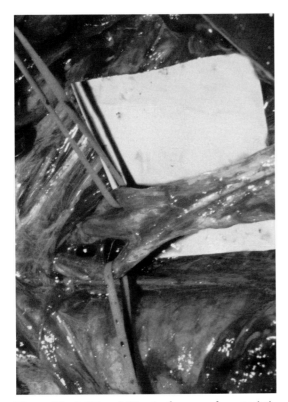

**Figure 12–4.** C5 and C6 spinal nerves characteristically combine to form the upper trunk. This is a useful landmark in supraclavicular and proximal plexus surgery. This patient had an additional major contribution to upper trunk from C4 (encircled by lower plastic loop), forming a prefixed brachial plexus.

arterioles and venules or small veins, and the vertebral artery is close by.

After a relatively short intraforaminal course, T1 exits its foramen and takes a transverse and somewhat curvilinear course laterally to meet C8. Both of these spinal nerves form the lower trunk (Figure 12–6). It is at this level that rami communicantes are most likely seen coming and going from spinal nerve. These rami and their ganglia form the cervical sympathetic chain, whose largest ganglion is usually found posterior to the vertebral artery close to the latter's takeoff from the subclavian artery.

## Trunks

The upper and middle trunks are the most readily identified portions of the supraclavicular plexus. The upper trunk is usually adherent to and sometimes partially covered by the anterior scalene muscle. With injury, sharp dissection is necessary along the medial edge of the trunk to dissect it away from the anterior scalene (Figure 12–7). Lateral dissection of the trunk is usually easier. As one proceeds distally along the lateral edge of the trunk, suprascapular nerve is encountered arising from the dorsolateral surface of the distal upper trunk, just as it forms anterior and posterior divisions more an-

**Figure 12–5.** Exposure of proximal left supraclavicular plexus viewed from the side. Anterior scalene has been resected. Lower Penrose drain is around the C5 spinal nerve and the proximal portion of the phrenic nerve. C6 is superior to this, and it's junction with C5 to form the upper trunk is readily seen. The phrenic nerve is also encircled by a plastic loop at the top left. The upper Penrose drain is around the junction of C7 to middle trunk. Nerve to subclavius muscle can be seen arising from the superior surface of the upper trunk (*left*) and taking its usual oblique course to the subclavius muscle.

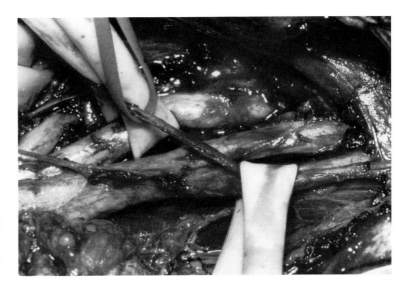

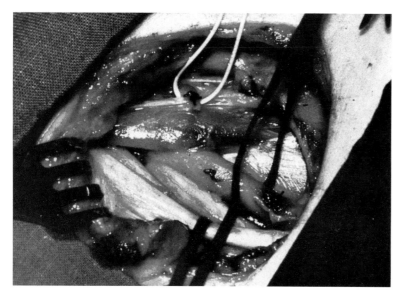

**Figure 12-6.** The right phrenic nerve is easily seen anterior to the scalenus anticus (white plastic loop). The right subclavian artery and plexus, however, are inclined at a much steeper angle than normal, so that the artery and lower trunk run upward and medially rather than in a more horizontal trajectory. Dark loop *(top right)* is around subclavian artery, whereas, bottom right, loop is around lower trunk. This was associated with a large cervical rib that displaced these structures laterally.

teriorly. In some cases, an anteriorly located branch to subclavius arises from the middle part of the upper trunk to run medially and somewhat obliquely to the subclavius muscle. Truncal divisions vary somewhat in their relation to the clavicle, depending on the positioning of the shoulder, neck, and head on the operating table. Some exposure of these structures is helped by placing folded sheets beneath the shoulder. The head is turned somewhat toward the opposite

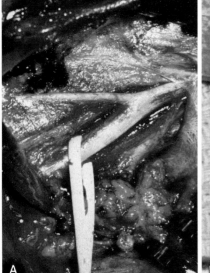
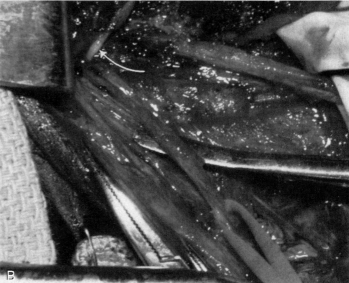

**Figure 12-7.** *(A)* Tracing this left phrenic nerve upward or posteriorly as it lies behind the prevertebral fascia on the front of scalenus anticus leads the surgeon to the C5 spinal nerve and upper trunk (surrounded by white plastic loop). This may be a useful maneuver in a heavily scarred plexus, because the locus of the C5 spinal nerve then defines the plane between scalenus anticus and medius. Dissecting downward in that plane defines the remaining spinal nerves of origin of the brachial plexus. The surgeon often has to dissect the C5 spinal nerve proximal to its contribution to the phrenic, and this is accomplished by dividing the muscle fibers of the scalenus anticus to reveal the anterior tubercles of the transverse processes of the C4 and C5 vertebrae. *(B)* Cervical plexus (beneath double-ended forceps) is seen coursing down in an oblique fashion from the region of the right C5 nerve root, whereas phrenic nerve *(arrow)* courses obliquely in a superior direction. If the surgeon tracks these branches proximally, their origin from C3 and C4 spinal nerve can be found. These branches can be used as lead-outs for some neurotization.

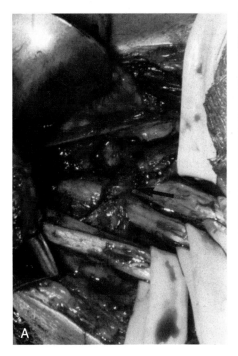
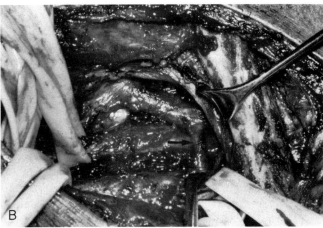

**Figure 12–8.** *(A)* Deep supraclavicular arterial and venous complex *(arrow)* originating from or terminating in subclavian vessels. These vessels cross left lower trunk *(below arrow)* and middle trunk *(below arrow)* to course beneath divisions of upper trunk *(bottom)*. Such vessels can bleed vigorously unless they are coagulated or tied off. *(B)* Subclavicular view of deep arterial origin of supraclavicular vessel *(arrow)* from subclavian artery. Clavicle is retracted superiorly by vein retractor.

side and elevated slightly above the chest level.[19] Sizable arterial and venous branches originating from or draining to subclavian vessels cross beneath the upper trunk divisions and are sometimes adherent to one or more of these elements (Figure 12–8). These constantly encountered vessels usually run across the distal middle trunk or its divisions and need to be either ligated or coagulated and divided for a complete dissection at both of these levels.

The middle trunk is found beneath the ante-rior scalene and is often covered by some muscular connections between the anterior and medial scalene or with scar tissue resulting from injury (Figure 12–9). The middle trunk is usually smaller in caliber than either the upper or lower trunk.

The distal middle trunk may on occasion blend into or be quite adherent to either the distal upper or the lower trunk, or occasionally to both. The posterior division of the middle trunk is usually relatively short and combines with

**Figure 12–9.** This dissection shows C7 to middle trunk exposed after resection of the anterior scalene muscle. Penrose drain is around the posterior division of this trunk just before it blends in with that of the upper trunk. Subclavian artery and origin of vertebral artery are seen superiorly. C5 and C6 (plastic loops) and upper trunk are seen inferiorly.

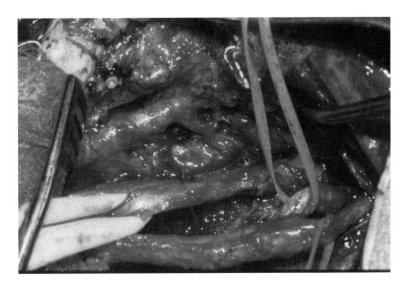

posterior divisions from upper and lower trunks to form posterior cord distal to the clavicle. The middle trunk anterior division combines with that from the upper trunk to form lateral cord, which, as a cord element, is usually formed before posterior cord but not as proximally as the medial cord.

The lower trunk is usually relatively short and lies somewhat behind the subclavian artery (Figure 12 – 10). Exposure is helped by skeletonizing enough of the inferior surface of the subclavian artery so that it can be gently elevated by a vein retractor. Metzenbaum scissors are then used to clear the medial edge of the lower trunk and proximal medial cord away from the vessel. This trunk is usually crossed by the same sizable artery and vein that involve more lateral middle and upper trunk divisions. Medially, vertebral artery ascends anterior to the level of the trunk and usually anterior to the T1 spinal nerve.

The posterior division of the lower trunk quickly blends with those divisions from the other trunks to help form posterior cord.[45] The bulk of the lower trunk proceeds directly through its anterior division to form the medial cord.

## Divisions

Although each trunk has an anterior and a posterior division as outlined above, they can blend with other divisions before forming cords (Figure 12 – 11). Sometimes one or more divisions trade back and forth several times.[42] In addition, the site at which cords begin distal to the clavicle can vary somewhat from patient to patient.

Separating divisions in cases in which there has been a stretch injury, gunshot wound, or prior vascular dissection can be quite difficult. The surgeon must work from trunks in a distal direction and cords in a proximal one to expose the divisions. By passing two moist and strung out $2 \times 4$ sponges beneath the clavicle with the help of a Munyon or curved hemostat, the clavicle can be shifted up or down. Subclavius muscle is sectioned or, more commonly, has a segment resected. If subclavicular vessels which run beneath the clavicle have not been ligated during the supraclavicular dissection, they are ligated or coagulated.

## Cords

These are named in relation to the axillary artery at the level of pectoralis minor (Figure 12 – 12). Lateral cord is usually superficial to the artery and is the first major neural element encountered as one begins dissection in the infraclavicular region. It tends to run somewhat obliquely over the artery from a medial to a lateral direction but sometimes is entirely lateral to the artery. It terminates in a contribution to the median nerve and an oblique takeoff running laterally to form the musculocutaneous nerve.

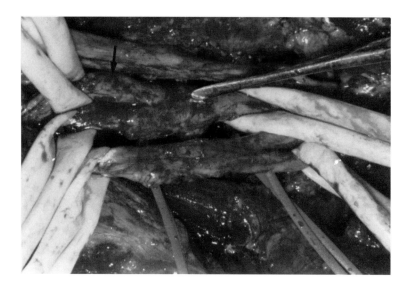

**Figure 12 – 10.** Exposure of left lower trunk (arrow) after mobilization of upper and middle trunks, which have been displaced laterally by Penrose drains.

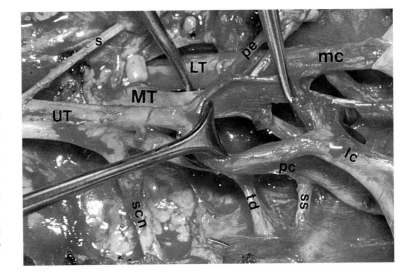

**Figure 12-11.** In this case, clavicle has been sectioned to expose divisions of trunks. lc = lateral cord; LT = lower trunk; mc = medial cord; MT = middle trunk; pc = posterior cord; pe = pectoral branches; s = nerve to subclavius; scn = suprascapular nerve; ss = subscapular (upper) nerve; td = thoracodorsal; UT = upper trunk.

The latter dives quickly into biceps/brachialis but usually gives off one or more coracobrachialis branches first.

The posterior cord is deep or posterior to axillary artery (Figure 12-13). A relatively small branch, the thoracodorsal, runs from its dorsal or posterior aspect almost directly posteriorly to supply the latissimus dorsi. The cord then divides into its two major branches, the axillary and the radial nerves. Several subscapular branches usually arise from the posterior cord or axillary take-off and run inferiorly and obliquely. After coursing inferiorly and slightly laterally, the axillary nerve dives down to reach quadrilateral space and eventually the deltoid muscle. The other posterior cord outflow is the radial nerve, which runs inferiorly towards the humeral groove to wind around the humerus. It passes over and sometimes through the leaves of the subscapularis muscle.[34] A very important anatomic landmark is the medial relation between the radial nerve and the profundus branch of the axillary artery. This can be used to locate the proximal radial and differentiate it from the more lateral axillary nerve.[24] It is especially important to maintain the profundus branch with either more proximal axillary or more distal brachial arterial occlusion.

Dissection in this area is difficult and requires patience. Care must be taken not to place severe

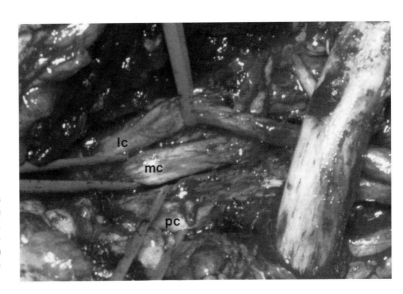

**Figure 12-12.** The three cords of the plexus. Lateral cord (lc) has been retracted superiorly, medial cord (mc) somewhat laterally, and posterior cord (pc) inferiorly and laterally. Clavicle is to the right.

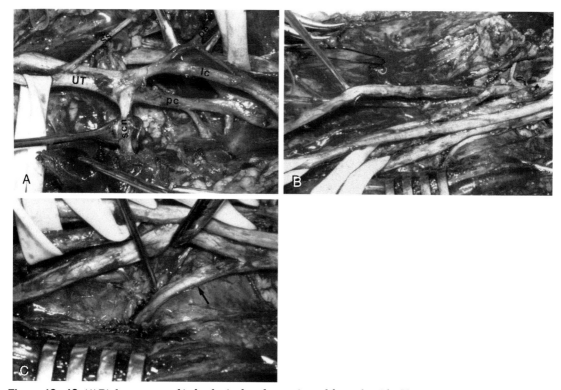

**Figure 12 – 13.** *(A)* Right supra- and infraclavicular plexus viewed from the side. Upper Penrose drain is around medial cord. Note rather lengthy lateral cord contribution to median. In this case, musculocutaneous nerve had a distal origin from the median complex. lc = lateral cord; pc = posterior cord; pe = medial pectoral branches; scn = suprascapular nerve; ss = subclavius branch; UT = upper trunk. *(B)* Infraclavicular plexus at a subclavicular level. Penrose to the far left is around distal median nerve. Penrose to the left of center is around axillary artery. Beneath or inferior to this Penrose is the radial nerve. Vein retractor is elevating ulnar nerve. *(C)* Closer view of course of axillary nerve *(arrow)* into quadrilateral space. Radial nerve is held slightly superiorly by the tips of the Metzenbaum scissors.

retraction against biceps/brachialis because musculocutaneous nerve runs a parallel but hidden course beneath the biceps muscle. If self-retaining retractors are to be used in this area, it is best to clear musculocutaneous nerve through upper biceps. Nerve can then be retracted anteriorly and laterally so that self-retaining retractors can be safely placed. Dissection also needs to extend around axillary and upper brachial artery and around the profundus branch. This permits their retraction so that the relation between the cords and nerves in this area can be adequately worked out. Variations are frequently found in the formation of musculocutaneous nerve and lateral cord branches to median and also in their relationship to medial cord branches to median.[21,22]

Lateral to axillary vein and somewhat in-

ferior to it is the medial cord, and, with injury, nerve can be quite adherent to vein. This requires careful dissection because holes in the vein are usually harder to repair than those in artery.

Medial cord sends a major contribution to median nerve which wraps around the medial and superior side of the axillary artery. On occasion, this contribution to median passes beneath the artery.[31] As this contribution is given off, so are the ulnar nerve and the lateral and medial antebrachial branches. These neural structures remain medial to brachial artery as they begin their descent down the upper arm. Stretch injury can change the positions of trunks, cords, and nerves and their proximal to distal positions in relation to the usual anatomic landmarks of the arm.

## CLINICAL EXAMINATION

A comprehensive clinical evaluation begins with an assessment of the shoulders, neck, and high back from behind with the patient erect. One can readily spot asymmetry of the shoulder girdles, dropped shoulder, or laterally rotated scapula.[2,15,36] In addition, the parascapular area is inspected for rhomboid atrophy, winging of the scapula, or atrophy of supraspinatus, infraspinatus, or deltoid. The mechanics of shoulder abduction and internal and external rotation of the upper arm can be viewed from behind, as can the response of latissimus dorsi to a deep cough.[38] If there is a question of diaphragmatic paralysis, the chest can be percussed from behind, matching inspiratory tympany with that on expiration. Then, standing at the patient's side, one can recheck internal and external rotation of the arm as well as adduction of the arm by the pectoralis and other muscles. Biceps/brachialis and brachioradialis can then be tested as forearm flexors and triceps as a forearm extensor. With the arm fully extended at the elbow, pronation and supination are tested, and then wrist extension and flexion.

Hand muscle function is best tested with both the subject and the examiner seated and facing one another. The patient's hands can be placed palm up on the knees for finger flexion testing and palm down on the knees or on a flat surface to test for extension. Each hand can then be held and manipulated to test for fine muscle hand intrinsic function, presence or absence of sweating, and sensory testing.

## DORSAL SCAPULAR NERVE PALSY

The function of the dorsal scapular nerve is to innervate muscles that pull the medial edge of the scapula upward and toward the midline (Figures 12–14 and 12–15). Injury to this nerve results in atrophy and weakness of the rhomboideus major and minor and can be observed as absence of bulk medial to the scapula and between that structure and the thoracic spinal col-

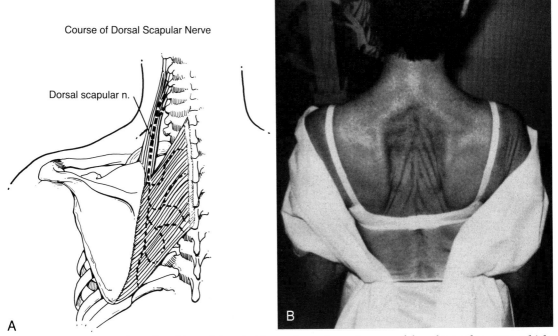

Course of Dorsal Scapular Nerve

Dorsal scapular n.

A

B

**Figure 12–14.** (A) Drawing of position of rhomboid muscles and usual course of dorsal scapular nerve, which arises from proximal C5 and C6 spinal nerves. Proximal course of dorsal scapular nerve is parallel to that of levator scapulae, which runs from cervical spine to superior and medial scapula. (B) Patient with bilateral rhomboid paralysis. (B, courtesy of Dr Michael Lusk, Naples, FL.)

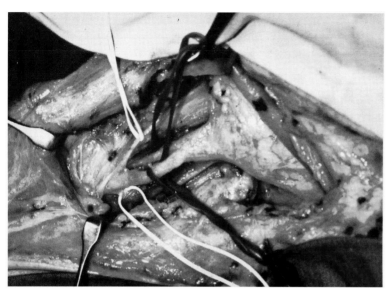

**Figure 12-15.** The right phrenic nerve has been dissected and mobilized (upper white plastic loop). This leads the surgeon to C5 and thence to C6 (dark plastic loops). This latter spinal nerve is attenuated as it flows over the edge of the transverse process. A proximal branch of C5 is the nerve to rhomboid (lower white plastic loop). Clinically, the patient had normal rhomboid function but no deltoid or biceps power. Supraspinatus and infraspinatus were paralyzed. Intraoperative stimulation of the phrenic nerve resulted in diaphragmatic contraction. As expected, stimulation of proximal C5 caused rhomboid and levator scapulae contraction, thus proving the integrity of the more proximal C5 spinal nerve. Somatosensory-evoked potentials could not be recorded by stimulating C6. Nerve action potentials could not be evoked by stimulating proximal upper trunk and recording from lateral and posterior cords. The massive neuroma (*on right*) of the distal upper trunk was therefore resected, and grafts were led from C5 to musculocutaneous and axillary nerves. A distal branch of cranial nerve XI was attached to the suprascapular nerve by a short graft. Two years later, the patient had 50% recovery of shoulder abduction and elbow flexion.

umn. It is most noticeable when the subject braces his or her shoulders as if at military attention. Another method of testing rhomboids is to have the patient place hands on hips and push back against pressure on one or both elbows. Loss produces some winging, lateral and slight downward displacement of the scapula, and a slightly awkward abduction of the shoulder. This abduction difficulty is, however, not as awkward as that seen with serratus anterior or trapezius paralysis. Because the nerve arises from the proximal intraforaminal portion of C5 and sometimes C6, loss of function from injury implies damage to the root or spinal nerve close to the spinal canal.

Levator scapulae runs between the transverse processes of the cervical vertebrae superiorly and the superior and medial angle of the scapula inferiorly (see Figure 12-15). This muscle receives neural input from C3, C4, and C5 and is usually spared with most plexus injuries and, of course, with accessory palsy. Thus, some ability to elevate the shoulder is usually present even with severe plexus or accessory palsy.

## LONG THORACIC NERVE PALSY

The long thoracic nerve arises from the proximal portions of the spinal nerves and innervates serratus anterior, which pulls scapula away from the midline and forward on the posterior chest area (Figures 12-16 and 12-17). This paralysis gives severe winging of the scapula, both at rest and with the shoulder flexed and the elbow fully extended. The latter is true whether the hand and arm push forward with the elbow flexed or with the elbow fully extended.[15] This differentiates it from the winging associated with spinal trapezius paralysis, in which winging is minimal when the elbow is fully extended and hand and arm push forward against resistance. With serratus anterior palsy, abduction of the shoulder is not smooth, particularly above the horizontal. If damaged in association with root or spinal nerve injury, long thoracic nerve palsy implies a very proximal loss.[29] This is particularly so for lesions involving C5, C6, and even C7, as well as C4 if it provides input to the long thoracic nerve.

Course of Long Thoracic Nerve

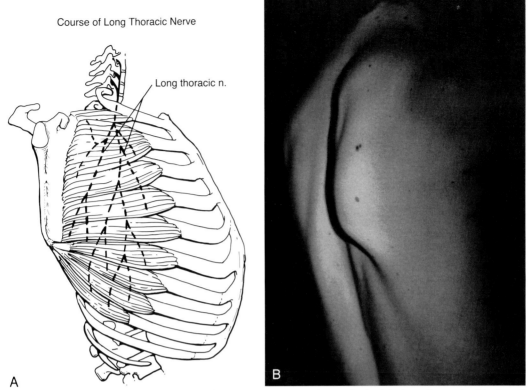

Long thoracic n.

A

B

**Figure 12–16.** *(A)* Lateral view of course of long thoracic nerve beneath clavicle (not shown in this drawing) and then over the lateral rib cage, where it branches at many levels to supply the serratus anterior. *(B)* Patient with long thoracic palsy and protrusion or winging of the right scapula.

## PALSY OF ACCESSORY (ELEVENTH CRANIAL) NERVE

Trapezius not only forms the posterior bulwark of the shoulder region, but its spinal portion provides major dorsal and medial support for the scapula. Muscle fibers used for shrugging the shoulder or pulling up the scapula can be roughly divided into medial, intermediate, and lateral divisions. Some accessory nerve lesions lateral to the sternocleidomastoid branch

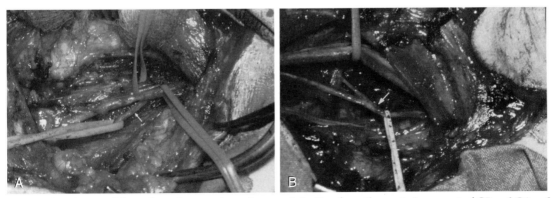

**Figure 12–17.** *(A)* Left long thoracic nerve *(arrow)* seen originating from the posterior aspect of C5 and C6 and running obliquely and posteriorly beneath upper trunk. Nerve then courses into the middle scalene muscle. *(B)* Bifid origin of a right long thoracic nerve *(arrow and white plastic loop)*. Upper trunk is retracted superiorly by the dark plastic loop.

may spare medial nerve or fibers, at times even some intermediate fibers, but always paralyze the lateral ones. The shoulder tends to drop or be carried lower than the contralateral normal shoulder. At times, the patient overcompensates and carries the injured shoulder higher than the normal one. Distance between the tip of the shoulder and the midline of the body usually appears shorter on the paralyzed side. With spinal segment loss of accessory nerve, the scapula wings and usually moves laterally with attempted abduction. The latter motion is unwieldy for the patient. Without the help of the spinal trapezius, abduction of the arm above the horizontal is difficult.

Unlike the winging seen with serratus palsy, that seen with loss of spinal trapezius is brought out best by having the patient push forward or across the chest with the elbow bent or partially flexed as opposed to pushing forward with the elbow fully extended.[36] The mechanics of shoulder abduction are severely affected by accessory paralysis. Some patients learn to substitute by rolling the forearm into a pronated position as abduction reaches the horizontal level. Despite loss of the whole trapezius, some elevation of the scapula and thus shrug of the shoulder can be gained through use of the levator scapula muscle, which runs from the superior border of the scapula to the lower cervical spinous processes.

It is rare to see paralysis of the sternocleidomastoid muscle as part of an accessory palsy. This is because branches to this large neck muscle come off proximally from the accessory nerve and run beneath that muscle to innervate it. These branches are deep and medial and are protected from most penetrating iatrogenic or spontaneous injuries. In addition, sternocleidomastoid muscle is also supplied by branches from C2, C3, and C4 spinal nerves. Further information about this important nerve is provided in the chapter devoted to it.

## SUPRASCAPULAR NERVE PALSY

The suprascapular nerve supplies both supraspinatus and infraspinatus and originates from the upper trunk of the plexus (Figure 12 – 18). The supraspinatus is readily observable along the superior border of the spine of the scapula. This muscle provides the first 20 to 30 degrees of abduction of the shoulder. This is best tested with the elbow fully extended. It works in concert with deltoid and parascapular muscles to provide shoulder abduction. If the deltoid is paralyzed, supraspinatus can be tested with gravity eliminated by placing the patient supine and asking the patient to attempt to abduct the outstretched arm away from the side. The infraspinatus is a large muscle located below or inferior to the spine of the scapula. It is the principal external rotator of the shoulder and thus the upper arm. External rotation is tested by flexing the patient's forearm at the elbow and holding the tip of the elbow against the patient's side, and asking him or her to externally rotate the

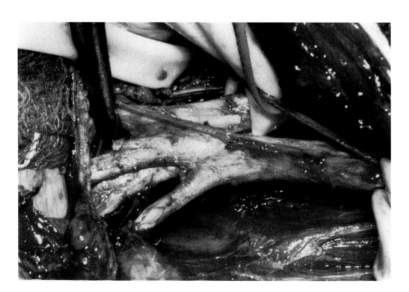

**Figure 12 – 18.** More distal left supraclavicular plexus showing origin of supraclavicular nerve and the anterior and posterior divisions of the upper trunk just to the right of the clavicle. Dissector is beneath the more distal middle trunk. Small caliber nerve at top is the phrenic; beneath or inferior to this lies nerve to subclavius muscle.

forearm and thus the humerus and shoulder joint laterally.

## AXILLARY NERVE PALSY

The axillary nerve arises from the posterior cord as it gives rise to the radial nerve (Figure 12–19; also see Figure 12–13C). The major input of this nerve is to the deltoid. Atrophy of this large and somewhat complex shoulder muscle is readily apparent on inspection, as is the dropped position of the head of the humerus. Loss affects abduction of the arm especially beyond 30 degrees from the horizontal. Motor loss may or may not be accompanied by sensory change over the cap of the shoulder. Sensory change is usually present in the relatively acute injury. Within a few weeks to months, descending cervical plexus fibers sprout or branch to supply sensation in this area, so that over time, loss, if present, is relative rather than absolute. With incomplete axillary nerve involvement or partial regeneration of the nerve to muscle, some deltoid contraction may be evident by inspection or palpation. Even a little function requires a good bit of reinnervation before the deltoid can overcome gravity, let alone pressure applied to the upper arm as abduction beyond 30 degrees is attempted.[30] Sometimes, the muscle mass of anterior deltoid contracts and yet the intermediate or posterior

muscle mass is poor. In this regard, some patients can substitute for lack of this muscle by initiating abduction by a well-developed supraspinatus and then using shoulder rotators as well as the long head of the biceps to gain a good deal of forward abduction of the arm.[42] Under these circumstances, the contracting biceps tendon is discernable and palpation of the deltoid itself shows it to be flaccid or to have minimal contraction.

With partial recovery, it is important to test the three major segments of the muscle — anterior, middle, and posterior. For example, it is difficult to gain coordinated recovery of the posterior deltoid muscle mass, and this must be tested by having the patient abduct the arm somewhat behind the plane of the body. Muscle must be not only inspected but palpated as the patient attempts to contract it, and this is best done with the patient standing or sitting erect in a chair.

## THORACODORSAL NERVE PALSY

The latissimus dorsi is one of the major adductors of the shoulder. The latissimus also extends the shoulder and medially rotates the arm. This large muscle innervated by the thoracodorsal nerve can also be palpated from behind (Figure 12–20). A deep cough should

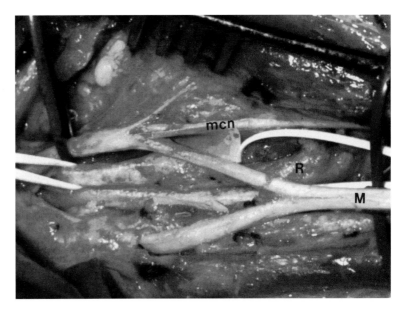

**Figure 12–19.** The medial (motor) and lateral (sensory) heads of the left median nerve (M) embrace the axillary artery. Tracing the lateral head proximally brings the operator to the origin of the musculocutaneous nerve (mcn) and a small twig destined for coracobrachialis. This patient suffered a posterior cord injury with loss of axillary and radial function. Plastic loops are passed above and below the neuroma in continuity involving posterior canal. Proximal portion of radial nerve (R) is still covered by scar. Origin of axillary nerve can be seen below the white loop, to the left.

Course of Thoracodorsal Nerve

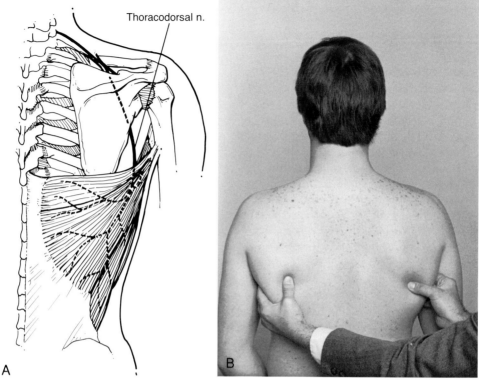

Thoracodorsal n.

A

B

**Figure 12–20.** *(A)* Course of the thoracodorsal nerve which originates from posterior cord of plexus and then travels inferiorly to innervate latissimus dorsi. *(B)* Testing patient for latissimus dorsi palsy. Because this is a branch of the posterior cord, a patient with wrist drop but intact latissimus has a lesion in radial nerve rather than posterior cord.

make it contract, and it is useful to place both hands on these muscles bilaterally and compare contraction. Another method of testing this muscle is to place the patient's extended and laterally abducted arm on the examiner's shoulder and ask the patient to push down on it. Muscle can be seen contracting in the posterior axillary fold, particularly the lower portion of the fold. Teres major resides in the high axillary fold and also serves as an adductor; it is innervated by proximal subscapularis branches of the posterior cord, axillary, or radial nerves. The three adductors of the arm are pectoralis, latissimus dorsi, and teres major.

and palpated as the elbow is brought down forcibly or against pressure to the side. The clavicular head is best tested by having the patient push down from a horizontal and anterior position of the arm with the elbow flexed.

After inspecting and testing these muscles, the examiner's attention is directed to the front of the patient's body. The neck is also inspected and palpated. Associated findings such as Horner syndrome, including ptosis, enophthalmos, miosis, or, less frequently, facial palsy should be looked for.[48] Scars in supraclavicular, infraclavicular, and axillary spaces should be inspected and palpated.

## PALSY INVOLVING PECTORALIS

This major large muscle has several segments or heads. The bulk of the muscle adducts the arm to the side of the chest and can be observed

## C5 SPINAL NERVE OR ROOT

Very proximal involvement of this nerve paralyzes rhomboids and weakens serratus anterior, so these functions should be tested as previously outlined. The C5 nerve supplies most of the suprascapular nerve's input to supraspinatus and infraspinatus. The latter muscle may also receive a little input from C6, so it may not be totally paralyzed with a C5 root lesion. Certainly, the deltoid muscle is paralyzed, because it almost always receives exclusive input from this spinal nerve. Sensory loss may be present over the cap or tip of the shoulder. Again, input or sprouting from the cervical plexus usually lessens this sensory deficit. Biceps/brachialis may also be weak, although this is a partial loss because C6 supplies this function as well.

## C6 SPINAL NERVE OR ROOT

This root provides input to biceps/brachialis, a function it shares with the C5 root. This muscle is best tested with the hand fully supinated so as to reduce elbow flexion by the brachioradialis. Tendon is seen to tighten over the flexor surface of the elbow, and the contracting muscle belly is most prominent at the midhumeral level. This root also supplies brachioradialis, which is a strong flexor of the elbow, especially when the hand is halfway between pronation and supination. It can be readily observed and palpated on the lateral aspect of the proximal forearm and elbow. C6 also supplies the supinator, a muscle deeply located in the proximal third of the forearm. Because biceps can also provide supination, true supinator function

should be tested by first extending or straightening out the elbow completely. The patient's hand is then placed in a pronated position and held by the examiner as the patient attempts to supinate it or turn it palm up. C6 can also supply some of the triceps, although the major input to this muscle is from C7. Outflow from C6, as from most of the roots, also contributes to the pectoralis, which is the major adductor of the arm. Latissimus dorsi, another adductor, is also weak or totally paralyzed with a C6 lesion.

Because upper trunk is formed by C5 and C6, loss with a complete lesion of this element includes loss to supraspinatus, infraspinatus, deltoid, latissimus dorsi, biceps/brachialis, brachioradialis and supinator. Partial lesions often produce loss of deltoid, whereas biceps/brachialis may be weak but not totally paralyzed. Variations at this level affecting function of muscles such as biceps or deltoid are much less common than at an infraclavicular level (Figure 12–21).

## C7 SPINAL NERVE AND MIDDLE TRUNK

The C7 root or spinal nerve forms all of the middle trunk, most of whose fibers go to the radial portion of the posterior cord through the posterior division. These fibers supply most of the triceps. This large muscle extends the forearm on upper arm. The examiner can gently

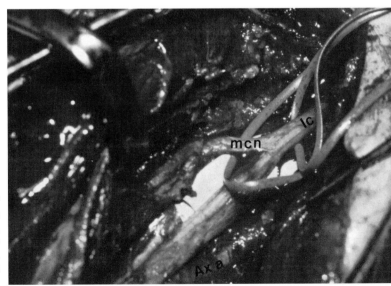

**Figure 12–21.** Origin of right musculocutaneous nerve (mcn) from lateral cord (lc). Axillary artery (Ax a) is seen inferior to median nerve, which was formed in part by the lc after it gave off the mcn.

grasp the muscle belly on the posterior upper arm and resist extension of the forearm with the opposite hand. To eliminate gravity for testing of this muscle as well as biceps, the patient can be placed supine and flexion and extension of the forearm gently resisted. Fibers from the posterior division of the middle trunk may also provide input to extensor carpi radialis, and sometimes to extensor carpi ulnaris as well. These muscles dorsiflex the wrist. The extensor carpi radialis does this in a radial direction and extensor carpi ulnaris in an ulnar direction. C7 may also provide some fibers to extensor communis or extensor pollicis longus, or both. Because of this, one or more digits may be weak or paralyzed in extension.

Nerve fibers going to the anterior division of the middle trunk are carried to the lateral cord and can supply the pronator teres as well as wrist and finger flexors. Loss in this distribution varies with C7 or middle trunk injury. C7 contributes primarily to muscles supplied by one or more other roots, so isolated injury to C7 often leads only to paresis rather than paralysis and may on occasion produce no discernable loss.

The pronator teres is tested with the elbow extended, holding the hand in a supinated position and rotating it against resistance into a palm down position. Wrist flexion and finger flexion can readily be tested but should be separated as to flexor superficialis and flexor profundus input.

## C8 SPINAL NERVE

Finger and thumb extensors as well as flexors to wrist and fingers receive input from this important root. It also supplies a variable amount of input to hand intrinsic muscles, sharing this function with the T1 root. Loss usually includes weakness or paralysis of extensors to thumb, forefinger, and long finger. Flexor profundi to the latter two digits are weak or paralyzed. Intrinsics are weak or paralyzed, especially thenar intrinsics such as abductor pollicis brevis and opponens pollicis. Testing procedures for these muscles are found in the chapters entitled "Ulnar Nerve" and "Median Nerve." Sensory loss or decrease is in the ulnar distribution and may involve the ring finger and even the little finger.

## T1 SPINAL NERVE

This root supplies hand intrinsics, especially those of the hypothenar eminence. This includes the abductor digiti quinti minimi and opponens digiti quinti minimi. Interossei, lumbricals, and adductor pollicis are weak or absent. Flexor profundi to the little and ring fingers may also be weak unless there is a predominant C8 input to these muscles. C8 is, however, more likely to supply flexor profundus input to the forefinger and long finger. The sensory field is again that of the little finger and sometimes the ring finger but may include skin over the hypothenar eminence and even sensory decrease on the ulnar side of the forearm.

## LOWER TRUNK

The anterior division of the lower trunk goes to the medial cord, which provides all of the ulnar nerve and input to the median nerve, especially to the thenar intrinsics and lumbricals to the forefinger and long finger.

The most reproducible loss with complete injury to this element is loss of all hand intrinsics, and this includes those in the ulnar and median distribution. With time there is obvious atrophy of interossei and muscles of hypothenar eminence and thenar eminence. There is a variable degree of finger and wrist flexor loss, especially to profundi. In addition, there may be some extensor loss because the posterior division of this trunk goes to the posterior cord, which supplies radial nerve. The portion of radial outflow most likely to be weak is that to extensor communis and pollicis longus.[19] In some patients, there may also be loss of extensor carpi ulnaris.[24]

## ELECTRICAL STUDIES OF BRACHIAL PLEXUS LESIONS

Although a thorough physical examination of the involved limb as well as the clinical examination of the patient as a whole are paramount, well-selected electrical and radiologic studies are usually of help for brachial plexus lesions.

## Special Electromyographic Studies

For supraclavicular palsies, the major question to be answered is how far proximal or medial the injury extends on the roots or spinal nerves. Special electromyographic (EMG) studies are of some help in this regard.[46] Nonetheless, the following electrical studies must always be interpreted in the context of the clinical findings and can never substitute, even in part, for a thorough clinical examination (Figure 12–22).

## Paraspinal Muscle Sampling

These large posterior-laminar muscles are supplied by posterior spinal branches that originate at a foraminal level, so denervation in their distribution implies proximal spinal nerve or root injury.[5] Because there is overlap in their input to muscle, even severe denervation does not necessarily mean that one or more plexus roots are not damaged more laterally and at a reparable level.[47] Not infrequently, C5, and sometimes also C6, has extraforaminal injury, and yet more proximal injury to C7, C8, and T1 can give extensive paraspinal denervational change. Nonetheless, widespread denervation of these muscles remains a relatively negative finding.

On the other hand, C3, C4, and at times also C2 may contribute to superior paraspinal muscles, so denervation may not be as widespread as one might think, even in the less common situation in which C5 or C6 or both are damaged quite proximally. Sampling must be done at a number of levels and by an experienced electromyographer.

## Serratus Anterior and Rhomboids

Although loss in these muscles is usually quite evident on clinical examination, sampling of their activity may be necessary. This is not an easy task because serratus is deep to the scapula and requires a very experienced electromyographer for its assessment. It is all too easy to place the tip of the EMG needle into an intercostal muscle. In the reverse sense, because the spinal segment of the trapezius overlies some of the rhomboids, the diagnostician has to be sure the needle is deep to this muscle before sampling is begun.

## Sensory Nerve Action Potential Recording

Presence of a sensory nerve action potential (sNAP) recorded at skin level along the dipole

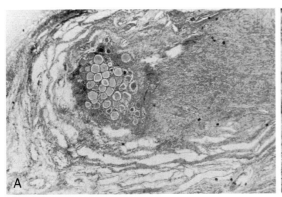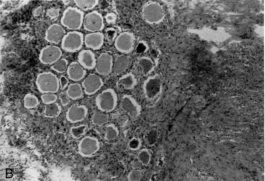

**Figure 12–22.** Histologic findings associated with proximal damage to spinal nerve(s). (A) Low-power view of Masson stain of section of a proximal spinal nerve. There is very little axonal structure; heavy scar is seen to the right and ganglion cells to the left. (B) Higher power view. Presence of ganglion cells indicated that spinal nerve had been pulled down into the foramen, and, thus, this element had preganglionic as well as postganglionic injury.

of a peripheral nerve such as ulnar, median, or radial suggests preganglionic injury of one or more dorsal roots[3,13,27]—providing loss is complete in the distribution of the nerve stimulated. If sensory loss is complete in either the ulnar or median distribution and yet a sNAP is recorded, this means one or more dorsal posterior roots feeding the nerve has been injured between the dorsal root ganglion and the spinal cord. Injury at this site does not lead to degeneration of the ganglion's more distal afferent fibers, so the nerve is still capable of conducting electrical impulses even though there is no central connection. Lack of a central connection can be shown especially at the operating table by stimulation of more distal spinal nerve and inability to record a somatosensory evoked potential or evoked cortical response from the spine or scalp[7,20,25,39] (Figure 12–23). Some clinicians have also suggested that the presence of a Tinel sign on percussion or deep palpation of the supraclavicular space when there is complete loss distal to this level indicates a central connection of at least some spinal nerve fibers.[8,32] Estimates for this number vary, but it may be as few as 100 fibers or so. Unfortunately, this is also the case when somatosensory and cortical response recordings are evoked, even by operative stimulation of spinal nerves after stretch injury. Such responses can be present even though only a few hundred fibers have a central connection.

Because each of the peripheral nerves usable for this type of study has three or more dorsal root contributions, the presence of a sNAP does not necessarily mean that all of the contributing roots are damaged at a preganglionic level.[24,41] Some attempt is made to get around this by stimulating distal fingers at sensory sites considered to be more precise for given roots. Little and ring finger digital nerves can be stimulated by ring electrodes to correspond with T1 and C8 dorsal roots, middle finger to correspond with C7, and forefinger or thumb to correspond with C6. The difficulty is that there is overlap peripherally in terms of input, especially to long finger, forefinger, and thumb. A sNAP recorded by stimulating the long finger and recording from the median nerve could be caused by a dorsal root lesion of C8 or even C6 rather than C7. A sNAP recorded by stimulating the forefinger and recording from median nerve could be caused by a dorsal root lesion of C7 in addition to or rather than C6. Stimulating little and ring fingers and recording from ulnar nerve is more certain for assessment of the C8 and T1 roots. Although controversial, there is in our experience neither a precise enough nor exclusive enough site to stimulate or record for a C6 distribution sNAP. In addition, neither axillary nerve nor suprascapular nerve can be stimulated precisely enough, let alone recorded from, to be certain of evaluation of the C5 root.[24]

Absence of a sNAP in the distribution of a nerve with plexus dorsal root input does not exclude preganglionic injury. If an injury is extensive enough, as frequently happens, it damages

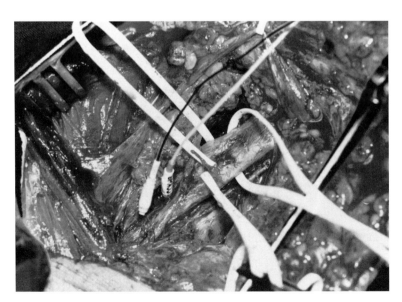

**Figure 12–23.** The integrity of spinal nerves can be checked by stimulation through electroencephalographic needles placed directly in proximal nerve. The recording of somatosensory-evoked potentials through posterior superior cervical skin electrodes or contralateral scalp electrodes indicates that at least the posterior rootlets of the spinal nerves are attached to the spinal cord and hence can be used, after transection, as proximal stumps for attachment to grafts in appropriate cases.

both the pre- and postganglionic segments of the root. In these cases, the sensory fibers do degenerate, and no sNAP is recorded even though root-level damage extends close to the spinal cord.

Although evidence of preganglionic injury to the dorsal root does not guarantee that the ventral root is damaged as severely and as closely to the spinal cord, it does strongly suggest it.[44]

## Other EMG Considerations

Sampling of other muscles may help the clinician work out the locus and extent of a plexus lesion or, in other cases, suggest the possibility of recovery even though there is no clinical evidence of this. For example, loss of deltoid and biceps/brachialis function may suggest an upper trunk lesion, but the latter is more certain if supraspinatus and infraspinatus are also denervated. These same muscles along with biceps/brachialis should be sampled when looking for early recovery after an upper trunk lesion. Even under favorable circumstances, the deltoid is slow in regaining input. The larger, more bulky biceps shows earlier electrical and clinical recovery.[13] With a complete upper trunk lesion, brachioradialis and supinator also lose input, and the electromyographer may decide to sample those muscles as well.

C7 and middle trunk lesions may display a variety of electrical findings. The triceps usually has denervational changes, although it may also receive input from C6 and, surprisingly often, even from C8. A similar problem exists with specificity if extensor muscles such as extensor carpi radialis and ulnaris, extensor communis, and extensor pollicis longus are sampled. These muscles usually receive C7 outflows, but often also have input from C8,[43] especially the extensor communis and extensor pollicis longus. A similar problem exists with sampling the flexor profundi: because of variable input from both C7 and C8, denervational changes within these muscles can suggest C8 or C7 injury or both. By comparison, lower trunk lesions cause loss in all hand intrinsics, including those of the thenar eminence. Clinical loss and electrical changes may also involve extensor communis and some of the flexor profundus system.[24,42] Unfortunately, the same is usually the case with medial

cord lesions, so it may be difficult for either the clinician or electromyographer to differentiate these two close but different levels.

After serious plexus injury, it may take many months for certain electrical signs of recovery to occur, and that undue delay while awaiting reversal of denervational change may make the timing for surgical repair inopportune. Nonetheless, with some injuries, recovery in the distribution of one or more elements may become evident in the early months. This makes repeated electrical as well as clinical study worthwhile.

# RADIOGRAPHIC STUDIES OF BRACHIAL PLEXUS INJURIES

## Plain Radiographs

The beginner in this field rapidly gains an appreciation of the value of these studies. Special attention should be given to the clavicle, scapula, shoulder joint including humeral bone, ribs, and the cervical spine. With blunt injury in which the plexus has been stretched, there is a high association with fracture and dislocation.[11] Despite this, there can often be severe plexus injury without any history of shoulder dislocation or radiographic presence of a fracture.[6] On the other hand, some fractures, especially those of the cervical spinal column, bode poorly in terms of reparability of the plexus. In addition, one cannot conclude that the fracture site localizes the level of the lesion.[10] Instead, the force fracturing the bone is often maximal at a site a distance from the plexus. Plexus damage is often proximal to the fracture site. Exceptions may be provided by complex depressed clavicular fractures, which can but do not always involve plexus maximally at that level.

Fracture-dislocations of the cervical spine are often associated with myelopathy but can also be associated with severe plexus stretch on one side or the other. If seen with either blunt or penetrating injuries, transverse process fractures augur poorly for the root or spinal nerve involved at that level. Damage usually extends proximally close to spinal cord on that element or adjacent ones and may not be reparable. With penetrating wounds and transverse process fracture, there may also be vertebral arterial injury. Associated vascular injury of this nature may not be evident without arteriography, and even a negative study does not completely rule out vascular injury. Fractures of the laminae of the vertebral column are more likely to be associated with myelopathy than those of the spinous processes, and vertebral body fractures bode poorly for reparability of roots at that level if loss is in their distribution and is caused by stretch/contusion.

Rib fractures can result from severe contusive blows to the chest as well as the plexus. These can be associated with pneumothorax or hemothorax as well as a usually severe and lengthy lesion to the plexus.

On occasion, a fracture can mimic a palsy because it prevents motion of a portion of the affected extremity. A good example was provided by a middle-aged woman who was referred for persistent "axillary palsy" some 7 months after she experienced a crushing injury to the shoulder. A humeral neck fracture had been treated for 7 weeks by a Velpeau type of sling. It was presumed healed, and, in addition, an electromyographer thought the deltoid showed denervational changes. When she was examined in New Orleans, she could not abduct her right shoulder beyond 10 degrees, and the deltoid muscle did seem somewhat shrunken but

not completely so. EMG needle sampling of the deltoid, however, showed no denervation. As a result, the right shoulder and arm were X-rayed with the arm at the side and then with it held abducted to 90 degrees by the technician. As can be seen in Figure 12–24, there was nonunion of this proximal humeral fracture and, as a result, the arm could not be effectively abducted. The shoulder was readily stabilized operatively by the orthopedist, and after a period of immobilization, almost full shoulder abduction was regained.

## Angiography and Venography

These studies are probably done more often than is needed in the management of plexus palsies.[44] Even so, we cannot be too critical of their use, particularly if penetrating injuries involving upper arm, shoulder, or neck are present. Angiography is certainly indicated if there is absence of a radial or carotid pulse, an expanding mass in the area of the wound, or presence of a bruit or a thrill in the area of the wound. Occlusion or vascular avulsion is usually localized as to level by an arteriogram because there is no filling beyond the injury site. Under these circumstances, collateral filling of more distal vessels is seen surprisingly early, es-

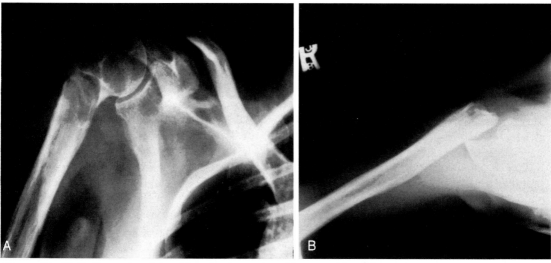

**Figure 12–24.** Radiographs of shoulder of patient referred because of "axillary palsy" and presumed paralysis of the deltoid following a humeral fracture thought to be healed. Inability to abduct the arm was due to malunion of a humeral fracture which was not very evident *(A)* until the arm was passively abducted and a radiograph *(B)* was taken in that position. (From Kline D and Hudson A: Acute injuries of peripheral nerves. *In* Youman J, ed: *Neurological Surgery.* Philadelphia, WB Saunders, 1990.

pecially with axillary-level lesions. In other cases, distal axillary and brachial vessels may be filled in a retrograde fashion through the profundus vessel.

Pseudoaneurysms are usually caused by a hole or laceration in the wall of the vessel which leads to a dissection by blood of tissues that invest artery. These lesions are seen with some gunshot wounds that involve the infraclavicular plexus and occasionally with a stab or glass wound to that area. Angiography cannot always be relied on to fill the aneurysm, because it is a false one and the site of leakage tends to seal off. More commonly, the intimal surface is irregular at the original site of the injury to the vascular wall.[24] As a result, the contrast column has partial interruption or appears irregular at this level. In about half of the pseudoaneurysm cases seen in our clinic, the preoperative angiogram was thought to be normal. In some cases, the diagnosis was suspected because of the presence of a pulsatile mass in the axilla or shoulder region with or without the presence of a bruit. In other cases, the lesion was discovered at the time of exploration for neural repair.

Less often, arteriography is indicated for vascular injury associated with stretch/contusion.[24,29] Associated vascular injury bespeaks a particularly severe stretch to the plexus, especially if it involves the subclavian artery. This is because a blunt or stretch injury involving vessels as well as plexus has usually severely distracted the shoulder and arm, resulting in a lengthy and proximal neural injury. This makes the probability of direct repair of a significant portion of the plexus lesion less likely than in one without vascular injury, but it does not completely exclude repair as a possibility. Sometimes, those repairing the vascular injury report their observations concerning the status of the plexus elements with regard to continuity or noncontinuity or obvious contusion or hemorrhage. More often, referral sources report one or more nerves being torn apart with one end seen but not the other, or nerves without a specific anatomic designation "running along and appearing bruised or hemorrhagic." Such reports should be weighed carefully but should not prevent neural exploration nor force it when it is too early to evaluate the regenerative ability of lesions in continuity.

Although frequently negative, arterial and venous angiograms are still widely used in patients with suspected thoracic outlet syndrome.[30] Venous and sometimes arterial injections are done, with the arm at the side and then with the arm abducted 90 degrees. Occlusion or constriction of flow suggests a thoracic outlet problem but seldom proves it outright. Such associated vascular abnormalities are more likely to be present if there are vascular as well as neural symptoms; presence of a bruit or thrill, especially with abduction; and, sometimes, a positive Adson test (see chapter entitled "Thoracic Outlet Syndrome").

A rare disorder is entrapment of axillary nerve near the quadrilateral space. This can be associated with posterior circumflex humeral artery or axillary arterial branch occlusion when the arm is hyperabducted and the axillary artery injected.[30] This is known as the quadrilateral space syndrome of Cahill. Patients have shoulder pain and paresthesias and sometimes a milder degree of shoulder abduction weakness than is seen with more severe axillary nerve injury. Palpation of the quadrilateral space by compression behind the posterior deltoid usually produces severe pain and tenderness. The symptoms are caused by neural compression of the axillary nerve with shoulder abduction rather than by vascular compression. Occlusion or narrowing of the circumflex humeral vessels is, nonetheless, a useful marker for the entity.

## Myelography

This is a diagnostic study primarily of use for stretch/contusion injuries in which there is a question of root avulsion.[6] Several early papers were seminal in the application of this technique to this injury.[33,35] Despite the more recent development of computed axial tomography (CAT) and magnetic resonance imaging (MRI) scans, such studies, even with subarachnoid placement of contrast, are not as valuable as a simple myelogram, because meningoceles can easily be missed unless the transverse slices are very thin. Presence of meningoceles on a root sleeve suggests but does not prove either avulsion of that root from the spinal cord or damage in continuity of the root very close to cord.[16,37] Presence of this finding on a root suggests but again does not prove that damage can also be quite proximal on other roots, particularly those adjacent to the level of the meningocele.[9] Proximal damage may be present even if there are no myelographic abnormalities at levels adjacent to one with a meningocele. On occasion, however, the root at the level of a meningocele is either quite intact or, less commonly, injured lateral to the intervertebral foramen.[23] Conversely, a root can be damaged close to cord or even avulsed from cord without a meningocele being present.[48] Thus, myelography for stretch injuries to the plexus has both a false-positive and a false-negative incidence. Despite this, the myelogram does provide some idea of how proximal the injury is. This in turn suggests the probability that in cases where meningoceles are present, especially on the lower roots, they will not be reparable. This does not mean that spinal nerves at a higher level, especially C5 and C6, cannot be repaired.

Other myelographic findings associated with root avulsion or very proximal stretch include widening of the cord from contusion or edema. For this reason, if a myelogram is done in the week or two after injury, a narrowing of the contrast column on one or both sides of the cervical gutter can be present with or without meningocele. The dye column in the gutter may be thicker than normal after several weeks because of spinal cord shrinkage. In still other cases, enough contrast may exit a damaged root sleeve to form a linear collection of contrast material at an epidural or subdural level. Thus, even if there is no myelopathy, presence of one or more findings such as these augurs poorly for repair of the roots, at least at the levels at which these abnormalities are seen.

Myelography can also be useful to help delineate plexus tumors involving spinal nerves or roots or to provide further assurance that those tumors involving more lateral plexus have not extended into the spinal canal. If such tumoral extension is the case, amputation or deformation of a root sleeve with or without compression of the cord itself can be seen.

In cases of presumed thoracic outlet syndrome, myelography, or CAT or MRI scans, with or without subarachnoid contrast, may be useful in excluding more proximal lesions such as cervical disc, tumor, or spondylitic disease.[44]

## CAT and MRI Scans

These studies have their greatest application for tumors either arising in plexus or secondarily compressing it.[12] Especially useful in this category is the MRI with contrast by gadolinium. Coronal slices of the neck and shoulder are most useful, especially if done bilaterally so that details on the affected side can be compared with those on the unaffected side. To date, not even MRI can show enough detail and change in plexus images to be of practical value for most injuries, although advances continue to occur, especially with the MRI and use of surface coil techniques.[14,44] CAT scans with metrizamide when positive at nerve root levels are nonetheless quite dramatic with stretch injuries.[28]

Unfortunately, those unfamiliar with the field of stretch injury to the plexus often try to substitute CAT or MRI scans for myelography. Even good cross-sectional studies with or without contrast such as metrizamide in the subarachnoid space, although interesting, seldom give more information than a thorough cervical myelogram with good anterior-posterior, oblique, and lateral views.[24,44]

Both CAT scan and MRI have been used to evaluate other tissues such as bone. Changes in bony relationships with motion of the shoulder and presumably the plexus are being studied with the MRI. This type of radiographic workup may have great applicability in the future for thoracic outlet syndromes, especially in cases in which there is not a more obvious radiographic abnormality such as a cervical rib or an elongated C7 transverse process.

## Bibliography

1. Abdullah S and Bowden RE: The blood supply of the brachial plexus. Proc R Soc Med 53:203–210, 1960.
2. Aids to the Examination of the Peripheral Nervous System. London, Bailliere Tindall, 1986.
3. Bonney G and Gilliat RW: Sensory nerve conduction after traction lesions of the brachial plexus. Proc R Soc Med 51:365, 1958.
4. Bowden REM, Abdullah S, and Gooding MR: Anatomy of the cervical spine, membranes, spinal cord, nerve roots, and brachial plexus. *In* Lord Brain and Wilkinson M, Eds: Cervical Spondylosis and Other Disorders of the Cervical Spine. Philadelphia, WB Saunders, 1967.
5. Bufalini C and Pescatore G: Posterior cervical electromyography in the diagnosis and prognosis of brachial plexus injuries. J Bone Joint Surg 51B:627–631, 1969.
6. Campbell JB: Peripheral nerve repair. Clin Neurosurg 17:77–98, 1970.

7. Celli L and Rovesta C: Electrophysiologic intraoperative evaluations of the damaged root in tractions of the brachial plexus. *In* Terzis JK, Ed: Microreconstruction of Nerve Injuries. Philadelphia, WB Saunders, 1987.

8. Copeland S and Landi A: Value of the Tinel's sign in brachial plexus lesions. Ann R Coll Surg 61:470, 1979.

9. Davies ER, Sutton D, and Bligh AS: Myelography in brachial plexus injury. Br J Radiol 39:362, 1966.

10. Dolenc V: Diagnosis and treatment of lesions of the brachial plexus and adjacent structures. Clin Neurosurg 11:110–127, 1983.

11. Drake CG: Diagnosis and treatment of lesions of the brachial plexus and adjacent structures. Clin Neurosurg 11:110–127, 1964.

12. Gebarski J, Glazer G, and Gebarski S: Brachial plexus: Anatomic, radiologic, and pathologic correlation using computed tomography. J Comp Asst Tomogr 6:1058–1063, 1982.

13. Gilliatt R: Physical injury to peripheral nerves, physiological and electrodiagnostic aspects. Mayo Clin Proc 56:361–370, 1981.

14. Gupta RK, Mehta VS, Banerji AK, et al.: Magnetic resonance evaluation of brachial plexus injuries. Neuroradiology 31:377–382, 1989.

15. Haymaker W and Woodhall B: Peripheral Nerve Injuries, 2nd Ed. Philadelphia, WB Saunders, 1956.

16. Heon M: Myelogram: A questionable aid in diagnosis and prognosis of brachial plexus components in traction injuries. Conn Med 29:260–262, 1965.

17. Hollingshead WH: Anatomy for Surgeons. Vol. 3: The Back and Limbs, 2nd Ed. Hagerstown, MD, Harper & Row, 1969.

18. Hovelacque A: Anatomie des nerfs craniens et rach, diens et du systéme grand sympathique. Paris, Doin, 1927.

19. Hudson AR and Trammer B: Brachial plexus injuries. *In* Wilkins R and Rengachary S, Eds: Neurosurgery. New York, McGraw-Hill, 1985.

20. Jones SJ: Diagnostic value of peripheral and spinal somatosensory evoked potentials in traction lesions of the brachial plexus. Clin Plast Surg 11:167–172, 1984.

21. Kaplan EB and Spinner M: Normal and anomalous innervation patterns in the upper extremity. *In* Omer GE and Spinner M, Eds: Management of Peripheral Nerve Problems. Philadelphia, WB Saunders, 1980.

22. Kerr AT: The brachial plexus nerves of man, the variation in its formation and its branches. Am J Anat 23:285, 1918.

23. Kewalramani LS and Taylor RG: Brachial plexus root avulsion: Role of myelography. Review of diagnostic procedures. J Trauma 15:603–608, 1975.

24. Kline DG, Hackett ER, and Happel LH: Surgery for lesions of the brachial plexus. Arch Neurol 43:170–181, 1986.

25. Landi A, Copeland SA, Wynn Parry CB, et al.: Role of somatosensory evoked potentials and nerve conduction studies in the surgical management of brachial plexus injuries. J Bone Joint Surg Br 62:492–496, 1980.

26. Leffert RD: Brachial Plexus Injuries. London, Churchill Livingstone, 1985.

27. Licht S: Electrodiagnosis and Electromyography, 3rd Ed. New Haven, CN, E Licht, 1971.

28. Marshall RW and DeSilva RD: Computerized axial tomography in traction injuries of the brachial plexus. J Bone Joint Surg 66B:734–738, 1986.

29. McGillicuddy J: Clinical decision making in brachial plexus injuries. Neurosurg Clin North Am 2:137–150, 1991.

30. McKowen HC and Voorhies RM: Axillary nerve entrapment in the quadrilateral space: Case report. J Neurosurg 66:932–934, 1987.

31. Miller RA: Observations upon the arrangement of the axillary artery and brachial plexus. Am J Anat 64:143–156, 1939.

32. Millesi H: Surgical management of brachial plexus injuries. J Hand Surg 2:367–378, 1977.

33. Murphey F, Hartung W, and Kirklin J: Myelographic demonstration of avulsing injury of the brachial plexus. Am J Epidemiol 58:102–105, 1947.

34. Pernkopf E: Atlas of Topographical and Applied Human Anatomy, Vol. 1, Head and Neck. Ferner H, Ed. Philadelphia, WB Saunders, 1980.

35. Robles J: Brachial plexus avulsion. A review of diagnostic procedures and report of six cases. J Neurosurg 28:434–438, 1968.

36. Seddon HJ: Surgical Disorders of the Peripheral Nerves. Baltimore, Williams & Wilkins, 1972.

37. Simond J and Sypert G: Closed traction avulsion injuries of the brachial plexus. Contemp Neurosurg 50:1–6, 1983.

38. Stevens J: Brachial plexus paralysis. *In* Codman EA, Ed: The Shoulder. Boston, T. Todd Co., 1934, pp 332–381.

39. Sugioku H, Tsuyama N, Hara T, et al.: Investigation of brachial plexus injuries by intraoperative cortical somatosensory evoked potentials. Arch Orthop Trauma Surg 99:143–151, 1982.

40. Sunderland S: Meningeal-neural relations in the intervertebral foramen. J Neurosurg 40:756–761, 1974.

41. Syneck V and Cowan J: Somatosensory evoked potentials in patients with supraclavicular brachial plexus injuries. Neurology 32:1347–1352, 1982.

42. Terzis J, Liberson W, and Maragh H: Motorcycle brachial plexopathy. *In* Terzis J, Ed: Microreconstruction of Nerve Injuries. Philadelphia, WB Saunders, 1987.

43. Warren J, Gutman NL, Figueroa A, and Bloor BM: Electromyographic changes of brachial plexus root avulsion. J Neurosurg 31:137–140, 1969.

44. Wilbourn A: Brachial plexus disorders. *In* Dyck P and Thomas PK, Eds: Peripheral Neuropathy, 3rd Ed. Philadelphia, WB Saunders, 1993.

45. Wolock B and Millesi H: Brachial plexus—applied anatomy and operative exposure. *In* Gelberman RH, Ed: Operative Nerve Repair and Reconstruction. Philadelphia, JB Lippincott, 1991.

46. Yiannikas L, Chahani B, and Young R: The investigation of traumatic lesions of the brachial plexus by electromyography and short latency somatosensory potentials. J Neurol Neurosurg Psychiatry 46:1014–1022, 1983.

47. Zalis A, Oester Y, and Rodriguez A: Electrophysiologic diagnosis of cervical nerve root avulsion. Arch Phys Med Rehabil 51:708–710, 1970.

48. Zorub D, Nashold B, and Cook W: Avulsion of the brachial plexus I: A review with implications on the therapy of intractable pain. Surg Neurol 2:347–353, 1974.

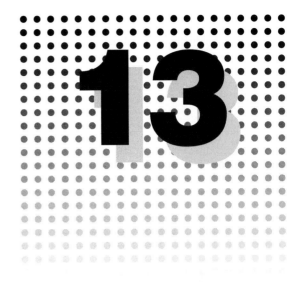

# Lacerations to
# Brachial Plexus

## SUMMARY

Lacerations were the most favorable serious plexus injuries to manage in our series. More than 60% of all elements involved by laceration and operated on reached a grade 3 or better recovery, and this figure included those thought to be unfavorable for repair, such as lower spinal nerve, lower trunk, and medial cord lesions. Analysis of data collected from complete transection as well as transections of a portion of the plexus in 47 patients indicated that acute repair with *sharp* injury was best, if it could be achieved. On the other hand, experience with *bluntly* transected plexus repaired acutely elsewhere was negative, so a delay of several weeks in repair of such lesions proved best. If bluntly transected elements are encountered acutely in the course of vascular repair, then stumps should be tacked down to maintain length. Delayed repair is more likely to be accomplished by grafts than by end-to-end repair, but results are less favorable than those seen with acute repair of sharp lesions or with end-to-end repair of blunt transections. This is, however, more associated with the severity of the blunt lesions and the length of the damage to the element rather than the delay in their repair. Despite a sharp or bluntly transecting mechanism for injury, 30 of the elements in this category were left in continuity. These lesions in continuity required intraoperative nerve action potential recording and based on this, either neurolysis, complete repair, or split repair.

## MANAGEMENT AND RESULTS OF BRACHIAL PLEXUS INJURIES

Although the majority of papers published concerning brachial plexus lesions focus on stretch and avulsion injuries, other injury categories deserve intensive discussion.[7,9] These categories include lacerations and focal penetrations involving the plexus, gunshot wounds, and a variety of mechanisms of injury from iatrogenic causes.[6] Proper management of these injuries usually produces better results than those seen with stretch injuries. Thus, careful and detailed management of these less frequently reported injuries is mandatory.

## LACERATIONS INVOLVING BRACHIAL PLEXUS

Laceration to the tissues surrounding the plexus has the potential to transect the entire plexus or, more often, a portion of it. Transecting injuries tend to be either sharp or blunt, and this observation has prompted either acute or delayed neural repair, depending on the mechanism of injury involved.[1,2,4,12,13] Mechanisms responsible for lacerations involving plexus in our series included injuries from knives and glass, which were classified as sharp, and those from auto metal fragments, fan or motor blades, and chain saws, which were classified as blunt (Figure 13–1). More focal penetrations of the neck or shoulder leading to plexus injury from mechanisms such as animal bites have been included under the blunt laceration category. One third of the laceration category injuries had been explored acutely because of clinically suspected or angiographically proven vascular injury. A variety of vascular lesions associated with penetrating injuries to the plexus have been described in the literature.[3,10,11,13] In this series, vascular injuries included partial or complete transection of major vessels and hematomas but did not include pseudoaneurysm or arteriovenous fistula. Knife wounds usually resulted from criminal acts perpetrated by others and inflicted with a kitchen or hunting knife (Figure 13–2). Glass injuries were caused by falls through glass windows and by exploding glass in factory or automobile accidents. In one instance, a storefront glass window collapsed on the patient's neck and shoulder when she leaned against it. The injuries from rotating propeller or fan blades were, in two cases, caused by automotive fan blades, but the majority were related to boat propeller and industrial propeller accidents. Three patients sustained chain saw injuries to the plexus, usually because

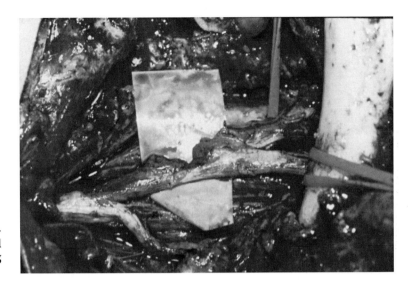

**Figure 13–1.** Partial transection of upper trunk by a shard of glass. A split repair using sural grafts was done.

the saw blade struck a knot in a limb and jumped back and severely lacerated the neck and all or a portion of the plexus. This gave a ragged and contusive tear to the plexus elements. Penetrating non-gunshot wounds were caused by shards of metal or, in several instances, by severe and deep animal bites, in one case by a bear and in several others by dogs.

## Management

In this subset of plexus injury, 47 patients with lacerations were examined at the Louisiana State University Medical Center, and 142 plexus elements were judged to be seriously injured. Of these 142 injured elements, 60 were determined to be sharply transected, 52 were bluntly transected, and 30 were found to be in continuity on surgical exploration. Most of these lesions in continuity could be treated several months after injury. Continuity was usually suspected because of a relatively high incidence of acute exploration for vascular injury and observations made on neural structures at that time.[5] Ten of these contused but not transected elements transmitted a nerve action potential (NAP) and had a neurolysis with recovery. Of the 20 requiring resection and repair, 7 had end-to-end suture, and 13 had replacement of their lesion in continuity with grafts. Recovery to a grade 3 or better level occurred in three fourths of these elements (Table 13–1).

If the mechanism of injury was determined to be sharp, repair was undertaken within the first 72 hours after injury if possible (Figure 13–3). Recovery was best in this subset, with 75% of the elements reaching a grade 3 or better level. Patients who were not referred in time to do this had 36 of their 60 sharply transected elements repaired secondarily. Graft repair was necessary in 26 of these because of stump retraction. Results with secondary suture (70%) were better than with grafts (50%) under these circumstances. Those with stump retraction, neuromatous and scarred stumps or both were more likely to require grafts rather than end-to-end suture.

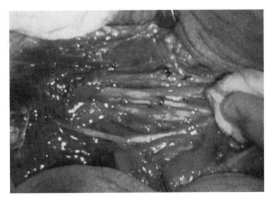

**Figure 13–2.** This supraclavicular plexus was totally transected by a knife. It has been repaired end-to-end relatively acutely. Stumps required minimal trimming, and repair was not under tension.

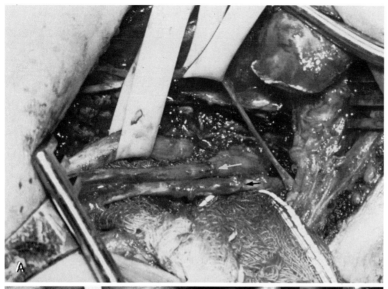

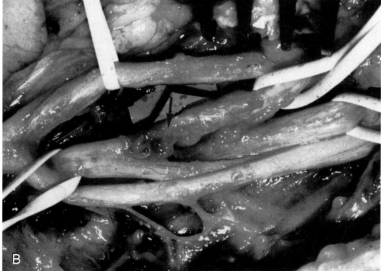

**Figure 13-3.** *(A)* These C5 *(black arrow)* and C6 *(white arrow)* spinal nerves had been transected by a knife wound at the point where they unite to form the upper trunk. They were repaired 4 hours after injury by end-to-end suture with 6-0 prolene. *(B)* Stab wound involving middle trunk of the plexus *(arrow)* and explored at 1 month. This lesion was resected and an end-to-end repair was done. This lesion could have been repaired acutely had there been the opportunity. See also color figure.

## TABLE 13-1
Lacerating Injury to Brachial Plexus Elements*

|  | One or More Elements in Continuity | Sharp Transection | Blunt Transection | Totals |
|---|---|---|---|---|
| Plexus cases (operated) | 11 | 18 | 18 | 47 |
| Plexus elements (operated) | 30 | 60 | 52 | 142 |
| Neurolysis/results | 10/9† | 0/0 | 0/0 | 10/9 (90%) |
| Primary epineurial suture/results | 0/0 | 24/18 | 0/0 | 24/18 (75%) |
| Secondary epineurial suture/results | 7/5 | 10/7 | 5/3 | 22/15 (68%) |
| Secondary graft/results | 13/10‡ | 26/13 | 47/22 | 86/45 (52%) |
| Total elements/positive results | 30/24 | 60/38 | 52/25 | 142/87 (61%) |

*Loss in the distribution of one or more plexus elements thought preoperatively to be complete loss.
†Grade 3 or better result in the distribution of an element.
‡Includes three split repairs where portion of lesion had a neurolysis and portion a graft.
Primary = repair within 72 hours of injury; secondary = delayed repair after several weeks.

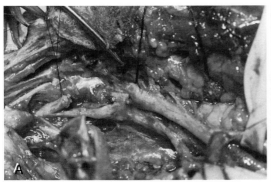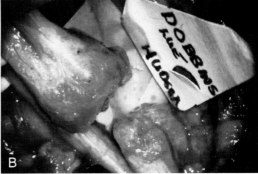

**Figure 13–4.** *(A)* Plexus transected bluntly and close to the clavicle, which was divided to provide this exposure. Most of the stumps have retracted. *(B)* More sharply transected plexus element in another patient.

Lacerations suspected to be blunt were repaired secondarily, if possible 2 to 3 weeks after trauma. Because of delay in referral or logistic or other scheduling difficulties, some were not done until several months after injury. Most blunt transections required graft repair because of stump retraction and the need to trim both stumps before a repair could be done (Figure 13–4). Fewer grafts might have been required if there had been an opportunity to "tack down" stumps to adjacent fascial planes to maintain length. Such an opportunity was sometimes present at the time of acute vascular repair, but unfortunately it was only used in two instances. Three (60%) of five sutures recovered, but only 22 (47%) of 47 graft repairs had positive results. Results were best if transection involved upper elements such as C5-C6, upper trunk, or lateral

or posterior cord injuries (Figure 13–5). However, two children, ages 6 and 10, with medial cord repairs gained substantial recovery in hand intrinsic muscle function, although this was not the case with adult injuries of this element or with similar injuries involving the lower trunk.

## Recommendations

Conclusions based on a study of this series of cases are relatively straightforward. First, even if loss is complete in the distribution of one or more elements of the plexus and the mechanism of injury is penetrating or cutting, continuity may be maintained in one or more elements with distal loss. In some cases, this is because of partial transection of the element or elements; in

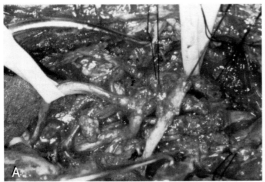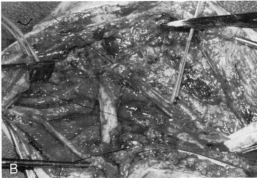

**Figure 13–5.** Transection of supraclavicular plexus caused by a chain saw. *(A)* Clavicle has been sectioned and ends are held apart by a Gelpi retractor. Trunks are to the right and cords to the left. Surgical exposure was made 1 month after injury because this was a blunt transection. An end-to-end repair was gained by trimming the proximal and distal stumps, with mobilization of the cord and cord-to-nerve segments and trunks to make up length. Sectioned clavicle was then pinned. In another chain saw injury, plexus was also totally divided, but repair was undertaken without section of the clavicle. Grafts, however, were necessary *(B)*.

others, it results from contusion without even partial division. If possible, these lesions are best treated in a delayed fashion so that NAP studies can be used to document presence or absence of regeneration or recovery (Figures 13–6 through 13–8).

Second, if the mechanism of injury is sharp, circumstances mandate early repair (within 72 hours after injury). Sorting out plexus injuries at the time of soft tissue or vascular repair is more straightforward than after delay and onset of scarring. Length is not lost to retraction, and an end-to-end repair can almost always be achieved after minimal trimming of each stump. As a result, outcome in this category is one of the best in the entire area of plexus injury, even for elements generally viewed as unfavorable for repair. Delay in referral led to secondary suture or was more likely to make grafts necessary in this category; such repairs did not fare as well as the primary end-to-end repairs.

Third, injury in which transection of one or more elements is thought to be caused by a blunt mechanism is best managed surgically after a delay of several weeks. This gives time for delineation of the extent of injury to both the proximal and distal stumps of the plexus so that both can be trimmed back to healthy tissue. With time, transected plexus stumps retract. Therefore, if acute exploration for vascular or soft tissue repair presents the opportunity, stumps should be tacked down to maintain length.[5,10] Then, at the time of secondary repair, end-to-end suture is more likely to be achieved. Grafts were often necessary in this subset, and

results were not as good as those for end-to-end suture either here or in the sharp transection category if repair was delayed (Figures 13–9 and 13–10).

If early operation for suspected vascular injury is done, it is very important to isolate and protect the neural structures, which are not only injured themselves but often adherent to the involved vessels.

## Results

Table 13–1 provides results for the three categories of injury under this subset. Averaged results are included for those elements with a poor prognosis for outcome as well as for those with a better one. Lesions found in continuity despite a transecting-type mechanism included 30 plexus elements in 11 cases. NAP recording across these lesions was positive in 13 elements. Ten of these had an external neurolysis, and nine recovered to a grade 3 or better level. Three had split repair, and each had acceptable recovery. Among those in which NAP recording showed no transmission beyond the lesion in continuity, seven elements had a secondary or delayed end-to-end suture, with five recovering, and ten had graft repairs, with seven recovering. Overall results in this category of lesions in continuity were favorable. Twenty-four of 30 elements reached grade 3 or better levels.

In the category of sharply transected lesions, referral or logistics were favorable for repair within 72 hours in 24 elements, and 18 (75%)

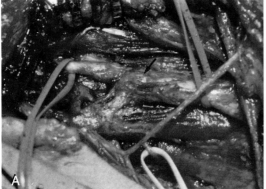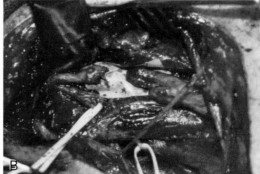

**Figure 13–6.** (A) Penetrating glass wound involving upper trunk (arrow) that left plexus in continuity. Darker loop to the left is around C5, and white loop is pulling a more superficial sensory nerve laterally. (B) Despite gross continuity, this was a complete lesion that did not transmit an NAP. As a result, it was resected, and in this photograph, stumps are awaiting a graft repair.

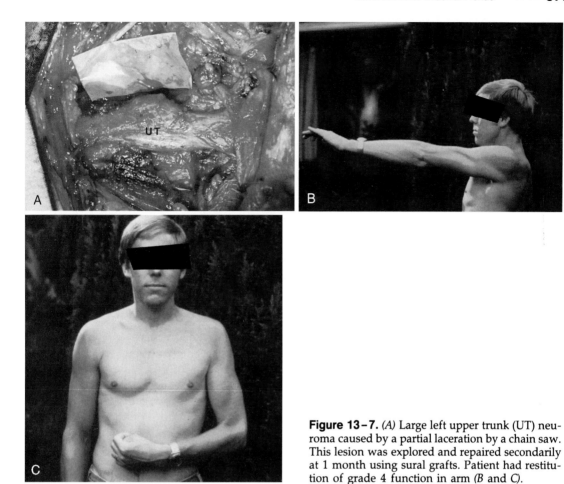

**Figure 13–7.** (A) Large left upper trunk (UT) neuroma caused by a partial laceration by a chain saw. This lesion was explored and repaired secondarily at 1 month using sural grafts. Patient had restitution of grade 4 function in arm (B and C).

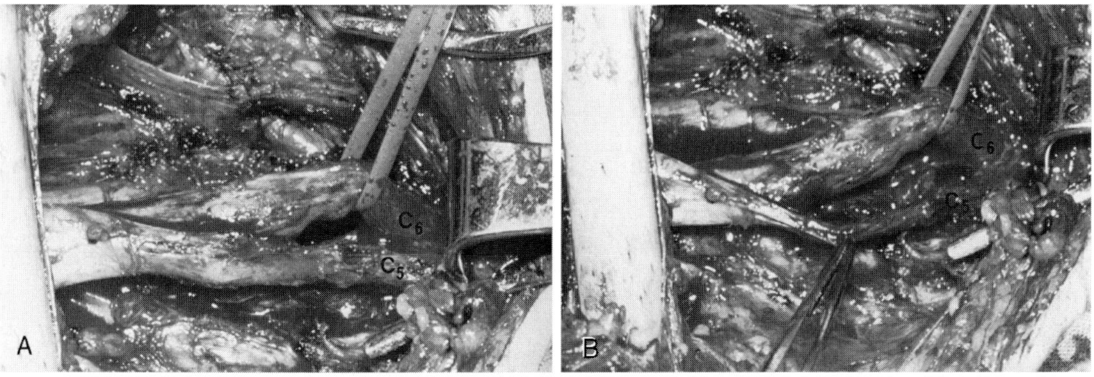

**Figure 13–8.** (A) Supraclavicular plexus involved by bear bite. This 15-year-old Boy Scout was attacked in his tent at night and had his scalp avulsed and also suffered a severe bite wound in the plexus. C5 inflow to upper trunk conducted a nerve action potential, but C6 did not and required replacement by grafts. He has had excellent upper trunk distribution recovery. (B) Shows some of C5 being split away from the upper trunk.

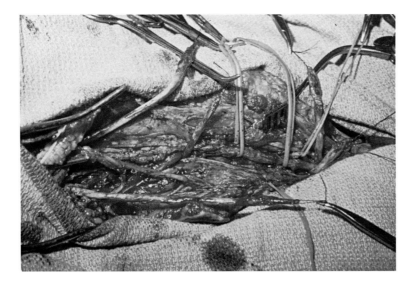

**Figure 13–9.** A sharp transection of the plexus at the cord level which was repaired in a delayed fashion but which might have been more readily done at the time of an acute arterial repair. An end-to-end suture of each element was obtained with help of both proximal and distal mobilization of the plexus.

recovered significant function (grade 3 or better). Usually because of delay in referral or transport, repair was postponed in 36 elements, and 20 (56%) recovered significant function. Seven of these had end-to-end suture, and 13 had graft repair. Overall recovery rate in this group was 63.3%; almost two thirds of the elements reached at least a grade 3 level.

Those lesions found to have blunt transection had delayed repair. Because of the retraction of stumps and the need to trim away neuromata, 47 of 52 lesions needed graft repair. Recovery to grade 3 or better after graft repair was 47%, and in this category as a whole, recovery was 48%.

In our series, the value of primary or acute repair in carefully selected and sharply transected cases is quite evident. This is not surprising, because these elements had a less severe up-and-down injury than the blunt transections. Nonetheless, elements sutured end-to-end in a delayed fashion, if this could be achieved, did almost as well. Graft repairs fared less well, but this, again, can be attributed to the fact that these were the more serious injuries.

On occasion, even a laceration to the brachial plexus can be mimicked by another type of injury, as seen in Figure 13–11.

### Case Summary—Laceration to Brachial Plexus

This 18-year-old, right-handed woman was stabbed from behind in the left paracervical area with a long knife. She immediately noticed absence of movement of the

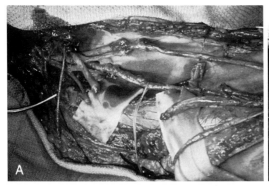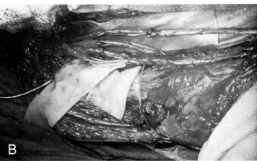

**Figure 13–10.** *(A)* Propeller injury which transected the plexus at the cord-to-nerve level in a blunt fashion. Clavicle is to the left, and hand is to the right. Loop surrounds the axillary-to-brachial artery segment, which had required acute repair. *(B)* Because of retraction as well as the need to trim stumps of neuromas, grafts were necessary when the injury was repaired at 3.5 months.

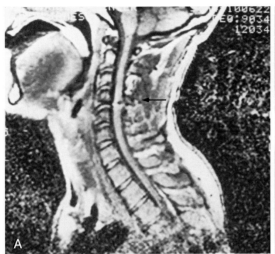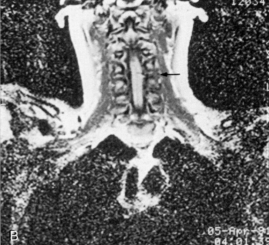

**Figure 13-11.** (*A* and *B*) Magnetic resonance images (MRIs) made of spinal cord 2 days after injury. This lesion mimicked a brachial plexus transection. Patient was stabbed in the supraclavicular region on the left side of the neck and then thrown from a speeding car, sustaining a closed head injury. When brought to the emergency room, he was unconscious but responded to pain by moving both legs and the right arm. The left arm was flaccid. The neck wound was explored. The track of the knife had run between the upper and middle trunks of the plexus without transecting either, and there was a linear punched-out entry through the left posterolateral lamina of the spine. Since there was no spinal fluid leak and this was a sharp wound, a laminectomy was not done. The MRIs were obtained 2 days later. Over the next week, the patient's level of consciousness and cooperation improved. It was then evident that he had a Brown-Séquard-like syndrome with mild but definite weakness as well as loss of touch and position sense in the left leg and loss of pinprick sensation in right leg, trunk, and most of the right hand and forearm.

shoulder girdle and loss of elbow flexion. The entrance wound was sutured at her local hospital. Cervical spine X-ray films and a CAT scan showed fracture of the left C5 and C6 transverse vertebral processes and some of the facet structure. Computerized tomographic myelography showed poor filling of the C6 root sleeve on the left.

When examined 3 months after injury, the patient had total paralysis of the left supraspinatus, infraspinatus, deltoid, biceps, brachioradialis, and supinator muscles. The remaining muscles of the left upper extremity were all functioning but somewhat weak. There was no Horner sign. Because of the proximal and complete injury of the C5 and C6 nerve roots, it was decided to explore the plexus by a posterior subscapular approach. Spinal nerves and trunks were exposed from behind. The elements were scarred but still in continuity, although the upper trunk was reduced to scarred threads of neurofibrous tissue. Extensive scar tissue was removed up to and into the neural foramina. During C4-5 and C5-6 foraminotomies, a lacerated vertebral artery was found occluded by organized clot and scar. The vessel ends were clipped and cauterized. The C5 and C6 roots were injured at their emergence from the dural sac. The C6 nerve root was scarred even medial to its dural exit, whereas some fascicular structure remained in the C5 root. Four sural nerve grafts, 3.8 cm long, were placed between the C5 root and the anterior and posterior divisions of the upper trunk.

The patient's postoperative period was uneventful. Examination at 14 months after repair revealed that the supraspinatus muscle was graded 3, the infraspinatus and deltoid muscles 1, and the biceps 2, but there was no brachioradialis muscle function. Subsequent follow-up evaluation at 3 years indicated further improvement in shoulder abduction (deltoid muscle grade 3 to 4) and forearm flexion (biceps and brachioradialis muscles grade 3). She could now use this arm to carry school books.

(Abstracted from Dubuisson A, Kline D, Weinstel S: Posterior approach to the brachial plexus. J Neurosurg 79:319-330, 1993.)

## Bibliography

1. Amine AR and Sugar O: Repair of severed brachial plexus: A plea to ER physicians. JAMA 239:1039, 1976.
2. Dunkerton MC and Boone RS: Stab wounds involving the brachial plexus. A review of operated cases. J Bone Joint Surg Br 70:566-570, 1988.
3. Galen J, Wiss D, Cantelmo N, and Menzoin J: Traumatic pseudoaneurysm of the axillary artery: Report of 3 cases and literature review. J Trauma 24:350-354, 1984.
4. Kline DG and Hackett ER: Reappraisal of timing for exploration of civilian peripheral nerve injuries. Surgery 78:54-65, 1975.

5. Kline DG: Perspectives concerning brachial plexus injury and repair. Neurosurg Clin North Am 2:151–164, 1991.
6. Kline DG and Judice D: Operative management of selected brachial plexus lesions. J Neurosurg 58:631–649, 1983.
7. Leffert RD: Brachial Plexus Injuries. New York, Churchill Livingstone, 1985.
8. Lusk M and Kline DG: Management of athletic brachial plexus injury. *In* Schneider R, Kennedy J, and Plant M, Eds: Sports Injuries: Mechanisms, Prevention, and Treatment. Baltimore, Williams & Wilkins, 1985.
9. Narakas A: The surgical management of traumatic brachial plexus lesions. Int Surg 65:521–527, 1980.
10. Nichols IS and Lillehei KO: Nerve injury associated with acute vascular trauma. Surg Clin North Am 68:837–852, 1988.
11. Robbs J and Naidoo K: Vascular compression of brachial plexus following stab injuries to neck (Ltr.). S Afr Med J 60:345–346, 1981.
12. Seddon H: Surgical Disorders of Peripheral Nerves. Baltimore, Williams & Wilkins, 1972.
13. Sunderland S: Nerves and Nerve Injuries. New York, Churchill Livingstone, 1978.

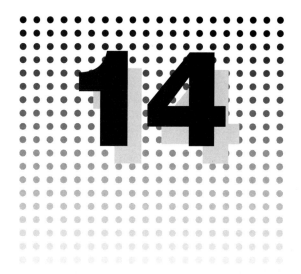

# Gunshot Wounds
# to Brachial Plexus

# SUMMARY

Operative experience with 90 gunshot wounds (GSWs) involving plexus and follow-up with 75 cases are reported in detail in this chapter. Only 6% of the plexus elements with complete loss distal to the lesion had total physical disruption in this category; the majority of GSWs left most plexus elements in continuity. Some of these lesions in continuity recovered spontaneously, but others showed no signs of reversal of loss or reinnervation after several months, and exploration and intraoperative nerve action potential (NAP) recording were performed. Some 48 of these elements had NAPs, indicating regeneration despite complete clinical and electromyographic loss distal to the lesion. Twenty-seven of these elements had no distal muscle response on stimulation and yet had a NAP across the lesion. These had a neurolysis, and more than 90% recovered to a grade 3 or better level. Many other elements (125 of 221) were not regenerating, and graft repair was usually required. Thus, maintenance of continuity did not ensure spontaneous recovery. Results with either end-to-end suture or graft repair were best with C5, C6, C7, upper and middle trunk, and lateral and posterior cord lesions. Recovery did occur in severe C8, T1, lower trunk, and medial cord injuries in continuity in which a NAP was recorded, but repair of these elements, whether by suture or graft, did not result in useful recovery except in several children. Reasons for nonoperation were incomplete loss in the distribution of multiple elements and improvement on follow-up during the early months after GSW. Less common reasons for conservative management included complete loss that reversed in the early months after injury, loss relegated to elements usually not helped by operative suture or graft repair, and referral 12 months or more after injury.

# GUNSHOT WOUNDS TO BRACHIAL PLEXUS

Next to stretch/contusion injuries, the largest category of injuries involving the brachial plexus is that of gunshot wounds (GSWs). At the time of war, there has been interest in reporting management of these intricate lesions.[4,7,17-20] Despite a sizable number of cases related to civil disturbance, there have been fewer cases of GSW involving plexus reported in times of relative world peace.[1,2,10,15,16] Nonetheless, management of civilian GSW injuries involving the plexus has changed since World War II.[5,8,13,21] Many injured elements, even though left in continuity, do not improve with time. Since the re-emergence of use of grafts for repair and the advent of intraoperative electrical techniques to evaluate lesions in continuity, successful repair is possible when indicated, and the necessity for repair or efficacy of neurolysis is more certain.[12]

Wounds in this civilian series were caused by handguns, shotguns, and rifles. Most wounds were from bullets, but some were from shell fragments. Even though many of the penetrating missiles were small, most had a relatively high velocity. Because soft tissue damage relates not only to missile or fragment size but also to the cube of its velocity, damage to nerve and other structures was extensive, just as with wartime injuries.[3,6,9] Included were 22-, 38-, 45-caliber, and even 470-magnum wounds. About half of the wounds were associated with crimes, and the rest were related to hunting accidents or, more frequently, to poor handling of weapons. About one sixth of these wounds were inflicted during unsuccessful suicide attempts.

Initial management of GSWs producing plexus-related palsy consisted of local wound care, administration of tetanus toxoid, and institution of antibiotics. Many patients had angiography in an effort to rule out vascular injury (Figure 14–1). This was often done even in the absence of any clinical signs of vascular compromise. In some cases, this was because there was a hospital or institutional policy that made angiography a requirement for any patient with a penetrating wound of the neck or shoulder. Conversely, not every patient having relatively acute exploration for suspected vascular injury

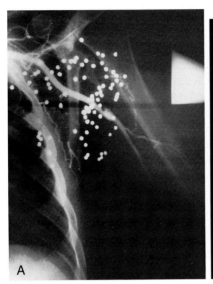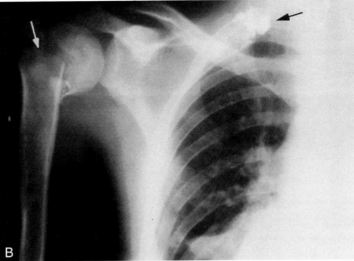

**Figure 14–1.** *(A)* Arteriogram done in a patient with a shotgun injury to the left brachial plexus. *(B)* Chest and shoulder radiograph in a patient with severe plexus palsy. Missile fragments are noted by black arrow and humeral fracture by white arrow.

had undergone prior angiography. In these six cases, persistent wound bleeding, usually of an arterial nature, expanding soft tissue hematoma, or absent radial pulse with or without other findings led to acute exploration.

The distribution of plexus injuries from GSWs managed at the Louisiana State University Medical Center is seen in Table 14–1. Seventy-five of the 90 operative cases had 2 or more years of follow-up. The number of elements evaluated intraoperatively is also included in this Table, as is the number of cases with total plexus palsy at each level.

## Associated Injuries

There was a high incidence of associated injuries and relatively acute operations for their repair. Heading the list was exploration for vascular repair (Table 14–2). Vascular repairs were in two categories. The first was the larger and included those explorations done, usually quite acutely, for suspected major vascular interruption. Indications included a penetrating wound of the neck, shoulder, or upper arm; absence of or diminished distal radial or brachial pulse; a cool hand; expanding mass or sizable hema-

**TABLE 14–1**
Gunshot Wounds to Brachial Plexus*

| Predominant Plexus Level | Total Cases | Operative Cases | Operative Cases with ≥ 2-year Follow-up† | Elements Evaluated Intraoperatively |
|---|---|---|---|---|
| Spinal nerve to trunk | 27 (6) | 21 (5) | 19 (4) | 49 |
| Division to cord | 35 (7) | 24 (6) | 21 (6) | 58 |
| Cord to nerve | 79 (9) | 45 (8) | 35 (6) | 114 |
| TOTALS | 141 (22) | 90 (19) | 75 (16) | 221 |

*Numbers in parenthesis refer to patients with complete loss of function of all elements at that level. Average interval between injury and operation was 17 weeks. Average length of follow-up was 46 months.
†From Kline DG: Civilian gunshot wounds to the brachial plexus. J Neurosurg 70:166–174, 1989.

**TABLE 14–2**

Injuries and Prior Operations Associated
With Gunshot Wounds to the Plexus

| Associated Injury or Prior Operation | Plexus— Operated (90 Cases)* | Plexus— Not Operated (51 Cases) |
|---|---|---|
| Vascular injury requiring repair | 30 | 8 |
| Chest tube placement | 6 | 1 |
| Thoracotomy | 8 | 1 |
| Orthopedic operation | 8 | 3 |
| Pseudoaneurysm removal | 6 | 0 |
| Sympathectomy for causalgia | 4 | 1 |
| Prior attempt at neural repair | 4 | 1 |
| TOTAL INCIDENCE | 66 | 15 |

*Adapted from Kline DG: Civilian gunshot wounds to the brachial plexus. J Neurosurg 70:166–174, 1989.

toma; persistent wound site bleeding; and progressive distal extremity swelling because of ischemia or venous insufficiency. In most of these cases, angiography performed before operation had demonstrated occlusion or vascular compromise. However, some wounds with suspected vascular injury as well as injury to nerve were explored acutely without preoperative angiography, usually because of persistent wound bleeding or expanding hematoma. Repairs to major arteries varied from simple suture to use of vein or synthetic graft replacement. The status of the plexus elements sometimes was noted but often was not. In a few cases, acute repair of transected neural elements was attempted, but as subsequent studies or operation suggested, this seldom led to a good result. In a few cases, transected elements were tacked down to adjacent fascial planes, and this appeared to be effective in maintaining the length of the neural structures. Unfortunately, secondary operation for plexus repair sometimes revealed that neural elements had been incorporated by suture into the vascular repair.

The second category of vascular injuries was less frequent, harder to diagnose, and not easy to treat. In this series, six pseudoaneurysms were found and operated on. Each was at a shoulder or axillary level (Figure 14–2). Diagnosis was usually suspected because of progressive pain and neural loss or, in two cases, because of the presence of a thrill and bruit and a palpable mass in the axillary region. In three of the six pseudoaneurysm cases, angiography was considered to be negative. In two more cases too recent to include in the tables, the diagnosis was not suspected preoperatively, angiograms were not done, and yet large aneurysms were encountered at the time of exploration for plexus repair.

If angiography was positive, it usually showed irregularity or roughening of a portion of the axillary artery, but not contrast fill of the aneurysm. At exploration, a large mass of variably organized and often encapsulated clot was found encircling axillary artery and displacing the cords and cord-to-nerve connections of the plexus (Figure 14–3). Dissection above, below,

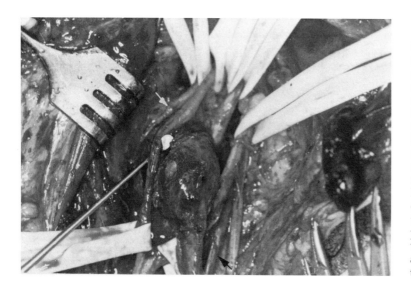

**Figure 14–2.** Pseudoaneurysm of axillary artery secondary to a gunshot wound. Dissector is beneath lateral cord contribution to median nerve. Medial cord contribution traveled beneath more distal axillary artery in this case. Ulnar nerve is marked by a black arrow and musculocutaneous nerve by a white arrow. This lesion severely stretched lateral and medial cord contributions to median and also the posterior cord. Most of the loss was reversed by removal of the aneurysm and neurolysis of the plexus.

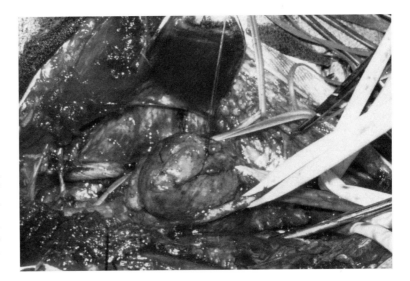

**Figure 14–3.** Large organized clot associated with another pseudoaneurysm caused by a gunshot wound. In this case, some of the cord and cord-to-nerve elements required repair after resection of the aneurysm.

and distally was required to isolate and gain control of proximal and distal axillary artery and the profundus vessel. The covering of the organized clot could then be opened after dissecting the neural elements free from its capsule. Repair of the vessel was usually straightforward. The vascular rent was oversewn in most instances but had to be patched by a piece of vein in two cases. One additional recent case has required interposition vein graft repair. Because four of the aneurysms were done in the early days or weeks after wounding, even intraoperative electrical studies could not predict the outcome for the elements that were in continuity but stretched and contused, so only a neurolysis could be done. In the two cases in which aneurysm was discovered several months after wounding, some of the involved elements had to be replaced with grafts, after nerve action potential (NAP) studies indicated lack of regeneration.

In a study completed and reported in 1989, 141 patients with GSWs involving the brachial plexus were evaluated (see Table 14–1).[12] In the 90 cases eventually operated on because of severe neural loss or pain, 30 vascular procedures had been done. This incidence was much lower for supraclavicular than for infraclavicular lesions and much higher in those requiring neural operations than in those not operated (only 8 of 51). Vascular grafts were placed in 24 of these cases and were either venous or synthetic in nature. Orthopedic procedures required in the early days after wounding included six for proximal humeral or glenohumeral joint fracture and several relatively acute repairs of comminuted clavicular fractures. Several other patients required clavicular stabilization at the time of neural repair, by either pinning or wiring. The severity of injury in this group of plexus patients is further borne out by the fact that eight required early thoracotomy and six others required placement of a chest tube.

## Pain Management

Management of pain was difficult in this series of cases. There were a few patients who had true causalgia, and these were either helped by repeated sympathetic blocks (2 patients), or they were helped temporarily by blocks (4 patients) but required cervical sympathectomy for more permanent relief. These patients with causalgia had severe pain and also autonomic disturbance, usually in the hand, but, more importantly, they could not stand to have the hand touched or manipulated even if their attention was distracted. Most of these patients had had a trial of phenoxybenzamine or similar sympatholytic agents and such management had failed. Others have had greater success with such a pharmacologic approach to causalgia associated with GSWs.[9,11]

More difficult to manage than the six patients with causalgia in this series were those with severe dysesthesias and often some degree of hyperpathia. These patients had severe neuritic pain rather than pain related to the sympathetic system. Nonetheless, manipulation of the sympathetic system had often been tried elsewhere but usually had failed. Some of these patients were helped by a combination of aggressive range of motion exercises, physical as well as occupational therapy, and use of amitriptyline and carbamazepine. The latter had to be gradually increased and often was not effective until dosages reached 1000 to 1600 mg per day. Pain of a neuritic nature and related complaints were most severe in the early months after wounding, and then they usually began to diminish rapidly with further time. Nonetheless, some patients had operation a number of months after wounding for pain of a non-causalgic nature in the hope that neurolysis and manipulation of the plexus would help their pain syndrome. Sometimes such an approach did just that, but 50% of the time, it did not.

An important step in the management of all cases was institution of range of motion exercises as early as possible. If paralysis was incomplete, more structured physical therapy was offered so that a regular system of exercise was instituted.

## Selection of Patients for Neural Operations

Because most civilian GSWs involving plexus do not transect elements but rather contuse, bruise, or stretch them, the majority of GSW

**TABLE 14–3**

Gunshot Wounds — Criteria
for Selection for a Neural Operation

A. Complete loss in the distribution of at least one element:
   1. No improvement clinically or by EMG in early months after injury.
   2. Loss should be in the distribution of at least one element usually helped by operation such as C5, C6, C7, upper or middle trunk, lateral or posterior cords or their outflows.
   3. Injuries with loss in lower element(s) only were not operated on. If there was also loss in other element(s) likely to be helped by operation, then they were repaired whenever possible.
B. Incomplete loss where pain could not be controlled pharmacologically. In addition, when completely injured elements were operated on, those elements incompletely injured were dissected out and also checked by NAP recordings.
C. Pseudoaneurysm, clot, or fistula involving plexus.
D. True causalgia requiring sympathectomy.

plexus cases were managed conservatively for 2 to 5 months (Table 14–3). A thorough baseline clinical examination was considered to be essential. Electromyographic (EMG) work-up was deferred for 3 to 4 weeks. Patients were then reevaluated on at least one occasion in subsequent months to see if there were clinical signs of reversal of loss or electrical evidence of reinnervation. For this reason, the average injury to operative interval was 17 weeks (Figure 14–4). Since most patients came from outside of the state of Louisiana for their initial evaluation and subsequent operation, these individuals could

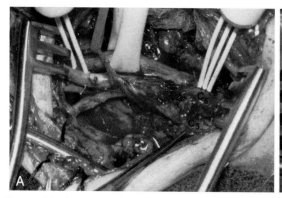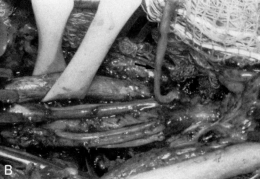

**Figure 14–4.** (A) Missile wound injury to C5, C6, and upper trunk. Function had not improved clinically or electrically by 5 months after wounding. Operative stimulation and recording showed only a small nerve action potential from a portion of the C6 outflow to upper trunk. This was split off and spared resection; the rest of C6 and all of C5 outflow to the upper trunk were replaced by grafts. (B) One graft (black arrow) remains to be attached distally. See also color figure.

not always be scheduled at 2 to 4 months, which was considered to be an optimal interval between injury and operation. The reason for neural operation was usually because loss in the distribution of one or more elements of the plexus failed to improve in the early months after injury; this occurred in 79 of the 90 operative patients. Pseudoaneurysm or clot compressing or involving plexus provided the major indication in six other cases. Five patients had operation despite incomplete loss in the distribution of each element at the level of involvement because noncausalgic pain was not responding to pharmacologic management.

Nonoperation was usually (in 34 of 51 cases) the result of incomplete loss in the distribution of each element that subsequently improved. Surprisingly, seven patients who initially had complete loss in the distribution of one or more elements, improved in the early months after injury and did not require operation. They progressed to a good spontaneous recovery. There were seven other patients with predominant lower element, C8, T1, lower trunk, or medial cord loss. Because these patients were adults, it was thought that operation for loss in that distribution would be unlikely to help. There were three additional patients who were referred a year or more after injury and for that reason were not considered reasonable candidates for operation.

## Operative Approach

Exposure of injured elements was usually performed by sharp dissection using a No. 15 blade on a long-handled, plastic knife-holder or by a long pair of Metzenbaum scissors. Dissections were done under some magnification, which was usually provided by 3.5-power eye loupes. Neural and vascular structures both proximal and distal to the injury site were exposed if possible. This permitted not only an optimal approach to the wound site but also placement of electrodes for operative stimulation and recording of NAPs. In patients with shotgun or high-power rifle wounds or extensive prior surgery for vascular or neural repair, a lengthy up-and-down exposure was necessary.

Injuries at the *supraclavicular level* were usually approached anteriorly through an oblique neck incision extending from the lateral border of the sternocleidomastoid muscle to the clavicle. Supraclavicular or transverse cervical vessels were isolated and ligated, supraclavicular fat pad was mobilized laterally, and anterior scalene region was totally dissected or skeletonized. Phrenic nerve, if still intact, was dissected out and mobilized medially so that the upper trunk could be dissected away from the anterior scalene (Figure 14–5). The anterior scalene muscle was usually resected so that C7 to middle trunk and the lower elements could be ex-

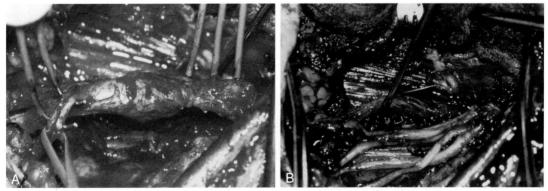

**Figure 14–5.** Severe injury to upper trunk caused by a gunshot wound. *(A)* At this point, C5 is being stimulated *(right)*, and recording electrodes are on supraclavicular nerve *(left)*. *(B)* There was no transmission through any portion of this lesion, so a graft repair was necessary. Middle trunk is retracted by instrument superior to the graft site.

posed. Exposure of divisions required dissection beneath the clavicle, ligation of subclavicular artery and vein, and usually resection of the subclavius muscle. By passing sponges around the clavicle, the latter could be pulled somewhat inferiorly to permit division-level dissection.

Generally, supraclavicular dissections were easier to accomplish than those below the clavicle. This was because subclavian artery and vein lay inferior to the majority of the dissection site and could be readily retracted with a vein hook. Below the clavicle, axillary artery, which was often injured or previously repaired, was at the core of the plexus lesion and had to be cleared and protected.

Injuries centered at an *infraclavicular level* were approached by splitting the pectoralis major muscle close to the deltopectoral groove. The deltopectoral vein was usually ligated as it crossed to reach axillary vein close to clavicle. Pectoralis minor muscle was divided or, for proximal infraclavicular lesions, retracted inferiorly by a Richardson retractor. Vessels overlying cords were coagulated or ligated and then divided. Subclavius muscle was divided, or, more commonly, a segment was removed. Clavicle could be mobilized somewhat and moved slightly superiorly by passing sponges beneath it and using them as slings to displace

clavicle superiorly. Again, as with the supraclavicular approach, subclavicular vessels were isolated. These vessels were ligated and divided, especially if dissection of the infraclavicular lesion required exposure of the divisions.

Self-retaining retractors such as an Adson were placed in either pectoralis minor or pectoralis major muscle on either side of the deltopectoral groove and opened to expose a broad expanse of the infraclavicular space. The initial element seen was lateral cord, usually lying superior and somewhat lateral to axillary artery. Because of the relatively high incidence of vascular injury associated with GSWs at this level, lateral cord as well as posterior and sometimes medial cord were adherent to vessels. Sometimes, one or more neural elements had been inadvertently incorporated into the vascular repair.

Dissection at an infraclavicular level for many GSWs was tedious and required great patience because of the need to skeletonize axillary artery and sometimes axillary vein (Figure 14 – 6). Rents or tears in these vessels often had to be repaired or re-repaired in the process of dissecting plexus elements away from vessels. Especially difficult was isolation of the posterior cord and then its distal course as it divided into axillary and radial nerves. Equally difficult was iso-

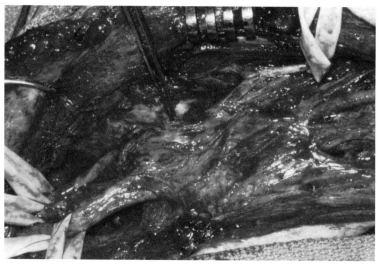

**Figure 14 – 6.** Severe scar involving cords of plexus and axillary vessels at an infraclavicular gunshot site. The initial operative step is isolation of axillary artery and, if necessary, axillary vein and major neural elements above and below the area of scar. Then each element is dissected out from the scar and, if not found to be transected, is electrically tested. Despite severe preoperative loss that was complete in the lateral and posterior cord distribution and incomplete in that of medial cord, each of these plexus elements transmitted nerve action potentials and were thus either regenerating well or only partially injured to begin with.

lation of branches coming off these elements if the posterior wall of the infraclavicular space was heavily involved in scar. Such branches included those to thoracodorsal, triceps, and subscapularis muscles.

Dissection was sometimes very difficult because of the intimate relationship of lateral and especially medial cord contributions to the median nerve as they wrap around or are adherent to the axillary artery. If there was physical continuity to musculocutaneous outflow from lateral cord into biceps/brachialis, dissection had to be precise, especially laterally. Small coracobrachialis branches run laterally from the lateral cord to the musculocutaneous nerve junction or very proximal musculocutaneous nerve and have to be spared whenever possible.

There were several cases in which GSWs involved roots very close to the spine. These patients were operated on by a posterior subscapular approach with resection of the first rib and exposure of the involved roots or spinal nerves medial to their dural exit.[14]

## RESULTS — GUNSHOT WOUNDS TO BRACHIAL PLEXUS

Only 6% of the elements operated on because of complete functional loss were found not to have some degree of physical continuity at surgery. Repair was obviously indicated for these elements and was done by grafts in most cases (12 of 14 transected elements). The more common finding was a lesion in continuity involving one or more elements, usually at one level and of variable length. Because operation was done in the early months after injury, it was necessary not only to stimulate above and below these lesions in continuity to see if distal muscle contraction could be gained, but also to attempt to record a NAP across the lesion (Tables 14–4 and 14–5). If any NAP was recorded beyond the lesion, it was usually not resected but instead had a neurolysis done. Exceptions were provided in four elements in which inspection suggested that a portion of the cross section of the injury was more severe or neurotmetic and a portion not so bad and probably responsible for the NAP. In these regenerating or only partially injured elements, the portion conducting a NAP was split away from that not conducting and spared resection. That portion not conducting was resected, and, because lesions in continuity caused by gunshot wounds tend to be lengthy, grafts were usually placed to accomplish a split repair.

In 125 of the 221 elements studied, no NAP was recorded, and the lesion was resected (Figure 14–7). End-to-end repair was obtained in only 26 cases. Graft repair was necessary in the other 99 cases because of the length of resection required.

The Louisiana State University Medical Center system for grading response for each element of the brachial plexus was used. This system takes into account proximal and distal muscle recovery as well as sensation in the hand if applicable. Function returning to grade 3 or better indicated a successful outcome for a given element.

Outcome was based on two or more years of follow-up in 75 of the 90 cases operated on. Table 14–3 shows the results listed by element and level in cases in which loss was believed clinically to be either complete or incomplete before operation. Most (94%) of the elements considered to have complete loss by physical examination were confirmed as having complete loss by preoperative EMG. Despite this, 48 elements in this category were found at operation to have evidence of early regeneration by NAP studies (Figure 14–8). As a result, these elements had neurolysis or, in four cases, a split repair. Twenty-one of these elements, when stimulated, had some degree of muscle contraction distal to the injury. Twenty-seven of the 48 elements in which a NAP was elicited did not have distal response to stimulation but nevertheless had an excellent outcome with either neurolysis or a split repair.

Most of the cases thought to have incomplete injury to elements were confirmed as such at the operating table. As can be seen from Table 14–3, there were, however, some exceptions. One C7 to middle trunk lesion did not transmit a NAP and required graft repair, as did one posterior cord lesion and one of the medial cord lesions which had a repair. Several medial and lateral cord elements contributing to the median nerve also did not have a transmitted NAP and required resection and repair.

As observed in an earlier but briefly summa-

## TABLE 14—4
Profile and Treatment Results in Gunshot Wounds in Continuity With Complete and Incomplete Loss of Function*

| Location of Injury | Complete Loss of Function | | | | | | | Incomplete Loss of Function | | | | | |
|---|---|---|---|---|---|---|---|---|---|---|---|---|---|
| | No. of Elements | NAP + | NAP − | Neurolysis (RESULT) | Suture (RESULT) | Graft (RESULT) | (?)Imp | No. of Elements | NAP + | NAP − | Neurolysis (RESULT) | Suture (RESULT) | Graft (RESULT) |
| Spinal Nerve to Trunk: | | | | | | | | | | | | | |
| C5-6 to Upper Trunk | 13 | 3 | 10 | 3/3 | 0/0 | 10/7 | 0/0 | 3 | 3 | 0 | 3/3 | 0/0 | 0/0 |
| C7 to Middle Trunk | 10 | 1 | 9 | 1/1 | 0/0 | 9/4 | 0/0 | 7 | 6 | 1 | 6/6 | 0/0 | 1/1 |
| C8-T1 to Lower Trunk | 12 | 3 | 9 | 3/3 | 0/0 | 8/2 | 1/0 | 4 | 4 | 0 | 4/4 | 0/0 | 0/0 |
| Division to Cord: | | | | | | | | | | | | | |
| Lateral | 9 | 3 | 6 | 3/3 | 1/1 | 5/4 | 0/0 | 11 | 10 | 1 | 10/10 | 1/0 | 0/0 |
| Medial | 13 | 5 | 8 | 5/4 | 1/0 | 14/4† | 3/0 | 7 | 7 | 0 | 6/6 | 0/0 | 1/1† |
| Posterior | 13 | 3 | 10 | 3/3 | 2/1 | 7/5 | 1/1 | 5 | 4 | 1 | 4/4 | 1/1 | 0/0 |
| Cord to Nerve: | | | | | | | | | | | | | |
| Lateral to Musculocutaneous Nerve | 10 | 3 | 7 | 3/3 | 2/2 | 5/5 | 0/0 | 3 | 3 | 0 | 3/3 | 0/0 | 0/0 |
| Lateral to Median | 28 | 10 | 18 | 9/7 | 5/4 | 14/9‡ | 0/0 | 3 | 1 | 2 | 1/1 | 2/2 | 0/0 |
| Medial to Median | 19 | 3 | 16 | 2/2 | 4/2 | 13/7† | 0/0 | 3 | 1 | 2 | 1/1 | 2/2 | 0/0 |
| Medial to Ulnar | 20 | 6 | 14 | 5/4 | 2/0 | 12/2† | 1/0 | 3 | 3 | 0 | 3/0 | 0/0 | 0/0 |
| Posterior to Radial | 16 | 7 | 9 | 6/6 | 2/2 | 8/4 | 0/0 | 4 | 4 | 0 | 4/4 | 0/0 | 0/0 |
| Posterior to Axillary | 3 | 1 | 2 | 1/1 | 1/1 | 1/1 | 0/0 | 2 | 2 | 0 | 2/2 | 0/0 | 2/2 |
| TOTALS | 166 | 48 | 118 | 44/40 | 20/13 | 105/54 | 6/1 | 55 | 48 | 7 | 47/44 | 6/5 | 2/2 |

*Results are given as total elements/number of elements recovering to grade 3 or better. Data does not include 14 elements found "blown apart" with a whole segment missing. NAP = nerve action potential distal to lesion;
+ = present; − = absent; (?)Imp = repair believed impossible because of lesion length.
†Includes one split or partial graft repair with grade 3 or better results.
‡Includes two split or partial graft repairs with grade 3 or better results.
From Kline DG: Civilian gunshot wounds to the brachial plexus. J Neurosurg 70:166–174, 1989.

**TABLE 14–5**

Results With Operations on Gunshot Wounds to Plexus—Elements
Found in Continuity*

| Type of Lesion | Nerve Action Potential | | Neurolysis | Suture | Graft | Impossible |
| --- | --- | --- | --- | --- | --- | --- |
| | **Present** | **Absent** | **Result** | | | |
| Lesions with complete loss (166) | 48 | 118 | 44/40 | 20/13 | 96/51† | 6/1 |
| Lesions with incomplete loss (55) | 48 | 7 | 47/44 | 6/5 | 2/2‡ | 0/0 |

*Results are given as total elements/number of elements recovering to grade 3 or better. Does not include 14 elements found apart with segment missing.

†Includes 5 split repairs with grade 3 or better results.

‡Includes one split repair with grade 3 or better result.

From Kline DG: Civilian gunshot wounds to the brachial plexus. J Neurosurg 70:166–174, 1989.

rized study of the first 46 GSWs to plexus operated on at LSUMC, results with repair were especially good for upper elements such as spinal nerves C5 and C6 and the upper trunk, lateral and posterior cords, and their outflows.[13] Nonetheless, it remained difficult to restore practical deltoid contraction, even though more proximal muscles such as supraspinatus and sometimes infraspinatus, and those more distal such as biceps-brachialis and even brachioradialis, often recovered function to grade 3 or better levels. Repairs of the C7 to middle trunk elements did not fare as well as upper element repairs: only four of nine graft repairs achieved a grade 3 or better. It was difficult to obtain recovery, particularly of good triceps function, although the patient usually substituted well for this loss by using gravity.

At a division-to-cord level, recovery of some triceps, brachioradialis, and even some wrist extension could usually be obtained with posterior cord lesions and with more distal posterior cord to radial lesions (Figure 14–9). In some cord-level cases, triceps branches were severely involved, and successful repair of these branches was difficult. Although there were several exceptions, it was also difficult to obtain useful finger or thumb extension with such proximal repairs of posterior cord and posterior cord to radial elements. By comparison, lateral cord and lateral cord to musculocutaneous nerve repairs gave almost uniformly good results (Figure 14–10). Even sensation in the median distribution of the hand returned to grade 4 levels in most lateral cord repairs. Some of these patients had flexor function spared to begin with or had recovery of some function from more proximal repair of median or ulnar out-

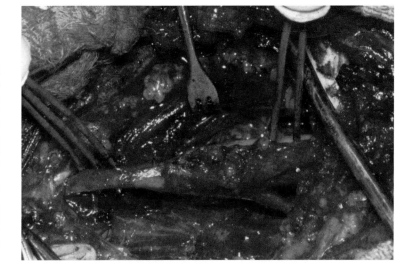

**Figure 14–7.** Gunshot wound involving upper trunk. C5 is being stimulated to the left, and recording electrodes are placed on the anterior division of the upper trunk to the right. This truncal lesion, which was exposed 3.5 months after injury, required resection and repair. Outcome was good. At 3.5 years, biceps graded 4 to 5, pronator, wrist, and finger flexors 3 to 4, and sensation in the median distribution 4. See also color figure.

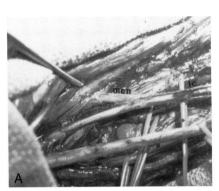
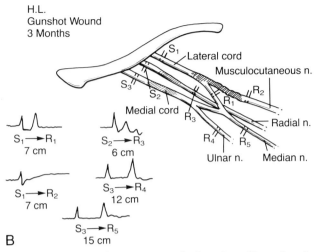

H.L.
Gunshot Wound
3 Months

**Figure 14–8.** (A) Gunshot wound at level of cords. The most serious damage was to the junction of lateral cord (lc) and musculocutaneous nerve (mcn). (Dissector tip points to entry of damaged mcn into biceps muscle.) No nerve action potentials (NAPs) transmitted along this segment, although they did transmit to median nerve. This segment of damage was resected and repaired by grafts. (B) Drawing of operative findings including NAP studies. Fortunately, medial cord, which was severely involved by preoperative clinical and electrical evaluation, transmitted a NAP ($S_3$ to $R_4$, $S_3$ to $R_5$). Posterior cord was less involved and, as expected, transmitted ($S_2$ to $R_3$). Because lateral cord transmitted to median ($S_1$ to $R_1$) but not to musculocutaneous ($S_1$ to $R_2$), its contribution to median was dissected proximally. Grafts were placed from lateral cord to musculocutaneous nerve only.

flows. These individuals were candidates for tendon transfer to substitute for wrist and finger drop.

Compared with the good results with repair of lateral cord and its outflows, results with C8, T1, medial cord, and medial cord to ulnar repairs were poor. On the other hand, medial cord to median nerve repairs fared surprisingly well, with four of six suture repairs and seven of 13 grafts recovering to grade 3 or better levels. In addition, a number of lesions involving lower elements or even medial cord were proved by NAP studies to be regenerating despite complete distal loss by clinical examination and EMG (Table 14–6). Eventual recovery with only neurolysis was excellent in this group of lower element injuries. Eleven of 13 recovered to grade 3 or better despite complete functional loss at the time of operation. The 16 patients with complete or nearly complete loss of func-

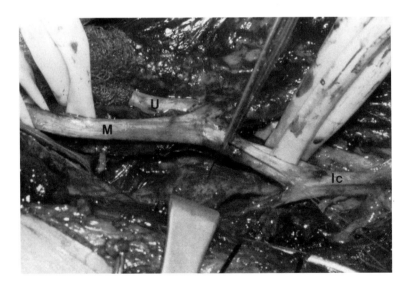

**Figure 14–9.** Severe lesion in continuity to posterior cord which did not transmit a nerve action potential (NAP) and required resection and graft repair. Musculocutaneous loss was also complete preoperatively, but this element had a NAP transmitted across the injury. It had a neurolysis done and is displaced inferiorly by the retractor. lc = lateral cord; M = median; U = ulnar. (From Kline DG: Civilian gunshot wounds to the brachial plexus. J Neurosurg 70:166–174, 1989.)

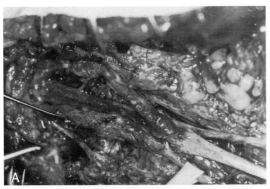

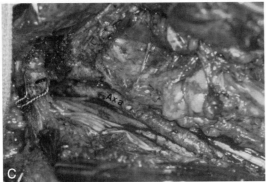

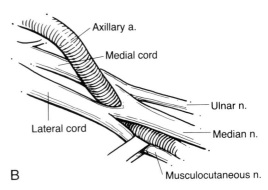

B

**Figure 14–10.** *(A)* This gunshot wound involved lateral and posterior cords. An arterial repair had been done acutely, and, unfortunately, the posterior wall of the artery was sewn to the lateral and some of the posterior cord. *(B)* The accompanying drawing depicts the major relationships of some of the plexus elements to the axillary artery. *(C)* The lateral cord segment required repair. Grafts are in place in lateral cord distribution. Clavicle had been divided because proximal suture site for the grafts was immediately below the clavicle. Ax a = axillary artery. (Reprinted in part from Kline DG, Judice DJ: Operative management of selected brachial plexus lesions. J Neurosurg 58:631–649, 1983.)

tion of all elements at the level of wounding did surprisingly well, at least in terms of upper element recovery, although repair of C8, T1, and their more distal outflows failed to restore useful hand function in these cases.

## Case Summaries — GSW Involving Plexus

### Case Number 1

This 55-year-old, right-handed warehouse manager was shot in the left shoulder by a 35-caliber pistol at close range. The bullet entered the supraclavicular space and

fractured the clavicle and the first two ribs. A shell fragment lodged in the posterior subscapular area. Initially, he had a flail arm. After angiography showed normal axillary and subclavian blood flow, the entrance wound was debrided at his local hospital to remove shell fragments and pieces of fractured clavicle.

When seen 6 weeks later, he had total paralysis of the supraspinatus, infraspinatus, deltoid, biceps/brachialis, triceps, brachioradialis, pronator teres, supinator, and wrist and finger extensor muscles. Wrist and finger flexion including the flexor pollicis longus muscle graded 2 to 3 and interosseus muscles graded 3, but there was no function of the lumbrical muscles of the hand or of thenar intrinsic muscles. There was sensory loss in the C5, C6, and C7 distributions, with relative sparing of C8 and T1.

**TABLE 14–6**
NAP Results and Percentage of Positive Results of Surgery for Gunshot Wounds to Brachial Plexus*

| | NAP Findings | | Operative Results | | | |
|---|---|---|---|---|---|---|
| | Present | Absent | Neurolysis | Suture | Graft | Repair Impossible |
| In continuity lesions with complete loss | 29% | 71% | 91% | 65% | 53% | 17% |
| In continuity lesions with incomplete loss | 87% | 13% | 94% | 83% | 100% | 0 |
| Transections | 0 | 0 | 0 | 50% | 64% | 0 |
| Elements thought to be favorable for repair | 30% | 70% | 96% | 69% | 66%† | 0 |
| Elements thought to be unfavorable for repair | 27% | 73% | 79% | 44% | 32%† | 0 |

*Based on grade 3 or better results. NAP = nerve action potential.
†Includes three split or partial graft repairs with grade 3 or better results.

Electromyography showed extensive denervational changes involving all muscles. The changes were most severe in the C5, C6, and C7 distributions. Exploration was performed almost 3 months after injury, through an anterior and supraclavicular as well as infraclavicular approach. The comminuted and callused portion of the clavicle was resected, and after extensive scar tissue was removed, the spinal nerves, trunks, and cords of the plexus were exposed. All elements were in continuity but scarred. No NAPs could be recorded by stimulating the C5, C6, or C7 nerves and recording from the anterior and posterior divisions of the upper and middle trunks. In addition, there was no distal muscle contraction on stimulation of these elements. On the other hand, stimulation of either C8 or T1 elicited a small amount of wrist flexion, and moderate-sized NAPs could be recorded from the medial cord. External neurolysis alone was performed on C8, T1, and their outflows. Portions of C5, C6, and C7 nerves and all of the upper and middle trunks were resected. Eleven grafts 5 to 6.4 cm in length were then placed from C5 to the suprascapular nerve, C5 to the lateral and posterior cords, C6 to the lateral and posterior cords, and C7 to the posterior cord and a portion of the medial cord. The clavicle was then wired together. Soft tissues were closed over a Penrose drain.

The drain was removed on the 3rd postoperative day, and the patient was discharged on the 7th day with instructions for physical therapy. He was seen on several occasions for follow-up evaluation. At 5 years postoperatively, muscle testing revealed the following results: supra- and infraspinatus muscles were graded 3 to 4, deltoid muscle 3, biceps/brachialis muscles 4, triceps muscle 3, pronation/supination 3, and wrist extension 4. Finger and thumb extension, however, were absent. Wrist and finger flexion graded 4, interosseus and lumbrical muscles graded 4, and thenar intrinsic muscles graded 3. Although touch and pinprick were decreased in the thumb, forefinger, and long finger, the patient could localize stimuli in these areas well. He considered a tendon transfer to improve finger and thumb extension because he was working and needed to use these functions. However, because he was able to work and use his arm and hand quite well, he did not wish to take time out to have this done. He has recovered to grade 4 for the C5, C6, and upper trunk repairs, and to grade 3 for the C7 and middle trunk repairs.

## Comment

This was a fortunate result from a very severe GSW to the plexus. If loss, especially that in the C5, C6, and C7 distribution or their outflows, does not improve spontaneously in the early months after wounding, exploration and intraoperative recordings are in order.

## Case Number 2

This 22-year-old, right-handed mechanic sustained a wound in the right shoulder from a shotgun blast at close range. Acutely, he required a subclavian to brachial artery extra-anatomic saphenous bypass graft and immobilization of the arm for a humeral fracture. Some voluntary contraction of the hand muscles was initially noted. Subsequent EMG showed complete denervation of the deltoid and biceps muscles as well as muscles innervated by radial and median, but only partial denervation of the hand intrinsic muscles.

Evaluation showed findings much as had been described from the referring institution. Supraspinatus and infraspinatus muscles were graded 3 to 4. Deltoid power was absent, as was biceps/brachialis and brachioradialis strength. The triceps muscle worked but was weak and graded 3. However, there was no finger, thumb, or wrist extension, and pronation and supination were absent. Wrist flexion was provided by the flexor carpi ulnaris muscle, which was weak (grade 3). Finger flexion was quite weak, although the profundi of the little and ring fingers were graded 2 to 3, as were the hand intrinsic muscles in the ulnar distribution. All median-innervated muscles had absent function, and there was hypoesthesia in the median and radial distributions and relative hypoesthesia in the ulnar distribution. These findings did not change over the next 6 weeks.

The patient underwent exploration of the infraclavicular plexus through an anterior approach some 5.5 months after wounding. The entire shoulder to upper arm area was found peppered with shot, and all elements were surrounded by heavy scar tissue. The pectoralis major and minor muscles were divided to provide adequate exposure. A segment of the lateral cord to musculocutaneous nerve was missing and was replaced by two sural grafts, each 5 cm in length. A longitudinal portion of the lateral cord to median nerve transmitted a small NAP, but the remainder did not. A split repair of the lateral cord was carried out so that a portion was replaced with a 5-cm graft, and the remainder of the element had a neurolysis. A large neuroma in continuity involving the posterior cord to radial nerve exhibited no NAP, was resected, and was replaced with three 6.4-cm sural grafts. The posterior cord to axillary nerve had a NAP, so only a neurolysis was performed. Despite heavy scarring around and some firmness in the medial cord and its outflows, NAPs could be recorded for all medial cord outflows except the medial cord to median nerve. After a thorough external neurolysis, an antebrachial sensory segment was fashioned into two 3.8-cm grafts which were placed from the medial cord to median nerve. Medial cord to ulnar nerve had only an external neurolysis done. The pectoralis major (but not minor) muscle was repaired, and the large wound was closed in multiple layers without a drain. The patient was given antibiotics postoperatively and remained afebrile. He was discharged to his referring facility for physical therapy on the ninth postoperative day.

The patient was seen on several occasions during the first postoperative year and was noted to have early recovery of deltoid function. He returned to work as a service station manager, using mainly his left arm with the right arm employed to assist the left. By 2 years postoperatively, biceps/brachialis power was 3 to 4 and pronation 4, and median and ulnar function had improved dramatically. Follow-up evaluation 6.5 years after injury indicated shoulder abduction to 110 degrees. Loss of axillary soft tissue restricted further abduction. Biceps, brachioradialis, and triceps function were excellent. There was excellent pronation and partial supination, and wrist extension graded 3 to 4. Finger and thumb extension were absent. There was a slight tendency to claw the fingers, but overall motor power grades for specific elements were axillary 4, lateral cord to musculocutaneous 4, lateral cord to median 4, medial cord to median 4, and posterior cord to radial 3 to 4. He now uses his right arm daily in his work, and this includes writing with his right hand even though it tires readily.

## Comment

If previous vascular surgery has resulted in a nonanatomic placement of a vascular graft, the surgeon must avoid injury to the graft. Repair of the pectoralis minor may compromise neural suture lines and is usually not done. By comparison, we carefully repair pectoralis major. Drains must be placed meticulously so as not to displace grafts by suction and must subsequently be removed with care for the same reason.

## Bibliography

1. Bateman JE: The Shoulder and Neck, 2nd Ed. Philadelphia, WB Saunders, 1978, pp. 565–616.
2. Binns JH and Wynn Parry CB: Successful repair of a complete brachial plexus lesion. Injury 2:19–21, 1970.
3. Black AN, Burns BD, and Zuckerman S: An experimental study of the wounding mechanism of high velocity missiles. Br Med J 2:872–874, 1941.
4. Brooks DM: Open wounds of the brachial plexus. J Bone Joint Surg Br 31:17–33, 1949.
5. Brown AK: Gunshot wounds then and now. J R Coll Surg Edinb 34:302–309, 1989.
6. Callender GR: Wound ballistics—mechanism of production of wounds by small arms, bullets and shell fragments. War Med 3:337–342, 1943.
7. Davis L, Martin J, and Perret G: The treatment of injuries of the brachial plexus. Ann Surg 125:647–657, 1947.
8. French LA: Clinical experience with peripheral nerve surgery with especial reference to the results in early nerve repair. MS Thesis, University of Minnesota, 1946.
9. Ghostine SY, Comair YG, Turner DM, et al.: Phenoxybenzamine in the treatment of causalgia. J Neurosurg 60:1263–1268, 1984.
10. Hudson AR and Dommissee I: Brachial plexus injury: Case report of gunshot wounds. Can Med Assoc J 117:1162–1164, 1977.
11. Jebara VA and Saade B: Causalgia: A wartime experience—report of twenty treated cases. J Trauma 27:519–524, 1987.
12. Kline DG: Civilian gunshot wounds to the brachial plexus. J Neurosurg 70:166–174, 1989.
13. Kline DG and Judice DJ: Operative management of selected brachial plexus lesions. J Neurosurg 58:631–649, 1983.
14. Kline DG, Kott J, Barnes G, et al.: Exploration of selected brachial plexus lesions by the posterior subscapular approach. J Neurosurg 49:872–880, 1978.
15. Leffert RD: Brachial Plexus Injuries. New York, Churchill Livingstone, 1985, pp. 131–139.
16. Nakaras A: The surgical management of brachial plexus injuries. In Daniels RK and Terzis JK, Eds: Reconstructive Microsurgery. Boston, Little, Brown & Co, 1977, pp. 443–460.
17. Nelson KG, Jolly PC, and Thomas PA: Brachial plexus injuries associated with missile wounds of the chest. A report of 9 cases from Viet Nam. J Trauma 8:268–275, 1968.
18. Nulsen FE and Slade WW: Recovery following injury to the brachial plexus. In Woodhall B and Beebe GW, Eds: Peripheral Nerve Regeneration: A Follow-up Study of 3,656 World War II Injuries. Washington, DC: US Government Printing Office, 1956, pp. 389–408.
19. Omer GE: Injuries to nerves of the upper extremity. J Bone Joint Surg 56A:1615–1627, 1974.
20. Seddon HJ: Surgical Disorders of the Peripheral Nerves. Baltimore, Williams & Wilkins, 1972, pp. 174–198.
21. Sunderland S: Nerves and Nerve Injuries, 2nd Ed. Edinburgh, Churchill Livingstone, 1978.

# Stretch Injuries to Brachial Plexus

## SUMMARY

Management of these frequently encountered lesions is one of the most controversial areas in medicine and surgery. As with other plexus lesions, it is most important to evaluate them in terms of complete and incomplete loss for each and every plexus element. Incomplete loss, significant sparing or early recovery can lead to a good spontaneous recovery in that element's distribution; however other, more seriously stretched or avulsed elements may not recover. Multiple signs of severe proximal injury and evidence supporting avulsion, particularly of C5, C6, and C7, argue against a successful direct repair of the plexus. However, there are limitations to the precision of some of these findings such as paraspinal denervation, positive sensory potentials, and even abnormal myelography. Nonetheless, we have followed a selective route and tried to study the value of direct repair for stretch injuries chosen for operation. Neurotization using the descending cervical plexus, the sternocleidomastoid branch of the accessory, or pectoral branches has been added sometimes to any direct repair possible. A separate series of patients from Canada having intercostal neurotization alone was also analyzed.

Grading recovery of function in plexus injuries where multiple elements were involved has been difficult, but an attempt has been made to do this using the Louisiana State University Medical Center system to gain some determination of the value of direct repair. C5, C6 distribution stretches have a relatively low incidence of avulsion, recover sometimes spontaneously, and surprisingly often include severe damage to C7. These injuries are excellent candidates for direct repair aided by neurotization with quite good results. C5, C6, C7 distribution stretches have more roots avulsed than do C5, C6 stretches, recover spontaneously with less frequency, and have a variable loss of wrist and finger movement. Nonetheless, some of these lesions are also good candidates for direct repair with acceptable results. C5 through T1 distribution stretches are difficult to help by direct repair, although almost 50% of those selected for operation regain some usable shoulder and arm function. There is an immense spectrum of presentations regarding reparability of roots or spinal nerves in the C5 through T1 stretches, and this affects outcome in a variable fashion.

Many infraclavicular-level stretch injuries do not recover spontaneously and require operation. As with the supraclavicular stretch injuries, it helps to sort out the various lesions by intraoperative nerve action potential recordings. Results with repair of lateral and posterior cords and their outflows, such as the musculocutaneous and axillary, are surprisingly good. As expected, medial cord recovery is poor if resection and repair are necessary. Repair of medial cord to median lesions is, however, useful in the majority of cases.

It is unusual for the suprascapular nerve to sustain isolated direct injury, but loss in its distribution is a frequent concomitant of C5, C6, and upper trunk injuries. Stretch injuries affecting both axillary and suprascapular nerves but not C5, C6, and/or upper trunk are also fairly common. The suprascapular portion usually improves with time and seldom requires repair although the axillary nerve sometimes does. Suprascapular entrapment also can and does occur relatively often, and ganglions can also form in the shoulder and compress this nerve. The suprascapular nerve enters the scapular area beneath the suprascapular ligament, and a relatively deep and lateral surgical exposure located superior to the scapular spine is usually required for section of the ligament. An alternative approach is a supraclavicular combined with an infraclavicular approach to the nerve, but this limits exposure of the nerve in the region of the scapula. Less frequently, nerve can be entrapped in the region of the scapular notch so that, on occasion, exposure of nerve on either side of the spine of the scapula has been necessary.

# INTRODUCTION

In spite of intense interest in and literature generated about brachial plexus injuries, and specifically those caused by stretch/contusion, in the last several decades, there is not unanimity concerning the management of these difficult problems. Some authors still believe that there is little indication for surgery, whereas others feel all cases should be operated on.[77] Some surgeons still urge relatively early amputation, at least for the flail or totally paralyzed arm.[49] Other clinicians, including ourselves, try to select those cases more likely to respond to plexus repair for operation.[36,37] There is also a diversity of operative procedures and combinations of them for such plexus palsies. Direct repair, usually with the help of grafts, is sought by a variety of approaches for roots or spinal nerves that can be repaired in this fashion.[1,4,39,46] Attempts at direct neural repair can also be combined with neurotization if other nerves, such as higher cervical roots, descending cervical plexus, accessory, phrenic, or intercostal nerves, are led to distal inputs with or without intervening grafts.[2,32,42,57] A few surgeons tend to prefer a neurotization procedure as the initial operation because more direct repair is either not possible or frequently fails.[13,20] Other surgeons utilize relatively early reconstructive procedures, such as fusion of glenohumeral joint which still permits some shoulder mobility, and, if possible, flexorplasty or pectoralis or latissimus dorsi transfer to provide some elbow flexion.[6,44,81]

Because there is such a diversity of opinion and variety of approaches available, we will first review a selected portion of the vast literature on stretch injuries before presenting our own results. The accompanying figures for the next section depict some of the different combinations of stretch injuries we have encountered and how they have been managed.

# BACKGROUND FOR STRETCH/CONTUSION INJURIES

The most common lesion of the plexus is that caused by stretch/contusion, usually secondary to motor vehicular accidents, particularly those involving motorcycles.[18,22] Not all such injuries are a result of vehicular accidents.[16] In a review of 39 patients with sports injuries involving the plexus, football was responsible for nine and bicycling for seven.[40] There were four skiing and sledding accidents, four equestrian injuries, seven water sport-related injuries, and eight injuries related to other sports such as wrestling, gymnastics, and golf. Regardless of the setting, the head and neck are usually forcefully pushed in one direction and shoulder and arm in another direction.[25,53] This results in severe stretch to soft tissues, including nerve and, less frequently, vessels[29,89] (Figures 15–1, 15–2, and 15–3).

Regardless of the mechanism of injury, a conservative, nonsurgical approach has usually been predominant. Leffert has nicely summarized the literature of the early 1900s.[43] These early authors included Thoburn, Kennedy, Clark, Taylor, Prout, A. S. Taylor, Forester, Sever, Jepson, and Stevens. Many of the cases reported were birth palsies, but some were adult traction injuries. Some success with surgery was reported, but as a whole, the limited outcomes were discouraging. On the other hand, it has always been obvious that spontaneous functional regeneration is limited with severe injuries and that the possibilities for reconstructive surgery are often small. Amputation can occasionally permit the use of a prosthesis.[61] Unfortunately, the amputees seldom use such devices, especially if amputation is done at a very proximal level. This makes this type of surgery only ablative in nature (Figure 15–4).

Some review of the last 40 to 50 years of literature regarding spontaneous recovery of function without surgery is necessary. In 63 cases injured by stretch reported by Barnes in 1949, 14 had only a C5 and C6 deficit, and 11 of these recovered some biceps and a little shoulder function in a spontaneous fashion.[5] In addition, 11 of 19 with C5, C6, and C7 root damage had some return of wrist and finger extension, biceps, and some shoulder abduction. Prognosis, however, was poor for complete palsies involving all the plexus elements, and the latter observation was confirmed by Bonney in 1959.[9] In his series of 19 patients with complete lesions of the entire plexus followed for 2 years, there was very little return of function. If recovery did occur, it was delayed for 12 to 24 months and was to proximal muscles only. Fifteen patients

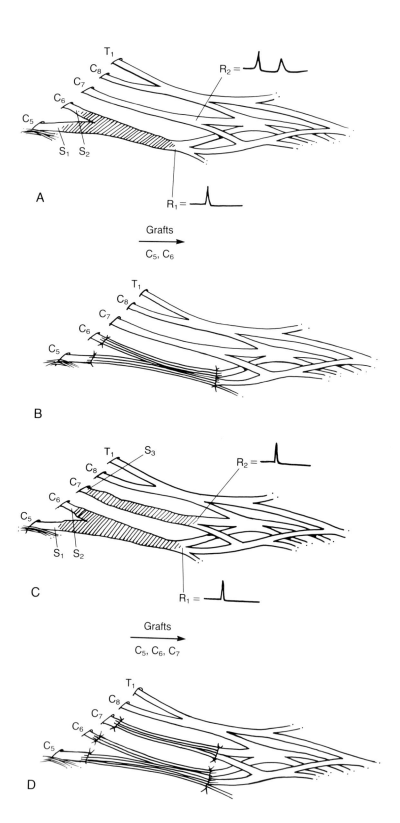

**Figure 15–1.** Two patterns of C5-C6 stretch injury that are fairly common. (A) Lesions in continuity extending from C5 and C6 through upper trunk did not transmit nerve action potentials but fortunately could be resected to healthy proximal tissue and replaced by sural grafts (B). In this example, C7 was found to be completely injured despite a clinical C5-C6 pattern of loss by physical and electromyographic examination (C). This occurred in one sixth of our C5-C6 cases. The repair is shown in D.

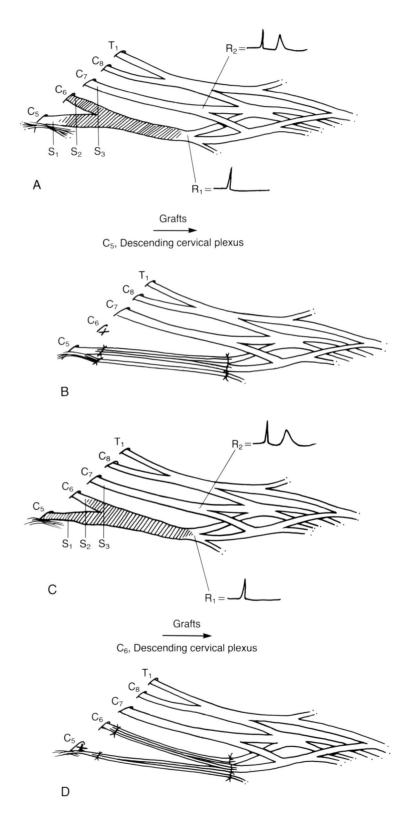

**Figure 15–2.** In the case depicted in *A*, no nerve action potentials were transmitted from C5-C6 to upper trunk divisions. However, C6 was not usable as a lead-out. As a result, descending cervical plexus was used as a lead-out for grafts, as well as the C5 spinal nerve *(B)*. In *C*, the situation was much the same, but here C5 was not usable as an outflow *(D)*. This is less frequently encountered than the scenario presented in *A* and *B*.

underwent exploration electively to determine prognosis. Each of the stretched elements was found to be in continuity, and no repairs were done. At that time, Bonney concluded that suture or grafting could be advised only if plexus was found to be torn apart and not if continuity was present. In 1962, P. E. Taylor found 90 stretch injuries reported in the literature and thought that 50 were adequate for study: 17 incomplete and 33 complete.[78] In the complete group, 60% regained no function at all.

Leffert and Seddon reviewed 31 closed brachial plexus injuries in which there was no fracture of the clavicle, swelling, or induration in the supraclavicular space; paralysis of muscles innervated by the dorsal scapular, suprascapular, or long thoracic nerves; or Horner syndrome.[45] In comparison with other series, this was a mildly injured group of patients with a predominately infraclavicular level of injury. The investigators, as a result, concluded that conservative management was in order. On the other hand, Alnot found that a number of infraclavicular lesions required operation.[3] Most cases done in his series involved posterior cord to radial nerve or axillary nerve, but a few involved lateral cord or lateral cord to musculocutaneous nerve or medial cord outflows.

Wynn Parry reported on a number of patients who were not operated on, but who were reexamined 5 or more years after injury.[84] In 36 patients treated conservatively who had complete C5 and C6 lesions, two thirds recovered some degree of elbow flexion and one third recovered some shoulder abduction (Figures 15–5 and 15–6). In 50 patients with complete C5, C6, and C7 lesions, one third recovered some degree of elbow flexion and some shoulder abduction. In 84 patients with complete C5 through T1 lesions, only 20% recovered elbow flexion, 16% elbow extension, and 7% finger flexion. From our perspective, however, spontaneous positive results do not seem to be quite this frequent. Perhaps this is because we are sent only the more serious cases. Those with very early recovery are probably treated conservatively elsewhere. This certainly seems to be the case with some series reported by neurologists. Nagano's figures on patients with postganglionic lesions of variable severity, reported in 1979, indicated good or excellent spontaneous recovery in more than 40% of patients.[54]

Unfortunately, in our experience, such is usually not the case if initial loss is complete in the distribution of two or more roots.

Yeoman and Seddon reported on patients with severe multiple-root injuries who had reconstructive orthopedic procedures.[87,88] Results were so poor that they recommended amputation and use of a prosthesis, even though Hendry was somewhat more optimistic about reconstructive orthopedic procedures in an earlier report.[27] On the other hand, Ransford and Hughes provided a 10-year follow-up on 20 patients with complete plexus palsies and noted that amputation did not relieve pain and that patients with prostheses seldom used them.[63] Nonetheless, a few authors still advocate early amputation for serious stretch injuries.[49]

In 1973, Zancolli and Mitre summarized their experience with latissimus dorsi transfer to substitute for biceps loss.[90] This and other muscle transfers have occasionally been useful if some function in the distribution of the plexus is spared to begin with or returns with time.[44,74] Experience with grafts for plexus lesions during the World War II period reported by Seddon and Brooks and by Nulsen and Slade gave some but not a great deal of encouragement for repair of these difficult lesions.[59]

Lusskin and Campbell urged a more aggressive approach for blunt injuries to the plexus than most earlier authors.[48] They indicated that neurolysis alone improved the outcome, as had Davis, Martin and Perrett, who reported on this procedure for penetrating wounds in 1947.[19] Lusskin and Campbell also recommended use of autografts.

A relatively aggressive but still selective approach was followed by Narakas.[55,56] Of 615 patients with stretch injuries, 237 were selected for operation. Four operations were for prognosis only, 4 were done on an emergency basis, 20 resulted in external neurolysis only, 13 had fascicular neurolysis, and 127 had autogenous, usually sural grafts placed. In 26 other instances, neurotization procedures using intercostal nerves were done, and 33 patients had such procedures as well as direct grafting of the plexus. Forty patients also had tendon transfers, 7 had a second operation, 18 had vascular repairs, and amputations were done in 8. What Narakas termed a good result occurred in 41% of his operated cases. Of the 143 patients with

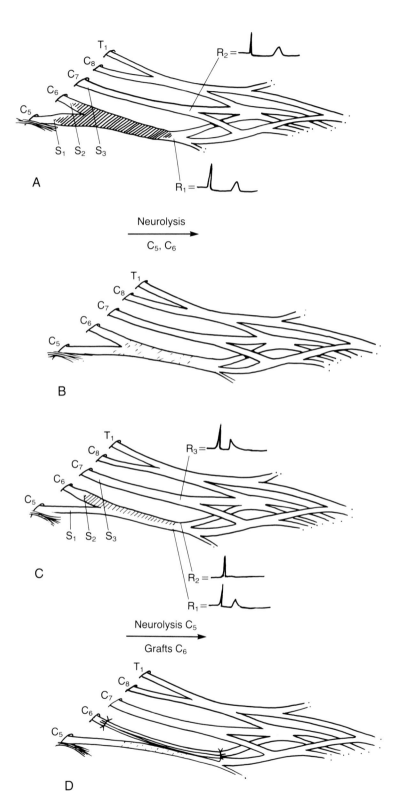

**Figure 15-3.** In *A*, C5-C6 to upper trunk (UT) elements were regenerating despite complete C5-C6 loss distally. C7 to middle trunk was not involved and had a normal nerve action potential. As a result, a neurolysis was done *(B)*. In *C* and *D*, a split repair of elements leading to and through UT is shown. In this case, C5 was completely spared from resection, whereas C6 through UT was replaced by grafts. In an occasional case, only that portion of C5 leading to suprascapular nerve will be found to be regenerating. It is then split off from the rest of UT and the C5 element, and the remaining damaged portion of C5 and UT is replaced by one or more grafts.

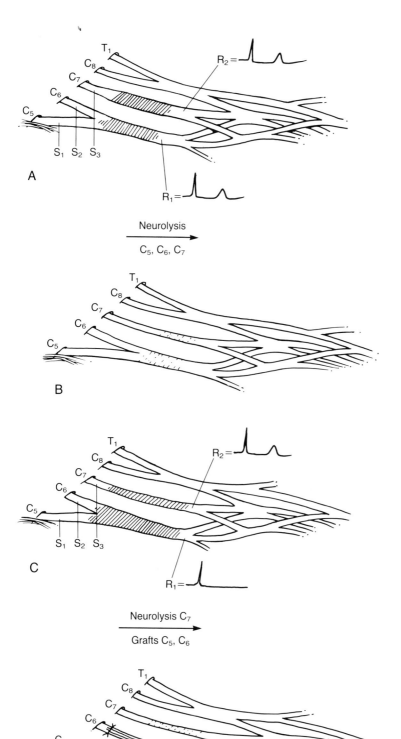

**Figure 15-4.** One pattern of injury and regeneration seen with C5, C6, and C7 injuries. *(A)* Adequate spontaneous regeneration occurred in all injured elements so a neurolysis was done *(B)*. Adequate regeneration was occurring only for C7 *(C)* in this case. Grafts were led from C5 and C6 to replace upper trunk (UT) *(D)*.

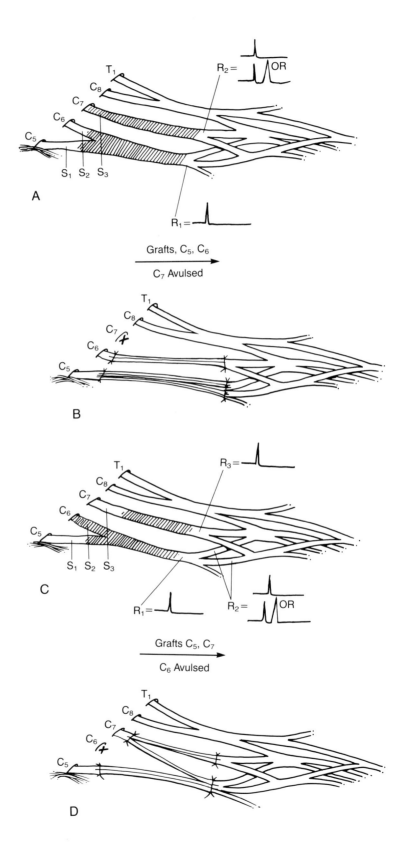

**Figure 15–5.** A fairly common pattern of operative findings with a C5, C6, C7 distribution injury (*A*). C7 was injured back to dura (NAP traces flat or showed preganglionic response), so grafts from C6 were led both to upper trunk (UT) divisions and to middle trunk (MT) division (*B*). C6 was damaged back to spinal dura (traces flat or preganglionic) (*C*); both C5 and C7 were used to contribute to the anterior division of UT as well as to their usual posterior division and MT division destinations (*D*).

supraclavicular lesions repaired by grafts who had 3 or more years of follow-up, only 15 had good results, and 30 had fair results. Narakas concluded that despite high magnification it was impossible to tell if scarred fascicles represented healed lesions or obstacles to regeneration, but intraoperative electrical recordings were not used. The author agreed with earlier suggestions that it was worthwhile to graft the pathways of the upper three roots, whereas grafts of pathways leading to the median nerve gave only fair or more often poor results. Repair of the lower elements, although giving flexor carpi ulnaris return, did not restore hand intrinsic function. Roughly one half of the patients having transfer of intercostal nerves, with or without sural grafts to the more distal portions of the plexus, benefitted from the surgery. However, they had improvement only in recovery of a single function, which was usually flexion of the forearm on the upper arm. More recently, Hentz and Narakas (1988) provided further useful data about their results with stretch injuries producing flail arms[28] (Figures 15–7 and 15–8).

Millesi reported on 54 stretch injuries operated on between 1964 and 1972.[51] He did not believe that myelography was useful, did not use intraoperative recording, and preferred operative exposure and direct microscopic inspection. Eighteen patients had a complete brachial plexus palsy caused by root-level lesions, with some of the roots avulsed and others with infraganglionic or lateral lesions suitable for graft repair. Twelve of these patients had lost physical continuity in all roots whereas six had some continuity, especially in the lower roots. Useful shoulder recovery occurred in 5 of 18, elbow flexion in 9, triceps alone in 4, and wrist and finger movement in 2. With complete lesions caused by more peripheral lesions, 6 of 13 had acceptable shoulder recovery, 7 had elbow function, and 5 had some degree of wrist and finger recovery. With partial palsy caused by variable root lesions, 3 of 10 recovered shoulder function, 7 elbow function, and 3 wrist and finger function. With partial palsies caused by more peripheral lesions, 7 of 10 patients obtained return of shoulder function, 8 of 9 recovered elbow function, 3 of 6, wrist, and 3 of 8, finger flexion. Millesi provided a partial update on his results in both 1984 and 1988 and consid-

ering the severity of these lesions his results remain excellent. He still relies on relatively early microscopic inspection of the elements to determine whether to resect those in continuity or not. Millesi also believes internal neurolysis improves function in some stretch injuries to the plexus. The latter tenet is not accepted by all and certainly has not been our experience.

In 1982, Sedel reported on 139 plexus injuries operated on between 1972 and 1980.[70] Sixty-three patients had enough follow-up for analysis, including 32 complete lesions involving all elements of the plexus and 31 incomplete ones. Repairs were done in 48 cases and neurolysis alone in 15. An attempt was made to compare operative results with those in a group of patients treated conservatively. Those patients operated on had higher grades of recovery. Most of these lesions were caused by traction, although one was caused by laceration, another by tumor resection, and one by iatrogenic injury. All roots and elements in continuity had only a neurolysis because intraoperative recording techniques were not used. His experience with transferring other nerves into more distal plexus was disappointing. Sedel updated some of this data in 1987.[69]

In 1983, Stevens and colleagues reported on 25 patients with plexus injuries operated on over a 32-year period.[76] Five of those repaired resulted from stretch/contusion, four complete to all roots and one incomplete. Partial recoveries were obtained in a few cases by transposition of intact proximal plexus elements into degenerated but noncorresponding distal elements without the use of grafts.

Various neurotization procedures have been described in which cervical plexus, accessory nerve, or intercostal nerves have been used as a proximal outflow to attach to sural grafts.[23,24,62,86] Results have been variable, although many authors remain optimistic about this type of approach.[12,20,66,82] Many workers have combined neurotization for spinal nerves not reparable with direct repair of spinal nerves where there is useful outflow. Results with such combined repairs appear better in those cases than in those of neurotization alone. Direct repair of the plexus may remain the first order of business, but neurotization is still often necessary.[38,86] Recently, MacKinnon advocated use of medial pectoral branches to neurotize musculo-

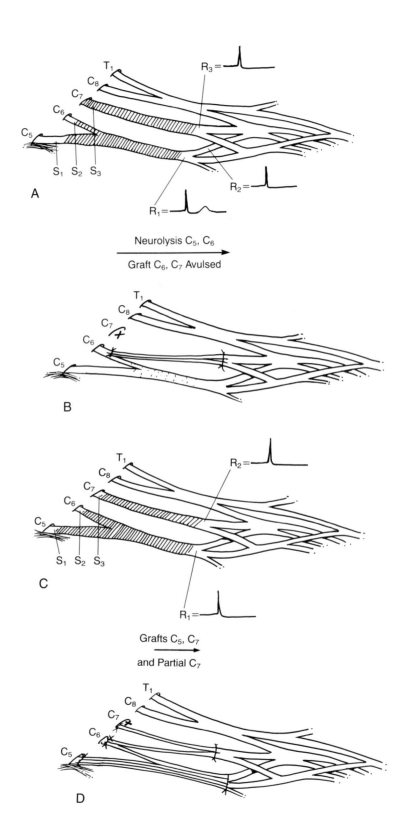

**Figure 15–6.** C5-C6 through upper trunk were regenerating; C7 was not regenerating and yet was damaged back to dura. *(A)* A portion of C6 was sectioned and used as a lead-out to middle trunk divisions. *(B)* An alternative procedure would be to use descending cervical plexus to do this. In *C*, none of the involved elements was regenerating, but only a portion of both C6 and C7 were usable as lead-outs *(D)*.

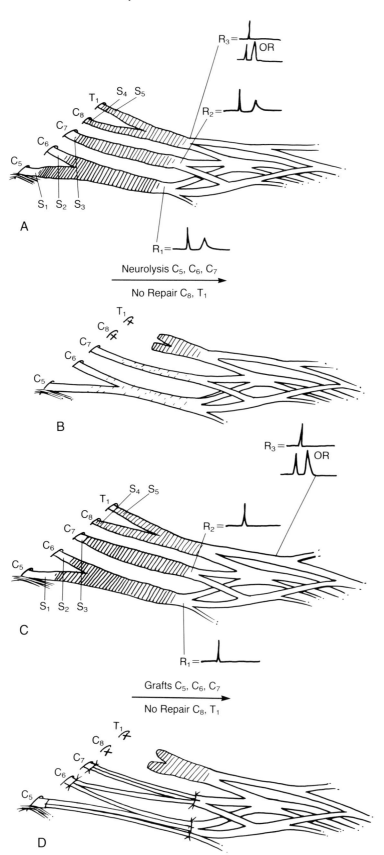

**Figure 15–7.** Two cases of C5 through T1 stretch injuries that produced flail arms. (*A* and *C*) C5, C6, and even C7 were regenerating (*B*) and could be spared resection, but C8 and T1 were not reparable (NAP traces flat or preganglionic in *A* and *C*). C5, C6, and C7 required graft replacement (*C*), whereas again C8 and T1 were not reparable (*D*).

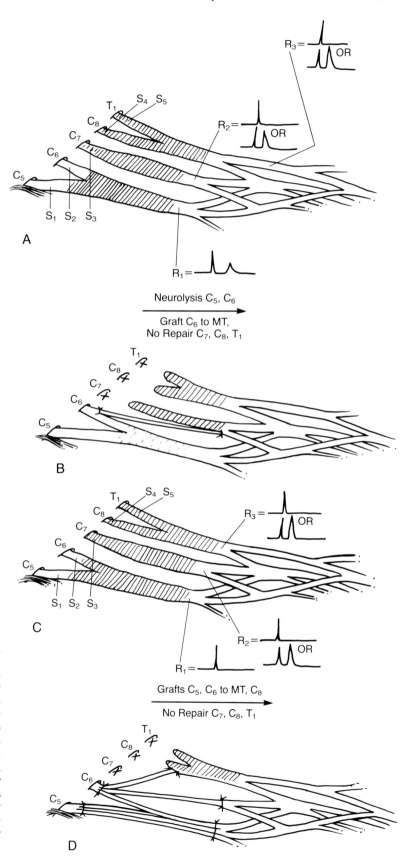

**Figure 15–8.** *(A)* Another relatively favorable set of circumstances with a C5 through T1 injury. Because C5-C6 through upper trunk had a regenerative nerve action potential, only a neurolysis was done. C7, C8, and T1 were irreparable *(B)*. Either descending cervical plexus or sternocleidomastoid branch of the accessory nerve can be added as a lead-out to C7 to middle trunk (MT) rather than using a portion of C6 as was done in this case. *(C and D)* Repair of C5 and C6 through to divisions or cords. Some of C6 has been led by grafts to middle trunk (MT) divisions and some by grafts to C8 and lower trunk. Again, direct repairs could be supplemented by lead-outs from descending cervical plexus and/or accessory nerve.

cutaneous nerve in C5-C6 lesions in which direct repair may not be possible.

There is little question that reconstructive and substitutive operations can be of value in some well-selected cases.[30,31] The difficulty with their use in the usual stretch injury is that there is often no muscle that works well enough to shift or move to provide substitution. Nonetheless, in cases in which loss remains complete in the C5-C6 distribution and yet C7 and lower root function are spared, a flexorplasty, in which either forearm flexors are slid proximally to originate above elbow or triceps is used to substitute for biceps, can be quite effective in restoring flexion of the arm.[15,35,50] Less frequently, recovery or sparing of enough pectoralis major or latissimus dorsi permits use of these muscles as a substitute for biceps/brachialis.[14,17] If, with upper root or spinal nerve damage, some forearm flexion can be regained but the shoulder remains paralyzed, then glenohumeral fusion of the shoulder can be done. This places the arm at

an effective partially abducted, forward flexed, and internally rotated position.[64,83] Muscle transfers, especially using extensions from the trapezius, have been tried to provide shoulder abduction, but usually with less success than with fusion.[26]

In some cases in which repaired stretch injuries either spare or recover some forearm and hand function, tendon transfers can be done particularly to improve wrist and finger extension (Figures 15–9, 15–10, and 15–11).[60,75,85]

In a series of 171 plexus injuries operated on between 1968 and 1980, 60 patients with stretch/contusion injury were reported by Kline and Judice in 1983.[39] The authors felt that it was important to follow each patient for 4 or 5 months before operation to look for clinical signs of recovery of function and, on electromyographic (EMG) evaluation, to search for evidence of reinnervation. As a result, cases with significant improvement in the early months

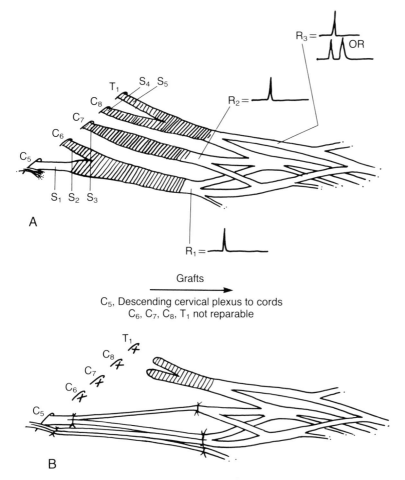

**Figure 15–9.** (A) An unfortunate but very common set of operative findings in patients with flail arms. Most of the plexus elements are not only injured back to dura but distracted more distally. Direct repair is, of course, limited and needs to be supplemented by neurotizations. In this case, grafts were led out from C5 and descending cervical plexus (B).

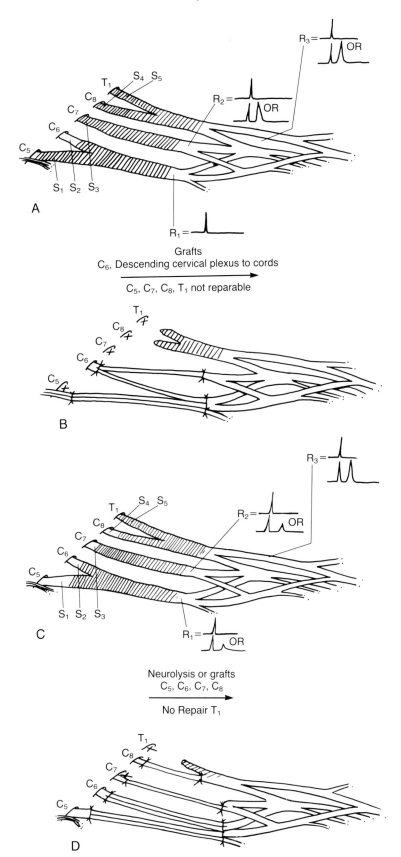

**Figure 15–10.** In *A*, even C5 was not usable as a lead-out, so grafts extended from C6 and descending cervical plexus to the cord level of the plexus *(B)*. NAP traces in distribution of C7, C8, and T1 were either flat or showed a preganglionic response. The pattern of injury in *C* is, unfortunately, infrequent. Either neurolysis (because of regenerative nerve action potentials) or grafts were possible for C5, C6, C8, and some of C7 *(D)*.

were not operated upon. At the time of operation for the more severe cases, intraoperative stimulation and recording techniques were used to ascertain whether injured elements required resection or were regenerating.

Patients were selected for operation because myelography showed absence of meningoceles at upper levels and because deficits persisted in the C5, C6, and usually C7 distributions. Those patients favorable for operation had intact proximal or medial muscles such as serratus anterior and rhomboids and had function of the diaphragm. Lack of significant paraspinal denervation by EMG and absence of sensory nerve action potentials (NAPs) from proximal median, radial, and ulnar nerves after stimulating distal nerves or fingers were also favorable factors. Positive sensory NAPs provided a relative contraindication to operation, at least at those root levels related to the nerves stimulated and recorded. Other relative contraindications included late referral or incomplete loss in the distribution of most of the elements. Similar criteria for selection for operation have been developed based on longer and more recent

experience and have been subsequently reported.[36,37]

As a result of this selective process, 148 stretched and contused elements that were surgically evaluated were reported in 1983 (Figures 15–12 and 15–13). The majority of elements operated on (114) were thought to be completely injured according to preoperative clinical and EMG testing. These cases were done by the classic anterior approach, although in the interim some were approached posteriorly if exposure of spinal nerves, especially lower ones close to dura, was desired.[41] Intraoperative NAP studies showed 31 of the spinal nerves to be regenerating or, in two cases, partially injured to begin with. These elements had only a neurolysis, and 26 recovered to a grade 3 or better functional level. Of the 58 elements that could be surgically repaired, only four could be repaired by direct suture, and two of these had significant recovery. Three elements had a split repair, in which a portion of the element received a neurolysis and a portion was replaced by grafts, and each recovered. Success with graft repair was slightly less than 50% and, sur-

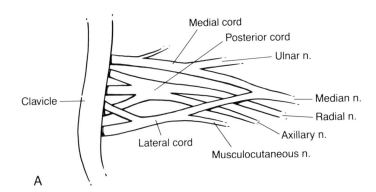

A

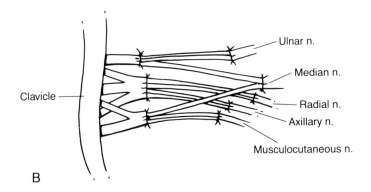

B

**Figure 15–11.** *(A)* Infraclavicular cord and cord-to-nerve level brachial plexus. *(B)* Entire plexus at cord and cord-to-nerve level is replaced by grafts. No attempt is made to repair input to antebrachial cutaneous nerves. Instead, they as well as sural nerves are used as donor grafts.

prisingly, compared well with patients having gunshot wounds to the plexus in cases in which grafts were necessary. This may be because a higher percentage of elements viewed as favorable for repair received repair in the stretch series than in the gunshot wound series.

Even after excluding stretch injuries thought not to be reparable, 25 elements in 12 cases were still not reparable because of medial or proximal root injury or damage over an excessive length. In only five patients was this true of all plexus elements. Partial repair was possible in the other seven cases. Nevertheless, histologic sections of the proximal faces of roots of several of these patients showed a mixture of heavy scarring with only fine axons and hundreds of ganglion cells. Such was also the case with several other patients in whom preoperatively it was considered that all the plexus was capable of repair by grafts from root to cord level. If heavy scarring and ganglion cells were seen, function did not result despite placement of technically satisfactory grafts.

In the five patients with total distraction of the plexus at a root level, three were not reparable either because of very proximal and severe root damage or because the gaps extended from the root level well down into the upper arm. In the other two patients, the upper roots could be used as lead-out for repair. Results were best in patients with C5, C6, and/or C7 lesions in whom myelography was normal or showed meningoceles only on one or more lower roots. Repair of upper elements by grafts resulted in biceps, brachialis, brachioradialis, and sometimes some degree of deltoid, supraspinatus/infraspinatus, and triceps function. Almost 40% of patients who preoperatively had complete loss in the distribution of all five roots gained partial recovery of upper root function after graft repair.

Bonney and associates published their experience with a small series of vascularized grafts to replace upper plexus elements.[10] The ulnar nerve was usually used because it was distal to a preganglionic injury involving the C8 and T1 roots. The authors were enthusiastic about their early results. At this time, their results seem no better than those more readily accomplished by use of nonvascularized sural interfascicular graft repairs. Support for the latter approach continues to grow, with relatively recent reports

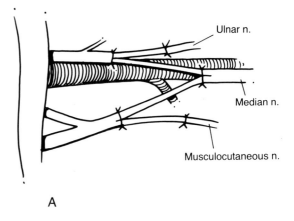

A

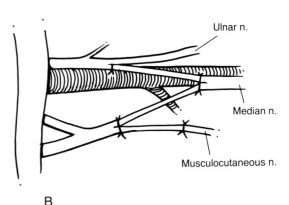

B

**Figure 15-12.** A fairly common scenario is partial infraclavicular stretch injury involving lateral and medial cords and their outflows with relative sparing of posterior cord. (A) Outflows to musculocutaneous, median, and ulnar nerves have received grafts from medial and lateral cords. In B both medial and lateral cord input to median required repair, but that to ulnar nerve did not.

from many European countries as well as Australia and New Zealand.[7,11,32,33,34,65,67,71,73]

Several investigators have looked at the fascicular anatomy of the various plexus elements in an attempt to make graft repair more specific.[8,72,79] The merits of such a microscopic approach, however, remain to be proven.

Central destructive lesions to brain or spinal cord can sometimes control the severe pain associated with some plexus stretch injuries.[47,68] Dorsal root entry zone lesions as advanced and practiced by Nashold and workers are, in their

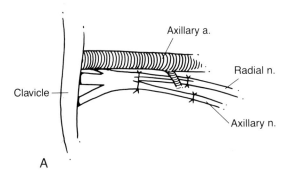

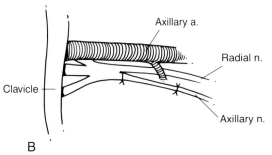

**Figure 15–13.** Posterior cord and one or two of its outflows can be damaged by stretch/contusion with relative sparing of lateral and medial cord structures. *(A)* Input to both radial and axillary nerves required replacement by grafts. *(B)* Input to axillary nerve only was replaced. Although it does occur, an isolated posterior cord to radial injury requiring repair is less common.

hands, relatively effective for the severe, unremitting pain seen with plexus stretches.[58] Most severe pain associated with plexus stretch injuries lessens or leaves altogether in the early months after injury. This pain can usually be

helped by institution of early physical therapy and especially range of motion exercises and use of carbamazepine and amitriptyline. Other cases associated with severe pain appear to be aided by operation on the plexus.[51,79] There are cases, however, in which the neuritic and at times phantom limb pain persists for several years or more, and then dorsal root entry zone lesions are indicated. There are potential complications such as paralysis and respiratory insufficiency, and their incidence varies according to the series presented.[80] This and other central procedures for pain should be done only in carefully selected patients.

Birth plexus palsies are also caused by a stretching and contusive mechanism. They will be taken up in a separate chapter because their management is even more controversial than that for adult stretch injuries.

## STRETCH INJURY RESULTS

Table 15–1 provides the overall postoperative grades at 18 or more months after operation in 204 supraclavicular stretch injuries. Included are 35 at C5 and C6, 47 at C5, C6, and C7, and 106 at C5 through T1 distributions. Follow-up on this group of patients was extremely difficult to obtain. These individuals were especially mobile, often had changed addresses, and did not always maintain contact with family, friends, or referring physicians. In addition, because at least 18 months of follow-up was desired, some operated patients were not far

**TABLE 15–1**

Overall Postoperative Grades* on Stretch-Injured Plexus Patients (LSUMC Series) (n = 204 Patients)

| Initial Loss | Postoperative Grade | | | | | | | | | |
|---|---|---|---|---|---|---|---|---|---|---|
| | 0 | 1 | 1 to 2 | 2 | 2 to 3 | 3 | 3 to 4 | 4 | 4 to 5 | Totals |
| C5/C6 (C) | 1 | 0 | 0 | 0 | 4 | 12 | 11 | 6 | 1 | 35 |
| C5/C6/C7 (C) | 1 | 0 | 0 | 0 | 6 | 18 | 13 | 6 | 3 | 47 |
| C5 to T1 (C) | 11 | 1 | 5 | 10 | 42 | 24 | 8 | 5 | 0 | 106 |
| C5 to C8 (C) | 0 | 0 | 0 | 0 | 0 | 1 | 1 | 0 | 0 | 2 |
| C6/C7/C8/T1 (C) | 0 | 0 | 0 | 1 | 0 | 2 | 1 | 0 | 0 | 4 |
| C7 to T1 (C) | 0 | 0 | 0 | 0 | 1 | 1 | 0 | 0 | 0 | 2 |
| C8 to T1 (C) | 2 | 1 | 1 | 0 | 0 | 0 | 0 | 0 | 0 | 4 |
| C8 to T1 (I) | 0 | 0 | 0 | 0 | 0 | 0 | 2 | 0 | 0 | 2 |
| C7/C8/T1 (I) | 0 | 0 | 0 | 0 | 0 | 1 | 1 | 0 | 0 | 2 |
| TOTALS | 15 | 2 | 6 | 11 | 53 | 59 | 37 | 17 | 4 | 204 |

C = complete or nearly complete loss; I = incomplete loss.
*Follow-up of 18 months or more postoperatively.

enough along to include. As a result, even though 362 patients with supraclavicular stretch palsies were operated upon during the same interval, sufficient follow-up was only available on 204 (see Table 15–1). We did better with follow-up on infraclavicular stretch injuries, which was available on 119 of 185 cases at 3 or more years of follow-up. Surgical approach to most of these lesions was an anterior one, as described in the chapter entitled "Gunshot Wounds to Brachial Plexus." A small number of stretch/contusive lesions had a posterior approach, as detailed at the end of this chapter.

Postoperative or recovery grades for the various patterns of supraclavicular stretch injuries operated on were initially calculated for each element, usually at root or spinal nerve level. These grades (ranging from 0 to 5) were then added together and averaged to obtain the overall grade. For example, if the postoperative grades in a patient with a C5 and C6 stretch injury were 3.5 in the C5 distribution and 4.0 in the C6 distribution, then the average would be 3.7, and the overall grade would be 3 to 4. If the initial lesion was a C5, C6, and C7 stretch injury and postoperative grades were C5 = 2, C6 = 4, and C7 = 3, then the average grade would be 3.

If elements were considered irreparable and no attempts were made to lead outflow from the proximal portions of other elements to those damaged or to neurotize them, then these elements were excluded from the calculations.

This situation usually applied to C8-T1 to lower trunk elements, so some of the grades in the flail arm series of operated patients reflect averaged grades for C5, C6, and C7 muscles. Despite this, we believe that the data accurately reflect the difficulties encountered in restoring neural function to the patient with a flail arm, because it was usually more difficult to repair or find outflows or substitutes for C7, C6, and sometimes C5 in the patients with C5-T1 lesions than in those with C5, C6, C7 or C5-C6 lesions. Patients having neurotization as their major procedure are analyzed separately (Table 15–2). The majority of stretch-injured patients selected for operation were done by a classical anterior approach. Most of the proximal stretch injuries required both a supraclavicular and infraclavicular anterior approach. Most cord and cord-to-nerve injuries were of course approached anteriorly. A few supraclavicular stretch injuries were done posteriorly. Patients having a posterior subscapular approach for repair of stretch injuries are included in Table 15–3.

## Results With Operated C5-C6 Stretch Injuries

There were 35 patients in this category. Most of the patterns of loss and the types of operative repairs used for this category are found in Table 15–4. Loss was complete in the C5-C6 distribu-

**TABLE 15–2**
Neurotization Procedures for Plexus Stretches and Outcomes
(University of Toronto Series) (n = 47 Patients)

| Donor Nerve | Recipient Nerve | Cases | Motor Outcomes | | | | |
|---|---|---|---|---|---|---|---|
| | | | Exc. | Good | Mod. | Poor | Bad |
| Intercostal | Musculocutaneous | 37 | 6 | 11 | 4 | 9 | 7 |
| | Axillary | 6 | — | — | 2 | 2 | 2 |
| | Median | 4 | — | — | — | — | 4 |
| | Radial | 1 | — | — | — | — | 1 |
| | Ulnar | 1 | — | — | — | — | 1 |
| Accessory | Suprascapular | 1 | — | 1 | — | — | — |
| | Musculocutaneous | 1 | — | — | — | 1 | — |
| | Axillary | 1 | — | — | — | 1 | — |
| | Median | 1 | — | — | — | — | 1 |
| | | | Sensory Outcomes | | | | |
| | | | Protective | | Not Useful | | Nil |
| Cervical Plexus | Median | 9 | 5 | | 3 | | 1 |
| Cervical Plexus | Ulnar | 11 | 6 | | 1 | | 4 |

Exc. = excellent; Mod. = moderate.

**TABLE 15-3**
Summary of Brachial Plexus Trauma Operated on Posteriorly* (n = 18 Patients)

| | Injury Mechanism | | |
| --- | --- | --- | --- |
| | Stretch/ Contusion | Laceration | Gunshot Wound |
| Number of Cases | 14 | 2 | 2 |
| Male/Female | 10/4 | 1/1 | 2/0 |
| Mean Age (yrs) | 31.5 | 26.5 | 22.5 |
| Neurologic Status | | | |
|   Severe pain | 2 | 0 | 1 |
|   Partial loss | 3 | 0 | 0 |
|   Complete loss of one or more elements | 11 | 2 | 2 |
| | (5 flail arms) | | |
| Associated Injury | | | |
|   Major vascular | 2 | 0 | 2 |
|   Fractured ribs, cervical spine | 1 | 1 | 0 |
|   Pneumothorax and spleen laceration | 1 | 0 | 0 |
|   Subdural hematoma | 1 | 0 | 0 |
| Mean Interval Between Trauma and Operation | 15 | 2 | 2 |
| Type of Repair | | | |
|   Neurolysis | 5 | 0 | 1 |
|   Direct suture | 0 | 1 | 0 |
|   Grafts | 9 | 1 | 0 |
|   Neurotization | 0 | 0 | 1 |
| Results | | | |
|   3 yrs after neurolysis (n = 5) | | | |
|     No recovery | 1 | 0 | 0 |
|     Grade 1 to 2 | 0 | 0 | 0 |
|     Grade 3 to 4 | 3 | 0 | 1 |
|   5 yrs after grafting (n = 8) | | | |
|     No recovery | 1 | 0 | 0 |
|     Grade 1 to 2 | 2 | 0 | 0 |
|     Grade 3 to 4 | 4 | 1 | 0 |
|   5 years after suture (n = 1) | | | |
|     Grade 3 to 4 | 0 | 1 | 0 |
|   Scapular winging | 1 | 0 | 0 |

*From Dubuisson A, Kline D, and Weinshel S: Posterior subscapular approach to the brachial plexus: Report of 102 cases. J Neurosurg 79:319–330, 1993.

tion and had persisted for 4 or more months in 34 of these 35 cases. Six patients who had a C5-C6 pattern of loss with no supra- or infraspinatus, and no deltoid, biceps, brachioradialis, or supinator function but intact function of the rest of the arm were found to have serious involvement of C7 root at the time of operation (Figures 15-14 and 15-15). In one of these cases, the root had been avulsed despite no clinical loss in the C7 distribution. In the remaining

**TABLE 15-4**
Operative Results of C5, C6 Stretch Injuries With Complete Loss Preoperatively (n = 35 Patients)

| Operation | No. of Patients | Results (Averaged) |
| --- | --- | --- |
| Grafts of C5 and C6* | 22 | grade 3 = 12 grade 3 to 4 = 5 grade 4 = 5 |
| C5 grafts, C6 avulsed, descending cervical plexus used† | 3 | grade 2 to 3 |
| C5 avulsed, C6 grafts, descending cervical plexus used | 1 | grade 4 |
| Neurolysis of C5 and C6 (positive nerve action potentials) | 7 | grade 3 to 4 |
| C5 neurolysis, C6 grafts | 2 | grade 3 to 4 |

*Five patients in this group had serious involvement of C7 despite a C5, C6 pattern of loss. One C7 was avulsed; the other four had no nerve action potentials and were resected and repaired by grafts. The resected C7 to middle trunk segments were neurotmetic by histologic examination.
†One patient in this subset had serious injury of C7 without a nerve action potential. This was resected and repaired by grafts to distal middle trunk divisions.

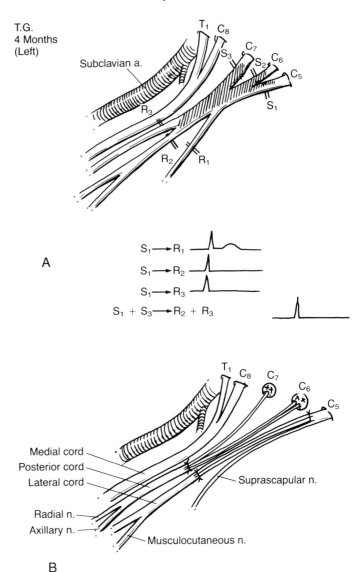

**Figure 15–14.** (A) This patient presented with typical C5 and C6 loss involving left arm. Function of triceps as well as wrist and finger extensors was excellent. Nonetheless, at the operating table, C7 was found to be severely injured. C5 to supraclavicular nerve was thought, based on nerve action potential studies, to be regenerating. The rest of C5 was used as a lead-out for grafts, but only a portion of C6 and C7 was usable (B). Postoperatively, there was no additional loss. About 1 in 6 patients with loss that appears clinically to be confined to C5 and C6 also have serious injury involving C7.

five cases, the root was in continuity but no NAP could be recorded. The C7 spinal nerve was resected in these cases, and a graft repair was done. Postoperatively, there was no increased loss and deficit remained in the C5-C6 distribution. Histologic examination of the resected roots showed them to be neurotmetic. One possible explanation was that these plexi were postfixed. Against this theory is that C5 and C6 were in each instance dissected out and at least at their dural exits had, as well as could be determined, normal volume. More likely as a theory is the occasional dominance of C8 input not only to wrist extensors but also to the triceps. These observations concerning C7 are im-

portant, for if it is not functional and yet not injured close to the spinal cord, it can be used to supplement lead-out from C5 and/or C6 by use of grafts.

In one patient with C5-C6 distribution loss, myelogram showed meningoceles at both the C5 and C6 nerve root levels. Nonetheless, C6, which was in continuity but had no NAP, was reparable but C5 was not. Descending cervical plexus was also used for lead-out to anterior and posterior divisions of upper trunk in this case. Those muscles in a C5 distribution gained only a grade 2 result, but those in the C6 distribution that had grafts from proximal root to upper trunk resulted in grade 4 recovery. Another pa-

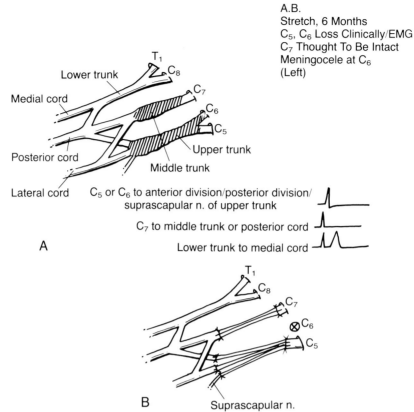

A.B.
Stretch, 6 Months
$C_5$, $C_6$ Loss Clinically/EMG
$C_7$ Thought To Be Intact
Meningocele at $C_6$
(Left)

**Figure 15–15.** (A and B) Another patient with an exact clinical pattern of C5 and C6 loss that clinically and by EMG was complete who was nonetheless found to also have complete injury to C7 at operation. If C7 to middle trunk had not been tested, the C7 outflow would not have been used to add to the graft repair.

tient with C5-C6 loss required 7.6-cm grafts for repair. Grafts could, however, be led out from both C5 and C6, and a overall grade 3 result in the distribution of both roots eventuated.

Most of the C5-C6 lesions selected for operation required graft repair. Nonetheless, there were seven cases in which both C5 and C6 roots had recordable NAPs despite being 4 to 8 months after injury with complete clinical and EMG loss (Figure 15–16). Six of these patients acquired grade 3 to 4 overall results with only neurolysis, and the seventh regained a grade 4 result. In another case, only neurolysis of C5 was necessary, but C6 required a graft repair. C5 was partially functional preoperatively, having graded 2. In this patient, C5 outflows regained a grade 4 result, and the grafted C6 achieved a 3 to 4 result by 36 months postoperatively. If these cases are taken out of the overall

results and the latter are recalculated for the repairs of input to the distal elements of both roots by grafts, 12 such patients gained a grade 3 result, 5 a grade 3 to 4 result, and 5 grade 4. This was despite the fact that three of the patients repaired by grafts had an avulsive injury of C6 that was irreparable. In two of these cases, lead-out from C5 was supplemented by neurotization using descending cervical plexus.

Although results were generally good with C5-C6 stretch repairs, recovery was not uniform in this distribution. Forearm flexion was almost always better than shoulder abduction. The latter was seldom good enough to raise the shoulder above the horizontal. Thus, it remains important to identify patients with early spontaneous recovery and spare them from surgery. Occasionally, very lengthy grafts are necessary (Figure 15–17). These appear to work better for biceps than deltoid recovery.

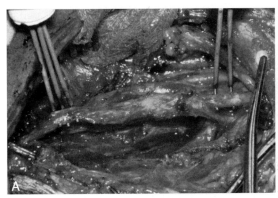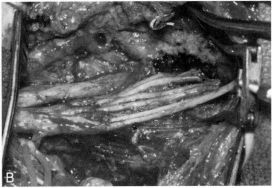

**Figure 15–16.** *(A)* Right C5 and C6 stretch injury extending into upper trunk. Clavicle is to the right. After exposing spinal nerves and more distal elements, nerve action potential recordings were done. Here C5 is being stimulated (to the *left*), and recording electrodes are on one of the upper trunk divisions (to the *right*). *(B)* Graft repair of another but left-sided C5-C6 stretch injury. Sural grafts run from an intraforaminal level of both C5 and C6 to distal upper trunk. Less injured or involved C7 to middle trunk is seen in the background. See also color figure.

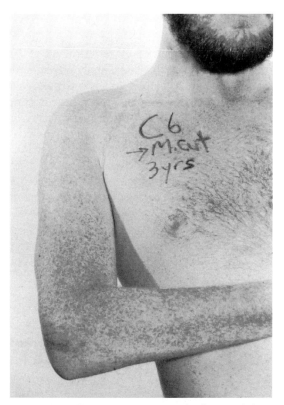

**Figure 15–17.** In severe upper spinal nerve injury over a length of plexus, a sural graft can sometimes be placed between C6 and the cut end of the musculocutaneous nerve. The grafts are led either superficial or deep to the clavicle. This patient obtained useful elbow flexion by 3 years after such a lengthy graft.

## Summary of C5, C6 Lesions

1. Distribution of loss is very predictable: supra- and infraspinatus, deltoid, biceps/brachialis, brachioradialis, and supinator.
2. Almost 30% regain significant function spontaneously. Signs of this are usually evident by 3 to 4 months after injury.
3. Despite apparent clinical and electrical sparing, C7 may be found to be seriously involved at operation. If C7 is resected because of an absent NAP in this setting, postoperative loss is not increased and yet C7 can be used to supplement the repair.
4. This is the most favorable group of serious stretch injuries to repair.
5. Direct repair of one or both spinal nerves is likely. Need for neurotization is less likely than with other injury patterns.

## Results of Operation on C5, C6, and C7 Stretch Injuries

The 47 patients in this category had not only a C5-C6 pattern of loss but lack of triceps and some weakness of wrist and sometimes finger extension. Loss was complete clinically and electrically in 35 cases. Partial function in nine cases was in the C7 distribution; in two instances there was some sparing of C6 and in one case some function in the C5 distribution. Three of the 47 patients operated on in this category had neurolysis not only because of physical continuity of the stretched elements but because of NAPs resulting from regeneration. This was despite the fact that loss clinically and electrically in their distribution was complete. One of these cases achieved an overall grade of 4 by 23 months, and another graded 3 to 4 by 30 months. The third patient achieved a grade 3 overall result by 28 months.

Most of the C5, C6, and C7 stretch injuries selected for operation required graft repairs (Figure 15–18). There were, however, important exceptions. If two of the three involved roots could have a neurolysis based on a positive NAP and despite complete clinical and electrical loss, results were also predictably good (Figure 15–19). For example, one patient achieved an overall grade of 3 by 19 months postoperatively despite the fact that C7 was avulsed and could not be directly repaired. Despite a positive NAP from C5 and C6, a portion of C6 was used as lead-out to anterior and posterior divisions of middle trunk and to those of the upper trunk. In a second case, both C6 and C7 had neurolysis but C5 required a graft repair. Grades for each root at 22 months were 3, giving an overall grade of 3. In a third patient, both C6 and C7 had a neurolysis and achieved a 3 by 18 months of follow-up, but graft repair of C5 only led to a trace of function in its distribution. Neurolysis of C6 and C7 in a fourth patient led to a 3 and a 4 grade, respectively, for these elements, and graft repair of C5 led to shoulder abduction against gravity. Follow-up was at 26 months only. One failure of neurolysis involved

the C7 root to middle trunk in a fifth patient who did recover level 2 to 3 function in a C6 root undergoing neurolysis and a level 3 result in a C5 root receiving a graft repair. In two additional cases, roots receiving a neurolysis had partial function to begin with, and then function usually improved further.

Where only one spinal nerve had a neurolysis, average recovery in that spinal nerve distribution was 3 to 4. Of the 15 cases of C5, C6, C7 loss operated on in which one spinal nerve only had a neurolysis, 10 of these elements initially had some degree of function. Grades of these spinal nerves as well as those having no function to begin with but having a neurolysis based on a positive NAP improved without exception over the several years during which these cases were followed. There were two instances in which improvement was to a grade of 3, and the remainder improved to grades of 4 (8 cases) or 5 (4 cases).

A second factor playing a large role in the outcome in these cases was the presence of avulsion injury extending to the level of the dura (Figure 15–20). This usually affected one root (13 instances). However, in two cases, such injury affected two roots. Under these circumstances, grafts were led from other spinal nerves (albeit close to spinal cord), not only to their distal connections but also to those in the territory of the avulsed roots. In two cases, such direct transfers were supplemented by neurotization using descending cervical plexus. In one of these cases, phrenic nerve was used as well.

If two spinal nerves or roots had been avulsed, transfers led to grade 3 and grade 4 results for roots C6 and C7 in one case with fol-

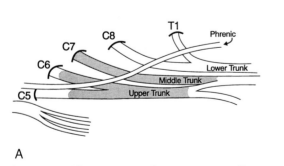
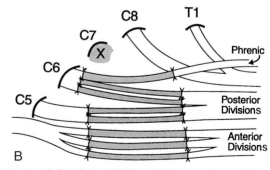

**Figure 15–18.** *(A)* Drawing depicting extent of lesion in patient with C5, C6, and C7 loss. C7 was not reparable, but C5 and C6 were *(B)*. Descending cervical plexus was also used to provide more lead-out for sural grafts which went to anterior and posterior divisions of upper and middle trunks. In this case, phrenic nerve was encased in scar, was further injured during the dissection, and was repaired by a graft as well.

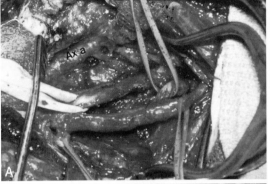
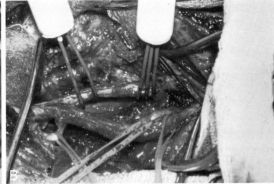
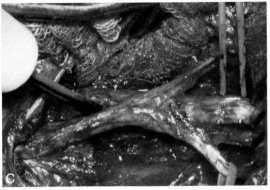

**Figure 15–19.** *(A)* Stretch injury involving left C5, C6, and C7 spinal nerves and their outflows. Ax a = subclavian artery. *(B)* Operative electrodes for nerve action potential studies are placed on C7 to middle trunk segments. *(C)* Exposure of C5, C6, upper trunk (UT), and divisions of UT in a patient with a right C5 to C7 stretch injury. Stimulating electrode is placed under the C6 spinal nerve and recording electrode on the anterior division of the UT. Loop displaces suprascapular nerve downward at right lower corner of photograph.

low-up to 62 months. In another case with two roots (C5 and C7) avulsed, follow-up only extended to 18 months because the individual was killed in an automobile accident. Recovery only graded 2 for the C5 and C7 distributions and 1 for C6, the root used to lead out grafts. In this case, C6 was also led to C5 and C7 outflows, and descending cervical plexus was mainly led to C5 outflows. It is possible that more recovery might have occurred had the patient lived longer.

If only one root was avulsed in the C5, C6, and C7 category, neurotization was not felt to be necessary. Instead, grafts were led out from

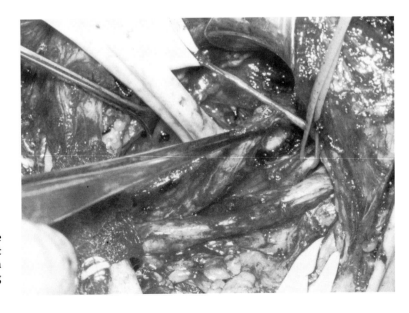

**Figure 15–20.** Meningocele beneath C7 root in a patient with a C5, C6, and C7 stretch injury. Forceps are elevating the C7 nerve root.

one or more of those roots damaged close to but not all the way to the spinal cord (Figures 15–21 and 15–22). Grafts were not only led distally to what the root normally innervated, but also to adjacent outflows whose proximal counterparts had been avulsed. C6 was the avulsed root in seven of these cases, and C7 was the avulsed root in six cases. Recovery in an avulsed root's distribution by transfer of grafts from other roots ranged from grades of 1 to 4, but averaged out to a grade of 2 to 3. Thus, avulsive root injuries usually lowered the overall grades for repair of C5, C6, and C7 injuries but not as much as expected before the data was analyzed.

Average grade for the 31 C5 spinal nerves repaired by grafts in the C5, C6, and C7 series was 2.4. There were 24 C6 spinal nerves repaired by grafts, and their average recovery was 2.7. Only 10 of the C7 roots were repaired by grafts, but they fared better, their average recovery being 3.2.

In the 25 cases in which avulsions were not present and yet grafts were used to lead out from one or more spinal nerves, overall case grades averaged 2.8. Fourteen of these cases had neurolysis of one or more roots because of positive NAPs. Results averaged 2.6 in the 16 cases in which one or more roots were avulsed and yet the remainder of spinal nerves either had graft repair or neurolysis depending on NAP studies. Of these cases, four had neurolysis of one or more roots. Thus, the percentage of spinal nerves having regenerative NAPs was twice as large in the cases without avulsion of one or more roots than in those with avulsion of one or more roots. Usually, roots having neurolysis based on positive NAP recordings recovered much better than those replaced by grafts or those neurotized from other sources.

## Summary of C5, C6, C7 Lesions

1. Loss involves triceps as well as shoulder muscles, biceps/brachialis, brachioradialis, and supinator. Loss of finger extension and flexor profundi is variable, as is degree of wrist extension weakness. In some patients, C8 input to these muscles is quite dominant.
2. There are a few cases of serious C5, C6, C7 injury but not many that improve spontaneously in the early months after injury. This number varies from series to series but approached 16% in our series.
3. Despite sparing of C8-T1 muscle function, opportunities for effective substitutive procedures are limited. For example, it is difficult to substitute for loss of shoulder and upper arm function. As a result, operation to attempt direct repair of the plexus with or without the addition of neurotization is usually indicated.
4. Direct repair of one or more elements frequently needs to be supplemented by neurotization using descending cervical plexus or a portion of the accessory nerve.
5. Outcome is usually best for biceps/brachialis, but imperfect return there can be af-

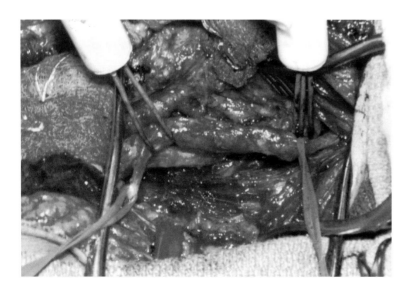

**Figure 15–21.** Recording on a severe stretch injury involving left C5, C6, and C7. Here, stimulating electrodes are on C6, and recording ones are on origin of supraclavicular nerve from upper trunk.

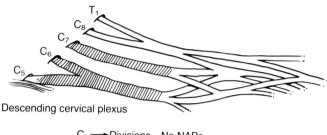

$C_5$, $C_6$ Loss (C)
$C_7$ Loss (I)
At 4 Months

Descending cervical plexus

$C_5$ ⟶ Divisions—No NAPs
$C_6$ ⟶ Divisions—( + ) NAP (Preganglionic)
$C_7$ ⟶ Middle trunk—( + ) NAP (Preganglionic)
$C_8/T_1$ ⟶ Lower Trunk—( + ) NAP (Healthy)

A

**Figure 15–22.** *(A)* Stretch injury involving proximal portions of C6 and C7 and more distal portion of C5. C8 and T1 were spared. *(B)* Despite avulsion at C6 and C7 levels, this was still a favorable injury for repair because lead-out was available from C5 as well as descending cervical plexus.

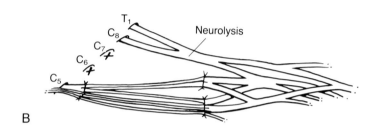

Neurolysis

B

## Results of Operation on C5-T1 Stretch Injuries

fected adversely by partial recovery of triceps. Supraspinatus recovery is usually better than that for deltoid.

These patients had flail or almost completely paralyzed arms. Criteria used to select these C5-T1 stretches for operation included preservation of rhomboid, serratus anterior, and diaphragmatic function. Patients with a meningocele of C4-C5, a cervical myelopathy, overwhelming medical problems, or who were eval-

uated by us a year or more after injury were excluded. Not unexpectedly, 251 of the 560 spinal nerves or roots evaluated at the operating table (Table 15–5) had proximal irreparable damage or were avulsed at the dural level. This was despite the fact that some attempt was made to select the more favorable patients for operation and to visualize the root or spinal nerve as close to the dural level as possible in these patients (Figures 15–23 and 15–24). On the other hand, despite this large number of avulsed and irreparable spinal nerves, an almost equal number were reparable or, in some instances, had a regenerative NAP. As can also be seen in Table 15–6, which shows the usual

**TABLE 15–5**
C5 to T1 Plexus Stretch Cases — Operative Findings or Treatment for Individual Roots in 112 Cases (n = 560)

| Number of Involved or Treated Roots | One | Two | Three | Four | Five | Total No. of Roots |
|---|---|---|---|---|---|---|
| Proximal irreparable damage or avulsion | 10 | 42 | 33 | 12 | 2 | 251 |
| Repaired by grafts | 16 | 36 | 40 | 6 | 4 | 252 |
| Split repair | 5 | 2 | 0 | 0 | 0 | 9 |
| Neurolysis (positive nerve action potential) | 8 | 12 | 2 | 0 | 2 | 48 |

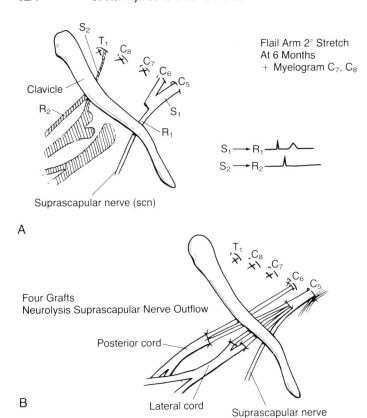

Flail Arm 2° Stretch
At 6 Months
+ Myelogram $C_7$, $C_8$

Suprascapular nerve (scn)

A

Four Grafts
Neurolysis Suprascapular Nerve Outflow

B

**Figure 15–23.** (A) Drawing of an unfortunately frequent set of findings at the operating table when the arm is flail. C5 to supraclavicular nerve was regenerating, but the rest of the supraclavicular plexus was torn as well as damaged back to spinal cord. (B) Grafts from C5 and some of C6 were 8 cm in length. When this case was done 10 years ago, other sources of lead-out or neurotization, such as descending cervical plexus or accessory branch to sternocleidomastoid, were not used, but they would be today.

operative findings in 112 patients with flail arms, C7, C8, and T1 roots were not reparable in 31 cases, and in 34 instances C8 and T1 were not. There were also 10 cases in which C5 was the only spinal nerve reparable by direct repair. These three patterns alone accounted for 201 of the 251 nonreparable roots.

Despite finding a large number of irreparable roots, graft repair of three or more spinal nerves was possible in 50 of the 112 C5-T1 cases (see Table 15–5). In another 36 cases, two spinal nerves could be repaired by grafts. Neurolysis, because of the presence of regenerative NAPs across and distal to root lesions, was done on one or more spinal nerves in 24 cases. Split repair, in which a portion of C5 or C6 and their outflows were repaired by grafts, was possible in nine roots in seven cases.

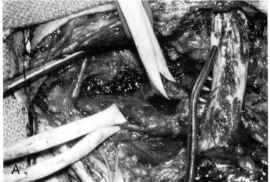

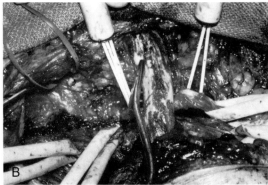

**Figure 15–24.** (A) Extensive stretch injury which has produced a flail arm. C5 and C6 to divisions of upper trunk did not conduct nerve action potential (NAP), nor did C7 to distal middle trunk. Lesion extended to cord levels. (B) Stimulation of lower trunk or C8 or T1 and recording from medial cord gave a rapidly conducting and relatively high amplitude NAP, indicating preganglionic injuries at these levels.

**TABLE 15-6**

C5 to T1 Stretch Injury Patterns Based on Operative Findings in 112 Cases (Usual Distributions)

| | No. Cases | Description |
|---|---|---|
| A. | 34 | C5, C6, C7 reparable or had neurolysis; C8, T1 not reparable |
| B. | 31 | C5, C6 reparable or had neurolysis; C7, C8, T1 not reparable |
| C. | 10 | C5 reparable or had neurolysis; C6, C7, C8, T1 not reparable |
| D. | 8 | All roots reparable (4 cases) or had neurolysis (2 cases) or both (2 cases) |
| E. | 6 | C5, C6, C7, C8 reparable or had neurolysis; T1 not reparable |
| F. | 2 | C6 reparable; C5, C7, C8, T1 not reparable |
| G. | 2 | No roots reparable directly nor responded to neurolysis |

**TABLE 15-7**

C5 to T1 Stretch Injury Patterns in 112 Cases (Unusual Distributions)

| | No. Cases | Description |
|---|---|---|
| A. | 4 | C5, C6, C8, T1 reparable or had neurolysis; C7 not reparable |
| B. | 3 | C5, C8, T1 reparable or had neurolysis; C6, C7 not reparable |
| C. | 2 | C5, C6, T1 reparable or had neurolysis; C7, C8 not reparable |
| D. | 2 | C5, C6, C8 reparable or had neurolysis; C7, T1 not reparable |
| E. | 1 | C5, C7, C8, T1 reparable or had neurolysis; C6 not reparable |
| F. | 1 | C5, C7, C8 reparable or had neurolysis; C6, T1 not reparable |
| G. | 1 | C5, C8 had neurolysis; C6, C7, T1 not reparable |
| H. | 1 | C5, C7 reparable; C6, C8, T1 not reparable |

Table 15-7 represents some of the more unusual distributions of reparable and irreparable loss. In four cases, C5, C6, C8, and T1 were reparable or had neurolysis but C7 was not reparable. In another three cases, C6 and C7 were not reparable, but C5, C8, and T1 were reparable or had a neurolysis. Still other variations can be seen in Table 15-7. This table serves to point out how diverse the patterns of both irreparable and reparable damage can be in patients with flail arms.

The C5-T1 lesions or flail arms were especially difficult to manage effectively. Restoration of function was often quite limited, even after an attempt was made to select patients for their operability. Although some restoration of shoulder abduction and flexion of the elbow

was obtained in approximately 40% of cases and some triceps function in 30%, these operations were salvage-like in nature (Figure 15-25). Useful wrist or finger motion was seldom obtained. In the few exceptions, presence of not only continuity but a non-preganglionic and regenerative NAP led to neurolysis of one or more lower elements and, because of spontaneous regeneration, some subsequent degree of useful recovery of hand function occurred. As can be seen in Table 15-1, only 31% of all C5-T1 patients gained an overall grade of 3 or better outcome. Most of the better grades came about because of shoulder and upper arm recovery and only a few because of recovery at wrist or finger levels.

Selection for attempted direct repair of the C5

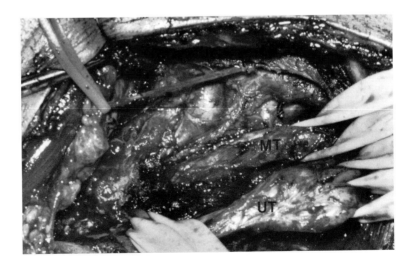

**Figure 15-25.** Stretch injury involving all elements within a heavily scarred supraclavicular space. Phrenic is retracted upward by the plastic loop; right upper Penrose is around thickened, scarred middle trunk (MT), and lower two Penroses are on the divisions of a very neuromatous upper trunk (UT).

**TABLE 15–8**

Preoperative to Postoperative Results If All Five Plexus Roots Either Had
Neurolysis, Graft Repair or Both (see D in Table 15–6)

| C5 | C6 | C7 | C8 | T1 | Follow-Up |
|---|---|---|---|---|---|
| 0 to 3 N | 2 to 4 N | 3 to 4 N | 2 to 4 N | 0 to 4 N | 19 mo |
| 0 to 4 N | 1 to 5 N | 0 to 4 N | 2 to 5 N | 0 to 4 N | 36 mo |
| 0 to 3 SP | 0 to 4 G | 0 to 3 G | 0 to 2 G | 0 to 0 G | 54 mo |
| 0 to 4 G | 0 to 4 G | 0 to 3 G | 0 to 0 G | 0 to 0 G | 51 mo |
| 0 to 4 G* | 0 to 4 G* | 0 to 2 G* | 0 to 0 G* | 0 to 0 G* | 24 mo |
| 0 to 2 G† | 0 to 4 G† | 0 to 0 G† | 0 to 0 G† | 0 to 0 G† | 20 mo |
| 0 to 1 G | 0 to 4 G | 0 to 2 G | 2 to 4 N | 3 to 4 N | 44 mo |
| 0 to 3 G | 0 to 3 G | 0 to 4 G | 3 to 5 N | 3 to 4 N | 30 mo |

G = graft; N = neurolysis; SP = split repair.
*Grafts 10 cm in length
†Grafts 15 cm in length

and possibly the C6 root was carried out if necessary. Cases operated on had rhomboid and serratus anterior function and did not have a meningocele at the C4-C5 level (involving C5 root or spinal nerve). As can be seen from Tables 15–6 through 15–13, C5 was either regenerating or was not regenerating but could usually be used to provide adequate lead-out for grafts at or after its dural exit (Figure 15–26). There were four exceptions. Two occurred in patients who were found at operation to have avulsion of this element at or proximal to the level of the dural exit of the root.

Two patients had avulsion of all the roots including C5 (see Table 15–6). Recovery did not ensue in either of these patients. In another two cases, C5, C7, C8, and T1 were avulsed but C6 was not. Some recovery was gained in these two cases by supplementing direct C6 repair with neurotization using descending cervical plexus and phrenic nerves as lead-outs for grafts.

If C5 was the only directly reparable root, as it was in 10 cases, recovery in the C5 distribution had overall grades that averaged only 2, and recovery in the C6 distribution averaged only 1.5. Grafts were led either from C5, or, in six cases, from descending cervical plexus and phrenic nerve, because C6 as well as other roots were not usable as lead-outs. Results in this subgroup for C7 distribution muscles that were neurotized by C5 or descending cervical plexus were even worse, averaging 0.7. An exception was provided by a youngster of 6 years of age who had grade 2 to 3 return in C5 muscles and grade 3 recovery in C6 and C7 muscles. There were two other patients who gained a grade 2 recovery in the C7 distribution.

A large subgroup of injuries had reparable or

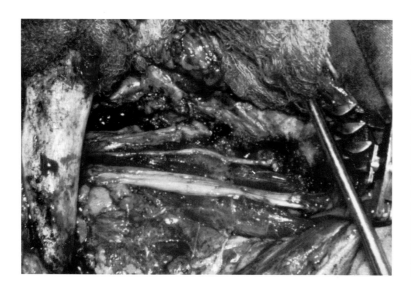

**Figure 15–26.** Grafts from C5 (3), C7 (1), C8 (3) and T1 (1) to cords in a 15-year-old with a flail arm due to a blunt, transecting, and stretch injury as a result of a motorcycle accident. Sural grafts were 12.7 cm in length and extended to the cord level. Acutely, a vein graft repair of the subclavian was necessary, but the patient had no restoration of the radial pulse. Follow-up over a 3.5-year period showed recovery of biceps, brachioradialis, and some supraspinatus and deltoid.

**TABLE 15–9**

Preoperative to Postoperative Results If C5, C6, C8, and T1 Were Reparable or Had Neurolysis But C7 Was Not Reparable* (see A in Table 15–7)

| C5 | C6 | C7 | C8 | T1 | Follow-Up |
|---|---|---|---|---|---|
| 0 to 2 G | 0 to 2 G | 0 to 2 AV | 3 to 4 N | 3 to 4 N | 28 mo |
| 0 to 2 G | 0 to 3 G | 0 to 3 AV | 3 to 5 N | 3 to 5 N | 32 mo |
| 0 to 2 G | 0 to 3 G | 0 to 2 AV | 0 to 0 G | 0 to 0 G | 36 mo |
| 0 to 2 G | 0 to 2 G | 0 to 2 AV | 3 to 4 N | 3 to 4 N | 19 mo |

AV = avulsion; G = graft; N = neurolysis.
*Grafts led out from C5 and C6 to distal C7 outflows (usually to the posterior cord) as well as to lateral cord.

regenerating C5 and C6 roots despite proximal avulsions of C7, C8, and T1 roots (Figures 15–27 and 15–28). These 31 cases formed the second largest subset of C5-T1 lesions selected for operation. If all 31 patients are summarized regardless of length of follow-up, average recovery in the C5 distribution was 2.2. Recovery averaged 2.3 in the C6 distribution and only 1.4 in the C7 distribution. In flail-arm patients with C5-C6 spinal nerve injuries that were reparable or regenerating after follow-up of 30 months and more, averaged C5 recovery was 2.7, and C6 recovered to 2.9 and C7 to 1.6. Looked at another way, 11 of 19 patients in this category with follow-up of more than 30 months achieved grades of 3 or more for C5- and C6-innervated muscles (Figure 15–29). One patient had a split repair of C5 to upper trunk with neurolysis of outflow to suprascapular nerve. Result in this patient's C5 distribution graded 4.

One flail-arm patient had neurolysis of both C5 and C6 because of the presence of regenerative NAPs. Neurolysis of the upper roots was supplemented by neurotization of distal middle trunk by descending cervical plexus. This patient, by 18 months postoperatively, had recovery of biceps/brachialis to a grade 3 to 4 level with shoulder muscles grading 2 to 3. Another patient who was 18 at the time had identical operative findings and an identical procedure and recovered C5 to grade 4, C6 to 3, and C7 to 1 to 2 by 24 months postoperatively.

The largest subset of C5-T1 stretch patients operated on were those with either regenerating or reparable C5, C6, and C7 roots and were found at the operating table (see Table 15–6). In these 34 cases, C8 and T1 were not reparable. This group was summarized for return in the distribution of various roots. C5 recovery averaged 2.4, C6 was 2.7, and C7 was 1.9. Only one patient had significant recovery in the C8 distribution, which was grade 2. In patients in this category who had 24 or more months of follow-up, C5 averaged 2.6, C6 was 2.9, and C7 remained 1.9. The data could be further analyzed in another way. In patients with 24 or more months of follow-up, 14 of 26 had recovery in both the C5 and C6 distributions averaging 3 or better. In seven of these same patients, C7 distribution recovery was 3 or better (Figure 15–30).

**TABLE 15–10**

Preoperative to Postoperative Results If C5, C8, and T1 Were Reparable or Had Neurolysis But C6 and C7 Were Not Reparable*
(See B in Table 15–7)

| C5 | C6 | C7 | C8 | T1 | Follow-up |
|---|---|---|---|---|---|
| 0 to 3 G | AV-3 | AV-2 | 3 to 5 N | 3 to 4 N | 38 mo† |
| 0 to 3 N | AV-2 | AV-3 | 0 to 4 N | 0 to 4 N | 34 mo |
| 0 to 3 G | AV-2 | AV-0 | 0 to 2 G | 0 to 2 G | 20 mo‡ |

AV = avulsion; G = grafts; N = neurolysis.
*Grafts were led from C5 and descending cervical plexus to distal outflows of C6 and C7 at a cord level.
†Grafts were placed to C6 and C7 inputs at the cord level as well as C5 input to cords. Grafts were 12.7 cm long.
‡Patient was only 3 years old when he sustained a flail arm as a result of a vehicular accident.

**TABLE 15–11**

Preoperative to Postoperative Results If C5, C6, and T1 Were Reparable But C7 and C8 Were Not Reparable*
(See C in Table 15–7)

| C5 | C6 | C7 | C8 | T1 | Follow-up |
|---|---|---|---|---|---|
| 0 to 2 G | 0 to 2 G | AV-0 | AV-0 | 0 to 1 G | 22 mo |
| 0 to 1 G | 0 to 1 G | AV-0 | AV-0 | 0 to 0 G | 60 mo† |

AV = avulsion; G = grafts.
*Grafts were led out from C6 to distal outflows of C7 and T1 to distal outflows of C8 at a cord level.
†Patient is considering amputation of his almost totally paralyzed arm.

**TABLE 15–12**

Preoperative to Postoperative Results
If C5, C6, and C8 Were Reparable But
C7 and T1 Were Not Reparable*
(See D in Table 15–7)

| C5 | C6 | C7 | C8 | T1 | Follow-up |
|----|----|----|----|----|-----------|
| 0 to 2 G | 0 to 4 G | AV-2 | 0 to 2 G | AV-0 | 48 mo |
| 0 to 2 G | 0 to 3 G | AV-2 | 0 to 0 G | AV-0 | 60 mo |

AV = avulsion; G = grafts.
*Grafts were led from C6 to C7 distal outflows and from C8 to T1 distal outflows at a cord level.

**TABLE 15–13**

Preoperative to Postoperative Results
in Patients With Either C5 Through C8
or C7 Through T1 Loss

| C5 | C6 | C7 | C8 | Follow-up |
|----|----|----|----|-----------|
| 0 to 2 G | 0 to 3 N | 0 to 3 N | 2 to 4 N | 20 mo |
| 0 to 3 G | 0 to 4 G | 0 to 4 N | 0 to 4 N | 36 mo |

| | C7 | C8 | T1 | Follow-up |
|----|----|----|----|-----------|
| | 3 to 4 N | 0 to 3 G | 0 to 2 N | 20 mo |
| | 3 to 5 N | 0 to 2 G | 0 to 2 G | 26 mo |

G = grafts; N = neurolysis.

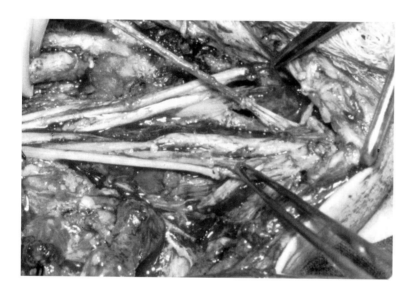

**Figure 15–27.** Graft repair of left plexus in a flail-arm patient. Lengthy grafts using sural nerve were led out from descending cervical plexus and C5 and C6 spinal nerves and sutured distally to lateral and posterior cords. C7 and C8 were damaged back to dura; T1 to lower trunk recordings showed a small nerve action potential, so only a neurolysis of this outflow was done. Forceps point to proximal suture sites for grafts.

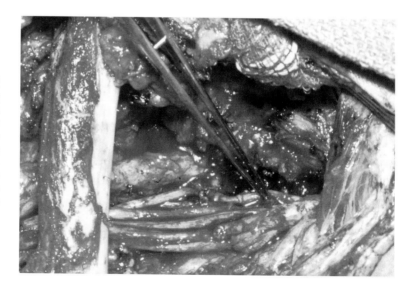

**Figure 15–28.** Placement of grafts from left C5, descending cervical plexus, and a portion of C6 to cord level just distal to the exposed clavicle. The patient had a flail arm. C7 was damaged back to spinal dura, so one C6 graft and one of the C5 grafts were led to middle trunk. Lower trunk is seen just above the grafts and in the middle of the photograph. It conducted typical preganglionic nerve action potentials so was not directly reparable.

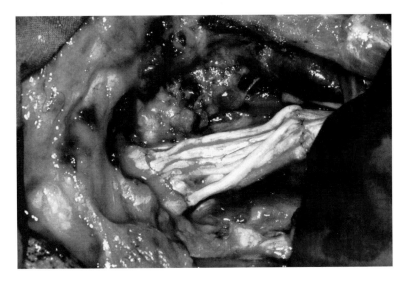

**Figure 15–29.** Graft repair in a patient with a flail arm as a result of a motor vehicle accident. Sural grafts were led from C5, C6, and descending cervical plexus to divisions of upper and middle trunk. C7 was not reparable, and C8 and T1 had preganglionic injury.

Three patients in the C5-T1 category of loss had neurolysis based on positive NAPs recorded from C5 or C6 or both, and recovery in their distributions was excellent. If split repair was possible, as occurred in two C5 roots in this series, recovery was also excellent. On the other hand, in two patients with relatively long grafts, 12.7 and 17.7 cm in length respectively, recovery was extremely poor.

In the six cases in which four spinal nerves were reparable or had neurolysis or both, results were generally good. In four of these cases, with

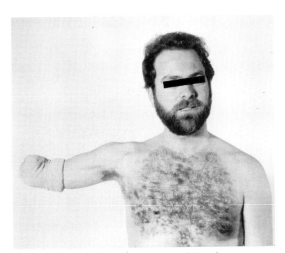

**Figure 15–30.** This man avulsed his lower roots and damaged his upper plexus in a motorcycle accident. The upper elements were repaired and the limb was subsequently amputated through the proximal forearm. Return of strong elbow flexion, some triceps function, and shoulder abduction allowed him to use a prosthesis very successfully.

24 months or more of follow-up, recovery in the C5 distribution averaged 2.6, in C6, 2.6, in C7, 2.8, and in C8, 1.0. There was no significant recovery that could be allocated to T1 alone. Three of these six patients had recovery of grade 3 or better in both the C5 and C6 distributions, but three of these six elements had split repair.

As might have been expected, recovery was also relatively good in the eight patients who could have either neurolysis or graft repair or both to all five plexus roots (see Table 15–8). If all five spinal nerves had neurolysis based on positive NAPs, recovery averaged 4 for both patients (Table 15–8 and Figure 15–31). Five of the ten elements evaluated operatively in these two patients had some degree of function preoperatively, and this averaged level 2. There were two patients in whom some elements had graft repair and some neurolysis, and thus all five roots had the potential for recovery. Average recovery for all elements for both of these patients was 3 to 4.

Graft repair of all five elements led to variable results (see Table 15–8). Even though grafts were 10 cm in length, significant recovery occurred in C5 and C6 distributions in one patient. Grafts 15 cm in length were not successful for C5, C7, C8, and T1 outflows but were for C6-innervated biceps in another patient. Follow-up on this individual has, however, only extended to 20 months postoperatively. In the other two patients in whom all elements were repaired by grafts, results in C5, C6, and also C7 distributions averaged 3 to 4.

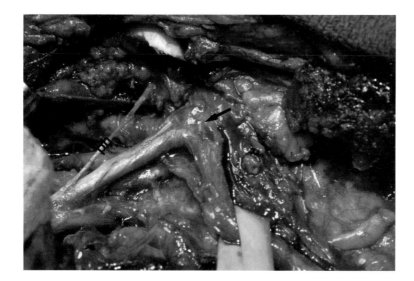

**Figure 15-31.** Stretched and distorted plexus *(arrow)* in a patient with a flail arm. Fractured and poorly healed clavicle was resected in this case. All elements conducted an operative nerve action potential, so only an external neurolysis of the plexus was done. ph = phrenic nerve.

Two patients had a combination of grafts and neurolysis. Both patients had graft repair of C5, C6, and C7 and neurolysis of C8 and T1 spinal nerves. The C8 and T1 roots in these cases had some function in their distribution preoperatively and improved significantly with neurolysis. Recovery in the C5, C6, and C7 roots in which grafts were done averaged 3.

Despite using criteria for selection for operability, 2 of the 112 patients had no reparable spinal nerves. (See G in Table 4.) There was of course no significant recovery in these two patients.

Table 15-7 depicts some of the less frequently seen patterns of involvement and repair in the flail-arm group of patients (Figure 15-32). Tables 15-9 through 15-12 give a breakdown on preoperative and postoperative grades, the procedure done on each root and its outflow, and length of follow-up in representative patients with a variety of injury and regenerative patterns.

## Summary of C5, C6, C7, C8 and T1 Lesions

1. This most frequent pattern of loss unfortunately produces a totally paralyzed or flail arm.
2. If loss in this distribution is severe or complete, incidence of spontaneous recovery of function is the lowest for all patterns of stretch.

3. This is difficult to help by either direct repair and/or neurotization, and these operations, either alone or together, are often only salvage-like in nature in this setting.
4. A combination of severe paraspinal denervation, positive sensory NAPs involving lower spinal nerve levels, or meningoceles at three or more levels, especially if upper levels are involved, stands against success with attempted direct repair. In such patients, the value of neurotization must be carefully weighed with these patients and their families.

## Other Stretch Patterns

The two patients with C5 through C8 loss were of interest, as were those two who had only C7, C8, and T1 loss (see Tables 15-1 and 15-13). Table 15-13 shows their preoperative and postoperative grades as well as the procedure done on each outflow. As might have been predicted, results were better in the C5, C6, C7, and C8 lesions than in the C7, C8, and T1 lesions.

There were 12 additional operative patients who had either partial loss to begin with or had only lower element, C8, and T1 loss (Figure 15-33). They have been excluded from this analysis. The C8-T1 repairs gave uniformly poor results in four cases; another two with partial loss improved, but might have improved without surgery also. In another two cases, loss was par-

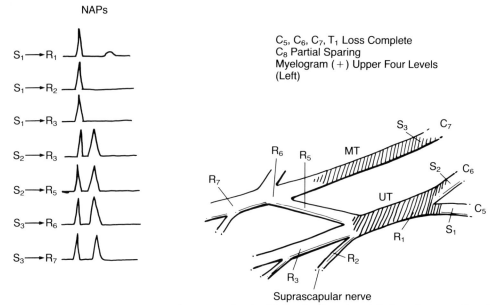

NAPs

$S_1 \longrightarrow R_1$

$S_1 \longrightarrow R_2$

$S_1 \longrightarrow R_3$

$S_2 \longrightarrow R_3$

$S_2 \longrightarrow R_5$

$S_3 \longrightarrow R_6$

$S_3 \longrightarrow R_7$

C5, C6, C7, T1 Loss Complete
C8 Partial Sparing
Myelogram ( + ) Upper Four Levels
(Left)

Suprascapular nerve

**Figure 15–32.** Flail arm with exception of some sparing in C8 distribution. As might have been predicted from the myelogram, most elements had preganglionic injury with large, rapidly conducted nerve action potentials. Despite this, some outflow from C5 to proximal upper trunk was regenerating. Patient subsequently had a shoulder fusion but refused an attempt to neurotize biceps by use of intercostal nerves.

tial in the C7, C8, and T1 distributions. Neurolysis in these cases was associated with some eventual recovery, but this again might have occurred without surgery. Graft repair of C6, C8, and T1, or C8 and T1 with neurolysis of C7 or C6 and C7 led only to significant recovery of C6 and proximal C8 innervational territories but not to recovery of fine muscle function (4 patients).

There are other systems for both grading recovery and tabulating patterns of loss and operative findings. Several examples of these are found in Table 15–14.

## NEUROTIZATION FOR BRACHIAL PLEXUS STRETCH INJURIES

Between 1972 and 1986, 47 patients seen at the University of Toronto underwent a variety of neurotization procedures for traumatic brachial plexus palsy with root avulsion (see Table 15–2). There were 42 males and 5 females. Age at injury ranged from 14 to 34 years

**TABLE 15–14**

P. L. Raimondi's (Lagano) Grading System for Plexus

| | |
|---|---|
| Shoulder | |
| Abduction | 5 points |
| External rotation | 5 points |
| Elbow | |
| Flexion | 5 points |
| Extension | 4 points |
| Wrist | |
| Flexion | 5 points |
| Extension | 5 points |
| Pronation/Supination | 5 points |
| Hand | 6 points |
| TOTAL | 40 points |

Narakus Method for Showing Status of Spinal Nerves or Roots After Stretch Injury Confirmed by Operation (With Added LSUMC Experience)

| Roots | Different Combinations | | | | | | | | | | | | |
|---|---|---|---|---|---|---|---|---|---|---|---|---|---|
| C5 | " | " | o | " | " | " | o | " | " | " | " | " | o |
| C6 | " | o | o | " | o | o | o | o | o | " | o | o | o |
| C7 | | | " | " | o | o | o | o | o | " | o | o |
| C8 | | | | | " | o | o | o | o | o | o |
| T1 | | | | | | " | o | o | o | o |

o = Avulsion; " = lateral distraction or incontinuity.

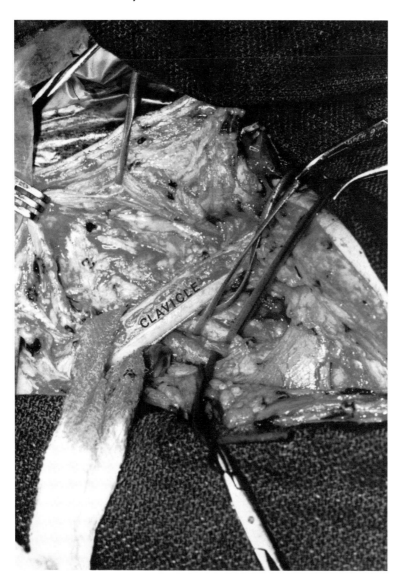

**Figure 15-33.** Lower trunk injury can be initially approached by an infraclavicular procedure. The shoulder is abducted and the artery and medial cord defined below the clavicle. Subsequently, the shoulder is abducted and the clavicle pulled down and forward by the encircling sponges, thus allowing the dissected vascular and plexus structures to be seen above the clavicle and followed medially in a safe fashion.

(mean 22 years). Most patients were injured in traffic accidents involving a motorcycle (28), a car (6), a bicycle (3), or as a pedestrian (2). Others were injured while skiing (2), waterskiing (2), or on a snowmobile (2). One patient tripped and fell, and another was struck by a falling tree. In 26 patients, the injury involved the dominant limb.

A standard protocol was used to assess all patients. After a detailed history and physical examination, plain radiographs of the cervical spine and shoulder girdle and clavicle, and a cervical myelogram were performed. This was followed by EMG of the limb and shoulder girdle musculature and motor and sensory nerve conduction velocity determinations. Angiogra-

phy was performed in two patients who had required emergency subclavian artery repair immediately after their injury. Patients finally underwent surgical exploration of the brachial plexus with intraoperative nerve stimulation and recordings as well as recording of somatosensory-evoked potentials to confirm root avulsion. Twenty-two patients had five roots avulsed, and avulsion involved four roots in 2 patients, three roots in 6, two roots in 15, and one root in 2 patients.

Neurotization procedures were offered to patients with root avulsion who were young, well-motivated, presented within 9 months of injury, and whose limb was in good condition. The majority of patients had intercostal nerves ex-

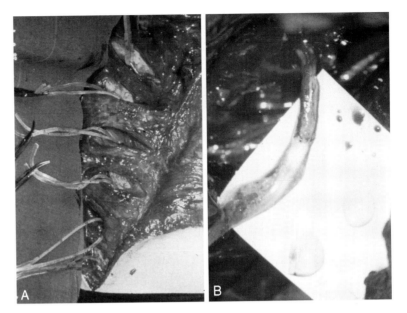

**Figure 15–34.** Intercostal neurotization to musculocutaneous and axillary nerves. *(A)* Intercostal nerves are isolated and sewn to sural nerve grafts. The graft bypasses the plexus, and the distal suture line is at the cut end of the recipient peripheral nerve *(B)*.

tended by grafts to musculocutaneous nerve (Figures 15–34 and 15–35). Some of these patients also had other neurotization procedures. Intercostal nerves were used as lead-outs to other nerves, as were accessory nerve and descending cervical plexus.

## RESULTS OF NEUROTIZATION (TORONTO SERIES)

There were no operative deaths and no significant morbidity after neurotization. Five patients developed small pneumothoraces after harvesting of the intercostal nerves, but all resolved spontaneously. There were no wound infections. None of the patients in this series was made worse by the procedure, and none developed a significant long-term pain syndrome.

The best results were achieved with neurotization of the musculocutaneous nerve with 21 (57%) of 37 patients obtaining useful elbow flexion (Figure 15–36; see Table 15–2). Outcome was correlated with the number of intercostal nerves used as donors. If three or four intercostal nerves were connected to the musculocutaneous nerve, the outcome was much more likely to be useful elbow flexion than if only two intercostal nerves were used. There was little difference in outcome whether three

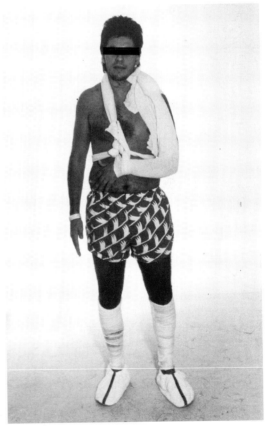

**Figure 15–35.** On the day after intercostal neurotization, the patient is out of bed. Dressings cover the wound of the initial plexus exploration, the lateral chest site of intercostal nerve surgery, and the donor sural nerve sites of both legs. Physical therapy commences 3 weeks later.

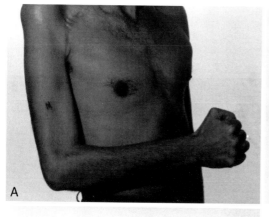

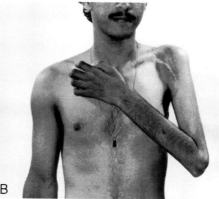

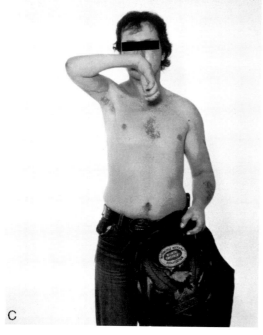

**Figure 15-36.** (A) Examination of a patient 2 years after intercostal neurotization for irreparable C5 and C6 injury reveals moderate elbow flexion augmenting useful hand function. (B) Although only a single lower root survived avulsion, another patient still felt that this degree of elbow flexion, following intercostal neurotization, was of use to him despite his severely limited hand function. (C) This patient avulsed all five roots on the right side. He regained sufficient elbow flexion on the right to carry his leather jacket (held in his normal left hand) over his flexed right forearm.

or four intercostals were used. There was no significant correlation between the length of the grafts, the interval from injury to surgery, or the age of the patient and outcome. Maximum recovery took up to 24 months in some patients. There were several patients in whom the musculocutaneous nerve was torn out of the biceps and thus intercostal neurotization of this nerve was impossible (Figure 15–37).

The restoration of active elbow flexion resulted in significant improvement in the functional abilities of these patients. Even in the presence of an anesthetic, immobile hand, active elbow flexion allowed the forearm to be used as a paperweight, as a platform on which

objects could be balanced, or as a hook from which they could be hung. The hand could be used to turn simple levers.

Intercostal neurotization of the radial, median, and ulnar nerves failed to restore useful function. Neurotization of the axillary nerve fared only slightly better. Using the spinal accessory as motor donor gave modest results, but the numbers are too small to allow definitive comment.

The sensory recovery after neurotization by the cervical plexus is also shown in Table 15–2. Protective sensation was restored to part or all of the hand and fingers in 11 instances (55%). In four other cases, a degree of sensibility returned

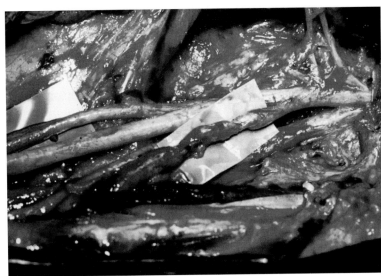

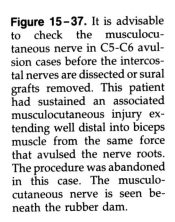

**Figure 15-37.** It is advisable to check the musculocutaneous nerve in C5-C6 avulsion cases before the intercostal nerves are dissected or sural grafts removed. This patient had sustained an associated musculocutaneous injury extending well distal into biceps muscle from the same force that avulsed the nerve roots. The procedure was abandoned in this case. The musculocutaneous nerve is seen beneath the rubber dam.

but was not sufficient to be adequately protective. We found no particular predictors of outcome for sensory recovery after neurotization.

None of the patients in this series requested amputation. A flail, anesthetic limb that is one's own seems preferable to an inanimate prosthesis. Thirty-seven patients returned to gainful employment, but only six returned to their preinjury occupations. The majority have resumed sports, and one even returned to motorcycle racing, the activity which led to her initial injury.

## PRESENT CRITERIA FOR SELECTING PATIENTS FOR POSSIBLE DIRECT REPAIR OF STRETCH-INJURED SUPRACLAVICULAR BRACHIAL PLEXUS

Not all patients with severe stretch injury involving the plexus can, at the present time, be helped by an operation. This is especially so if direct repair is preferable and if neurotization is not to be used in an attempt to restore function.

For the usual case with serious paralysis of the plexus, we evaluate the patient as early as

possible. This includes grading any residual motor or sensory function in the extremity and obtaining a baseline EMG at 3 or 4 weeks after injury. Special attention is given to assessing proximally innervated muscles such as paraspinal muscles, rhomboids, serratus anterior, and supraspinatus. In addition, it is most important to define how complete the injury and loss are to each element of the plexus involved. Significant, incomplete loss in the distribution of an element, usually improves with time, but complete loss often does not. In addition to radiographs of associated bones such as spine, scapula, clavicle, ribs, and shoulder joint including humerus, a chest film is important to note the relative positions of the diaphragms. The patient is usually followed for about 3 to 4 months with periodic clinical and electromyographic examinations. If significant function does not begin to recover, then the patient has a myelogram if that has not already been done.

The patient is then operated on if there are not too may stops or negatives to exploration and if there is a possibility of direct repair of at least a portion of the plexus at levels favorable for repair, which are usually C5, C6, C7, and their more distal outflows. One advantage to a delay of several months in exploring stretch injuries to the plexus relates to the fact that often there is physical continuity to one or more of the plexus elements. These elements have not been avulsed from the spinal cord or distracted more laterally but require time for even adequate spontaneous regeneration to occur if it is to occur. Even direct intraoperative recordings cannot with certainty exclude adequate regeneration in these elements with lengthy lesions in continuity until 3 to 4 months from the time of injury. Such a delay has to be balanced against the advantage provided by earlier repair. The problem with earlier surgery is that even intraoperative electrical techniques have difficulty assessing fairly the need for resection. In addition, those cases capable of spontaneous recovery in the distribution of one or more elements may have them prematurely resected and replaced by grafts if operation is done too early. In any case, maintenance or recovery of a good range of motion in all involved joints is paramount while awaiting operation.

There are some "stops" or findings which make the possibility of direct repair less likely. The presence of one stop should seldom prevent exploration, although serious spinal cord injury at the plexus level usually does. Such findings, especially if multiple, usually make direct repair with significant outcome less likely (Table 15–15). Nonetheless, if there is doubt, it is probably better to explore these lesions. The opportunities for other reconstructive or neurotization procedures are not very good in most patients, or only help one portion of the paralyzed limb. Unfortunately, direct repair may

also not lead to enough return to muscles to make them usable for transfer. This is because the yield in terms of significant muscle power is relatively low, especially when an attempt is made to reinnervate a flail arm.

Winging of the scapula as a result of long thoracic nerve palsy and serratus anterior loss suggests a very proximal lesion of C5, C6, and C7 spinal nerves. The long thoracic nerve usually arises from the distal intraforaminal portion of C6 but can also receive proximal spinal nerve branches of C5 and sometimes C7 or even C8. For a similar reason, rhomboid paralysis suggests a proximal spinal nerve lesion of C5 and C6 because the dorsal scapular nerve has a proximal intraforaminal origin from these structures. It is unusual, however, for these losses to be present unless there has been severe scapular or thoracic dissociation. Even though the phrenic arises usually from C3 and C4 spinal nerves, it may have input from C5 and, in any case, is adherent and often incorporated into a portion of C5 as the latter exits its foramen. If the diaphragm is paralyzed and thus elevated and yet the injury is blunt and nonpenetrating to the neck and supraclavicular plexus, relatively proximal damage to C5 is often present. If C5 is damaged proximally, so may be C6 and even C7, and yet these are the very levels responding best to direct repair if it can be achieved.

Another clinical finding suggesting a proximal level of injury is the presence of Horner syndrome. This suggests but does not prove proximal involvement of the T1 and frequently the C8 spinal nerve also. There is a false-positive and false-negative incidence of correlation of Horner syndrome with the nonreparability of T1 and C8 spinal nerves. Like meningoceles on a myelogram, though, this finding usually means a proximal and thus irreparable lesion at these lower levels. Nonetheless, the presence of Horner syndrome does not necessarily mean that more proximal spinal nerves such as C5, C6, and C7 are not more laterally injured and thus reparable. Similar arguments can be marshalled for and against the value of myelography in this setting, and these have been summarized earlier in the chapter. Similarly, sensory NAP recordings, which can provide evidence of preganglionic injury fairly effectively in lower

**TABLE 15–15**
Relative Stops for Direct Repair
of Plexus

Evidence of proximal spinal nerve injury at multiple levels, especially the upper levels; included is extensive paraspinal denervation by electromyelogram, rhomboid, serratus anterior, or diaphragmatic paralysis.

Sensory nerve action potentials elicited by stimulation of and recording from multiple peripheral nerves.

Presence of pseudomeningoceles at multiple spinal nerve levels, especially the upper levels.

Presence of extensive fractures of the cervical spine or serious cervical myelopathy.

Injury limited to the C8-T1 spinal nerves or their outflows.

Referral of the patient a year or more after injury.

Most cases in which there has been scapular or thoracic distraction, especially if there has been subclavian arterial avulsion, do not usually have reparable plexus elements.

spinal nerves such as C8, T1, and sometimes C7, are not usable to evaluate either C5 or C6, and yet these are the spinal nerves of the plexus we would like to know the most about.

## COMPLICATIONS OF OPERATIONS ON STRETCH/CONTUSION INJURIES TO BRACHIAL PLEXUS

Complications included phrenic paralysis, which in most instances reversed in time but did persist beyond a year in three cases. Two patients required a chest tube postoperatively, and three others had thoracentesis. Serious wound infection was not seen in this category of injuries. All patients received perioperative and postoperative coverage by antibiotics and were sent home on an antibiotic for 7 days. Several seromas were aspirated in the early postoperative period and fortunately did not recur. One patient required aspiration of a collection of lymph, and the wound subsequently healed with the help of a compressive dressing. Two patients collected cerebrospinal fluid at their wound sites, and these resolved by recurrent local aspiration and compressive dressing.

In the earlier years of this series, the clavicle was sometimes divided. Despite fixation, malunion occurred in several instances. In the last 15 years, the clavicle has been cleared of soft tissues, encircled by sponges, and drawn up superiorly and then down inferiorly to complete the necessary dissection of plexus beneath it. Bleeding from the vertebral artery at a foraminal level led to its surgical occlusion in five cases; in other instances the bleeding was stopped by use of the bipolar forceps and oxycel cotton. Vertebral occlusion, if necessary, was usually tolerated well. In a case too recent for inclusion in this series, vertebral occlusion led to a delayed cerebellar and brain stem stroke, possibly caused by embolization. The patient had undergone prior occlusion of an ipsilateral carotid cavernous fibula by a balloon technique, and the internal carotid had subsequently occluded. What role that might have played in this complication is unclear at this point.

## OPERATIVE RESULTS WITH INFRACLAVICULAR STRETCH AND CONTUSIVE INJURIES

These cord and cord-to-nerve lesions had a higher incidence of associated injuries than the supraclavicular stretch injuries. Axillary artery injury, shoulder dislocation or fracture, and humeral fracture were especially prevalent. On the other hand, because of a more distal locus, shoulder function was sometimes spared completely or at least in part. As can be seen from Table 15–16, however, this was not always the case. Isolated axillary palsy or one associated with other cord or cord-to-nerve injuries was quite common. Tables 15–16 and 15–17 also depicts the common patterns and combinations of involvement seen with infraclavicular stretch injuries.

Unlike gunshot wounds involving plexus at an infraclavicular level, injury was less focal and thus less likely to be restricted to one level of the plexus elements alone. In other words, damage was seldom restricted to cords alone and more likely to extend from divisions to cords to more distal nerves. As might be expected, such damage sometimes began at a divisional level and extended a variable distal distance along peripheral nerves. If repair was necessary in such instances, results were, as expected, not good because of the length and severity of the lesion in continuity.

**TABLE 15–16**

Infraclavicular Stretch Injuries — Common Patterns or Associated Nerve Lesions

| No. Cases | Description |
|---|---|
| 33 | Posterior cord to axillary alone |
| 14 | All elements including axillary |
| 11 | All elements except axillary |
| 11 | Posterior cord and axillary |
| 7 | Axillary and suprascapular |
| 4 | All elements except posterior cord |
| 3 | Lateral to musculocutaneous nerve alone |
| 3 | Lateral and medial cord to nerves |
| 2 | Lateral to musculocutaneous nerve and also posterior cord injury |

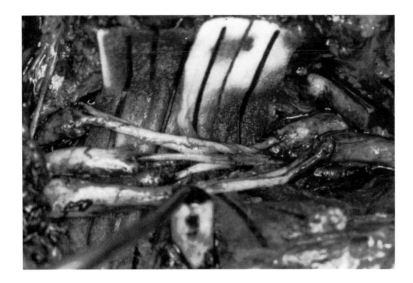

**Figure 15-38.** This plexus stretch injury was associated with a fracture of the clavicle as a result of a fall from a horse. Lesions extended from trunks to cords and were resected and replaced with grafts. Trunks are to the left and cords to the right.

## Cord Lesions

If injury was primarily at a divisional-to-cord or cord level alone, then lesions for purposes of analysis were categorized as those to "cords" (Figures 15-38, 15-39, and 15-40). If injury extended beyond cord to peripheral nerve level, they were placed in the "cord-to-nerve" category. Stretch injuries involving cords were less common than those involving cords to nerves (see Table 15-17). In the 27 cases involving primarily the cords of the plexus, 10 involved lateral, medial, and posterior cords, 6 medial and posterior, 5 lateral and medial, 3 lateral and posterior, and 3 a single cord alone. Table 15-17 depicts the larger numbers of elements in the distribution involved by stretch at a cord or cord-to-nerve level.

Outcomes in 64 operated cord elements in 27 cases were calculated. As in the gunshot wound series, elements in the lateral cord distribution, including musculocutaneous nerve to biceps,

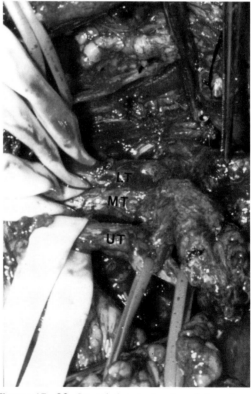

**Figure 15-39.** Stretch/contusion involving plexus at a divisional-to-cord level. Not surprisingly, this required a graft repair. LT = lower trunk; MT = middle trunk; UT = upper trunk.

**TABLE 15-17**
Number of Injured Infraclavicular
Elements Operated at Each Level

| No. Elements | Description |
|---|---|
| 18 | Lateral cord |
| 26 | Medial cord |
| 20 | Posterior cord |
| 44 | Lateral cord to musculocutaneous nerve |
| 39 | Lateral cord to median |
| 29 | Medial cord to median |
| 38 | Medial cord to ulnar |
| 52 | Posterior cord to radial |
| 67 | Posterior cord to axillary |
| 333 | Total Elements |

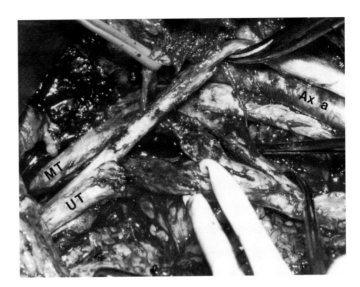

**Figure 15–40.** This unusual stretch injury involved only the posterior divisions of all three trunks. These elements did not transmit nerve action potentials, were resected, and were then replaced by grafts. Loss was to the deltoid and to all of the muscles in the radial distribution. Ax a = axillary artery; MT = middle trunk; UT = upper trunk. See also color figure.

lateral cord to median outflow to proximal median-innervated forearm muscles, and median distribution sensations, did well (Tables 15–18 and 15–19). Despite several extensive lesions requiring lengthy grafts, overall grades in the graft category were 3.8 (Table 15–18), and the average was 3.9 for all types of repairs to lateral cord, including two sutures and three split repairs. Neurolysis based on NAP recordings gave the expected excellent outcome. Grades averaged 4.6 if NAPs were recorded and if function was partial and neurolysis was done. If

function was completely out and yet a NAP could be recorded across the lesion, outcome averaged 4.2.

By contrast, outcome was not nearly as good with the medial cord stretch injuries. Graft repair of seven elements gave an average result of 1.2 and suture of two elements gave a 2.2 average grade. If split repair could be done, as it was in four cases, results were better and averaged 3.6. If regeneration or partial sparing could be shown by operative NAP studies, neurolysis alone gave an average recovery of 3.9. Thus,

**TABLE 15–18**
Infraclavicular Plexus Stretch Injuries*

| | Cases With Initial Partial Function and Neurolysis/ Result | Cases With Complete Loss and Neurolysis/ Result | Cases With Complete Loss and Suture/ Result | Cases With Complete Loss and Grafts/ Result | Cases With Complete Loss and Split Repair/ Result | Repair Impossible/ Result |
|---|---|---|---|---|---|---|
| **Cords** | | | | | | |
| Lateral | 3/4.6 | 4/4.2 | 2/4.3 | 6/3.8 | 3/4.0 | 0 |
| Medial | 8/4.1 | 3/3.5 | 2/2.2 | 7/1.2 | 4/3.6 | 2/0 |
| Posterior | 5/4.5 | 4/3.8 | 2/3.6 | 5/3.0 | 3/3.5 | 1/0 |
| **Cords to Nerves** | | | | | | |
| Lateral to Musculotaneous | 7/4.7 | 8/4.0 | 0 | 29/3.8 | 0 | 0 |
| Lateral to Median | 14/4.5 | 8/3.5 | 1/4.0 | 14/3.0 | 0 | 2/0 |
| Medial to Median | 6/4.7 | 11/4.1 | 1/4.0 | 9/3.0 | 0 | 2/0 |
| Medial to Ulnar | 14/4.2 | 11/3.1 | 1/0 | 8/1.4 | 1/2.3 | 3/0 |
| Posterior to Radial | 16/4.8 | 5/3.3 | 1/0 | 27/2.7 | 2/3.5 | 1/0 |
| Posterior to Axillary | 10/4.7 | 11/4.7 | 1/3.0 | 44/3.5 | 1/4.0 | 2/0 |
| Totals Cases/Results | 83/4.5 | 65/3.8 | 11/2.8 | 149/3.2 | 14/3.3 | 13/0 |

*Number of cases/averaged grade of recovery achieved.

**TABLE 15–19**

Average Grades for Neurolysis and Repair by Element Category*

| | No. of Elements Operated | Neurolysis Grades | Repair Grades | Overall Grade |
|---|---|---|---|---|
| **Cords** | | | | |
| Lateral | 18 | 4.4 | 3.9 | 4.1 |
| Medial | 24 | 3.9 | 2.1 | 2.9 |
| Posterior | 19 | 4.1 | 3.9 | 4.0 |
| **Cords to Nerves** | | | | |
| Lateral to Musculocutaneous | 44 | 4.3 | 3.8 | 4.0 |
| Lateral to Median | 37 | 4.1 | 3.1 | 3.7 |
| Medial to Median | 27 | 4.3 | 3.1 | 3.9 |
| Medial to Ulnar | 35 | 3.7 | 1.4 | 3.0 |
| Posterior to Radial | 51 | 4.4 | 2.7 | 3.4 |
| Posterior to Axillary | 63 | 4.3 | 3.4 | 3.7 |
| Average Grade | | 4.1 | 3.1 | 3.6 |

*Overall grades are averaged for each category: 0 = poor to 5 = excellent.

when operating on lesions in continuity involving medial cord, it is especially important to be certain that resection is necessary or, conversely, that it is not.

Posterior cord lesions did not do as well as lateral cord ones, but they certainly did much better than medial cord lesions. This was despite the fact that their dissection was often complicated by adherence or incorporation of the element to a vascular repair site. In this setting, there was a need to spare or dissect out axillary and radial nerves for repair along with any retained triceps branches. Graft repair of five injured posterior cords gave an average result of 3.0. Split repairs fared somewhat better, achieving an averaged grade of 3.5 (see Table 15–18). Neurolysis based on positive NAPs averaged 4.1 (see Table 15–19) and, as expected, was once again better for those elements having partial function than those in which function was entirely gone but adequate regeneration was proven (Table 15–18).

## Cord-to-Nerve Lesions

Outcomes in 267 operated elements in 92 cases were studied in this category. Dissections usually extended from clavicle well down into upper arm and required preservation of major vascular structures including axillary artery, profundus artery, and axillary veins wherever

possible. Despite the need for such extensive dissection, outcomes seemed to justify these procedures (see Tables 15–18 and 15–19). Once again, it was especially important to assess each lesion in continuity by operative NAP recordings.

## Lateral Cord to Musculocutaneous Nerve

Overall average grade for outcome in this group of elements was 4.0. Not unexpectedly, neurolysis gave the better results, averaging 4.5, but 7 of those 15 having neurolysis had some biceps contraction before their operation. Nonetheless, those eight with absent biceps preoperatively and yet a recordable NAP indicating good regeneration had an average grade of 4.0. Averaged outcome for 29 graft repairs in this category was 3.8. This was despite the inclusion of two cases in which grafts were 12.7 and 15.2 cm in length and, as a result, recovery was extremely poor (Figure 15–41).

## Lateral Cord to Median Nerve

Another favorable category for gaining recovery was injuries involving lateral cord to median nerve elements. In 38 cases, 22 had neurolysis. Fourteen had partial function in this distribution, with some pronator teres and wrist and finger flexion function before surgery.

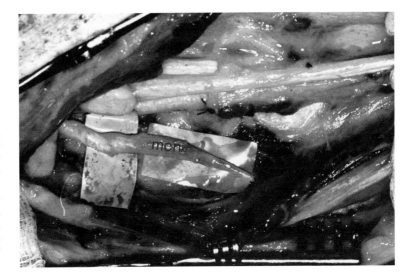

**Figure 15–41.** Most isolated musculocutaneous nerve (mcn) stretch injuries occur near the take-off from the lateral cord. On occasion, the injury also extends close to the entry point into biceps. Only a few small fascicles were found in this attenuated nerve. The clinical result was poor after graft repair.

Eight had a NAP across their lesion despite absence of distal function (Figure 15–42). Recovery in this latter group averaged 3.5. In the former group, in which function was partial to begin with, recovery averaged 4.5. As expected, those with partial function to begin with regenerated to a level superior to those without any function at the time of surgery. Regeneration was nonetheless excellent in those patients with complete distal loss if intraoperative NAPs were present across the lesions. Graft repairs for 14 lateral cord to median nerve lesions had averaged results of 3.0 (Figure 15–43). There were also two cases in which lengthy (>15 cm) avul-

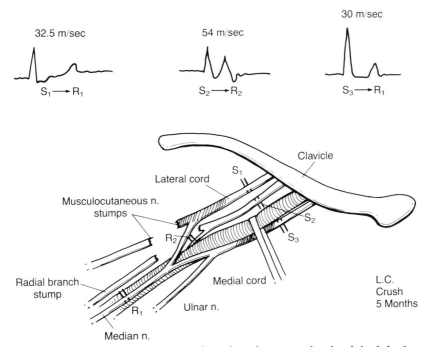

**Figure 15–42.** Drawing of contusive injury to cords and cord-to-nerve levels of the left plexus. Musculocutaneous nerve had been distracted, as had radial nerve just distal to the triceps branches. Fortunately, lesions in continuity involving lateral cord to median nerve and medial cord transmitted nerve action potentials and did not need resection. Grafts were used to repair lateral cord to musculocutaneous and posterior cord to radial nerves. NAPs were recorded from lateral cord to median (S1 to R1), posterior cord to triceps branch (S2 to R2), and medial cord to median (S3 to R1).

sive or stretch injury extending from lateral cord to median nerve precluded repair. As expected, no recovery occurred in these two cases.

### Medial Cord to Median Nerve

Even if only some function was spared initially, or if a NAP was recordable despite complete loss, this was a surprisingly good category or subset of element injury, not only for spontaneous recovery but also for recovery after repair. The latter usually included grafts.

Those 17 patients having partial function in this category and having neurolysis based on a positive NAP across the lesion recovered to an average grade of 4.5. Function was gauged to be absent preoperatively, and yet a NAP could be recorded in 11 cases. Neurolysis was done in these cases, and the average outcome was graded as 4.1.

In the nine cases in which function was completely absent preoperatively and a repair of this element could be done, outcome averaged 3.0. There were two cases in which the length of the injury extended from the medial cord well

distal on the median nerve to elbow level, and this precluded any effective repair. Another case had this portion of the infraclavicular plexus totally avulsed, and it could not be repaired.

### Medial Cord to Ulnar Nerve

As might be expected, this was a difficult element to manage with success. Graft repairs did not work very well. If neurolysis could be done because of partial sparing of function or because of a positive NAP despite absence of distal function, results were acceptable.

If function was partially spared in the distribution of this element, as it was in 14 cases, outcome was good and graded an average of 4.2. If loss was complete and yet a NAP was recorded, as it was in 11 cases, average grade was 3.1. Results in those nine patients in whom repair by graft or suture was attempted averaged only 1.4. Extensive up-and-down damage in two cases and total avulsion of this portion of the plexus in another precluded even graft repairs.

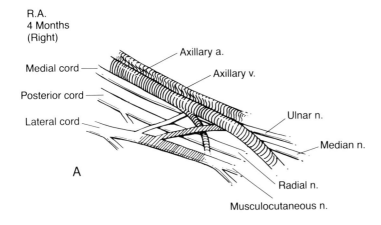

R.A.
4 Months
(Right)

Axillary a.
Medial cord
Axillary v.
Posterior cord
Lateral cord
Ulnar n.
Median n.

A

Radial n.
Musculocutaneous n.

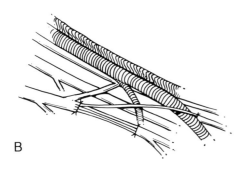

B

**Figure 15–43.** (A) Drawing of lateral cord injury involving outflow to musculocutaneous and median nerves. These lesions in continuity did not transmit nerve action potentials and were replaced by grafts. (B) This was a very favorable infraclavicular stretch injury for repair, and, as a result, recovery was good.

## Posterior Cord to Radial Nerve

There were 51 elements in this category operated on for stretch/contusion. In 16 cases, there was some function to begin with. As expected, NAPs across these lesions were positive and, with neurolysis and time, results had an average grade of 4.8. If function was absent but a NAP was recorded across the lesion, as it was in five instances, the average grade was 3.3. Despite evidence of regeneration at the operating table, these relatively low grades reflect the difficulty in regaining functional reinnervation of finger and thumb extensors.

If repair was necessary because of absence of a NAP, as it was in 30 posterior cord to radial elements, average grade was 2.7. This included two split repairs and one suture with the expected good results but also two cases in which grafts were 12.7 and 15.7 cm long, respectively, with the expected poor results. Also included was one case in which repair was thought to be impossible. If these cases are excluded, average recovery after graft repair of this element was 3.4.

## Posterior Cord to Axillary Nerve

These 65 operated elements included 33 that were unassociated with other serious plexus element damage. (See *D* in Table 15 – 20). These represented isolated axillary palsies caused by stretch (Figures 15 – 44, 15 – 45, and 15 – 46). If function was partial and neurolysis only was done, as in two cases, graded recovery was a 4. If function was absent but adequate regenera-

tion was shown by intraoperative NAPs, average grade was 3.5 (4 cases). If either suture, grafts, or split repairs were done in isolated axillary palsies (26 cases), grades averaged 3.5. This included one case in which distal axillary nerve was avulsed from deltoid, and grafts that were sutured or "dead ended" directly into muscle and gave no result. In another case, length of the lesion (15.7 cm) was thought to preclude repair, and, as expected, there was no recovery.

There were seven posterior cord to axillary palsies associated with suprascapular nerve palsy (see A in Table 15 – 20). In each case, suprascapular loss was either partial (4 cases) or had a recordable NAP across the lesion at operation (3 cases). Supraspinatus and infraspinatus recovered to a satisfactory level in all cases. Despite this, five of these combined lesions required graft repair of the axillary nerve. Results in grafted axillary nerves in this subset averaged 3.2. The other two cases had neurolysis and recovered quite well. On rare occasion isolated C5 stretch injury mimicked combined axillary and suprascapular stretch injuries (Figure 15 – 47).

Not too unexpectedly, 11 of the axillary palsies were associated with posterior cord or posterior cord to radial palsy (see B in Table 15 – 20). Axillary nerve had graft repair in seven of these cases; average result was 3.7. If neurolysis of the axillary nerve could be done, as it was in three cases, results averaged 4.3.

Another 14 axillary lesions were associated with more widespread infraclavicular stretch injuries (see C in Table 15 – 20). In seven cases in which axillary had partial function to begin

**TABLE 15 – 20**
Various Axillary Lesions (n = 65)

| | Cases With Initial Partial Function and Neurolysis/ Result | Cases With Complete Loss and Neurolysis/ Result | Cases With Complete Loss and Suture/ Result | Cases With Complete Loss and Grafts/ Result | Cases With Complete Loss and Split Repair/ Result | Repair Impossible/ Result |
|---|---|---|---|---|---|---|
| A. Axillary associated with suprascapular | 0 | 2/4.0 | 0 | 5/3.2 | 0 | 0 |
| B. Axillary associated with posterior cord | 1/4.0 | 2/4.5 | 0 | 7/3.7 | 0 | 1/0 |
| C. Axillary with other lesions | 7/5.0 | 3/3.7 | 0 | 4/3.0 | 0 | 0 |
| D. Axillary alone | 2/4.0 | 4/3.5 | 1/3.0 | 24/3.5 | 1/4 | 1/0 |
| TOTALS | 10/4.7 | 11/3.8 | 1/3.0 | 40/3.4 | 1/4 | 2/0 |

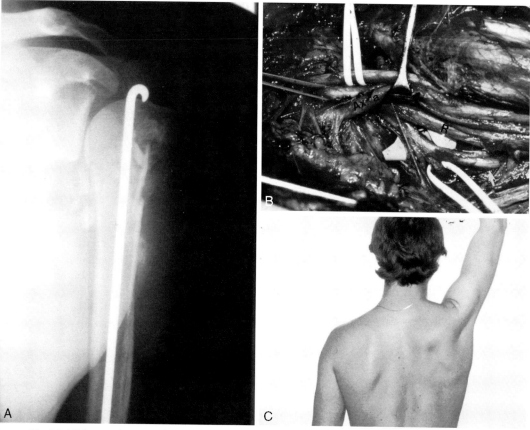

**Figure 15–44.** *(A)* Severe humeral fracture associated with a complete axillary palsy which was present before placement of rod. *(B)* Dissection of axillary nerve and subscapularis branch *(white loop)* below the radial nerve from an anterior approach. Radial nerve (R) is seen originating from posterior cord; vein retractor is on axillary artery (Ax a). *(C)* Recovery of function in deltoid after graft repair.

with and a NAP was recordable across the lesion, the average result was 5.0. If loss was complete but at operation a NAP could be recorded, as in three cases, outcome graded 3.7. Grafts to the axillary nerve were required in four other cases associated with other infraclavicular lesions. Average results in these cases were at a 3.0 level. In one instance, severe avulsive injury resulted in 10-cm grafts extending from proximal posterior cord to distal axillary nerve. No significant recovery occurred in this case. The same was true for posterior cord to radial and medial cord to ulnar repairs with grafts of the same length. On the other hand, lateral cord to musculocutaneous repairs over a similar length led to at least grade 3 function of the biceps.

It is to be re-emphasized that results of repair

of stretch injury to axillary nerve alone can be seen in D in Table 15–20 (see also Figure 15–48).

## Summary of Infraclavicular Stretch Injuries

1. These injuries are less frequent than supraclavicular ones, but loss can be as severe.
2. There is a high association with fractures and serious vascular injuries.
3. Some of these injuries improve spontaneously, but many do not and thus require surgery.
4. Operations can be technically more demanding than those in the supraclavicular region because there is a need to skeletonize large vessels such as axillary and proximal

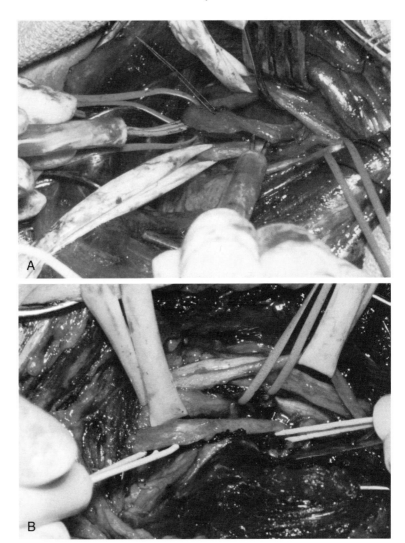

**Figure 15–45.** *(A)* Nerve action potential (NAP) testing of axillary nerve injured by stretch/contusion. This lesion had no NAP across the lesion and required resection and a graft repair. *(B)* NAP testing of another stretched axillary nerve with complete loss of deltoid for 5 months. This lesion conducted a NAP and had only neurolysis.

brachial arteries which often have had prior repair.

5. Results of suture and graft repair are relatively favorable for lateral and posterior cord and their outflows. Usually, repair of medial cord to median nerve also gives acceptable results.

6. Results of repair of medial cord and medial cord to ulnar nerves are poor. If resection is not needed in this distribution because of recordable NAPs across a lesion in continuity, then outcome from spontaneous regeneration can be surprisingly good.

7. Sometimes, outflow to shoulder and triceps is spared with more distal cord lesions, and then the patient can be rehabilitated to a better level of function than the patient with a flail arm caused by an infraclavicular lesion.

## Selection of Infraclavicular Stretch Injuries for Operation

Operation is indicated for many of these lesions because recovery is not assured without it. Patients were usually followed for 3 to 5 months before operation. This usually permitted recovery from the frequently associated vascular and orthopedic injuries and time for adequate soft tissue coverage if that had been disrupted by the original injury. Those selected for operation did not show early and significant

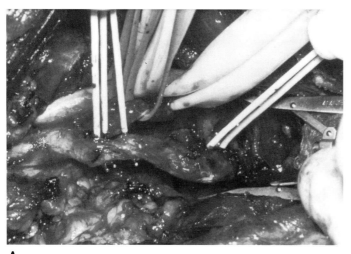

**A**

A.J.
5 Months
(Right)

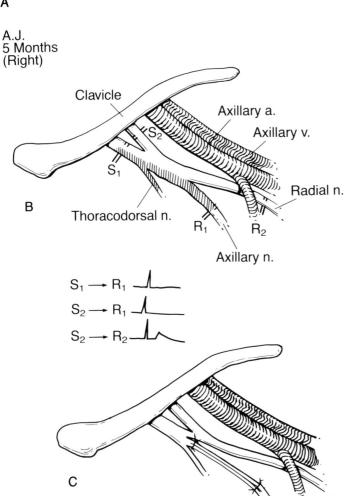

Clavicle

Axillary a.

Axillary v.

$S_2$

$S_1$

Radial n.

**B**

Thoracodorsal n.

$R_1$

$R_2$

Axillary n.

$S_1 \rightarrow R_1$

$S_2 \rightarrow R_1$

$S_2 \rightarrow R_2$

**C**

**Figure 15–46.** *(A)* Axillary stretch injury 5 months after a vehicular accident. No nerve action potentials were evoked. Stimulating electrodes are to the left and recording ones to the right. A graft repair was necessary. In *(B)* the lesion began in posterior cord and extended into axillary nerve, so a relatively lengthy graft repair was necessary. *(C)* Antebrachial cutaneous nerve was used for the graft repair.

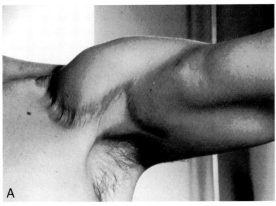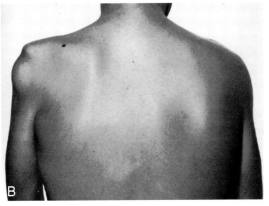

**Figure 15–47.** *(A)* Return of deltoid function and bulk 2.5 years after axillary nerve grafts 5 cm in length were placed. *(B)* The wasted left rhomboid, supraspinatus, and infraspinatus muscles indicate that the shoulder subluxation resulting from deltoid palsy is caused by a very proximal C5 spinal nerve or root injury and not an axillary stretch injury.

clinical or electrical reversal of loss. Operation was more likely to be selected if loss persisted in the distribution of one or more elements which could potentially be helped by operation, particularly if repair was necessary. Actually, this usually included most of the infraclavicular elements. The major exceptions were patients in whom the major deficit was in medial cord and medial cord to ulnar loss, where loss was mild or nonexistent in other cord distributions.

## Complications of Infraclavicular Stretch Injury

Operation often had to be done despite the fact that vascular repair pre-existed. Often, vascular repair had included placement of a graft from subclavian or axillary artery to brachial artery. In these cases especially, the vessels had to be carefully dissected out and preserved or re-repaired. As a result, these were difficult dissections. Usually, re-repair could be done by the operating service, but there were three cases in which repeat vascular repair was necessary within 72 hours of the infraclavicular plexus surgery. These cases were done by our vascular surgery service.

Other complications included wound infection in three cases. These infections were superficial and responded to local wound care and antibiotics. A Penrose drain was usually placed at the time of operation, but in one case, a persistent seroma required drainage. Three patients had increased deficit postoperatively, but in two of these it was in the lateral cord distribu-

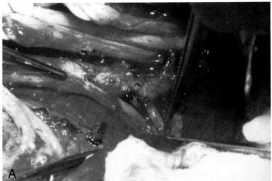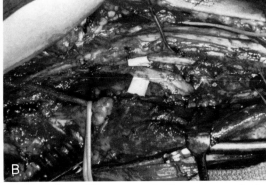

**Figure 15–48.** *(A)* Dissection of axillary nerve away from circumflex axillary artery. Axillary artery and other cord-to-nerve level plexus elements lie superior to the axillary nerve. *(B)* Neuroma of axillary nerve with rubber dam beneath it. Radial nerve lies superiorly in this dissection.

tion, and in both cases this improved spontaneously with time. The third patient had increased radial distribution loss and with time had improved triceps, brachioradialis, and wrist extension function, but finger and thumb extension remained poor.

## POSTERIOR APPROACH TO THE BRACHIAL PLEXUS

Most of the operations done for injury in this series involved an anterior approach to the plexus. In a few selected cases in which injury was very close to the spine or was predicted to be intraforaminal, a posterior subscapular approach was used (see Table 15–3). In these injuries operated on posteriorly, the facet joint over involved spinal nerves was usually removed by a Kerrison rongeur or a high speed drill. The root could be more readily traced to its dural exit and thus sometimes more readily repaired by a posterior approach than if an anterior approach had been used.[41] In several cases in which injury was caused by laceration or gunshot wound, the posterior subscapular approach also permitted a repair which would have been most difficult from an anterior approach. Both gunshot wounds to plexus operated on posteriorly had a complete deficit at a spinal nerve level, and both patients had undergone prior anterior operations for vascular repair. The two lacerated plexus injuries operated on posteriorly were suspected to have transection of one or more spinal nerves close to their dural exit.

### Traumatic Plexus Injuries Operated Posteriorly

Eighteen patients were operated on posteriorly for traumatic brachial plexus palsy. There were 13 males and 5 females in this subset. Patient age ranged from 19 months to 61 years (mean age of 28 years). In 14 patients, the injuries were secondary to stretch/contusion trauma. Injury resulted from automobile or motorcycle accidents in eight cases, iatrogenic stretch/contusion trauma from a transaxillary operation in three cases, football injury in one, snowmobile accident in one, and birth-related stretch injury in one. Two injuries were caused

by laceration: one from a stab wound and the other from transection by a scalpel during transaxillary first-rib resection. Two patients sustained a gunshot wound to the plexus.

Preoperatively, 15 patients presented with a complete deficit in the distribution of one or more plexus elements. Five of these patients had a flail arm. An incomplete but severe and persistent deficit was present in the other 10 patients. Patients were operated on because of persistence of complete denervation in the distribution of at least one plexus element or because of severe pain, or both.

At operation, 10 patients were found to have ruptured or transected elements or absence of NAPs across a lesion in continuity. After resection of these lesions, sural grafts were placed. Neurolysis with removal of scar tissue was performed on one or more elements in six patients because of the presence of regenerating axons proven by NAP recordings. The patient with birth injury was explored at 19 months after injury because of complete C5-C6 loss. NAPs were recorded from the upper trunk divisions after stimulation of both C5 and C6, so only a neurolysis was performed. Recovery in this distribution began 1 year later, and follow-up evaluation at 11 years of age shows acceptable shoulder and arm function. Neurotization using the descending cervical plexus was performed in one patient with a gunshot wound to the plexus in whom the proximal plexus elements were found impossible to repair. In another patient, an iatrogenic laceration of the C8 nerve root was treated 2 weeks after injury by end-to-end anastomosis.

Eight of ten patients with graft repair had a follow-up period of at least 5 years: one patient underwent amputation of a painful flail arm, one recovered strength to only grade 1, another to 2, and five to a level of 3 or better. Five of six patients treated by neurolysis had a follow-up period of at least 3 years: one patient made a poor recovery, three had a good recovery and one an excellent recovery. The patient with end-to-end suture of the C8 root after an iatrogenic laceration recovered to grade 3 strength in that distribution by 5 years postoperatively. One patient with a stab wound involving the dural level of C5 and C6 roots which was partially repaired by grafts has made a good recovery to date. No follow-up evaluation is available for the patient who underwent the neurotization procedure.

## Operative Technique

### Positioning of the Patient

The patient is turned to a lateral decubitus position and rolled to a prone position, which brings the operative side close to the edge of the operating table. Rolls are placed laterally under the anterolateral chest wall and transversely beneath shoulders and the manubrium of the chest. Upper extremity on the operative side is partially abducted and flexed forward at the shoulder. The arm is then flexed at the elbow and placed in a padded Mayo stand at a level below that of the operating table (Figure 15–49). Elbow, wrist, and hand are wrapped with protective pads. The operating table is then tilted up 20 degrees or so or in a reverse Trendelenburg position to allow further abduction of the shoulder and the scapula. Head is turned toward the operative side and placed on a well-padded donut or on several folded sheets, taking care to keep pressure off the orbits and to maintain the airway. The contralateral arm is padded at the elbow and placed to the side.

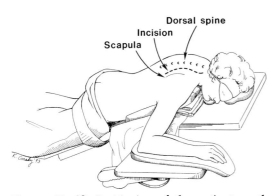

**Figure 15–49.** Positioning of the patient on the operating table for subscapular approach to the plexus. Rolls are placed under the chest and transversely beneath the shoulders. The arm is abducted at the shoulder, flexed at the elbow, padded, and placed on a Mayo stand. The head is turned toward the operative side and placed on a donut. The operating table is placed in a reverse Trendelenburg position 15 to 20 degrees above the horizontal axis.

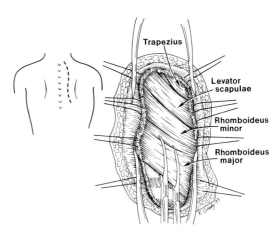

**Figure 15–50.** Diagram on left shows line of parascapular incision. On the right, the trapezius muscle has been sectioned and a portion of the rhomboid muscles are about to be sectioned between two long Kelly clamps. Divided muscle edges are marked on both sides by suture for subsequent closure. Note position of levator scapulae which sometimes needs to be divided as well.

### Surgical Exposure

A curvilinear skin incision is made centered between the thoracic spinous processes and the medial edge of the scapula (see Figure 15–49, upper center). This incision tends to protect the spinal branch of the accessory nerve and the ascending branch of the transverse cervical artery, which course close to the medial vertebral border of the scapula. The spinal or inferior portion of the trapezius muscle is divided along the entire length of the skin incision, and the edges are marked at intervals with suture for later approximation. Beneath the trapezius lie the levator scapulae muscle superiorly, the rhomboideus minor muscle somewhat intermediately, and the rhomboideus major muscle somewhat inferiorly (Figure 15–50). All three of these muscles insert on the medial border of the scapula. A Kelly clamp is used to dissect beneath them midway between the scapula and the spine. By dividing muscle away from the edge of the scapula, the deeper dorsal scapular nerve and ascending branch of the transverse cervical artery are protected. Segments of muscle are clamped and sectioned between two clamps, beginning inferiorly and proceeding superiorly. If the rhomboid muscles are thick, they are divided into two layers. Each of the edges is marked with heavy suture. Paired sutures of heavy Vicryl (polyglactin 910) are placed behind each clamp and tied. The needles are left attached and the ends fastened to adjacent drapes so that subsequent approximation of divided muscle is as accurate as possible. As dissection approaches the neck, the thicker portion of the trapezius muscle can be split somewhat in a medial direction and, if necessary, the levator scapulae muscles can be clamped, divided, and marked by sutures as well. Occasionally, some of the serratus posterior muscle is also sectioned.

After division of muscles, the posterior chest wall is exposed. The surgeon then sees a relatively avascular plane beneath the scapula and with gloved fingers can create a plane between the shoulder blade and chest wall. One blade of a medium self-retaining chest retractor is placed beneath the scapula and the other is inserted into the paraspinous muscle mass. A length of the paraspinal mass can be split down to the posterior chest wall to permit firm placement of the medial blade of the thoracic retractor. The retractor is opened as the limb on the Mayo stand is lowered or the operating table is elevated to provide further abduction and external rotation of the scapula.

Ribs are then palpated. Running the fingers superiorly and downward over the second rib permits palpation of the first rib. Sharp dissection of intercostal muscles on the caudal side of the rib and the scalene muscles on the cephalad side, as well as use of an Alexander periosteal elevator and Doyen rib dissectors, helps to clear the rib of soft tissues (Figure 15–51). The first rib is removed extraperiosteally, from the costotransverse articulation posteriorly to the costoclavicular ligament anteriorly.

Leksell rongeurs or sometimes a rib cutter are used to resect the rib. Periosteum is then resected. Subperiosteal resection of the posterior portion of the second rib is sometimes useful in exposing the first rib in very large patients or for large tumors extending into the mediastinum. Bone edges should be carefully manicured and waxed to minimize injury to pleura or surrounding tissues. The posterior and middle scalene muscles are released from their insertions and are resected to their origin from the transverse spinous processes. The roots or spinal nerves and the trunks of the brachial plexus are exposed after removal of these muscles superi-

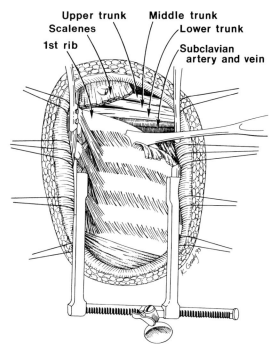

**Figure 15–51.** A self-retaining chest retractor is placed beneath the scapula laterally and embedded in the paraspinous muscles medially, then gradually opened as the arm is further abducted by lowering the Mayo stand or raising the operating table. The scalene muscles have been detached from the superior surface of the first rib, and a periosteal dissector is used to remove intercostal muscles from the inferior rib surface. Early exposure of the subclavian vessels and the trunks of the plexus is seen.

orly (Figure 15–52). The roots and divisions are further exposed by following the trunks medially and then laterally. The extraspinal course of the nerve roots is dissected back to the spine. Some elevation and retraction of the paraspinous muscle mass exposes lateral posterior spine overlying the intraforaminal course of the spinal nerves.

A Weitlaner retractor can be placed on the second rib and in the superior soft tissues of the neck to open up the supraclavicular space posterior to the plexus. A malleable chest retractor can be placed over the apical pleura to protect it as the posterior portion of the first rib is removed between the T1 and C8 nerve roots. The lower trunk is then isolated from the underlying subclavian artery and exposed circumferentially. Dissection of the plexus can then proceed medially along its spinal nerves and laterally

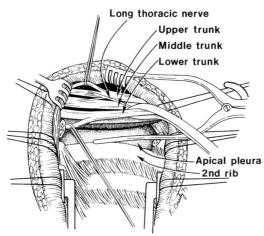

Long thoracic nerve
Upper trunk
Middle trunk
Lower trunk
Apical pleura
2nd rib

**Figure 15–52.** After resection of the first rib and scalene muscles, one blade of a Weitlaner or similar retractor is placed against the superior surface of the second rib and the other blade in the superior soft tissues of the neck. Paraspinal muscles are retracted by a large rake so as to expose the spinal nerves or roots. If necessary, either Kerrison rongeurs or a high-speed drill can be used to remove overlying facets to provide exposure of roots close to their dural exits.

along its truncal divisions. The middle trunk is isolated next and, if necessary, the upper trunk. The long thoracic nerve is visible as it originates from the posterior aspect of the C6 or sometimes C5 and C7 spinal nerves, and can be protected.

With this exposure, the phrenic nerve is anterior to both the upper trunk of the brachial plexus and the anterior scalene muscle, which is usually not divided during this procedure. Nerve roots or spinal nerves are dissected free in a circumferential fashion. The use of Penrose drains around the various elements, including the roots, to gently retract them helps in the dissection. If indicated, intraoperative NAP recordings can then be obtained. Lateral dissection can extend to divisions, but it is difficult to gain much exposure of the cord level of the plexus with such a posterior approach.

If necessary, the facet joint can be removed using a high-speed drill or Kerrison rongeurs to expose the intraforaminal course of the spinal nerve. In most cases, the nerve can be traced to its dural exit by careful bites with a rongeur, keeping the rongeur footplate on top of the nerve but not compressing it. The vertebral artery lies anteriorly, so the roots can be readily

unroofed without fear of serious bleeding. More laterally, the subclavian artery is anterior and inferior to the lower trunk of the brachial plexus, and the subclavian vein is anterior to both. Both vessels are identified early in the dissection and can be readily dissected away from the lower trunk and its divisions and easily protected. If more than two facet joints are removed, the area of bone removal is filled in with methyl methacrylate.

After such a plexus procedure, it is important to achieve meticulous closure of the wound by approximation of the divided but previously marked muscles. Anatomic reapproximation of the different muscle planes of the greater and lesser rhomboid muscles, as well as most of the spinal portions of the trapezius and levator scapulae muscles, is necessary. Good hemostasis must be obtained. A Penrose drain is sometimes placed with one end deep to the muscle closure and superior to the apical pleura. The other end of the drain is then brought out posteriorly through a separate stab wound. Any pleural rents must be repaired. The integrity of the pleural repair is tested by filling the wound with saline and having the anesthetist perform a Valsalva test. A chest tube is seldom needed. The reader is referred to the recently published report of Dubuisson, Kline, and Weinshel[21] for further information.

## Iatrogenic Plexus Injuries

Operations or other medical procedures resulting in brachial plexus injury are not uncommon (Figure 15–53). The consequences may be severe, particularly if the injury is either ignored or not corrected in a timely fashion. The list of operations or medical maneuvers done on or around the neck and shoulder is a large one. We have evaluated and attempted to correct a variety of different injuries to the plexus caused by iatrogenic mechanisms. This has included division of plexus or a plexus element by scalpel, scissors, or rongeur; crush or traction injury caused by a hemostat or a retractor or by hyperabduction of the shoulder; compression injury from the surgeon or assistant leaning on the patient; suture or bone hardware in or around the plexus; clot or pseudoaneurysm resulting from angiography; and even injection injuries.

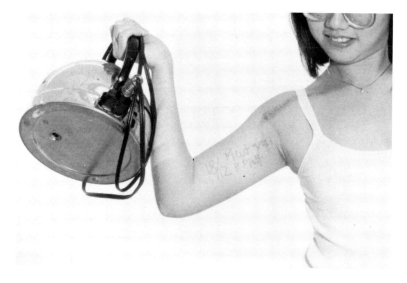

**Figure 15–53.** This gymnast suffered an iatrogenic injury to the musculocutaneous nerve during an anterior shoulder repair. Eighteen months after graft repair of the musculocutaneous nerve, she had regained useful elbow flexion.

Whenever possible, we used the same criteria to select patients for surgery and to time operations as used for other plexus lesions caused by noniatrogenic transection and stretch, contusion, or compression. Because of the nature of these injuries and the referral logistics involved, acute repair of surgically sharp plexus transections was seldom possible (Figure 15–54). Exceptions were provided by an occasional local case in which transection of one or more plexus elements was recognized and help was sought by the operating surgeon while the patient was still anesthetized. Outcomes were best in these cases, but it must be kept in mind that these were sharply divided plexus elements that were ideal candidates for primary end-to-end repair. If one or more bluntly transected or torn ele-

ments were found in such a case, the contused stumps were tacked down to adjacent fascial levels; a secondary delayed repair was then done several weeks later when stumps could be more accurately trimmed back to healthy tissue. Some of these lesions required graft repair, as did some sharp as well as blunt injuries referred for repair after some delay of time (Figure 15–55).

Most of the iatrogenic injuries to plexus were blunt and led to lesions in continuity. If clinical or electrical improvement did not occur in the early months postoperatively, then the plexus was explored and intraoperative NAP and stimulation studies were usually used to make a decision for or against resection and repair (Figure 15–56). Unfortunately, some categories of op-

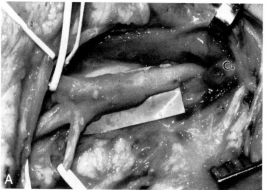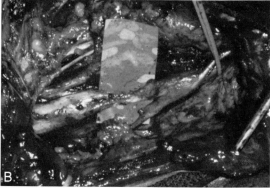

**Figure 15–54.** (A) Relatively sharp section of C5 spinal nerve with a scalpel during the course of a scalenotomy for thoracic outlet syndrome. Proximal stump of C5 is seen to the right, and suprascapular nerve and divisions of the plexus are seen to the left at the time of a delayed repair. (B) Inadvertent supraclavicular plexus injury during the course of a neck dissection led to this bluntly shredded element.

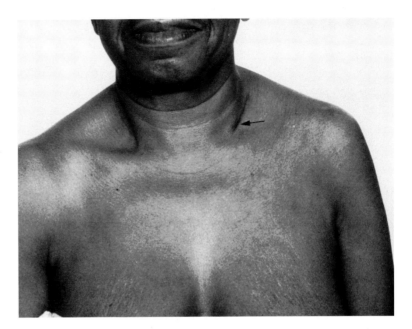

**Figure 15–55.** A left "scalenotomy" was performed on this patient who suffered from carpal tunnel syndrome. Postoperatively, the patient could neither abduct the left shoulder not flex the left elbow. The upper trunk had been accidentally divided and subsequently required repair by sural grafts.

erative complications of the plexus frequently involved C8, T1, and lower elements and their outflows such as medial cord, proximal ulnar, and, less frequently, proximal median nerves. As might be expected, gaining practical results in these categories was very difficult. Functional results even with careful repair were poor if associated with thoracic outlet operations, such as transaxillary first rib resection, in which the iatrogenically injured elements were usually lower trunk or medial cord. Despite these functionally poor results, repair, if indicated by exploration and intraoperative electrical studies, was still worthwhile if the lesion was accompanied by severe neuritic pain. Cleaning up the operative site and resection of the iatrogenic lesion often reduced the pain.

If suture was found to be encircling or in a plexus element, removal without resection and repair of the involved nerve sometimes helped but often did not unless a NAP could be transmitted beyond the lesion (Figure 15–57). If orthopedic hardware or manipulation directly involved an element in a patient selected for operation because of persisting severe loss, repair of that element rather than neurolysis was usually necessary although not always possible (Figure 15–58).

One subset of 11 patients thought to have thoracic outlet syndrome had undergone 13

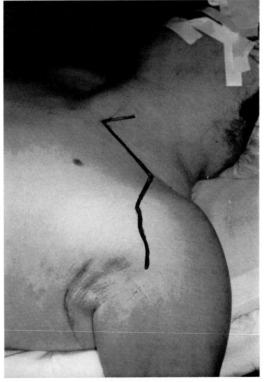

**Figure 15–56.** Planned skin incision for a supraclavicular and infraclavicular plexus exploration marked out before draping the patient. In this case, the patient had sustained a plexus injury as a result of transaxillary resection of the first rib. The surgical scar for that operation can be seen in the patient's axilla.

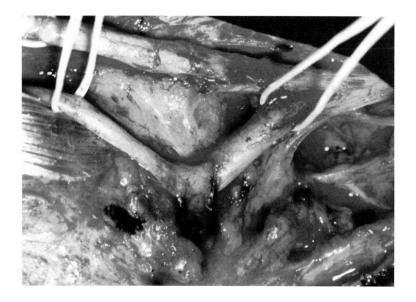

**Figure 15–57.** Kinking and distortion of left axillary nerve by a suture. Radial nerve lies above the axillary nerve. (Proximal is to the right and distal is to the left.) Note swelling of the nerve proximal to the point of distortion. The segment of nerve involved by suture did not transmit a NAP and required resection. Nerve was then repaired.

prior operations done elsewhere, including 11 transaxillary and 2 supraclavicular plexus dissections. These patients had mild to moderate deficits postoperatively. These are discussed in more detail in the chapter entitled "Thoracic Outlet Syndrome." The pertinent features of these cases are nonetheless summarized for this chapter.

Symptomatology included recurrence of pain in all patients. Pain was associated with mild to moderate neurologic deficit in nine patients; the EMG tracings were normal in eight, and one showed partial denervation of the C8- and T1-innervated muscles. In one patient, a cervical rib was shown on radiographic films. In each of these 11 patients, a posterior operation was performed to further decompress the brachial plexus. Spinal nerves and plexus trunks were treated with neurolysis. Residual first ribs and, in one case, cervical rib were resected. Scar tissue was usually found involving the lower elements of the plexus. In three cases, residual bands or fascial edges of medial or minimus scalene muscle also appeared to compress the lower plexus elements. Most patients had abnormal NAP studies across the lower elements and more normal conductions and amplitudes on the upper elements. Follow-up evaluations

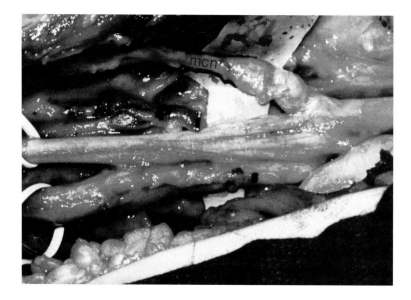

**Figure 15–58.** In this case, a good bit of the right musculocutaneous nerve (mcn) had been avulsed from the biceps during a Putti-Platt operation. This made a useful repair of this element difficult. Less involved plexus elements are seen below musculocutaneous nerve (mcn).

were available for 10 patients (mean follow-up period 3.3 years). Nine had improvement in pain, and the one whose pain was unchanged underwent repeat neurolysis through an anterior approach with only partial improvement. Most of those patients with a preoperative mild deficit had some improvement in function on follow-up evaluation, as did three of those with a moderate deficit. The other patients did not show progression of their deficits on follow-up examination.

Another three patients who had undergone transaxillary first-rib removal for thoracic outlet syndrome sustained severe injury to the plexus requiring repair. These cases are considered earlier in the chapter under traumatic brachial plexus injuries operated upon by a posterior subscapular approach.

Information concerning irradiation plexitis and patients selected for plexus operation can be found in the chapter entitled "Tumors Involving Nerve."

Blood clots, pseudoaneurysms, and arteriovenous fistulae involving other nerves as well as plexus have been discussed in other chapters. These complications usually involved infraclavicular plexus. Results were best if they were identified early and if plexus could be decompressed without the need for resection and repair (Figures 15–59 and 15–60).

## SUPRASCAPULAR NERVE ENTRAPMENT AT LEVEL OF SCAPULAR NOTCH

Entrapment, stretch injury, tumor, or ganglion cyst in this area prompts this seemingly straightforward but difficult surgical exposure. Patients may or may not have a history of trauma or injury. Not infrequently, they are weight lifters, gymnasts, or heavy construction workers who strain their shoulder and have severe scapular and parascapular pain for a period of time. Pain associated with this disorder, particularly in the early weeks, can be quite severe. This may be because of compression of suprascapular nerve fibers destined for the glenohumeral and acromioclavicular joints or because of atrophy of the supraspinatus and infraspinatus. In either case, as quickly as the pain originates and as severe as it is, it usually suddenly disappears after denervation has proceeded. Then, the patient notes difficulty with initial abduction of the upper arm (supraspinatus) and external rotation of the shoulder (infraspinatus) or, in some cases, infraspinatus loss only. Inspection of the posterior shoulder at this point usually reveals atrophy of the spinati.

EMG sampling shows denervational changes in supraspinatus and infraspinatus, with changes in the latter usually being more severe

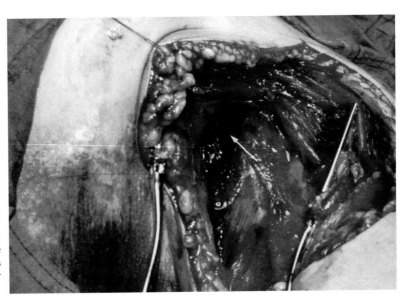

**Figure 15–59.** Blood clot at the level of the axilla *(white arrow)* as a result of an angiographic study. A compressive neuropathy of the plexus was reversed by relatively early evacuation of the clot.

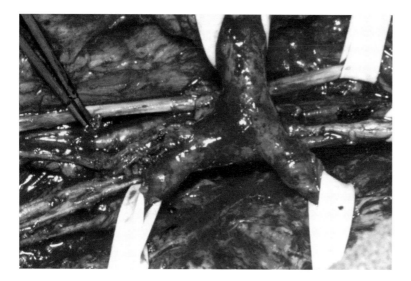

**Figure 15–60.** Compressive lesion to cords of the plexus secondary to construction of an axillary arteriovenous fistula for renal dialysis. Scar beneath the fistula and involving lateral and medial cords was severe. Fortunately, these elements conducted NAPs and were helped by neurolysis. The fistula had to be preserved because other extremity sites for dialysis had been exhausted.

and widespread than in the former. Delayed conduction from stimulation at the Erb point and recording from supraspinatus or infraspinatus muscles may be demonstrable. Normal latencies from the Erb point to supraspinatus have a relatively large range, from 1.7 to 3.7 msec, so it is best to compare the affected side with the contralateral, asymptomatic side.

If suprascapular nerve is involved by brachial plexitis, there is usually other loss in the distribution of the brachial plexus or accessory nerve.

The suprascapular involvement in such cases is not helped by surgery.

## Operative Approach

The patient with a suprascapular neuropathy can be operated on in either the supine or prone position. This is a difficult operation because the entrapment point is at the depth of the exposure (Figures 15–61 and 15–62). Preferred is an ini-

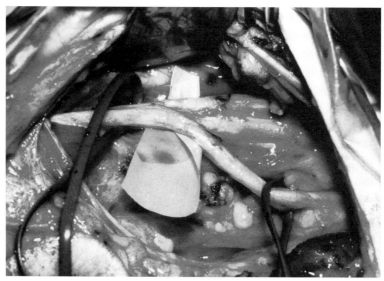

**Figure 15–61.** The right suprascapular nerve (loop to the right) leaves the upper trunk (loop to the left) as that structure starts to divide into its anterior and posterior divisions. As the suprascapular nerve runs laterally, it goes beneath or deep to the inferior belly of the omohyoid and beneath the trapezius. The nerve then runs through the suprascapular notch, where it lies beneath transverse scapular ligament. Dissection to that level becomes difficult with an anterior approach because the surgeon is crowded more and more by the clavicle in front and the upper border of the scapula behind. Even though the transverse scapular ligament (suprascapular ligament) can be sectioned by an anterior procedure, the lesion is more easily approached from behind.

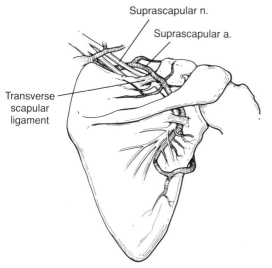

**Figure 15–62.** Drawing of course of suprascapular nerve and artery as viewed from behind. Usual entrapment site is beneath the transverse scapular ligament (suprascapular ligament). Occasionally, the nerve can be entrapped at or distal to the level of the scapular notch. The usual loss under those circumstances involves the infraspinatus with sparing of supraspinatus function.

tial supine positioning and then elevation of the head and thorax to about 45 degrees with elevation of the top of the operating table. Folded sheets are placed beneath the interscapular area, and the head is supported by a donut. In this position, the spine of the scapula and the supraspinatus and infraspinatus muscles are accessible if the surgeon stands at the head of the operating table. A transverse incision is made superior and anterior to the spine of the scapula and carried well toward the tip of the shoulder (Figure 15–63). After dissection through the subcutaneous layers, supraspinatus muscle fibers are either split transversely or separated from the superior aspect of the scapular spine and retracted to expose underlying nerve and vessels. The region of the notch of the scapula is much more lateral than anticipated, so dissec-

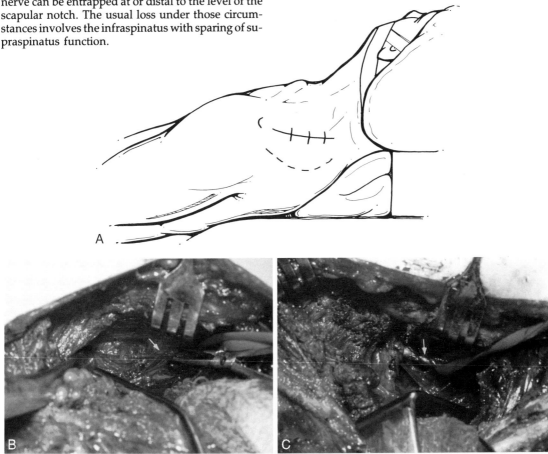

**Figure 15–63.** (A) Positioning of patient and planned incision for exposure of left suprascapular nerve by a posterior approach. (B) Curved hemostat placed under ligament (*white arrow*) and superior to suprascapular nerve on the right side. Supraspinatus has been split in the direction of its fibers to gain this exposure. (C) Loop is around suprascapular nerve (*white arrow*) after release of the ligament on the right side.

tion must be continued laterally to reach it. The scapular notch is not always readily palpable without splitting or separating some of the supraspinatus muscle fibers from scapular spine. Nerve is found at quite a depth — 8 to 10 cm. It takes a somewhat oblique course, running on top of dorsal superior scapular bone and angling from a medial locus anteriorly to a lateral one posteriorly. Nerve can be encircled with a Vasoloop or narrow Penrose drain and traced proximally. The usual area of entrapment is where the nerve passes beneath the ligament. The latter must be divided to free the nerve. We also like to clear more distal nerve as it runs around the lateral edge of the scapular spine and through its notch.

In this park bench–like position, the more distal suprascapular nerve can also be exposed inferior to the spine. Here, a portion of infraspinatus whose fibers run in a longitudinal fashion to the superior surface of the scapular spine needs to be detached transversely from the spine, leaving a cuff to sew back to. Then, some of the superior and lateral infraspinatus is swept away from the inferior surface of the scapular spine to expose the lateral spine of the scapula

from below. Both the supraspinatus and infraspinatus muscle-splitting approaches have had to be used in the same patient in several cases. In these instances, tumor, usually a ganglion cyst, had compressed nerve in the notch region and was situated both above and below this structure as well as in it (Figure 15–64).

## Results

Results in 20 spontaneous entrapment cases have been quite satisfactory. Several additional patients had ganglion cysts involving the nerves in this region removed with good results. Decreased pain and increased shoulder mobility have been almost uniformly obtained. Function of the supraspinatus usually recovered to a better level than that of the infraspinatus, but the latter usually reached a grade of 3 to 4. Exceptions were provided by three additional patients who had the onset of their palsy associated with scapular fracture. Here, recovery of function was not as good, although pain seemed to be helped in two of the three cases operated on.

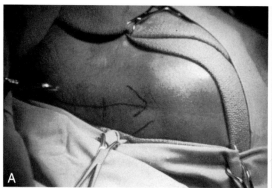
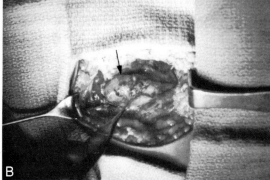
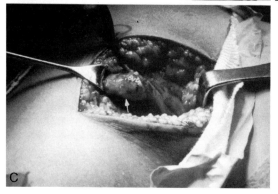

**Figure 15–64.** (A) Outlined incision line for posterior approach to ganglion involving suprascapular nerve. Incision runs parallel to and a little superior to spine of scapula and should extend laterally to the acromion-scapular junction. (B) Ganglion (*black arrow*) involving right suprascapular nerve exposed by splitting supraspinatus muscle parallel with the spine of the scapula. (C) Ganglion cyst (*white arrow*) involving right suprascapular nerve in another patient.

# Bibliography

1. Allieu Y, Privat J, and Bonnel F: L'exploration chirugicale et le traitement des paralysies du plexus brachial. Paris, Reunion annuelle de la Societe Francaise de Neurochirurgie, 1980.
2. Allieu Y, Privat JM, and Bonnel F: Les neurotisations par le nerf spinal (nerf accessorius) dans les avulsions radicularis du plexus brachial. Neurochirurgie 28:115–120, 1982.
3. Alnot J: Infraclavicular lesions. North Am Clin Plast Surg 11:127–131, 1984.
4. Alnot J, Jolly A, and Frot B: Traitement direct des lesions nerveuses dans les paralysies traumatiques du plexus brachial chez l'adult. Int Orthop 63:82–90, 1981.
5. Barnes R: Traction injuries of the brachial plexus in adults. J. Bone Joint Surg Br 31:10–16, 1949.
6. Barr JS, Freiberg JA, Colonna PC, and Pemberton PA: A survey of end results on stabilization of the paralytic shoulder. Amer Orthop Assn report. J Bone Joint Surg 24:699–710, 1942.
7. Birch R: Traction lesions of the brachial plexus. Br J Hosp Med 32:140–145, 1984.
8. Bonnel F: Microscopic anatomy of the adult human brachial plexus: An anatomical and histologic basis for microsurgery. Microsurgery 5:107–117, 1984.
9. Bonney G: Prognosis in traction lesions of the brachial plexus. J Bone Joint Surg Br 41:4–35, 1959.
10. Bonney G, Birch R, Jamieson A, et al.: Experience with vascularized nerve grafts. North Am Clin Plast Surg 11:137–142, 1984.
11. Brophy BP: Supraclavicular traction injuries of the brachial plexus. Aust N Z J Surg 48:528–532, 1978.
12. Brunelli G: Neurotization of avulsed roots of the brachial plexus by means of anterior nerves of the cervical plexus. Int J Microsurg 2:555–558, 1980.
13. Brunelli G and Monini L: Neurotization of avulsed roots of brachial plexus by means of anterior nerves of cervical plexus. Clin Plast Surg 11:149–152, 1984.
14. Carroll RE and Kleinman WB: Pectoralis major transplantation to restore elbow flexion to the paralytic limb. J Hand Surg 4:501–507, 1979.
15. Carroll RE and Hill NA: Triceps transfer to restore elbow flexion. A study of 15 patients with paralytic lesions and arthrogryposis. J Bone Joint Surg 52A:239–244, 1970.
16. Clancy WG, Brand RL, and Bergfield JA: Upper trunk brachial plexus injuries in contact sports. Am J Sports Med 5:209, 1977.
17. Clark JP: Reconstruction of biceps brachialis by pectoralis muscle transplantation. Br J Surg 34:180, 1946.
18. Davis DH, Onofrio BM, and MacCarty CS: Brachial plexus injuries. Mayo Clin Proc 53:799–807, 1978.
19. Davis L, Martin J, and Perrett G: The treatment of injuries of the brachial plexus. Ann Surg 125:647–657, 1947.
20. Dolenc V: Intercostal neurotization of the peripheral nerves in avulsion plexus injuries. Clin Plast Surg 11:143–147, 1984.
21. Dubuisson A, Kline D, and Weinshel S: Posterior subscapular approach to the brachial plexus. Report of 102 cases. J Neurosurg 79:319–330, 1993.
22. Fletcher I: Traction lesions of the brachial plexus. Hand 1:127–136, 1969.
23. Friedman AH, Nunley JA, Goldner RD, et al.: Nerve transposition for restoration of elbow flexion following brachial plexus avulsion injuries. J Neurosurg 72:59–66, 1990.
24. Friedman AH: Neurotization of elements of the brachial plexus. Neurosurg Clin North Am 2:165–174, 1991.
25. Frykholm R: The mechanism of cervical radicular lesions resulting from stretch and forceful traction. Acta Chir Scand 102:93–96, 1957.
26. Harmon PH: Surgical reconstruction of the shoulder by multiple muscle transplantations. J Bone Joint Surg, 32A:583–586, 1950.
27. Hendry AM: The treatment of residual paralysis after brachial plexus injury. J Bone Joint Surg 31B:42–49, 1949.
28. Hentz V and Narakas A: The results of microneurosurgical reconstruction in complete brachial plexus palsy. Orthop Clin North Am 19:107–114, 1988.
29. Highet J: Effect of stretch on peripheral nerve. Br J Surg 30:355–369, 1942.
30. Hoffer MM, Braun R, Hsy J, et al.: Functional recovery and orthopedic management of brachial plexus palsies. JAMA 264:2467–2470, 1981.
31. Hovnanian AP: The treatment of residual paralysis after brachial plexus injury. J Bone Joint Surg 31B:42–49, 1949.
32. Hudson AR and Trammer B: Brachial plexus injuries. *In* Wilkins R and Rengachary S, Eds: Neurosurgery. New York, McGraw-Hill, 1985.
33. Jamieson A and Hughes S: The role of surgery in the management of closed injuries of the brachial plexus. Clin Orthop 147:210–215, 1980.
34. Kawai H, Kawabuta H, Masuda K, et al.: Nerve repair for traumatic brachial plexus palsy with nerve root avulsion. Clin Orthop Related Res 237:75–86, 1989.
35. Kettlecamp DB and Larson CB: Evaluation of the Steindler flexorplasty. J Bone Joint Surg 45A:513–517, 1963.
36. Kline DG: Perspectives concerning brachial plexus injury and repair. Neurosurg Clinics of North Am 2:151–164, 1991.
37. Kline DG: Selection of brachial plexus cases for operation. *In* Samii M, Ed: Peripheral Nerve Lesions. Berlin, Springer-Verlag, 1990.
38. Kline DG and Hudson AR: Coaptation of anterior rami of C3 and C4. (Letter). J Neurosurg 75:667–668, 1991.
39. Kline DG and Judice DJ: Operative management of selected brachial plexus lesions. J Neurosurg 58:631–649, 1983.
40. Kline DG and Lusk M: Management of athletic brachial plexus injuries. *In* Schneider R, Kennedy J, and Plant M, Eds: Sports Injuries—Mechanisms, Prevention and Treatment. Philadelphia, Williams & Wilkins, 1985.
41. Kline DG, Kott J, Barnes G, and Bryant L: Exploration of selected brachial plexus lesions by the posterior subscapular approach. J Neurosurg 49:872–880, 1978.
42. Kotani T, Toshimu Y, Matsuda H, Suzuki G, et al.: Postoperative results of nerve transposition in brachial plexus injury. Orthop Surg Tokyo 22:963, 1971.
43. Leffert RD: Brachial Plexus Injuries. London, Churchill Livingstone, 1985.
44. Leffert RD: Reconstruction of the shoulder and elbow following brachial plexus injury. *In* Omer G and Spinner M, Eds: Management of Peripheral Nerve Problems. Philadelphia, WB Saunders, 1980.
45. Leffert RD and Seddon H: Infraclavicular brachial plexus injuries. J Bone Joint Surg Br 47:9–22, 1965.
46. LeJune G, LeClerq D, Carlier A, et al.: Direct microsurgical treatment of brachial plexus lesions. Acta Chir Belg 82:251–260, 1982.
47. Levy WJ, Nutklewicz A, and Ditmore M: Laser-induced dorsal root entry zone lesions for pain control. J Neurosurg 59:884–886, 1983.

48. Lusskin R, Campbell J, and Thompson W: Post-traumatic lesions of the brachial plexus. J Bone Joint Surg 55A:1159–1176, 1973.
49. Malone JM, Leal JM, Underwood J, et al.: Brachial plexus injury management through upper extremity amputation with immediate postoperative prosthesis. Arch Phys Med Rehabil 63:84–91, 1982.
50. Mayer VL and Green W: Experiences with the Steindler flexorplasty at the elbow. J Bone Joint Surg 36A:775, 1954.
51. Millesi H: Brachial plexus injuries—management and results. Clin Plast Surg 11:115–120, 1984.
52. Millesi H: Brachial plexus injuries: Nerve grafting. Clin Orthop Related Res 237:36–42, 1988.
53. Milton GW: The mechanism of circumflex and other nerve injuries in dislocation of the shoulder and the possible mechanism of nerve injury during reduction of dislocation. Aust N Z J Surg 23:4, 1953.
54. Nagano A: Brachial plexus injuries: Prognosis of postganglionic type. Orthop Surg 30:1534–1536, 1979.
55. Narakas A: Brachial plexus surgery. Orthop Clin North Am 12:303–323, 1981.
56. Narakas A: The surgical treatment of traumatic brachial plexus lesions. Int Surg 65:521–527, 1980.
57. Narakas A: Thoughts on neurotization or nerve transfers in irreparable nerve lesions. Clin Plast Surg 11:153–159, 1984.
58. Nashold BS and Ostahl RH: Dorsal root entry zone lesions for pain relief. J Neurosurg 51:59–69, 1979.
59. Nulsen FE and Slade WW: Recovery following injury to the brachial plexus. In Peripheral Nerve Regeneration: A follow-up study of 3,656 WW II Injuries. Washington, DC, US Government Printing Office, 1956.
60. Omer GE: Tendon transfer for reconstruction of the forearm and hand following peripheral nerve injuries. In Omer GE and Spinner M, Eds: Management of Peripheral Nerve Problems. Philadelphia, WB Saunders, 1980.
61. Perry J, Hsu J, Barber L, and Haffer M: Orthoses in patients with brachial plexus injuries. Arch Phys Med Rehabil 55:134, 1974.
62. Ploncord P: A new approach to the intercostobrachial anastomosis in the treatment of brachial plexus paralysis due to root avulsion: Late results. Acta Neurochir 6:281–290, 1982.
63. Ransford AO and Hughes SP: Complete brachial plexus lesions. A ten-year follow-up of twenty cases. J Bone Joint Surg Br 59:417–420, 1977.
64. Richards RR: Operative treatment for irreparable lesions of the brachial plexus. In Gelberman RH, Ed: Operative Nerve Repair and Reconstruction. Philadelphia, JB Lippincott, 1991.
65. Rorabeck CH and Harris WR: Factors affecting the prognosis of brachial plexus injuries. J Bone Joint Surg 63B:404–407, 1981.
66. Samardzic M, Gruzicic D, Antunovic V, et al.: Reinnervation of the avulsed brachial plexus using the spinal accessory nerve. Surg Neurol 33:7–12, 1990.
67. Samii M: Use of microtechniques in peripheral nerve surgery: Experience with over 300 cases. In Handa H, Ed: Microneurosurgery. Tokyo, Igaku-Shoin, 1975.
68. Samii M, Kohmura E, Khalil H, and Matthies C: Dorsal root entry zone coagulation for control of intractable pain due to brachial plexus injury. In Samii M, Ed: Peripheral Nerve Lesions. Berlin, Springer-Verlag, 1990.
69. Sedel L: The management of supraclavicular lesions: Clinical examination, surgical procedures, results. In Terzis J, Ed: Microreconstruction of Nerve Injuries. Philadelphia, WB Saunders, 1987.
70. Sedel L: The results of surgical repair of brachial plexus injuries. J Bone Joint Surg. Br 64:54–66, 1982.
71. Sharpe E: The operative treatment of brachial plexus paralysis. JAMA 66:876–880, 1981.
72. Slingluff CL, Terzis JK, and Edgerton M: The quantitative microanatomy of the brachial plexus in man: Reconstructive relevance. In Terzis J, Ed: Microreconstruction of Nerve Injuries. Philadelphia, WB Saunders, 1987.
73. Solonen K, Vastamaki M, and Strom B: Surgery of the brachial plexus. Acta Orthop Scand 55:436–440, 1984.
74. Steindler A: Kinesiology of the Human Body. Springfield, IL, Charles C Thomas, 1955.
75. Steubdker A: Muscle and tendon transplantation of the elbow. In Thomson JE, Ed: Instruction Course Lecture on Reconstructive Surgery, Vol 2. Chicago, American Academy of Orthopedic Surgeons, 1944.
76. Stevens C, Davis D, and MacCarty C: A 32-year experience with the surgical treatment of selected brachial plexus lesions with emphasis on reconstruction. Surg Neurol 19:334–345, 1983.
77. Sunderland S: Nerves and Nerve Injuries. Baltimore, Williams & Wilkins, 1972; See also Nerve Injuries and Their Repair: A Critical Appraisal. London, Churchill Livingstone, 1991.
78. Taylor PE: Traumatic intradural avulsion of the nerve root of the brachial plexus. Brain 85:579–602, 1985.
79. Terzis J: Microreconstruction of Peripheral Nerve Injuries. Philadelphia, WB Saunders, 1987.
80. Thomas DG, Jones SJ: Dorsal root entry zone lesions (Nashold's procedure) in brachial plexus avulsion. Neurosurgery 15:966–968, 1984.
81. Tsuyama J, Hara T, and Nagano A: Intercostal nerve crossing as a treatment of irreparably damaged brachial plexus. In Noble J and Galusko C, Eds: Recent Developments in Orthopedic Surgery. Manchester, England, Manchester University Press, 1987.
82. Tuttle H: Exposure of the brachial plexus with nerve transplantation. JAMA 61:15–17, 1913.
83. Wilde AH, Brems JJ, and Broumphrey FR: Arthrodesis of the shoulder: Current indications and operative technique. Orthop Clin North Am 18:463–472, 1987.
84. Wynn Parry C: The management of traction lesions of the brachial plexus and peripheral nerve injuries to the upper limb: A study in teamwork. Roscoe Clarke Memorial Lecture. Injury 11:265–285, 1980.
85. Wynn Parry CB: Rehabilitation of the Hand. London, Butterworths, 1981.
86. Yamada S and Peterson G: Coaptation of the anterior rami of C3 and C4 to upper trunk of the brachial plexus for cervical root avulsion. J Neurosurg 74:171–177, 1991.
87. Yeoman P: Cervical myelopathy in traction injuries of the brachial plexus. J Bone Joint Surg Br 50:253–260, 1968.
88. Yeoman P and Seddon H: Brachial plexus injuries. Treatment of the flail arm. J Bone Joint Surg Br 31:493–500, 1961.
89. Yoshimura M, Amaya S, Tyujo M, et al.: Experimental studies on the traction injury of peripheral nerves. Neuro Orthop 7:1–7, 1989.
90. Zancolli E and Mitre H: Latissimus dorsi transfer to restore elbow flexion: An appraisal of eight cases. J Bone Joint Surg 55A:1265–1272, 1973.

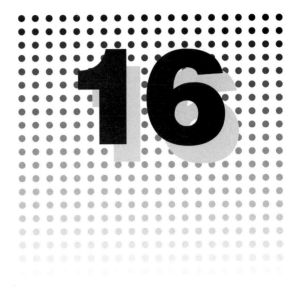

# Birth Palsies

## SUMMARY

Management of birth palsies is certainly the most controversial topic in nerve surgery at the present time. As a subset of plexus injuries, their management is undergoing great change and will probably continue to do so. Historically, it has always been clear that the stretch injury occurring at birth is less severe than those caused by the usually large, accidental forces affecting the adult plexus. It also appears that infants and children may have greater ability to regenerate in a useful fashion or rehabilitate their own limbs. A trend begun by Tassin and Gilbert's work suggests that if the biceps, a C6- and partially C5-innervated muscle, does not recover by 3 months, surgery with resection of the stretched plexus elements should be done. In their view, this permits earlier operation for the more severe cases and leads to better results than a later operation or more conservative management. Our own approach is more conservative, based on the analysis of a panel of patients who have been followed for quite a few years in most cases. From this analysis, it is apparent that many infants who do not begin to recover biceps until 4 to 9 months postpartum nevertheless progress to an acceptable, spontaneous recovery. The majority of these patients make a better recovery than we would have predicted had surgical resection and graft repair of the plexus been done. Those patients selected for surgery because of failure to recover function that could potentially be helped by operation did recover some function even if operated on 9 or more months postpartum. Patients in this series who did was either quite severe and involved the proximal portions of elements that do not do well with repair, even in infants. It would, however, be incorrect to conclude that no birth palsies are candidates for surgery, although their numbers are fewer than would be the case if lack of biceps recovery by 3 months were the major criterion to select them for operation. In this series of birth palsies, 6 infants were operated on after 9 months of age. Our assumption to date is that these infants are able to respond to repair at a postpartum interval much greater than 3 to 4 months of age. We also believe that the works of Gilbert, Tassin, and others have stimulated a long-overdue renewal of interest in this problem and are welcome additions to the literature.

Birth palsy is a special category of stretch/contusive injury to the brachial plexus and, as such, deserves individual analysis. Although the mechanisms leading to stretch of the plexus in infants are similar to those involved in vehicular and sports accidents in adults and older children, the forces are usually less.[15] There are exceptions to this, and the birth-related flail arm may not always recover with or without surgery.[1,14] As a group, though, spontaneous recovery in these birth-related palsies is considerably better than in the adult.[3,5,6,28] There is also the perception that spontaneous regeneration after injury in the very young is much more successful than in the adult. Distances required for regrowth are relatively short, and the infant or child tends to move and use the arm more than a similarly affected adult. As a result, management of these injuries remains controversial. Some workers favor an early and aggressive approach.[7,16,24,30] Other clinical investigators advise a totally conservative, nonsurgical management, and some, including ourselves, elect a very selective surgical approach for this disorder.[19,27] To our knowledge there have not been any prospective, controlled studies to prove either the value of early surgery or that of operation on large numbers of these infants.[4]

In the early 1900s, literature concerning birth palsies was, for the most part, descriptive.[6,19,35] Erb described the upper plexus stretch injury and Klumpke the lower. This was followed by a period in which case reports provided some detail about operative attempts at repair.[31] A variety of reconstructive efforts, especially for residual shoulder deformity, continue to be valuable for this disorder.[12,21,37,40] Vigorous physical therapy, even in these very young patients, has always been advocated.[8,19,36] For the most part, modern writers condemned operations on the plexus until Gilbert and Tassin's work which suggested the efficacy of early operative intervention and repair by grafts.[9,34] Gilbert has stressed the importance of biceps return in deciding whether or not to operate in infants.[10] He and others have promulgated a 3-month rule and advocate surgical replacement of the plexus if the infant's biceps has not recovered by 3 months of age.[24] These observations have prompted a renewal of interest in operative correction, especially by use of grafts, but occasionally by more direct repair.[2,5,17,23,25,35]

Factors favoring origin of birth plexus palsies include excessive weight gain by the infant's mother, a small maternal pelvis, shoulder dystocia, a breech or legs-first presentation, a need to use forceps for delivery, and a large neonate, especially one weighing more than 9 pounds.[11,22,31] Associated neonatal central nervous system damage is probably higher in this group of infants than in neonates in general.[29] Congenital malformations can occasionally also play a role. Hydrocephalus may produce a large head, making delivery difficult. Labor may be poor if the infant already has brain damage, and this may make the need for forceps or other manipulation more likely. Often, in addition to the brachial plexus palsy, the infant is born with a poor Apgar score. Despite these associations, birth palsy involving plexus can occur in the absence of these factors. It can also occur even though caesarean section is done. In general, though, the forces involved are less than in the older child or adult thrown from a vehicle. This, as well as the youth of the patient, may lead to the relatively better prognosis for plexus injury seen in the infant.[26] Our impression, and that of others, is that with improved prenatal and obstetric care, the incidence of this disorder has decreased in the last 30 years.[13,20,32] Nonetheless, birth palsy still occurs and requires skillful and informed management. In addition, in some cases, the severity of the injury approaches that seen in the adult stretch palsy where presumably larger forces are in play (Figure 16–1).

## REVIEW OF LSUMC PANEL AND PATIENTS

Over a 17-year period, we have seen 76 infants or children with birth palsies at the Louisiana State University Medical Center. Fifty-eight of these patients have had one or more

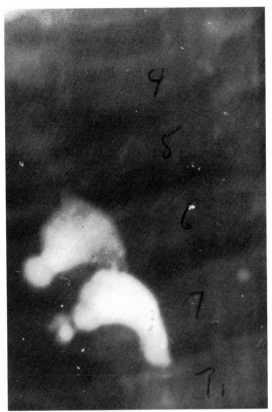

**Figure 16–1.** Infant myelogram showing two relatively large meningoceles at C6-C7 (seventh root) and C8-T1 (eighth root).

years of follow-up. One of the patients was born with a bilateral stretch palsy similar to the one seen in Figure 16–2. Some 80% of these patients have been seen at two or more intervals and thus form a reasonable group for analysis (Table 16–1). There were 43 cases with two or more years of follow-up and 58 cases with one or more years of follow-up. Analysis of these cases was especially valuable from the standpoint of formulating a prognosis and designing management. In addition to clinical evaluation, each patient had one or more electromyographic studies done (Figure 16–3).

Included were eight patients seen at 10 to 15 years of age (Table 16–2). Seven of these patients had Erb-Klumpke paralysis and a flaccid arm at birth. In the six patients managed without operation, deltoid and thus full abduction of the shoulder remained absent in two. Supination and hand intrinsics were poor in two instances. There was variable wrist and finger flexion and extension in several patients. One

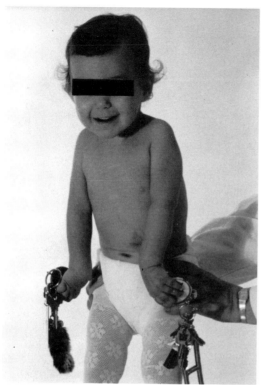

**Figure 16-2.** A 1-year-old child with bilateral birth palsies. Note externally rotated arms with paralysis, predominantly in the C5, C6, and C7 distributions.

**TABLE 16-2**

## Birth Palsies—Grades in Older Patients

M.H. — Age 15—Erb-Klumpke—Flaccid at birth.
S/I 3, D 0, Bic, 3 to 4, Tric 1, Pron 2 to 3, Supin 0, Wr Ext 2 to 3, F Ext 0, Wr Fl 3, F Fl 2 to 3, Ints 0

W.M. — Age 14—Erb-Klumpke—Flaccid at birth.
S/I 3 to 4, D 3 to 4, Bic 4, Tric 2, Sup 3, Wr & F Ext 0, Wr & F Fl 2 to 3, Ints 0

J.L. — Age 13 Erb-Klumpke—Flaccid at birth.
S/I 2 to 3, D 0, Bic 4, Tric 4, Supin 4, Wr & F Ext 4, Wr & F Fl 4, Ints 4

M.B. — Age 12—Erb-Klumpke—Flaccid at birth.
S/I 4, D 4, Bic 5, Tric 3, Supin 3, Wrist Ext & Fl 2 to 3, F Fl 2 to 3, F Ext 0, Ints 1

P.P. — Age 14—Erb-Klumpke—Flaccid at birth.
S/I 3 to 4, D 4, Bic 4, BR 3, Tr 5, Supin 4, Wr & F Fl and Ext 4 to 5, Ints 4

D.D. — Age 13—Erb-Klumpke—Slt finger motion at birth.
S 3, I 2, D 3, Biceps/BR 3 to 4, Tric 3, Supin 3 to 4, Wr Ext & Fl 3, F Ext 2, F Fl 4, Ints 4

*L.K. — Age 11—C5, C6, C7 (C), C8, T1 (I); *neurolysis at 9 months of age.*
S/I 3, D 3 to 4, Bic/BR 3 to 4, Tric 4, Supin 3, Wr &F Fl & Ext 4, Ints 5

S.S. — Age 10—Erb+ at birth—C5, C6 (C), C7 (I).
S/I 4, D 4, Bic 4, Tric 4, Pron 4, Supin 3, Wr & F Fl & Ext and Ints 5

---

Bic = biceps; BR = brachioradialis; (C) = complete loss; D = deltoid; F Ext = finger extension; F Fl = finger flexion; (I) = incomplete loss; Ints = hand intrinsic muscles; Pron = pronator; S/I = supraspinatus/infraspinatus; Slt = slight; Supin = supinator; Tric = triceps; Wr Ext = wrist extension; Wr Fl = wrist flexion. Muscles graded on a 0 to 5 basis.
*Operated on.

---

Erb-Klumpke patient had excellent recovery of shoulder and arm function but very little wrist or finger function. Overall results, however, were good. Although the affected limbs were smaller than the contralateral limbs in two of the patients, they were quite functional and were used well despite their residual deficits. Especially impressive was the breadth and strength of the return, not only in biceps but usually also in triceps and forearm muscles.

One patient, followed until 11 years of age, had neurolysis of the plexus at 9 months of age

**TABLE 16-1**

## Birth Palsies—LSUMC Series 1975-1992

A — 76 cases evaluated*
B — 58 cases with 1 or more years follow-up
43 at 2 or more years
33 at 3 or more years
18 at 5 or more years
(8 patients evaluated at 10 to 15 years of age)
C — 6 patients operated on (8%)
— Plus, one patient scheduled for operation (9%)

---

*One infant had bilateral palsy.

---

because of persistent severe C5, C6, and C7 distribution loss. Fortunately, the C8- and T1-innervated muscles had partial function from the early months of life. Nerve action potential (NAPs) were recorded from all elements, and the eventual result was quite good. It could be argued that this recovery may have occurred without operation, although the C5, C6, and C7 elements had a neurolysis and were cleared of scar tissue. The principal effect of the operation was to ascertain that the elements in question were adequately regenerating.

The ten patients followed until they were 5 to 7 years of age were also of interest. Table 16-3 shows the degree of spontaneous recovery seen in seven of these patients. Results were quite satisfactory, with the principal deficient areas being lack of full shoulder abduction in three instances. In two of these patients, part of the difficulty was caused by winging of the scapula, related either to rhomboid or trapezius paresis. There was poor hand-intrinsic function in two (one of these had a Klumpke paralysis at birth), and poor supination in two.

**TABLE 16–3**
Birth Palsies—Spontaneous Recovery by 5 to 7 Years of Age

| Age (Yrs) | Initials | Initial to Subsequent Grades by Element | | | | Comments |
|---|---|---|---|---|---|---|
| | | C5 | C6 | C7 | C8-T1 | |
| 5 | CB | 0 to 2–3 | 0 to 3 | 0 to 3 | 0 to 4 | Erb-Klumpke<br>Winging scapula<br>Rhomboid loss |
| 5 | EC | 0 to 4 | 0 to 3–4 | 0 to 3–4 | 2 to 4 | Erb-Klumpke<br>Lacks smooth shoulder abduction |
| 5 | CC | 0 to 2 | 0 to 4 | 0 to 3 | 4–5 to 4–5 | Erb-Klumpke<br>Winging scapula<br>Trapezius loss<br>Poor supination |
| 5.5 | DS | 0 to 3 | 0 to 4 | 0 to 3 | 0 to 2 | Erb-Klumpke<br>Makes only a partial fist |
| 6 | RH | 5 to 5 | 5 to 5 | 2 to 4 | 0 to 1 | Klumpke with slight recovery |
| 6.5 | RS | 0 to 4 | 0 to 5 | 3 to 5 | 5 to 5 | Erb+ with good recovery |
| 7 | HL | 0 to 3 | 0 to 5 | 2 to 4 | 5 to 5 | Erb+<br>Lacks smooth shoulder abduction<br>Supination poor |

There were three cases reaching the 5-year-old group who were operated upon earlier in life (Table 16–4). Two were Erb-Klumpke cases and one a pure Erb. In the Erb-Klumpke cases, loss was severe in the entire plexus distribution, whereas in the Erb case it was, of course, in the C5-C6 distribution. The three cases were operated on at 12, 18, and 36 months of age, respectively, and followed for 2.5 to 4 years postoperatively. Follow-up data was thus collected at 30, 42, and 48 months postoperatively. Surgery was especially helpful for persistent C5-C6 loss, even if grafts were necessary. As a result, postoperative recovery was fairly good in that distribution. Recovery occurred in the C7 distribution as well as that of C5-C6, but not in the C8-T1 distribution. Looked at another way, late

operation, in part because of late referral but also because we usually follow birth palsies for 9 to 12 months before considering surgery, has given good results so far, at least in these three cases.

Table 16–5 summarizes five cases followed for 4 or almost 4 years past onset of birth palsy. Even by 4 years, results were quite good in both the Erb cases. One of these had neurolysis because of lack of deltoid function by 2 years of age. Biceps had begun to contract at 3 months of age in this patient. In the intervening 2 years since operation, deltoid has returned and grades 3. The other three cases were Erb-Klumpke cases. One had sensory NAPs from all peripheral nerves, indicating preganglionic injury at least at C7, C8, and T1, and another had severe

**TABLE 16–4**
Birth Palsies—Comparison of Initial to Operative Results by 5 to 6 Years of Age

| Age (Yrs) | Initials | Preoperative to Postoperative Grades by Element | | | | Comments |
|---|---|---|---|---|---|---|
| | | C5 | C6 | C7 | C8-T1 | |
| 5 | WB* | 0 to 3 | 1 to 4 | 0 to 3 | 1 to 1–2 | Erb-Klumpke<br>Grafts at 18 months of age |
| 5 | RC* | 0 to 3 | 1 to 3 | 0 to 3 | 0 to 0 | Erb-Klumpke<br>Neurolysis at 12 months of age |
| 6 | AR* | 0 to 2–3 | 0 to 3 | 4 to 5 | 5 to 5 | Erb<br>Grafts C5-C6 at 36 months of age |

*Operated patient

**TABLE 16–5**

Birth Palsies

Spontaneous and Operated/Recovery by 4 Years of Age

| | | Initial to Subsequent Grades by Elements | | | | |
|---|---|---|---|---|---|---|
| Age | Initials | C5 | C6 | C7 | C8-T1 | Comments |
| 4 | BL | 0 to 2–3 | 0 to 4–5 | 2 to 4 | 5 to 5 | Erb+ |
| | | | | | | No biceps until 5 months of age |
| 4 | MM | 0 to 0 | 0 to 3 | 0 to 1–2 | 0 to 0 | Positive sensory NAPs all nerves |
| 4 | CP* | 0 to 3 | 3 to 4 | 3 to 5 | 5 to 5 | Erb+ |
| | | | | | | Neurolysis at 24 months of age |
| 3.9 | SR | 0 to 2–3 | 0 to 3 | 0 to 3 | 0 to 0 | Horner syndrome |
| | | | | | | Biceps recovery at 7 months of age |
| 3.7 | ML | 0 to 3 | 0 to 3 | 0 to 1–2 | 0 to 0 | Brain damage, shunt, triceps recovery on |
| | | 0 to 3 | 0 to 4 | 0 to 3 | 0 to 0 | electromyogram |
| | | | | | | Bilateral birth palsy |

*Operated patient

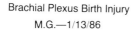

Brachial Plexus Birth Injury
M.G.—1/13/86

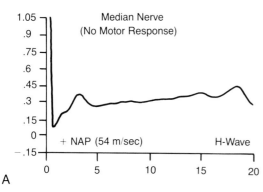

A

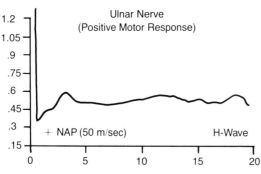

B

**Figure 16–3.** Sensory potentials recorded from both median *(A)* and ulnar *(B)* in a patient with a brachial plexus birth injury. In this case, there was relative sparing of C8 and T1 function, and thus ulnar stimulation gave both a nerve action potential (NAP) and a positive motor response. By comparison, the median nerve, although giving a positive NAP, gave no motor response, suggesting C7 or C6 preganglionic injury, or both.

brain damage as well as bilateral plexus injuries. A less complicated Erb-Klumpke case (initials SR) although having a Horner syndrome and no recovery of biceps until 7 months of age, has had a good deal of spontaneous recovery by 4 years.

Table 16–6 summarizes in tabular form the Louisiana State University Medical Center experience with ten cases followed out to 3 years of age. The Erb and "Erb +" palsies did well, including, to date, the one operated on and requiring grafts. As might have been predicted, the Erb-Klumpke cases recovered well spontaneously in C5-C6 and some C7 muscles. Major deficits outstanding by 3 years remained scapular winging in two patients, supinator weakness in three, lack of full shoulder abduction in three, and hand-intrinsic loss in four. Based on birth palsies followed longer, however, some further recovery can occur for 5 to 6 years after injury. This has to be tempered by the fact that most of the spontaneous recovery that occurs in these patients takes places by 3 years of age.

There are a number of patients in this panel who are between the ages of 1 and 3. To date, most are recovering well spontaneously. One Erb-Klumpke patient, however, has been scheduled for surgery because of continued absence of C5-C6 recovery by 9 months of age. Other Erb-Klumpke patients have shown significant upper plexus recovery as seen in Figure 16–4. Some of these patients still have poor C7 distribution function and most retain poor hand intrinsic function.

Of note is the fact that in a number of these

**TABLE 16–6**
Birth Palsies Followed Until 3 Years of Age—Summary of 10 Patients

| No. of Cases | Description | Result |
|---|---|---|
| 2 | Erb palsy | Both had excellent spontaneous recovery—shoulders abduct to 120° to 150° and good biceps function in both. |
| 2 | Erb+ (C5, C6, C7) palsy | Both recovered spontaneously to overall grades 4 and 3 respectively. |
| 1* | Erb+ palsy operated at 14 months with grafts to C5 and C6 and neurolysis C7 | Grades 2 to 3 for C5, 3 for C6, and 4 for C7 muscles. |
| 5 | Erb-Klumpke | Good function recovered to C5, C6, & some C7 muscles; major residual deficits to date include winging of scapula (2 cases), some supinator difficulty (3), lack of full shoulder abduction (3), and hand-intrinsic loss (4). |

*Operated case

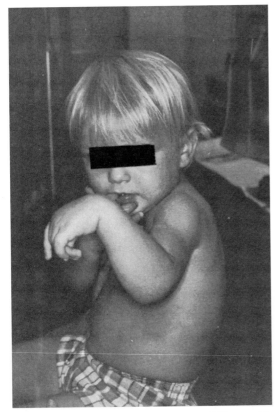

**Figure 16–4.** Youngster who is 3 years old born with an Erb-Klumpke palsy. Shoulder and upper arm function returned, but loss is still severe in C7, C8, and T1 distribution. Wrist and fingers could be flexed but not extended. Hand-intrinsic function also remained poor. (See Table 16–6 under Erb-Klumpke cases.)

patients upper plexus recovery is occurring even though biceps did not begin to contract until 4 or more months after delivery. Thirty of the 70 patients not operated on in this series had delay in recovery of biceps beyond 3 months of age.

## DISCUSSION

Outcomes in this series should be compared with those of Tassin, who followed 44 children with birth palsy and without a brachial plexus operation for almost 34 years.[34] Fourteen of these patients had good (M3) recovery. In these children, there was M3 recovery of deltoid as well as biceps in the first 3 months after delivery. In another 11 patients, recovery was nearly complete by 10 years. These youngsters had a Mallet IV shoulder and arm (Figure 16–5). They could abduct the arm to above 90 degrees, could place the hand with ease behind their head, could externally rotate the shoulder more than 20 degrees, could place the hand behind the back to the T12 level or higher, and could bring the hand to the mouth. Most of these patients had some biceps contraction by 3 months of age and usually a strong biceps by 5 or 6 months of age. Eight of these patients were thought to need disinsertion of subscapularis, and two had either teres major or latissimus dorsi transfers to improve function. In the other 19 patients reported by Tassin, 12 obtained a Mallet III level

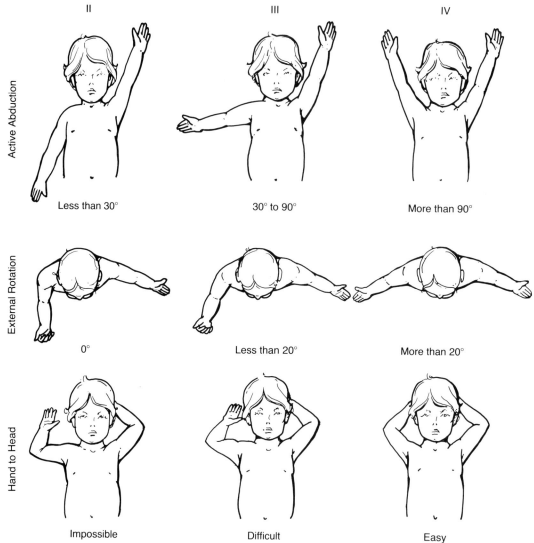

**Figure 16–5.** Grading system as proposed by Mallet. The Mallet system grades the amount of usable abduction and external and internal shoulder rotation, as well as the child's ability to reach the mouth with the hand. Affected limb is the child's right arm on the reader's left. (Adapted from Gilbert A and Tassin JL: Obstetrical palsy: A clinical, pathologic, and surgical review. *In* Terzis J, Ed: Microreconstruction of Nerve Injuries. Philadelphia, WB Saunders, 1987.)

and 7 a Mallet II level. If there was some biceps return at 3 months of age or less, the subsequent evolution of biceps function was thought to be slow in this group. Supination remained poor in most, as did internal rotation of the shoulder, although the latter is of little functional consequence.

The Mallet system for grading is a functional one for most C5-C6 functions; most of the LSUMC patients reached a Mallet III or IV level. A relatively large percentage of our cases improved spontaneously. Such improvement was not always evident in the early months but,

when it occurred, was more obvious in many by 9 to 12 months of age. Because the majority of lesions in our series were Erb-Klumpke (C5-T1), we chose to grade the results by element. Even though results by spontaneous regrowth were good, there were clearly failures, too. Whether or not the failures of spontaneous recovery could have been improved by surgery cannot be stated. The cases that were selected for surgery were operated on between 9 and 36 months of age and yet had acceptable results.

Gilbert evaluated 230 birth palsies over a 5-year period.[9,10] If biceps did not contract by 3

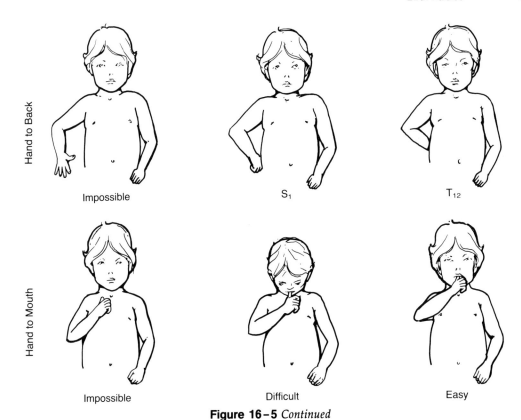

Hand to Back

Impossible          $S_1$          $T_{12}$

Hand to Mouth

Impossible          Difficult          Easy

**Figure 16–5** *Continued*

months, the infants were operated on, and with this criterion 114, or almost 50%, had surgery. This is a much higher operative rate than reported in most other series. Myelography was used in many but not all cases. There were said to be 14 false-positives and 3 false-negatives in the 79 myelograms analyzed. Average time of myelography was 4 months after birth. Forty of the 114 operated cases had their surgery on plexus at 4 or more months of age. Operatively, although evoked cortical potentials were used to study root-to-spinal-cord connections, NAP recording of root-to-division and to plexus cord-level segments to ascertain presence or absence of regeneration was not done. Only 24 patients had total paralysis of the plexus when operated upon. This differs from the LSUMC series, in which the majority of infants have had Erb-Klumpke palsies.

Sixty-two infants in Gilbert's series had C5-C6 loss and 19 had C8-T1 loss. As expected, the C5-C6 (Erb) patients did better in terms of shoulder and biceps recovery than the C5-T1 (Erb-Klumpke) patients. Also as expected, C5 and C6 levels were often reparable, but C8-T1

levels, because of avulsion, seldom were. Using the Mallet system of grading, 10 cases with initial C5-C6 (Erb) loss and having 2 or more years of follow-up were available. Three reached a grade IV level, five a grade III level, and two a grade II level. Among the C5-T1 (Erb-Klumpke) patients, five were available for follow-up at 3 years; three had a Mallet III level and two a Mallet II level. In Gilbert's experience, one half of the patients having graft repair of C5 and C6 achieved normal or near normal shoulder function, whereas none that he was following without operation did so spontaneously. As reported, Gilbert's operative results were excellent. Operative deltoid motor grades of M3 occurred in 22% of the patients at 1 year, in 46% at 2 years, and in 64% at 3 years. Biceps recovery to the M3 level in one subset of his series was 34% at 1 year, 67% at 2 years, and 72% at 3 years. Some of his operative patients also had disinsertion of subscapularis to correct excessive internal rotation of the shoulder. Use of trapezius transfer and other transfers as advocated by Zancolli and others in an attempt to substitute for shoulder abduction was less successful.[39] On the other hand, forearm procedures to improve excessive supination or pronation were more successful.[38,40] His analysis also indicated that patients operated on after 9 months of age did not do as well as those operated on earlier because of "fixed" deformities. By contrast, fixed deformities in the LSUMC series were not seen until the children were much older.

It is apparent from the LSUMC series that use of the biceps as a bellwether to predict the need for surgery is not as promising as initially believed. A significant number of infants did not have recovery of biceps until 4 to 9 months of age and yet had subsequent spontaneous recovery which was acceptable. As a result, we favor a more selective and, if needed, later operation for birth palsies. At the present time, we try to make a decision for or against operation at 9 to 12 months of age. The principal determinant is whether complete loss of function persists for this period in the distribution of one or more plexus elements that can be helped by operation. Thus, the findings in the distribution of C5, C6, and C7 and the upper and middle trunks are very important. Also of great importance is the observation that, unlike the adult plexus, the neonate's or young infant's plexus appears to respond and regenerate despite a substantial delay between injury and operation.

We also favor the use of intraoperative electrical testing, including NAP recording to help make the decision whether to resect stretched elements or not. Electromyography can suggest reinnervation after only a few hundred fibers have reached muscle, and, on occasion, simple stimulation, even used directly on an element at the operating table, can produce muscle function if only a portion of the fiber population has reached muscle. Sometimes, such electrical findings do not lead to satisfactory eventual function in this age group. On the other hand, presence of NAPs hinges on thousands of fibers 5 to $6\mu$ or greater in diameter between stimulating and recording sites. In other cases, NAP recording can confirm presence of preganglionic injury because a relatively high amplitude and rapidly conducted response is recorded. Such medial or proximal injury can be further confirmed by inability to record evoked cortical responses.

One of the major conclusions reached from this study was that many of these palsied children had acceptable spontaneous outcomes despite the fact that biceps recovery did not begin until 4 to 9 months after birth. The majority of patients described in this section were managed without surgery. They constitute another "benchmark" of the natural history of this disease, against which the results of a more aggressive surgical approach can be measured. Nonetheless, the renewal of surgical interest in this difficult disorder is a welcomed change, and those promoting it deserve much credit. Guidelines for management of this difficult disorder will thus, we believe, continue to evolve in future years.[4,6,17,18,26,27]

## Bibliography

1. Adler B and Patterson RL: Erb's palsy: Long-term results of treatment in eighty-eighty cases. J Bone Joint Surg Am 49:1052–1064, 1967.
2. Alanen M, Halonen JP, Katevuo K, et al: Early surgical exploration and epineurial repair in birth brachial palsy. Z Kinderchir 41:335–337, 1986.
3. Bennett GC and Harrold AJ: Prognosis and early management of birth injuries to the brachial plexus. Br Med J 1:1520–1521, 1976.
4. Bodensteiner J, Rich K, Landau W: Early infantile surgery for birth-related brachial plexus injuries: Justification requires a prospective controlled study. J Child Neurol 9:109–110, 1994.
5. Boome RS and Kaye JC: Obstetric traction injuries of the brachial plexus. Natural history, indications for surgical repair and results. J Bone Joint Surg Br 70:571–576, 1988.
6. Brown K: Review of Obstetrical Palsies: Non-operative Treatment. In Terzis J, Ed: Microreconstruction of Nerve Injuries. Philadelphia, WB Saunders, 1987.
7. Dol'nitzkii OV: Microsurgical operation on the brachial plexus in children. Klin Khir 6:22–25, 1980.
8. Eng GD, Kock B, and Smokvina MD: Brachial plexus palsy in neonates and children. Arch Phys Med Rehabil 59:458–464, 1978.
9. Gilbert A and Tassin JL: Obstetrical palsy: A clinical pathologic and surgical review. In Terzis J, Ed: Microreconstruction of Nerve Injuries. Philadelphia, WB Saunders, 1987.
10. Gilbert A, Razabonic R, and Amar-Khodja S: Indications and results of brachial plexus surgery in obstetrical palsy. Orthop Clin North Am 19:91–105, 1988.
11. Gordon M, Rich H, Deutschberger J, et al.: The immediate and long-term outcome of obstetric birth trauma: I —Brachial plexus paralysis. Am J Obstet Gynecol 117:51–56, 1973.
12. Green WT and Tachdijian MD: Correction of the residual deformities of the shoulder in obstetrical palsy. J Bone Joint Surg 45A:1544–1549, 1963.
13. Greenwald AG, Schute PC, and Shively JL: Brachial plexus birth palsy: A 10-year report on the incidence and prognosis. J Pediatr Orthop 4:689–692, 1984.
14. Hardy AE: Birth injuries of the brachial plexus. J Bone Joint Surg Br 63:98–99, 1987.

15. Hudson AR and Trammer B: Brachial plexus injuries. *In* Wilkins R and Rengachary S, Eds: Neurosurgery. New York, McGraw-Hill, 1984.

16. Kawabata H, Masada K, Tsuyuguchi Y, et al.: Early microsurgical reconstruction in birth palsy. Clin Orthop 215:233–242, 1987.

17. Laurent JP, Schenaq S, Lee R, et al.: Upper brachial plexus birth injuries. A neurosurgical approach. Concepts Pediatr Neurosurg 10:156–162, 1990.

18. Laurent J, Lee R: Birth-related upper brachial plexus injuries in infants: Operative and non-operative approaches. J Child Neurol 9:111–117, 1994.

19. Leffert RD: Congenital brachial palsy. *In* Brachial Plexus Injuries. New York, Churchill Livingstone, 1985.

20. Levine MG, Holroyde J, Woods JR, et al.: Birth trauma: Incidence and predisposing factors. Obstet Gynecol 63:792–795, 1984.

21. Mallet J: Paralysies obstetricales du plexus brachial. Traitement des sequelles. Rev Chir Orthop 58 (Suppl):166–172, 1972.

22. McFarland LV, Ruskin M, Daling JR, et al.: Erb-Duchenne's palsy: A consequence of fetal macrosomia and method of delivery. Obstet Gynecol 68:784–788, 1986.

23. Metaizeau JP, Prevot J, and Lascombes P: Les paralysies obstetricales: Evolution spontanée et resultats du traitement précoce par microchurchie. Ann Pediatr (Paris) 31:93–102, 1984.

24. Meyer RD: Treatment of adult and obstetrical brachial plexus injuries. Orthopedics 9:899–903, 1986.

25. Narakas A: Brachial plexus surgery. Orthop Clin North Am 12:303–323, 1981.

26. Piatt JH: Neurosurgical management of birth injuries of the brachial plexus. Neurosurg Clin North Am 2:175–185, 1991.

27. Piatt JH, Hudson AR, and Hoffman HJ: Preliminary experiences with brachial plexus exploration in children: Birth injury and vehicular trauma. Neurosurgery 22:715–723, 1988.

28. Rossi LN, Vassella F, and Mumenthuler M: Obstetrical lesions of the brachial plexus. Natural history in 34 personal cases. Eur Neurol 21:1–7, 1982.

29. Sjoberg I, Etrichs K, and Bjerre I: Cause and effect of obstetric (neonatal) brachial plexus palsy. Acta Paediatr Scand 77:357–364, 1988.

30. Solonen KA, Telaranta T, and Ryoppy S: Early reconstruction of birth injuries of the brachial plexus. J Pediatr Orthop 1:367–373, 1981.

31. Soni AL, Mir NA, Kishan J, et al.: Brachial plexus injuries in babies born in a hospital. An appraisal of risk factors in a developing country. Ann Trop Pediatr 5:69–71, 1985.

32. Specht EE: Brachial plexus palsy in the newborn. Incidence and prognosis. Clin Orthop 110:32–34, 1975.

33. Tan KL: Brachial palsy. J Obstet Gynecol Br Commonwealth, 80:60–62, 1973.

34. Tassin JL: Paralysies obstetricales du plexus brachial: Evolution spontanée resultats des interventions reparatrices précoces. Thesis, Université Paris VII, 1983.

35. Terzis JK, Liberson WT, and Levine R: Our experience in obstetrical brachial plexus palsy. *In* Terzis JK, Ed: Microreconstruction of Nerve Injuries. Philadelphia, WB Saunders, 1987.

36. Wickstrom J: Birth injuries of the brachial plexus: Treatment of defects in the shoulder. Clin Orthop 23:187–192, 1962.

37. Wickstrom J, Haslam ET, and Hutchinson RH: The surgical management of residual deformities of the shoulder following birth injuries of the brachial plexus. J Bone Joint Surg 37A:27–36, 1955.

38. Zancolli E: Paralytic supination contracture of the forearm. J Bone Joint Surg 49A:1274–1275, 1967.

39. Zancolli E: Classification and management of the shoulder in birth palsy. Orthop Clin North Am 12:433–457, 1981.

40. Zyaoussis AL: Osteotomy of the proximal end of the radius for paralytic supination deformity in children. J Bone Joint Surg 45B:523–525, 1963.

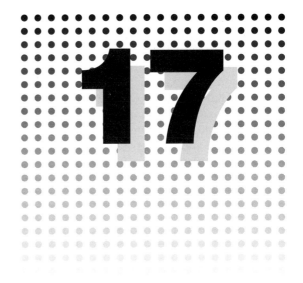

# Thoracic Outlet
# Syndrome

# SUMMARY

The controversial diagnosis of thoracic outlet syndrome (TOS) could more properly be termed a brachial plexus compression or irritation syndrome. TOS is also a diagnosis of exclusion. A thorough workup of neck, shoulder, and arm structures remains the key to such a diagnosis. Nonetheless, based on our personal experience, TOS is an entity that does truly exist even though it may be overdiagnosed and overoperated on. Observations and results of surgery in 95 patients, 7 of whom were thought to have bilateral TOS, are presented. There were three categories of patients: those with spontaneous onset of symptoms unrelated to trauma, those with symptoms associated with trauma, and those who were thought by other physicians to have had TOS and were operated initially elsewhere with either failure of relief, increased symptoms, or sometimes loss of plexus function. Some of these previously operated patients had upon reoperation inspection of the plexus from a posterior subscapular approach, and some from a more classic anterior supraclavicular approach. Intraoperative nerve action potential (NAP) recordings were done on spinal nerves and spinal nerves to trunks and plexus divisions in 70 instances. Intraoperative electrical abnormalities were found in 62 cases. These abnormalities included reduction not only in NAP amplitude, but also in NAP conduction velocity, especially in recordings made from T1 and C8 to lower trunk. These electrical abnormalities were particularly striking in a subset of 13 patients who had Gilliat-Sumner hand and thus seemingly spontaneous onset of muscle wasting and weakness. Less frequently, abnormalities were found in C7 to middle trunk recordings.

Based on this experience, it would seem that most TOS abnormalities involve neural elements located close to the spine. As a result, inspection and external neurolysis of spinal nerves or roots is the operation of preference for true TOS. In cases in which structural abnormalities other than obvious cervical ribs or prior operative damage to plexus were thought responsible for irritable or compressive lesions, these appeared to be soft tissue rather than bony. Included were hypertrophied or thickened medial edge of middle scalene, scalenus minimus, or Sibson fascia. Nine of the patients in this series had sustained serious plexus injury as a result of prior TOS operation and required operative repair. Our own complications included winging of the scapula, phrenic paralysis, and pneumothorax or hemothorax.

# INTRODUCTION

Thoracic outlet syndrome (TOS) has been popular to write about but remains both confusing and difficult to manage. TOS is a diagnosis of exclusion; there are neither single findings nor tests available that are diagnostic of it. Even combinations of findings, whether clinical or electrical, are not diagnostic.[13,54] This should make the selection of patients for both diagnosis and surgery with TOS symptoms rigorous and quite selective. Those selected should have an obvious brachial plexus compression/irritation syndrome. In addition, surgery when elected should be done by experienced operators.[48,60] Judging from the treatment complications seen in individuals who were labeled as TOS and

sent to us for corrective surgery, this is not the case. Recognition of these truths, however, will not eliminate this entity. There will still be patients whose symptoms, and at times findings, suggest this diagnosis and in whom no other cause for their difficulties can be found.[33,35] It is probably true that patients with these symptoms have been operated on too often.[58] But, well-selected patients are sometimes helped by decompressive operations on the thoracic outlet.[4,7,44] And although conservative nonoperative management does not always work, conservative management should be tried in most cases.[39,51]

Most clinicians would agree that anatomic variations such as cervical rib or an elongated lower cervical transverse process can be associated with bands or abnormal origins of scalene muscles that may lead to compression or, with repetitive motion of the shoulder, to a friction injury to a portion of the plexus.[1,9,46] In some cases, these bony abnormalities and their associated soft tissue abnormalities can be associated with neural loss as well as pain.[14,62] Less definite in terms of structural abnormalities is the more common situation, in which there are no anatomic variations seen radiologically and yet the patient has shoulder and arm pain and perhaps even paresthesias in the ulnar distribution. Some have pointed to the relationship of the first rib to that of the clavicle and the plexus, suggesting compression of the latter between the bony elements.[3] Others have related the anatomy of the scalenes, particularly the anterior scalene, to the plexus and possible TOS.[26,29,37] In addition to cervical ribs or an elongated transverse process, Bonney pointed out that a hypertrophic suprapleural membrane (Sibson fascia) can trap lower elements, particularly if "a deep part runs behind subclavian artery and in front of lower trunk from seventh cervical transverse process to the first rib."[2] Other clinicians have described a variety of soft tissue abnormalities, such as bands originating from scalenes or their origins and inserting on the ribs, as the cause of TOS (Table 17–1).[32,40,53]

## CLINICAL APPRAISAL

Workup for TOS must exclude the more common diagnoses. The differential diagnoses include cervical disc and spondylitic disease, tumor originating from or compressing the plexus or more peripheral nerves (e.g., Pancoast tumor), ulnar or median nerve entrapment, and brachial plexitis.[14,21] Presentation may be related to vascular symptoms such as aching pain, easy fatiguability, or coldness in the hand after exercise and repetitive use.[28] Severe vascular compression can lead to thrombosis and even secondary embolism with distal gangrene.[10,47] However, incidence of the vascular type of outlet compression is very low compared with the number with neural symptoms.[36] The latter may include paresthesias, burning pain, weakness, or tiring as the limb is used, especially in an elevated position, and sometimes actual loss of function. There is occasionally a case in which both vascular and neural symptoms coexist, but most are neural alone, a fact that decreases the importance of a positive Adson test or presence of a bruit or even a thrill.[19,55] A positive Adson or Roos test is not a consistently detected finding, nor is the presence of a thrill or bruit in the supraclavicular or infraclavicular region.[66] A positive Adson test can be present in asymptomatic patients, as can subclavian artery or vein occlusion in hyperabduction.[12] On the other hand, a positive Adson ipsilateral to the symptoms, coupled with other findings suggesting TOS, can be significant. Hyperabduction syndromes are associated with use of the arms above the head. Compression or friction of the cords beneath the insertion of pectoralis minor into coracoid process is probably responsible. A positive Adson may or may not be present. In the neural form of TOS, paresthesias are usually in the ulnar distribution. Pain can be in shoulder, upper arm, forearm, or hand, but some symptoms are usually found in the ulnar distribution, because C8 to T1 and lower trunk are the usual structures compressed by a fascial band or scalene origins.

Motor loss, when present, involves hand intrinsic muscles, but not exclusively those innervated by the ulnar nerve. Thenar intrinsic muscles such as abductor pollicis brevis, flexor pollicis brevis, and opponens pollicis can be weak and atrophic, as can hypothenar muscles, interossei, lumbricals, and adductor pollicis. This is known as a Gilliatt-Sumner hand (Figure 17–1). Occasionally, thenar intrinsic loss can occur without ulnar-innervated

**TABLE 17–1**

Potential "Band" or Fascial Edges Affecting Plexus in Thoracic Outlet Syndrome

Type I — Tip of cervical rib to first dorsal rib
Type II — Elongated C7 process to first dorsal rib (anterior border of middle scalene)
Type III — Neck of first dorsal rib to scalene tubercle crossing concave margin of rib (Roos)
Type IV — Anomalous connection between middle and anterior scalenes
Type V — Scalenus minimus, between plexus and artery to first dorsal rib
Type VI — Scalenus minimus or Sibson fascia
Type VII — Fascial condensation of anterior border of anterior scalene beneath subclavian vein

From Luoma A and Nelems B. Thoracic outlet syndrome. Thoracic surgery perspective. Neurosurg North Am 2(1):187–226, 1991.

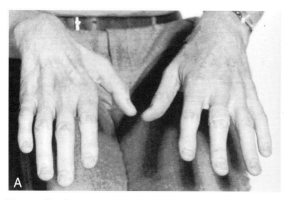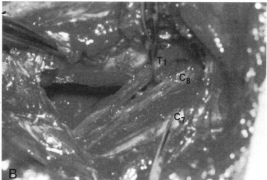

**Figure 17 – 1.** *(A)* Bilateral C8-T1 loss is worse on the patient's right side than on the left. *(B)* Plexus in a patient with a Gilliatt-Sumner hand whose spinal nerves and trunks were exposed by a posterior subscapular approach. In this photograph, the plexus is viewed from the head looking toward the posterior chest wall. Nerve action potentials (NAPs) recorded by stimulating T1 and C8 and recording from lower trunk were of very small amplitude and conducted at less than 30 msec. Stimulation of more healthy-appearing C7 and recording from the middle trunk gave a higher amplitude NAP that conducted at 60 msec.

intrinsic loss, as pointed out by Gilliatt and colleagues.[14,15]

For the patient without a background of prior injury to the shoulder or neck or prior operation to decompress the thoracic outlet, there seems to be a spectrum of symptoms as well as operative findings.[18,38,59] Symptomatology can vary, from the patient with the neurologically obvious Gilliatt-Sumner hand to one with pain and paresthesias only with elevation and use of the arm, in whom the Adson or Roos maneuvers may or may not be positive and yet there is no discernible neurologic loss and no electrical abnormality.[50] Although the EMG may show denervational and conductive changes in the patient with an obvious Gilliatt-Sumner hand, electrical abnormalities are both sparse and inconstant in the much larger group of patients suspected of having TOS and yet having no hand intrinsic muscle atrophy. Despite this fact, there continues to be a large interest in the electrodiagnostic work-up of potential TOS patients.

## ELECTRODIAGNOSTIC STUDIES

Noninvasive electrodiagnostic studies are not specific for TOS because there is not an accurate stimulating or recording site to or from plexus on either side of the clavicle.[9,23] Wilbourn has also cast doubt on the validity of earlier published reports of evoked abnormalities thought to be associated with TOS.[61] A stimulus applied at the Erb point, which is the junction of the clavicle and the lateral border of the sternocleidomastoid muscle, can stimulate either spinal nerves or trunks at variable loci. This can make measurements to distal recording sites inaccurate enough to affect conduction calculations seriously, even if the normal side is compared with the symptomatic side. Even if one could be certain that an element was stimulated at a given precise point, there is no assurance that this would be proximal to the level of compression, which can vary from case to case and, in our experience, is usually at a spinal nerve or spinal nerve to trunk level rather than more laterally.[27]

Stimulation distally and recording over plexus, or what is termed a peripheral somatosensory study, is possible,[17,52,65] but interpretation of results can be misleading. Plexus recording sites are not precise enough for accurate conduction studies unless needles are placed through soft tissues and directly into plexus elements. Again, however, it is difficult to place recording electrodes proximal to the usual entrapment sites involved in true TOS. Recording spinal somatosensory-evoked potentials after distal stimulation offers the disadvantage that cervical disc or degenerative disease simulating or complicating TOS can affect nerve root function and produce prolonged latencies for these as well as evoked cortical response recordings.

More distal electrical studies, particularly of the ulnar nerve, may show reduction in motor and sensory conductions and decreased sensory nerve action potential (NAP) amplitudes, but can often be normal.[5,16] Some view abnormal sensory and motor conductions from ulnar nerve, coupled with abnormal median motor but normal median sensory conductions, as indicating TOS.[8,58] Such studies can also be used to exclude the diagnosis of ulnar entrapment at the elbow or wrist, and similar studies of the median nerve can also usually exclude carpal tunnel syndrome.[8,31]

The afferent and efferent limbs of F waves traverse the thoracic outlet, and these values may be prolonged, particularly if compared with the unaffected side of the patient.[9,23] Nonetheless, such an abnormality is not specific for TOS because root disease caused by disc injury, spondylosis, or even more central tumor can result in similar changes. For similar reasons, somatosensory studies when recording sites are over spine or contralateral cerebral cortex, although their results may be abnormal, are insufficient to pin down the diagnosis, let alone the site of thoracic outlet compression. Locus of the distal stimulating site may be fairly precise, but the recording locus is not. Electromyography is of use to document muscle denervational patterns, and particularly to document progression and thus the need for surgical intervention.[14,28]

We manage the majority of patients referred with a diagnosis of TOS in a conservative fashion. Patients only come to surgery if clear-cut brachial plexus irritation or compression is diagnosed and conservative treatment has failed. Marginal cases require repeat consultative visits to thoroughly exclude other diagnoses and to allow the surgeon to gauge the psychological makeup of the patient.

## SURGICAL APPROACHES

Cervical ribs are usually excised through an anterior neck approach, dividing the anterior scalene to expose the extra rib and the middle scalene and lower roots and trunks[19] (Figure 17–2). Some large cervical ribs and accompanying soft tissues in the LSUMC series have been excised through a posterior subscapular

approach. Scalenectomy has been used in the past for TOS, and there has been some return of interest in this approach in recent years.[42,45] It has been suggested that first rib excision may not be necessary for the relief of TOS.[49] The most popular current approach for first rib resection if there is not an anatomic variation shown by radiologic study is a transaxillary approach.[30,43,56,63] Although this is a very expeditious operation providing the surgeon has had proper training and experience, it is an approach that does not provide direct visualization of the plexus. Indeed, plexus and vascular structures usually have to be retracted or swept away from the rib as it is resected. Some surgeons have even advocated both first rib excision and scalenectomy for TOS.[41,42] We do not advocate first rib resection as treatment for TOS, and we have seen more than 40 patients with significant brachial plexus (usually lower trunk) injury after first rib resection.

Most TOS patients can be operated on by an anterior supraclavicular approach. A portion of anterior scalene is resected, and this permits direct inspection of lower spinal nerves or roots as well as trunks.[25] They can be directly manipulated and freed of any constrictive or irritative structures. The plexus level of divisions to cords is freed by dissecting beneath the clavicle and, when necessary, displacing clavicle inferiorly. With this approach, at least in our hands, the first rib is not resected.

A number of the earlier patients operated on had had prior transaxillary first rib resection with retention of the posterior third of the first rib and either recurrence of the syndrome or surgical damage to the plexus. In these cases, we used the posterior subscapular approach as suggested by Clagett, who adapted it from a thoracoplasty approach used in the past for tuberculosis[6,27] (Figure 17–3). Others reported favorable results on a variation of this approach for TOS.[24] Such an approach permits direct inspection of the spinal nerves at the point at which they exit from their intervertebral foramina and distal to a point at which divisions form cords. It is a larger operative procedure than transaxillary first rib resection, and there is a 5% incidence of postoperative winging of the scapula. Nevertheless, the procedure has yielded good results in this difficult group of patients and has since also been used in some pa-

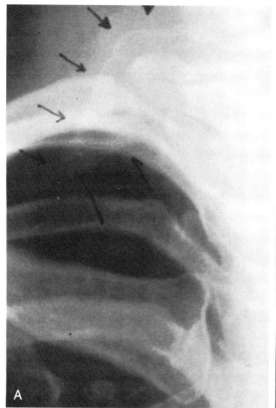

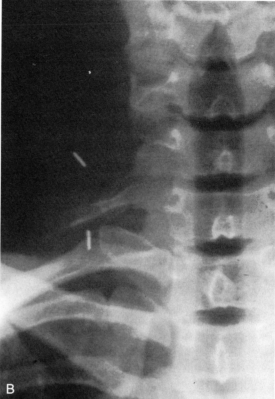

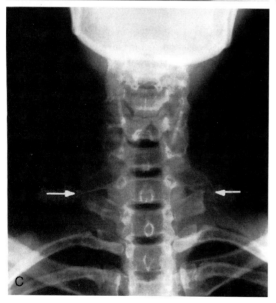

**Figure 17 – 2.** *(A)* Large cervical rib in a patient with symptoms of thoracic outlet syndrome (TOS). *Arrows* outline the extra rib. *(B)* Partially resected cervical rib in another patient whose TOS symptoms did not reverse after the initial operation. At the time of reoperation, medial scalene was still attached to the tip of the cervical rib. Note presence of metallic clips. *(C)* Radiograph of a patient who had elongated transverse processes of C7 vertebra *(arrows)* and who had bilateral first rib resection and yet recurrence of symptoms.

tients with TOS who did not have prior operations.

Direct intraoperative stimulation and recording studies can be done during either an anterior or posterior operation because the neural elements, including proximal roots or spinal nerves, are directly exposed.

An excellent trilogy of review papers has been published on the topic of surgery for TOS, and the student of TOS can make good use of them.[4,32,59] What follows in this text are observations on cases operated on that had predominantly neural symptoms rather than vascular ones. Based on the background of each case,

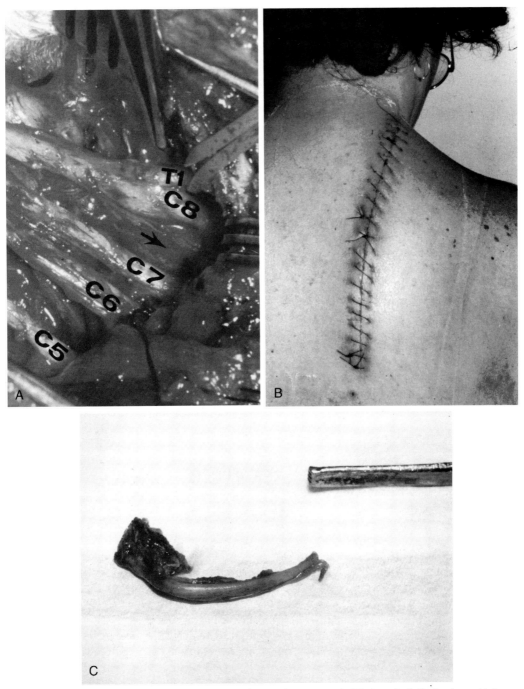

**Figure 17–3.** (A) Plexus exposed from a posterior subscapular approach. The cervical rib site *(arrow)* is between C8, T1, and C7 and has deformed junction of C8 and T1. (B) Incision (sutured) used for a posterior subscapular approach to the plexus. (C) A resected cervical rib specimen from another patient.

there are three categories of neural TOS. The first category has TOS-like symptoms that are spontaneous in onset. The second has similar symptoms and findings, but there is a background of trauma or injury to the shoulder or neck. The third category has had a prior attempt to relieve TOS symptoms by operation which has failed or has resulted in increased symptomatology or serious loss of function.

For approximately the last 15 years, we have

attempted intraoperative NAP recording on the plexus elements of a number of patients in each of these three categories.[27] These included, in the first category or spontaneous group, patients with deficits such as Gilliatt-Sumner hand as well as those in both the first and second category without neurologic loss but with neural symptoms. Some but not all of these patients had relatively minor electromyographic or conductive findings such as distal ulnar slowing. Abnormalities recorded included plexus NAPs of decreased conduction velocity or amplitude or both. The most striking finding was that these conductive and amplitude changes began close to the spine on the spinal nerves or roots or at a root-to-truncal level, but not at a divisional level or division-to-cord level, where the lateral third of the rib is located. The other striking finding related to these studies was that the abnormal electrical findings were most marked on the lower roots or spinal nerves C8 and T1. Usually, the most abnormal conductive studies were on T1; the next most often occurred on C8, whereas usually C7 and almost always C5 and C6 roots had more normal conduction and amplitudes.

Exceptions were provided by a few cervical rib patients in whom abnormalities on C7 were also sometimes found. Changes in NAP amplitude and conduction were greatest on C8 and T1 elements in those patients with Gilliatt-Sumner hand but were also seen in patients without apparent distal loss. Those patients with hand-intrinsic atrophy, including ulnar and median intrinsics, always had recordable abnormalities from C8 and T1 roots. Similar electrical abnormalities were seen in TOS patients with a prior history of trauma, and even more frequently in those with prior operation for TOS. However, there were some patients without neurologic deficit who did not have significant electrical intraoperative abnormalities. Some of them seemed nevertheless to be helped by operation, although the success rate was less in this group than in those who had intraoperative NAP abnormalities.

If bands, fascial edges, or scar were found impinging on elements, conductive abnormalities across these potentially constrictive or irritative points were usually found. On the other hand, conductive abnormalities were also seen in patients in whom obvious sites of compression were less evident, even at the operating table. Almost always, however, the constrictive structures and the conductive abnormalities occurred on proximal plexus elements. Both the structural and electrical changes were distant from the first rib and were associated with soft tissue structures such as bands, fascial edges associated with medial scalene, or Sibson fascia.

The message is clear from these studies that first rib resection without division of soft tissues around the lower roots and without neurolysis of these elements may fail to relieve TOS. If the first rib is to be removed, then it needs to be taken near its origin, and soft tissue structures related to it require division at a proximal or medial level. It is preferable to shift the focus from removal of the first rib, which does not seem to be the offender in TOS, to the soft tissue structures surrounding, investing, and potentially compressing the proximal plexus elements.

Bony abnormalities may be present but are not required for true TOS to be present. Such abnormalities include not only a cervical rib but often an elongated transverse process of C7 (Figures 17–4 and 17–5). These anatomic variants displace the takeoff or course of scalene muscles and make it more likely that they will compress or, with motion, irritate plexus roots and sometimes trunks. Again, the abnormalities are close to the spine and not in the lateral thoracic outlet. Compressive or irritative bands or fascial edges can, however, also be present without these bony abnormalities.

Intraoperative NAP recordings tended to be even more dramatic in the group of patients who had prior operations for TOS. This was especially so if there had been inadvertent operative trauma to the plexus. This usually involved lower plexus, but there were even exceptions to this in which all elements had been inadvertently injured. For example, one patient who had had prior scalenectomy by laser required graft repair of most of the plexus because of absence of recordable NAPs across the lesions in continuity. Over the years, 12 patients who had had prior first rib resection or scalenectomy were referred to LSUMC with complete injury in the distribution of one or more plexus elements. Two were reoperated on because even though loss was in the C8 and T1 to lower trunk and medial cord distributions, associated pain was manageable, and repair, because of dis-

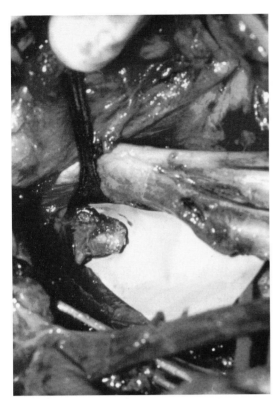

**Figure 17–4.** Plexus retracted away from the tip of cervical rib beneath a rubber dam. An anterior approach was used. Medial scalene muscle and a fascial band have been removed from the tip of this bony abnormality. The bony protrusion was then removed with a rongeur.

tance involved between injury and repair site and the nature of the fine muscles to be reinnervated, appeared contraindicated. Other patients with lower element loss had graft repair of these damaged elements because of severe pain along with their palsy, and sometimes pain was helped by such a repair. This was especially so if C7 and its middle trunk outflow required repair, because recovery in that distribution was better than that in the C8 and T1 distribution.

TOS remains difficult to diagnose and even more difficult to treat successfully.[14,44,57,58] It is clear, however, that there are cases with TOS-like symptoms or findings that can be helped sometimes by surgery. It is also clear, based on intraoperative NAP studies, that most patients with neural symptoms sustain plexus change at a relatively proximal level, so that whatever is done should include that level (Figure 17–6). In our opinion, such an operative procedure should include direct inspection and neurolysis

or freeing up of the lower spinal nerves 360 degrees around and should expose plexus close to the spine.

## OPERATED TOS CASES

### Patient Population and Symptoms

For the purpose of this study, patients thought to have TOS who were operated on and who had at least 1 year of follow-up were included. Table 17–2 provides the demography of this patient category. There were 95 patients who had 102 operations by our service either by an anterior or a posterior subscapular approach. Eighty-eight patients had unilateral symptomatology, and seven had bilateral symptoms and required bilateral operations. There was a female predominance because only 42 of the 95 patients were male. Age range varied from 11 years to 70 years of age with more than one half of the patients presenting between 30 and 40 years of age. Nonetheless, 13 operations were done in patients who were quite young, between 11 and 20 years of age, and 12 were done in patients older than 50 years of age.

There was a prior history of trauma to shoulder and neck in 32 of the operative cases. Forty-seven operations were done on plexus in

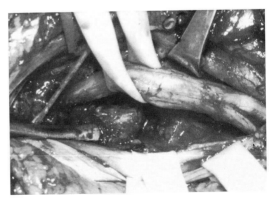

**Figure 17–5.** Elongated process of C7 vertebra exposed beneath C7 spinal nerve to the middle trunk area in a patient with TOS. Lower trunk is retracted slightly by vein retractor at the top of the picture. Discoloration due to the irritative/compressive lesion can be seen on the underside of the trunk. See also color figure.

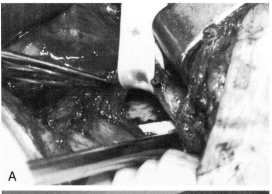
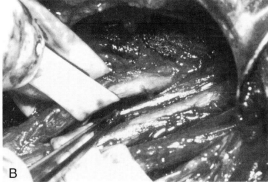
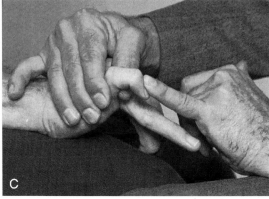

**Figure 17–6.** *(A)* View of a fibrous edge to medial scalene in a patient with left-sided thoracic outlet syndrome (TOS). This somewhat oblique band lay behind the C8 to T1 junction with lower trunk and must have been a source of irritation to it. *(B)* Fibrous edge of medial scalene beneath lower trunk of the plexus. This raphe of tissue is shown grasped by fine-toothed forceps. *(C)* Muscle most likely to be weak in a patient with true TOS. This is the lumbrical for the little or fifth finger.

cases in which there had been prior first rib or cervical rib resection, scalenectomy, or plexus neurolysis. Some of these patients had a prior history of trauma, and some did not. There were, however, 42 instances in which there was no significant history of trauma or prior operation near the plexus.

Pain and paresthesias were the principal complaints in 84 instances. In the other 18 instances, sensory or, more often, motor deficit, particularly in the intrinsic hand muscles, was the presenting complaint. Twelve of these presentations were because of a Gilliatt-Sumner hand, and one additional patient had primary thenar wasting and weak thumb movements.[15] Only one of the patients with a Gilliatt-Sumner hand had a cervical rib, although three other patients did have an elongated transverse process of C7.

## Prior Operations

The complexity of this subset of patients is reflected by Table 17–3. The 95 patients had undergone a total of 80 operations performed prior to our TOS surgery. Some of these patients had had multiple prior operations. For example, several patients had had prior excision of the first rib as well as a carpal tunnel release or ulnar transposition, or both. Others had had a prior supraclavicular scalenectomy along with transaxillary resection of the first rib or, in a few cases, anterior supraclavicular neurolysis of the plexus as well as first rib removal.

The operation performed most often before referral was transaxillary first rib excision. This was done once in 33 patients and twice in three more patients. Seven patients had prior attempts at cervical rib removal. Sixteen patients had prior attempts to treat TOS-like symptoms by either carpal tunnel release or ulnar neurolysis and transposition. However, 48 of the 95 patients had no prior operations in the vicinity of the plexus. Although some of these patients had undergone more peripheral neural procedures, their initial operative approaches to the plexus were made by ourselves. This encompassed 52 operations, because four of these individuals required bilateral procedures for TOS.

**TABLE 17–2**
Thoracic Outlet Syndrome

| | | | |
|---|---|---|---|
| A. | Unilateral TOS patients | | 88 |
| | Bilateral TOS patients | | 7 |
| | Total patients operated | | 95 |
| | Total operations on the plexus | | 102 |
| | Anterior supraclavicular plexus dissections | | 38 |
| | Posterior subscapular approach to plexus | | 64 |
| B. | Gender | Males | 42 |
| | | Females | 53 |

C. Age Ranges of Patients (yrs)

| Age | No. of Operations |
|---|---|
| 10–20 | 13 |
| 20–30 | 19 |
| 30–40 | 47 |
| 40–50 | 11 |
| 50–60 | 9 |
| 60–70 | 3 |

| | | |
|---|---|---|
| D. | Pain and paresthesias | 84 |
| | Prior first rib, cervical rib, or plexus operation | 47 |
| | Prior history of trauma to shoulder or neck | 32 |
| | Progressive deficit with serious loss of hand muscles (Gilliatt-Sumner hand) | 13 |

**TABLE 17–3**
Prior Operations — Thoracic Outlet Syndrome

| Operation | Subsequent Anterior Approach (n = 38) | Subsequent Posterior Approach (n = 64) |
|---|---|---|
| Transaxillary first rib operation × 1 | 11 | 22 |
| Transaxillary first rib operation × 2 | 1 | 2 |
| Cervical rib removal | 2 | 5 |
| Scalenectomy | 2 | 2 |
| Anterior neurolysis | 2 | 1 |
| Thrombectomy | 0 | 1 |
| Sympathectomy | 0 | 2 |
| Cervical laminectomy | 0 | 2 |
| Anterior cervical fusion | 1 | 2 |
| Pulmonary lobectomy | 0 | 2 |
| Plate to clavicle | 1 | 2 |
| Ulnar transposition | 4 | 3 |
| Carpal tunnel release | 6 | 3 |
| Needle biopsy of plexus | 1 | 0 |
| TOTALS | 31 | 49 |

## Operative Findings

Table 17–1 outlines some of the potential sites for a supraclavicular level of entrapment or impingement thought to be responsible for TOS and described in the literature. Bony abnormalities are not listed but included cervical rib and elongated C7 transverse process; this was seen in 15 of our 102 operated cases. Fusion of the first and second ribs was seen in another case, and bony callus secondary to fracture of rib or clavicle and involving plexus was seen in three of our cases.

Table 17–4 summarizes our gross operative findings. If there had been prior operation for TOS, scar involving plexus often made certain identification of entrapment or irritative sites difficult. Cervical ribs in symptomatic patients without prior operation were usually found to have displaced scalene edges or bands running from the cervical rib to the first rib. These findings were thought to be responsible for the TOS symptomatology. If cervical ribs had been incompletely resected, these soft tissue abnormalities were usually present but mixed in with the scar of the prior operation, making their certain identification difficult. The presence of residual first rib from prior operation was often associated with adhesions, which usually encompassed the T1 root but sometimes C8 as well. Clear-cut bands or fascial edges involving plexus elements were nonetheless identified in

**TABLE 17–4**
Gross Operative Findings

| Finding | Anterior Approach (n = 38) | Posterior Approach (n = 64) |
|---|---|---|
| Cervical rib | 3 | 5 |
| Residual cervical rib | 2 | 4 |
| Residual first rib | 2 | 8 |
| C7 elongated with or without band or displaced scalene | 10 | 5 |
| Medial scalene bands | 12 | 7 |
| Other bands (scalenus minimus or anterior scalene) | 7 | 8 |
| Sibson fascial band | 3 | 3 |
| Tight or taut plexus element(s) | 3 | 23 |
| Scar involving plexus element(s) | 10 | 27 |
| Prior serious operative injury to plexus | 4 | 5 |

40 of the 102 operations. Included were 30 patients who had not had prior operation on or near the plexus and who did not have a background of injury to neck or shoulder. In another 26 operations, one or more plexus elements appeared tight or taut without a readily identifiable anatomic source for this observation. As might be predicted from the frequency of prior operations, especially transaxillary resection of the first rib, scar investing one or more elements was a frequent finding.

Unfortunately, there were nine cases in which prior operation had led to serious plexus injury (Figures 17–7 and 17–8). Neuromas in continuity, transection, and intraneural scar formation were seen in these cases (Table 17–4). Several of these patients had severe neuritic pain associated with their injuries, but none had true causalgia.[20,57] Despite the iatrogenic nature of these injuries, it was thought important whenever possible to try to correct the abnormality in as timely a fashion as possible.[22,60] In two of these patients, transections of a lower root or trunk were repaired secondarily by

grafts. In the seven other cases, lesions in continuity were evaluated by NAP studies. This led to graft repair of one or more elements in four cases and a split graft repair in one. The group requiring graft repair included one patient who had sustained lengthy injury to all trunks associated with use of a laser during scalenectomy. Another patient sustained upper trunk injury during scalenectomy, had NAPs across the lesion on stimulation of C6 but not C5, and had a split repair of the upper trunk. The C6 outflow was traced through the upper trunk and maintained, whereas the C5 portion of the trunk had replacement by grafts. The other lesions in continuity requiring repair involved the lower trunk or medial cord and required replacement by grafts.

Another patient had severe posterior cord to radial loss after first rib resection and at exploration 6 months postoperatively had a lengthy lesion extending from posterior divisions of the lower and middle trunks to posterior cord and proximal radial nerve. Fortunately, the complex transmitted a NAP, so only a neurolysis was

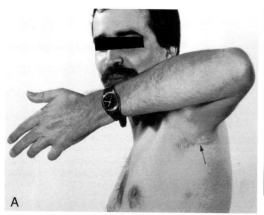

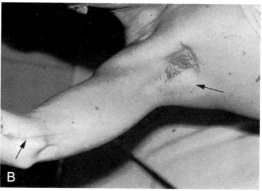

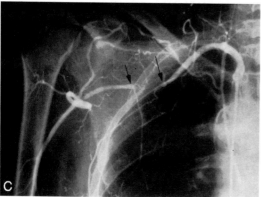

**Figure 17–7.** (A) Patient with thoracic outlet syndrome who had transaxillary resection (TAR) of the first rib (arrow) with resultant ulnar distribution palsy. (B) Another patient had carpal tunnel release, ulnar transposition, then TAR of the first rib. The last operation was associated with a pneumothorax, and a lower trunk injury resulted. (C) An axillary artery injury (arrows) associated with TAR.

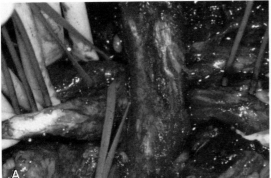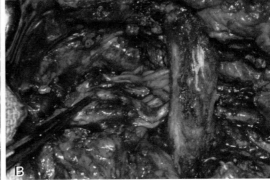

**Figure 17-8.** *(A)* An injury to the entire plexus as a result of use of a laser during a scalenectomy. Most of the plexus did not transmit an operative nerve action potential. *(B)* Most of the plexus extending from trunks to cords had to be replaced with sural grafts.

done, and she has recovered some innervation to triceps, brachioradialis, and some wrist extensors over a 3-year period.

If upper elements required repair, results were good, but most patients required lower element repair. Although their pre-repair pain seemed to be helped, recovery in the C8 and T1 distribution of hand intrinsic muscles was limited. If finger extension or flexion was paralyzed or weak preoperatively, some recovery of these functions was gained by lower element repair. Three other patients had long thoracic or suprascapular nerve injury which required repair, but since plexus was not secondarily decompressed, they were not included in this series of 102 operations.

## Intraoperative NAP Recordings

After neurolysis of the plexus, we did NAP recordings in 70 of the 102 operations (Table 17-5). Fine tripolar electrodes were placed around each spinal nerve root and were used to stimulate. Responses were recorded from the midportion of each trunk by bipolar electrodes. Amplitudes and conduction velocities recorded from lower trunks were compared with those recorded from middle and, in most cases, upper trunks. In eight cases, amplitude and conduction data recorded from lower elements was comparable to that recorded from middle or upper trunks. There were, however, 62 other operative cases in which distinct electrical abnormalities were recorded.

In 47 of the cases in which intraoperative recordings were done and found to be abnormal, there had been no prior operation on or close to the plexus. Seventeen of these cases had a prior history of injury to neck or shoulder and 30 did not. In an additional 15 cases, there had been prior operations close to or on plexus, usually transaxillary resection of the first rib. The most frequent abnormality recorded was decreased amplitude or absence of a NAP on stimulating the T1 root and recording from the lower trunk (Figure 17-9). Decreased amplitudes were also

## TABLE 17-5

NAP Recordings Performed on Thoracic Outlet Syndrome Patients Intraoperatively*

| | No. of Recordings |
| --- | --- |
| Abnormalities found in 62 patients | |
| Decreased amplitude T1 to L.T. | 38 |
| Decreased C.V. T1 to L.T. | 32 |
| Flat T1 NAP trace | 7 |
| Decreased amplitude C8 to L.T. | 26 |
| Decreased C.V. C8 to L.T. | 21 |
| C7 to M.T. abnormality | 8 |
| NAPs abnormal on all elements | 1 |
| NAP studies performed on seven patients with serious injury secondary to prior TOS surgery | |
| (−) NAPs = Grafts | 4 |
| (+) NAPs = Neurolysis | 1 |
| (+) and (−) NAPs = Split or partial graft repairs | 2 |

C.V. = conduction velocity; L.T. = lower trunk; M.T. = middle trunk; NAP = nerve action potential; (+) = positive; (−) = negative.
*70 patients had these studies; in 8 patients, they were normal.

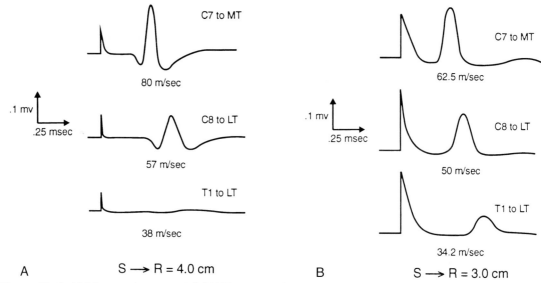

**Figure 17–9.** *(A)* Nerve action potential (NAP) tracings show a very small and slow response *(bottom tracing)* recorded from T1 to lower trunk (LT) in a patient with thoracic outlet syndrome (TOS). The response from C8 to LT was probably abnormal also, especially compared with the one recorded from C7 to middle trunk (MT). *(B)* NAP tracings in another patient with spontaneous TOS. Trace is also abnormal from T1 to LT, but less so from C8 to LT, and again that from C7 to MT is more normal.

usually associated with decreased conduction velocity if an NAP was present at that site. Next in frequency were abnormalities in C8 to lower trunk recordings. There were also eight instances in which the C7 to middle trunk recordings showed abnormality. Not unexpectedly, those patients with prior TOS surgery on or near the plexus and resultant lesions in continuity usually had absent NAPs across injured elements.

The recordings suggested that the conductive abnormality, whether associated with a history of injury, prior surgery, or TOS of spontaneous onset, was a proximal one close to the spine. The data further suggested that operations designed for TOS should reach close to the midline and that direct inspection of the neural elements, and preferably external neurolysis of them, may be the optimal procedure.

## Operative Results

Table 17–6 depicts the results in 102 operations on 95 patients. Pain and paresthesias were helped in most cases (Figure 17–10). In nine patients serious residual pain persisted, and in three of these cases, another operation either on plexus or by implantation of a dorsal column

**TABLE 17–6**
Results in 102 Thoracic Outlet Syndrome Operations on 95 Patients

| | Result | Anterior Approach (n = 38) | Posterior Approach (n = 64) |
|---|---|---|---|
| A. | No pain/paresthesias | 21 | 33 |
| | Partial improvement— pain | 14 | 25 |
| | Serious residual pain | 3 | 6 |
| | Required another operation for pain | 1 | 2 |
| B. | Mild motor deficit improved | 5 | 9 |
| | Mild motor deficit unchanged | 3 | 2 |
| C. | Severe motor deficit improved | 3 | 3 |
| | Severe motor deficit partially improved | 6 | 10 |
| | Severe motor deficit unimproved | 3 | 7 |
| D. | New deficit produced | 0 | 1 |
| | Pleural opening | 3 | 4 |
| | Chest tube | 0 | 2 |
| | Postop Thoracentesis | 2 | 3 |
| | Phrenic paresis | 3 | 1 |
| | Wound infection | 0 | 1 |
| | Scapular winging | 0 | 4 |
| | Chylothorax | 1 | 0 |
| | Subsequent diagnosis of syrinx | 0 | 1 |
| | ? Diagnosis of amyotrophic lateral sclerosis | 0 | 2 |

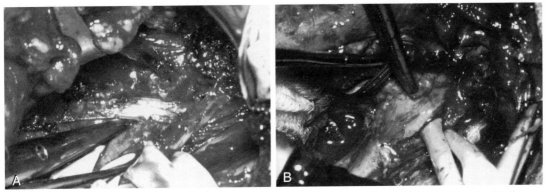

**Figure 17–10.** *(A)* Hypertrophied Sibson fascia passing across junction of C8 and T1 in a patient with thoracic outlet syndrome. *(B)* Scar surrounding lower elements of plexus and associated with previous resection of first rib.

stimulator was tried elsewhere. Presenting motor deficits were improved in some patients. If the deficit was severe and in the distribution of C8-T1, as it usually was, it was difficult to reverse (Figures 17–11). Severe deficit in 26 instances either remained unchanged or only partially improved postoperatively. By comparison, mild motor deficit improved in 14 of 19 instances. In both categories, loss or decreased function involving finger extension or flexion improved more than hand-intrinsic muscle loss. Despite this observation, a number of patients did improve intrinsic function by one or two grades. This involved, with descending frequency, hypothenar, thenar, interosseous, and lumbrical muscles. Two patients with progressive loss of hand function despite operative de-

compression of the plexus were later thought to have amyotrophic lateral sclerosis. Both of these patients had had TOS operations prior to our procedure.

Complications were not frequent but are worth noting. Pleura was opened in seven cases; if this occurred, it was then sewed shut as the anesthetist gave the patient a Valsalva maneuver. In only two cases were chest tubes necessary postoperatively because of persisting hemopneumothorax. Several other patients did, however, require thoracentesis in the early postoperative period. Phrenic paresis with diaphragmatic elevation occurred four times. This improved over a period of months and initially was managed by intermittent positive-pressure breathing treatments and incentive spirometry.

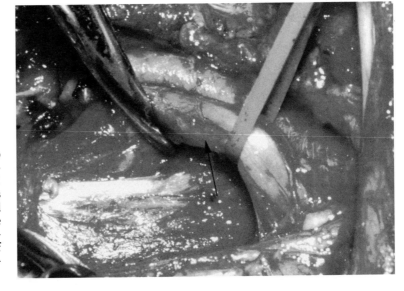

**Figure 17–11.** Fibrous edge to medial scalene which had irritated junction of C8 and T1 with lower trunk. The latter is being elevated by a loop and Metzenbaum scissors, and the arrow points to the area of irritation and some thickening of epineurium on its inferior surface.

It produced minimal to no symptoms in three of the four cases. Scapular winging, despite an attempt to carefully close rhomboids and spinal trapezius, occurred in four of the operations done posteriorly. This decreased abduction of the arm above the horizontal and, fortunately, was temporary in two of the cases.

The one wound infection was treated by local debridement, irrigation, and antibiotics, and the wound healed by secondary intention without reoperation. The one patient with chylothorax had a prior anterior operation on the left. This was treated by thoracentesis and a compressive dressing to the area of the neck wound and, fortunately, did not recur.

Table 17–7 summarizes a group of 48 TOS patients having 51 posterior subscapular operations and divided into three categories: spontaneous TOS, post-traumatic TOS, and TOS with prior operation on the plexus. These cases were carefully selected for this procedure. Outcomes were fairly comparable in each of the three categories, although serious deficit associated with prior operation on or near the plexus was difficult to reverse by another operation. Somewhat surprising was the fact that electromyographic abnormalities were found more often in patients with apparent spontaneous onset of TOS than in those with post-traumatic TOS.

## Conclusions

The authors believe there is a need for operation on selected patients with TOS symptoms (Table 17–8). The diagnosis can be entertained only after careful exclusion of other causes of neural compression or irritation. Cases must be carefully selected for operation. Both the structural abnormality and its electrical correlates are close to the spine at a root or spinal nerve-to-trunk level. Direct inspection and a complete external neurolysis of neural elements, especially the lower areas, is at present the procedure we favor.

At the present time, we use the posterior sub-

**TABLE 17–7**
Thoracic Outlet Syndrome Cases Operated Posteriorly*

|  | Spontaneous TOS | Traumatic TOS | TOS and Prior Operation |
|---|---|---|---|
| Patients | 25 | 12 | 11 |
| Posterior Operations | 27† | 12 | 12‡ |
| Male/Female | 12/13 | 7/5 | 2/9 |
| Mean Age (yrs) | 35 | 40 | 33.5 |
| Prior Neural Operations | 2 CTR | 1 CTR | 11 TAR |
|  | 2 ulnar | 2 ulnar | 2 supracl. pl. |
|  | transpositions | transpositions | 1 CX laminect. |
| Clinical Presentation |  |  |  |
| Pain | 27 | 6 | 12 |
| Mild deficit | 8 | 6 | 3 |
| Moderate deficit | 7 | 2 | 6 |
| Severe Deficit | 8 | 0 | 0§ |
| Electromyograms With Denervation |  |  |  |
| (C7, C8, or T1 distribution) | 13 of 24 | 2 of 12 | 1 of 9 |
| Cervical Rib | 5 | 0 | 1 |
| Elongated C7 Transverse Process | 4 | 1 | 0 |
| Abnormal Intraoperative NAPs | 12 of 16 | 5 of 9 | 6 of 10 |
| Number with Follow-Up | 23 | 11 | 10 |
| Average Years of Follow-up | 4.6 | 3.3 | 3.3 |
| Postoperative Status |  |  |  |
| Good results | 19 | 8 | 9 |
| Unchanged | 4 | 3 | 1 |
| Scapular winging | 0 | 1 | 1 |

CTR = carpal tunnel release; CX laminect. = cervical laminectomy; NAPs = nerve action potentials; Supracl. Pl. = dissection supraclavicular plexus; TAR = transaxillary rib removal; TOS = thoracic outlet syndrome.

*From: Dubuisson A, Kline D, and Weinshel S: Posterior subscapular approach to the brachial plexus. Report of 102 patients. J Neurosurg 79:319–330, 1993.

†Two patients had bilateral operations.

‡One patient had a bilateral operation.

§Three other patients with severe loss after prior TAR for TOS are included under traumatic plexus injuries.

## TABLE 17–8
### Thoracic Outlet Syndrome — Conclusions

1. True thoracic outlet syndrome (TOS) *does* occur.
2. Thorough exclusionary work-up remains the key to the diagnosis.
3. Both the structural abnormality and its electrical concomitants are very close to the spine.
4. True TOS is a soft tissue and not a bony disorder.
5. Operative procedures for TOS which do not get close to the spine may fail.
6. Most abnormalities involve neural elements, so direct inspection and complete external neurolysis of neural elements appear indicated.

scapular approach for TOS if there has been prior first rib excision and there is a significant remnant of rib left attached to the spine, if there is a large cervical rib, or if there has been prior significant injury to lower elements. Although the complication of winged scapula is infrequent, it can occur. With experience, the anterior approach can provide good access to lower elements, particularly in fresh, previously unoperated cases. The anterior approach can also be complicated by pleural opening or phrenic paresis, but it does provide a somewhat better view of the effect of any constricting bands or scar on neural elements. Whether performed anteriorly or posteriorly, a thorough and proximal neurolysis of spinal nerves as well as trunks seems to be in order for true TOS patients.

## Case Summaries — Thoracic Outlet Syndrome

### Case Number 1

A 54-year-old woman presented with a 2-year history of weakness in hand muscles. She first noted atrophy of the right thenar eminence and had pain in the base of the thumb. Computed tomography showed a smooth bulge of the C6-C7 disc. There was a prior history of right middle lobectomy for a localized carcinoma with no evidence of recurrence. On examination, her loss was confined to hypothenar, thenar, interosseous, and lumbrical muscles, which graded 2 to 3. An Adson test was normal, as was a chest radiograph, but the transverse process of C7 was elongated bilaterally, especially on the right. Ulnar and median nerve stimulation at the wrist gave no hand-intrinsic motor function, and evoked muscle action potentials recorded from intrinsic muscles were quite small in amplitude.

Under general anesthesia and with the patient in a prone position, a posterior subscapular approach to the

plexus was done. The elongated C7 transverse process was resected. Several bands of connective tissue running between C7 transverse process and first rib appeared to entrap and compress both C8 and T1 spinal nerves. These were divided, and the posterior and lateral portion of the first rib was removed.

NAP recordings evoked by stimulation of C5, C6, and C7 and recording from upper and middle trunks gave sizable responses, conducting at 66 to 77 m/sec. Recordings from lower trunk after stimulation of C8 and T1 gave very small, barely recordable NAPs, conducting at 20 to 27 m/sec. She did well postoperatively, and by follow-up at 4 years, hand intrinsics graded 3 to 4 and she was free of pain. There was mild winging of the scapula, but she had no trouble with abduction of the shoulder. She is able to work as a certified public accountant.

### Comment

Plain radiographs of the cervical spine and imaging studies may show mild degenerative changes and yet the etiology for symptoms may be more laterally located TOS or even distal entrapment. A step in the posterior approach to the plexus is first rib resection, unless that has been done before. Despite this either scar or other soft tissue abnormalities can be responsible for the plexus element compression or irritation as was so in this case.

### Case Number 2

A 36-year-old woman complained of vague tingling in her hand and pain running down her arm. She thought this pain was aggravated when she worked overhead. The patient consulted a physician who released her left carpal tunnel. In retrospect, it was apparent the patient had some weakness of her abductor pollicis on the affected side, but many of the characteristic features of carpal tunnel syndrome were absent, and the patient had not had any electrophysiologic studies undertaken before surgery. The patient improved for a few weeks, and then returned to her former state. Imaging studies of her lower cervical spine showed no abnormality. The patient was advised to have her first rib resected, and this was done through the axilla 1 year after the onset of symptoms. After the patient recovered from the anesthetic, she noted that her hand was quite numb, but she was told this was a minor problem and that it would soon go away. Subsequent examination revealed that the patient had significant atrophy of both the thenar and hypothenar eminences on the affected side. This was not present before the rib resection. The clinical examination was suggestive of a severe lower trunk injury. Re-exploration was suggested, but this was postponed a further 3 months. Eventually, the patient came to supraclavicular exploration, and a severely injured lower trunk was found, just proximal to the divisions. In addition, two large bands were found and divided. These bands were compressing the junction of C8 and T1 at a point close to the tips of the transverse processes. A neurolysis was undertaken because NAPs of small amplitude could be obtained across the lesion. When seen some 3 years later, the patient had improved her hand function somewhat but still had a significant deficit.

### Comment

Tingling in the hands and vague discomfort in the upper limbs are common complaints. Hypochondriasis can be an underlying factor. Carpal tunnel surgery should only be undertaken after the diagnosis has been established with certainty. It is also unwise to advise surgery for TOS unless there are clear-cut symptoms and signs, and unless conservative management has failed. The latter should include a well-thought-out program of exercise and training to improve posture. This should include close work with a good physical therapy team. The diagnosis of TOS is made after all other conditions are excluded, and on the basis of a positive history and physical examination.

Transaxillary first rib resection is a standard operation, but we have treated a number of patients with significant neurologic deficits caused by complications of this operation. We prefer the supraclavicular approach, in which all of the compressive structures close to the cervical spine can be easily visualized and managed. Cervical ribs or elongated transverse processes can be dissected out with due care given to protection of the elements of the brachial plexus. The complications of the transaxillary operation observed by us include direct injury to the lower trunk or medial cord in the majority of cases. On occasion, injury to the lower plexus elements has followed vascular injury during first rib resection, which resulted in very rapid application of clamps, some of which involved the neural elements.

There are several additional syndromes similar to TOS that deserve mention.

# HYPERABDUCTION SYNDROME

The diagnosis of this syndrome is made by exclusion, and the treatment, which is usually conservative, precludes visual confirmation of the pathologic changes that might be seen at operation.[21] The existence of the syndrome, and the fact that it does qualify as an entrapment syndrome, is confirmed by the striking similarities of arm positioning required in the occupations of Mayfield's 14 patients in whom this diagnosis was made and the ablation of their signs and symptoms as a result of changing occupations.[34,35] The etiology for this infrequent condition is usually repetitive abduction of the arm rather than true hyperabduction which would lead of course to dislocation of the shoulder.

The mechanical basis underlying this syndrome was described by Wright.[64] It is compression of the brachial plexus and axillary artery and vein when the arms are held in constant abduction. The compression occurs at the point at which the tendon of the pectoralis minor muscle inserts onto the coracoid process of the scapula. Indeed, the process acts as a fulcrum around which the nerves and vascular structures are tightly constricted. Wright arrived at this conclusion by deductive reasoning and substantiated his conclusions by cadaver dissections.[64] In his dissections, he also demonstrated that the costoclavicular space became narrowed by the rolling motion of the clavicle induced by the extremes of abduction. He had anticipated using ablation of the radial pulse by hyperabduction of the arms as a diagnostic test for the syndrome but abandoned the idea after he noted bilateral ablation of the radial pulse in 82% of 150 symptomless, young subjects to whom this maneuver was applied. Apparently, this fact escaped Adson and Coffey's attention when they suggested the same maneuver as a diagnostic test for the then so-called scalenus anticus syndrome.[1]

The hyperabduction syndrome is singular in that there are no constitutional abnormalities leading to its initiation or evolution. It is, rather, a matter of occupations in which unusual arm positions, maintained for varying lengths of time, cause a normal contiguous structure to impinge on and constrict normal nerves, arteries, and veins. Although the flow of axoplasm and blood is impeded for short periods of time, there is apparently no permanent damage to the neurovascular bundle. All 14 of Mayfield's patients recovered after they were prevented from working with the arms in hyperabduction. The question of whether the signs and symptoms are caused by the impedance to the flow of blood or of the axoplasm, or both, may only have a partial answer. Most cases have, of course, abnormal nerve conduction. On the other hand, fatigability of the arms could be construed as being caused by insufficient blood flow.

Eight of Mayfield's patients were laborers who worked on ceilings as painters or plasterers, and the remainder were mechanics who regularly lay on their backs on dollies under automobiles with their arms hyperabducted as they worked.[34] All of them noted, after prolonged work of this type, fatigability of their arms accompanied by paresthesias of the thumbs and index fingers. Occasionally, the latter spread to involve the middle fingers, which perhaps indicates involvement of the middle trunk of the brachial plexus.

Signs and symptoms rarely progressed beyond this point, were ameliorated or absent during vacation periods, and disappeared after the patients changed occupations and began sleeping in halters designed to prevent unconscious hyperabduction. In this group, the diagnostic sign of any validity was the reproduction of symptoms on extreme abduction of the arm, combined with percussion or deep palpation over the brachial plexus at the point at which the pectoralis minor tendon inserted onto the coracoid process.

# COSTOCLAVICULAR SYNDROME

In 1943, Falconer and Weddell noted that soldiers complained of numbness in their arms when they stood at attention wearing loaded knapsacks attached to their persons by straps that crossed the clavicles.[11] Apparently, this was not malingering, for large groups of soldiers experienced these same sensations in similar circumstances or on prolonged marches if they were carrying knapsacks of similar load and construction. It was the contention of these authors, which they confirmed by anatomic dissections, that weight applied to the clavicle caused it to ride down on the first rib and, in doing so, compressed the brachial plexus and neighboring blood vessels between them. They also noted that in normal, symptom-free subjects, forceful backward dislocation of the shoulders sometimes produced the symptoms and ablated the radial pulse, and that the Adson maneuver of stretching the scalenus anterior muscle did not affect this pulse if the point of compression was at costoclavicular junction.

Hudson's group found 15 cases of this syndrome, and in each of them, a fracture of the clavicle and excessive callus formation was an antecedent clinical event.[67] The portions of the brachial plexus that were compressed varied, the degree of compression ranged from partial to complete, and these facts dictated the extent and severity of the clinical symptoms. Because of the nature of the antecedent cause, these patients sought attention early, and the symptoms rarely had progressed beyond paresthesias and pain in the expected nerve distribution. There was little or no evidence that compression of vascular structures played any part in the evolution of the symptoms.

Treatment has consisted of wide excision of the clavicular callus, and the results have been good. In retrospect, however, it would seem that the operation of choice would be posterior or transthoracic excision of the first rib. The rib resection would release the brachial plexus and subclavian artery from compression while avoiding any skeletal instability that might accompany excision of the clavicle.

## Bibliography

1. Adson A and Coffey J: Cervical rib: A method of anterior approach for relief of symptoms by division of scalenus anticus. Ann Surg 85:839–857, 1927.
2. Bonney G: The scalenus medius band: A contribution in the study of thoracic outlet syndrome. J Bone Joint Surg Br 47:268–272, 1965.
3. Bramwell E and Dykes HB: Rib pressure and the brachial plexus. Edinburgh Med J 27:65–88, 1921.
4. Campbell J, Waff N, and Dellon A: Thoracic outlet syndrome: Neurosurgical perspective. Neurosurg Clin North Am 2(1):227–233, 1991
5. Cherrington M: Ulnar conduction velocity in the thoracic outlet syndrome. N Engl J Med 294:1185–1189, 1976.
6. Clagett OT: Research and proresearch: Presidential address. J Thorac Cardiovasc Surg 44:153–166, 1962.
7. Dale WA: Thoracic outlet compression syndrome. Critique in 1982. Arch Surg 117:1437–1445, 1982.
8. Daube JR: Nerve conduction studies in thoracic outlet syndrome. (Abstract). Neurology 25:347, 1975.
9. Dawson D and Hallett M: Entrapment Neuropathies, 2nd Ed. Boston, Little, Brown & Co, 1990.
10. Eden K: Vascular complications of cervical ribs and first thoracic rib abnormalities. Br J Surg 27:111–139, 1939.
11. Falconer M and Weddell G: Costoclavicular compression of the subclavian artery and vein: Relation to the scalenus anticus syndrome. Lancet 2:539–543, 1943.
12. Geroudis R and Barnes R: Thoracic outlet arterial compression: Prevalence in normal persons. Angiology 31:538–541, 1980.
13. Gilliatt RW: Thoracic outlet compression syndrome. Br Med J 1:1274–1275, 1976.
14. Gilliatt RW: Thoracic outlet syndrome. *In* Dyck P, Thomas P, and Lambert E, Eds: Peripheral Neuropathy. Philadelphia, WB Saunders, 1984.

15. Gilliatt RW, Le Quesne PM, Logue V, and Sumner AJ: Wasting of the hand associated with a cervical rib or band. J Neurol Neurosurg Psychiatry 33:615–624, 1970.

16. Gilliatt RW, Willison RG, Dietz V, and Williams IR: Peripheral nerve conduction in patients with a cervical rib and band. Ann Neurol 4:124, 1978.

17. Glover JL, Worth RM, Bendick PJ, et al.: Evoked responses in the diagnosis of thoracic outlet syndrome. Surgery 89:86–93, 1981.

18. Greep JM, Lemmors HA, Roos DB, and Urschel HC, Eds: Pain in the Shoulder and Arm: An Integrated View. The Hague, Martinus Nijhoff, 1979.

19. Hardy R and Wilbourn A: Thoracic Outlet Syndrome. In Wilkins R and Rengachary S, Eds: Neurosurgery. Baltimore, McGraw-Hill, 1985.

20. Horowitz SH: Brachial plexus injuries with causalgia resulting from transaxillary rib resection. Arch Surg 120:1189–1191, 1985.

21. Hudson A, Berry H, and Mayfield F: Chronic injuries of nerve by entrapment. In Youmans J, Ed: Neurological Surgery, 2nd Ed. Philadelphia, WB Saunders, 1983.

22. Hudson A, Kline D, and MacKinnon S: Entrapment neuropathies. In Horowitz N and Rizzoli H, Eds: Postoperative Complications of Extracranial Neurological Surgery. Williams & Wilkins, 1987.

23. Jerrett SA, Cuzzone LJ, and Pasternak BM: Thoracic outlet syndrome. Electrophysiologic reappraisal. Arch Neurol 41:960–963, 1984.

24. Johnson CR: Treatment of thoracic outlet syndrome by removal of first rib and related entrapments through posterolateral approach: A 25-year experience. J Thorac Cardiovasc Surg 68:536–545, 1974.

25. Kempe LG: Operative Neurosurgery, Vol. 2. New York, Springer-Verlag, 1970.

26. Kirgis H and Reed A: Significant anatomic relations in the syndrome of the scalene muscles. Ann Surg 127:1182–1201, 1948.

27. Kline D, Hackett E, and Happel L: Surgery for lesions of the brachial plexus. Arch Neurol 43:170–181, 1986.

28. Kopell HP and Thompson WL: Peripheral Entrapment Neuropathies. Baltimore, Williams & Wilkins, 1976.

29. Lawson FL and McKenzie KG: Scalene syndrome. Can Med Assoc J 65:358–361, 1951.

30. Leffert R: Thoracic outlet syndrome. In Gelberman R, Ed: Operative Nerve Repair and Reconstruction. Philadelphia, JB Lippincott, 1991.

31. Licht S, Ed: Electrodiagnosis and Electromyography, 3rd Ed., Baltimore, Williams & Wilkins, 1961.

32. Luoma A and Nelems B: Thoracic outlet syndrome: Thoracic surgery perspective. Neurosurg Clin North Am 2(1):187–226, 1991.

33. Mackinnon S and Dellon A: Surgery of the Peripheral Nerve. New York, Thieme Medical Publishers, 1988.

34. Mayfield F: Neural and vascular compression syndromes of the shoulder girdle and arms. In Vinken P and Bruyn G, Eds: Handbook of Clinical Neurology, Vol. 7. Amsterdam, North Holland, 1970, pp. 430–446.

35. Mayfield F and True C: Chronic injuries of peripheral nerves by entrapment. In Youmans JR, Ed: Neurological Surgery. Philadelphia, WB Saunders, 1973, pp. 1141–1161.

36. Nelson RM and Davis RW: Thoracic outlet compression syndrome. Ann Thorac Surg 8:437–451, 1969.

37. Ochsner A, Gage M, and DeBakey M: Scalenus anticus (Naffziger) syndrome. Am J Surg 28:669–695, 1935.

38. Pang D and Wessel H: Thoracic outlet syndrome. Neurosurgery 22:105–121, 1988.

39. Peet RM, Henriksen JD, and Anderson TP: Thoracic outlet syndrome. Evaluation of a therapeutic exercise program. Mayo Clin Proc 31:281–287, 1956.

40. Pollak EW: Surgical anatomy of the thoracic outlet syndrome. Surg Gynecol Obstet 150:97–103, 1980.

41. Qvarfordt PG, Ehrenfeld WK, and Stoney RJ: Supraclavicular radical scalenectomy and transaxillary first rib resection for the thoracic outlet syndrome. A combined approach. Am J Surg 148:111–116, 1984.

42. Roos DB: The place for scalenectomy and first rib resection in thoracic outlet syndrome. Surgery 92:1077–1085, 1982.

43. Roos D: Thoracic outlet syndromes. Update 1987. Am J Surg 154:568–572, 1987.

44. Roos D: The thoracic outlet syndrome is underrated. Arch Neurol 47:327, 1990.

45. Sanders RJ, Monsour JW, Gerber WF, et al.: Scalenectomy versus first rib resection for treatment of the thoracic outlet syndrome. Surgery 85:109–121, 1979.

46. Sargent P: Lesions of the brachial plexus associated with rudimentary ribs. Brain 44:95–124, 1927.

47. Scher LA, Veith FJ, Haimovici H, et al.: Staging of arterial complications of cervical rib: Guidelines for surgical management. Surgery 95:644–649, 1984.

48. Schlesinger EB: The thoracic outlet syndrome from a neurosurgical point of view. Clin Orthop 51:49–52, 1967.

49. Stallworth JM, Quinn GJ, and Aiken AF: Is rib resection necessary for relief of thoracic outlet syndrome? Ann Surg 185:581–592, 1977.

50. Sunderland S: Nerves and Nerve Injuries, 2nd Ed. Edinburgh, Churchill Livingstone, 1978.

51. Swift TR and Nichols FT: The droopy shoulder syndrome. Neurology 34:212–215, 1984.

52. Synek VM: Diagnostic importance of somatosensory evoked potentials in the diagnosis of thoracic outlet syndrome. Clin Electroencephalogr 17:112–116, 1986.

53. Thomas GI, Jones TW, Stavney LS, and Manhas DR: The middle scalene muscle and its contribution to the thoracic outlet syndrome. Am J Surg 145:589–592, 1983.

54. Thoracic outlet compression syndrome. (Editorial). Br Med J 1:1033, 1976.

55. Tindall S: Chronic injuries of peripheral nerve by entrapment. In Youmans J, Ed: Neurological Surgery, 3rd Ed. Philadelphia, WB Saunders, 1990.

56. Urschel HC Jr and Razzuk MA: Management of the thoracic outlet syndrome. N Engl J Med 286:1140–1143, 1972.

57. Urschel HC and Razzuk MA: The failed operation for thoracic outlet syndrome. The difficulty of diagnosis and management. Ann Thorac Surg 42:523–525, 1986.

58. Wilbourn A: The thoracic outlet syndrome is overdiagnosed. Arch Neurol 47:328–332, 1990.

59. Wilbourn A: Thoracic outlet syndromes: A plea for conservatism. Neurosurg Clin North Am 2(1):235–245, 1991.

60. Wilbourn A: Thoracic outlet syndrome surgery causing severe brachial plexopathy. Muscle Nerve 11:66–74, 1988.

61. Wilbourn A and Lederman R: Evidence for conduction delay in thoracic outlet syndrome is challenged (letter). N Engl J Med 310:1052–1053, 1984.

62. Wilson S: Some points on the symptomatology of the cervical rib with special reference to muscular wasting. Proc R Soc Med 6:133–141, 1913.

63. Wood VE, Twito R, and Versha JM: Thoracic outlet syn-

drome: The results of first rib resection in 100 patients. Orthop Clin North Am 19:131–146, 1988.

64. Wright J: The neurovascular syndrome produced by hyperabduction of the arm. Am Heart J 29:1–19, 1945.

65. Yiannikas C and Walsh JC: Somatosensory evoked responses in the diagnosis of thoracic outlet syndrome. J Neurol Neurosurg Psychiatry 46:234–240, 1983.

66. Youmans CR and Smiley RA: Thoracic outlet syndrome with negative Adson's and hyperabduction maneuvers. Vasc Surg 14:318–329, 1980.

67. Young MC, Richards RR, and Hudson AR: Thoracic outlet syndrome with congenital pseudoarthrosis of the clavicle: Treatment by brachial plexus decompression, plate fixation and bone grafting. Can J Surg 31:131–133, 1988.

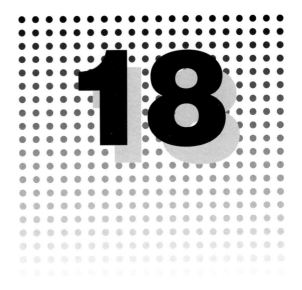

# Accessory Nerve

## SUMMARY

Most injuries involving this nerve are iatrogenic in origin, and the most common complicating operation is lymph node biopsy. Other iatrogenic causes in the series of 84 cases reported herein included tumor excision, carotid endarterectomy, face lift surgery, and irradiation. There were 20 cases caused by stretch/contusion, stab or glass wounds, and gunshot wounds. It is extremely important to differentiate scapular winging caused by accessory palsy from that caused by long thoracic or dorsal scapular palsy. Forty-four patients with accessory palsy required operation. About one third had lesions in continuity and required nerve action potential recordings, with subsequent neurolysis or resection and repair. End-to-end repair was done after lesion resection or if nerve was already either pulled apart or transected (13 cases). Grafts were used in 18 cases. Usually it was possible to utilize nearby sensory nerves for this purpose, but because of extensive scarring in the neck, the sural nerve had to be harvested and used in seven cases. Neurotization using C2 and C3 outflows or burial of grafts from proximal accessory directly into muscle was less successful. All seven patients having a neurolysis based on presence of a nerve action potential had a grade 3 or better recovery, and 25 (75%) of 33 having a suture repair recovered well. Only 2 of these patients, however, reached a full grade 5 recovery.

Extracranial injuries to the eleventh cranial (accessory) nerves are unusual but do occur.[2,6] The leading cause is iatrogenic and operative. Most cases are associated with lymph node biopsy, but, as can be seen from Table 18–1 as well as in the literature, other associated operations include excision of neck tumors, carotid endarterectomy, plastic surgery procedures, and irradiation[7,8,13] (Figure 18–1).

Although more commonly spared in stretch injuries involving neck or shoulder, this nerve can be stretched either in association with plexus stretch or in a more solitary fashion. Penetrating wounds from knives, glass, or gunshot wound can occasionally involve this nerve. Even less frequent is a more spontaneous onset which may or may not involve compression,[3] physical exertion, or, as in this series, a solitary case of Hansen disease and a probable plexitis case involving the accessory nerve.

Historically, accessory palsy has also been associated with tuberculosis or scrofula of the neck and with vascular ectasias involving the nerve in the neck.[4,5] In the past, the accessory nerve was routinely sacrificed as part of a radical neck dissection, but in more recent years, many surgeons have been sparing this nerve during such dissections.[1,14]

Table 18–1 lists the causes responsible for 84 accessory palsies in a series seen at LSUMC. The most frequent mechanism for injury was iatrogenic, and 42 of these were related to lymph node biopsy. There were, however, 20 injuries caused by stretch, laceration, and gunshot wound.

**TABLE 18–1**

Causes of Accessory Palsy (n = 84)

| Cause | No. of Cases |
|---|---|
| Iatrogenic Causes | |
|   Lymph node biopsy | 42 |
|   Tumor excision | 14 |
|   Carotid endarterectomy | 1 |
|   Plastic face lift | 1 |
|   Radical neck surgery | 1 |
|   Irradiation | 1 |
| Traumatic Causes | |
|   Stretch | 13 |
|   Laceration | 6 |
|   Gunshot wound | 1 |
| Other causes | |
|   Compression | 1 |
|   Weight lifting | 1 |
|   Hansen disease | 1 |
|   Plexitis | 1 |

Abstracted from Donner TR and Kline DG: Extracranial accessory nerve injury. Neurosurgery 32:907–911, 1993.

## SURGICAL ANATOMY

Rootlets making up the accessory nerve arise from both the lower medulla and the upper, usually four, segments of the cervical spinal

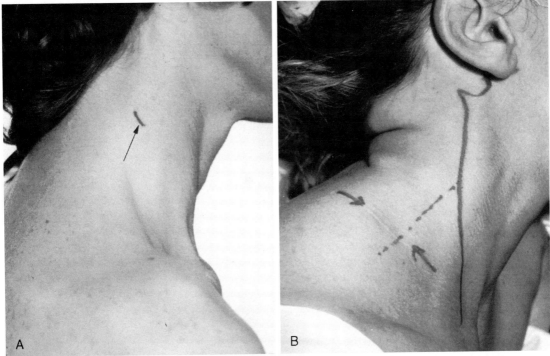

**Figure 18–1.** *(A)* A small lymph node biopsy incision resulted in severance of cranial nerve XI. *(B)* A lower incision in another patient caused a distal injury to the accessory nerve. Arrows drawn on skin point to scar from incision used to remove the lymph node. The solid line drawn on the skin outlines the lateral border of the sternocleidomastoid; the dotted line shows the usual course of the accessory nerve. Some suspensory trapezius function from accessory nerve branches proximal to the injury site was retained in this patient.

cord. The cervical rootlets ascend the ventral spinal canal to join the medullary descending rootlets. They form the accessory nerve, which exits the skull through the jugular foramen. Below the base of the skull, accessory nerve lies lateral to the internal jugular vein. The nerve then courses either anterior or posterior to the internal jugular vein. Then, the nerve lies behind the stylohyoid and digastric muscles. The nerve then tunnels beneath the more proximal sternocleidomastoid (SCM) muscle, which it innervates. This junction is also shared by spinal branches from C2, C3, and sometimes C4, so even complete injury to proximal accessory nerve does not give paralysis of the SCM.

The accessory runs from beneath the posterior or lateral border of SCM, usually at a point one fourth to one half of its length from mastoid eminence to clavicle. It is in close juxtaposition to the great auricular nerve which wraps around the lateral border of SCM to course cephalad. The accessory nerve is almost always cephalad to the great auricular nerve, and the two nerves

together form an important landmark. The course of the accessory nerve can also usually be judged by palpating the C2 transverse process beneath SCM and then projecting a straight line from there to the tip of the shoulder.

The accessory nerve then courses somewhat obliquely across the posterior triangle, where it lies on the surface of the levator scapula muscle. On reaching the superior portion of the trapezius, it branches to innervate this muscle. It supplies short branches to supply the trapezius along the superior and posterior border of the neck and longer branches to descend into the thoracic or what some authors term the spinal portion of the muscle.

In some cases, branches from C2 or even C3 spinal nerves may supplement input to trapezius, especially the lower or spinal portion of that muscle.[11,12] The majority of the evidence points strongly to the fact that the main motor supply to the trapezius muscle is by the eleventh cranial nerve. Certainly, by the time the nerve is seen in the posterior triangle, it is, in our experience, the sole source of motor supply to the trapezius. Regardless of whether it has picked up contributions from the cervical plexus before entering the posterior triangle, if the accessory nerve is injured in that area, the patient will have a major trapezius motor loss. The nerve to serratus anterior arises from C5, C6, and C7 spinal nerves. The main physical contribution is often from the posterior surface of the C6 spinal nerve. The confluence of these three spinal nerves often occurs within the substance of scalenus medius before the named nerve emerges in the lower portion of the posterior triangle. Thus, it is virtually impossible selectively to injure the nerve to serratus anterior through an incision placed directly over the course of the accessory nerve in the posterior triangle unless, of course, the plexus itself is seriously injured. Contrariwise, it is extremely easy to injure the accessory nerve through an incision placed directly over the course of that nerve.

One of the key points relating to the anatomy of the accessory nerve in the posterior triangle is the fact that it is covered only by skin and the investing fascia of the neck. It is therefore very exposed to operative injury. Cervical lymph nodes often immediately abut on the accessory nerve. Lymph nodes may lie deep to the plane of the accessory nerve, so that the nerve, in its course through the posterior triangle, runs through lymph node–bearing adipose tissue. This anatomic relation underlies the fact that the most common cause of iatrogenic accessory nerve injury seen by us is cervical lymph node biopsy (Figure 18–2).

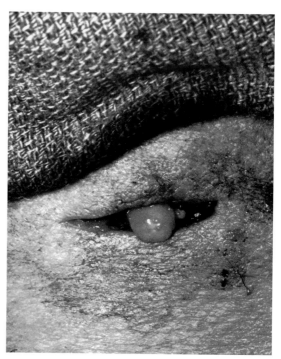

**Figure 18–2.** A small posterior triangle incision for a lymph node biopsy just missed cranial nerve XI. The nerve lay in the depths of the wound just beneath the lymph node, which was somewhat adherent to it.

## CLINICAL FINDINGS

Onset of this palsy is usually associated with pain, presumably because of atrophy of this relatively large shoulder and back muscle. The tip of the shoulder droops, and this may produce traction on soft tissues of the neck, including nerves which may also be responsible for or contribute to the pain. This is variously described as a dragging or pulling sensation in the neck and can be associated with arm pain and occipital as well as posterior neck discomfort.

Patients may well ascribe their initial postoperative abnormal symptoms to the operation, such as a lymph node biopsy, itself. It is not un-

usual for a patient to delay recognition that something is seriously wrong for a few days or weeks. Pain may not be noticed for several weeks until the patient attempts to resume household tasks requiring normal shoulder activity. Progressively, the patient notices a decrease in strength of the affected arm and difficulty in such daily tasks as combing hair, putting on a shirt or blouse, and raising the arm above the horizontal plane.

With severe or complete palsy, the scapula wings and the patient, in addition to shoulder droop, notes inability to abduct the arm in a smooth fashion, especially above the horizontal (Figure 18–3). Pushing forward with the elbow flexed or across the chest against resistance accentuates the winging. On the other hand, pushing forward against resistance with the arm extended forward does not produce severe winging, as it would with long thoracic palsy. Some patients learn that with abduction in a lateral direction, they can turn the hand from a palm down to palm up direction and gain some further abduction above the horizontal. Others

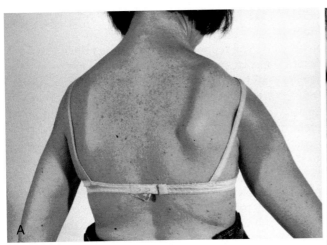

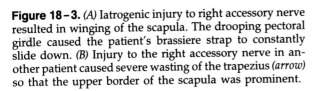

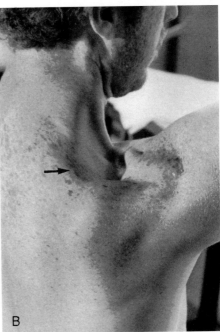

**Figure 18-3.** (A) Iatrogenic injury to right accessory nerve resulted in winging of the scapula. The drooping pectoral girdle caused the patient's brassiere strap to constantly slide down. (B) Injury to the right accessory nerve in another patient caused severe wasting of the trapezius (*arrow*) so that the upper border of the scapula was prominent.

learn to throw or toss their arm out in abduction and use the force of the initiation of abduction to carry the arm past the horizontal, despite their winging and lateral rotation of the scapula.

Shrug of the shoulder is poor, although levator scapula can substitute for this in a variable fashion, especially for more medial shoulder function. More medial trapezius may also contract because branches to this portion of the muscle may arise from a more proximal portion of the accessory beneath SCM and thus be spared with the usual more lateral nerve injury. Simple inspection shows atrophy of the superior portion of the trapezius and some, but usually not complete, winging of the scapula. This winging is not as severe or as complete as is seen with serratus anterior loss. Mild wasting of supra- and infraspinatus is a common accompaniment of a wide range of disorders of the shoulder joint, including trapezius palsy. The appearance of this sort of scapular muscle wasting should not mislead the examiner to an incorrect diagnosis of brachial plexus injury, amyotrophy, or suprascapular nerve injury.

Loss of trapezius function results in lack of coordinated trapezius/serratus anterior function, which is required for rotation of the scapula during the final 90 degrees of shoulder abduction. This may be the main complaint expressed by the patient. Supraspinatus and deltoid abduct the humerus to the 90-degree position, but further abduction requires rotation of the scapula. This rotation is primarily brought about by the combined action of trapezius and serratus anterior. Deltoid and supraspinatus functions are retained, but these muscles have the disadvantage of working from an unstable base and, in addition, the crucial component of scapular rotation is severely impaired by the weakness or paralysis of trapezius. A stable scapula is essential to serve as a platform for function of short muscles around the shoulder joint. The lack of scapular stability which follows trapezius palsy thus results in alteration of coordinated function of the short muscles and hence of fluent shoulder movement. Very characteristically, patients complain of sudden "clunking" of the scapula during attempted circumduction of the shoulder. The upper border of the scapula is often prominent if the patient is viewed from the opposite side, and there is a characteristic flattening of the tissues immediately behind the clavicle on the affected side, compared with the normal side.

After a few weeks, electromyography (EMG) shows denervational changes in the trapezius.

There may be some relative sparing of medial fibers, but with severe lesions there is seldom sparing of intermediate or more lateral muscle innervation. By comparison, EMG study of SCM seldom shows denervational change[2,9] (Figure 18–4). Needle studies of the spinal portion of the muscle are difficult to do because rhomboideus major and minor are just deep to the more inferior portion of the trapezius and levator scapula to the more superior part of it.

If reinnervation occurred spontaneously in this series, its onset was usually delayed for 3 to 9 months. As with other muscles, early electrical signs included presence of nascent units and usually a simultaneous decrease in the intensity of fibrillations and denervational potentials. The muscle is usually reinnervated from above down. Only very clear-cut evidence of significant reinnervation should be allowed to delay surgical exploration.

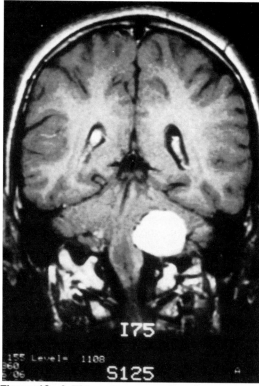

**Figure 18–4.** This patient was referred as a case of peripheral eleventh nerve injury. Clinical examination and EMG, however, revealed absent sternocleidomastoid function on the same side, and a magnetic resonance scan revealed the true site of the eleventh nerve compression.

## OPERATION

The reoperation follows the principles of any nerve exploration. It is usually appropriate to add vertical limbs to the previously placed skin-crease horizontal incision. Reflection of the two triangular flaps thus created allows the posterior or more lateral border of the SCM to be cleared and the anterior border of the trapezius to be displayed. The transverse cervical and greater auricular nerves serve as guides. These branches of the cervical plexus are usually easily found during the initial stages of the dissection, because they curve around the posterior border of SCM. The proximal stump of the accessory nerve is usually found approximately 1 to 2 cm above or superior to these nerves. The usual pattern is that of a single nerve trunk with branches running a short distance to the anterior border of the trapezius. If the nerve injury is distal to a branch, every effort must be made to conserve that function. On occasion, the main trunk may appear to divide, and, once again, all functioning elements must be preserved.

As a general principle, it is, as with other nerve injuries, appropriate to dissect out nerve proximal and distal to the lesion, subsequently working toward the main pathology. In accessory nerve injuries in the posterior triangle, this is a difficult maneuver. Often a mixture of scar and adipose tissue occupies the upper part of the posterior triangle between the posterior border of the SCM and the anterior border of the trapezius. The dissection under the operating microscope or loupes may occupy a considerable period of time as the dissector distinguishes cervical plexus and other sensory branches to the skin of the neck and periaural regions running medially from the area of the trapezius muscle, and the damaged accessory nerve (Figure 18–5). The operation is hampered if the vertical limb placed at the medial extent of the previous horizontal incision is not extended sufficiently high. A variable voltage nerve stimulator helps locate the proximal stump because it causes SCM contraction. The searching electrode may accidentally directly stimulate levator scapulae or cervical branches to it and this occurrence should not be misinterpreted as evidence of trapezius contraction.

The surgeon should be at pains to preserve even wisps of nerve tissue emanating from the

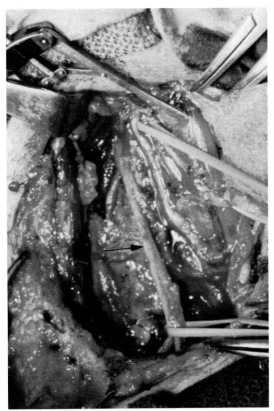

**Figure 18-5.** Dissection of an injured accessory nerve which is marked by single arrow. Plastic loop to the right is around some of the adjacent cervical sensory nerves.

branches indicating motor entry points. The proximal nerve runs between sternomastoid and cleidomastoid, and the neuroma may be found enmeshed in adipose and fibrous tissue or, less frequently, as a well-defined and smoothly outlined proximal neuroma bulb.

The proximal and distal stumps are prepared in standard fashion after the appropriate electrophysiologic and microsurgical appraisal of the lesion. Although the greater auricular nerve is an excellent donor nerve, we have sometimes used sural nerves for grafting purposes. The graft should be placed in a relaxed fashion to allow movement of the patient's neck postoperatively and to allow for shrinkage of graft substance (Figures 18-6 and 18-7). If a lesion in continuity is found, the standard electrical and microscopic criteria are utilized to decide for or against resection after an external neurolysis has been performed. If direct stimulation of the nerve results in trapezius contraction (i.e., in a situation in which none was seen on clinical examination), then the procedure is terminated, because this feature is consistent with an excellent prognosis. Attempts should be made to obtain nerve action potentials (NAPs) across the lesion. Sometimes this may be difficult because the distance available between proximal and distal electrode placement may be short.

proximal accessory stump, because the difficulty with this operation may be that of defining an appropriate distal stump. The operator may have to search through the scar tissue on the anterior border of the trapezius to find fascicles or

## RESULTS

Patients selected for operation usually had complete or nearly complete loss of trapezius with denervation by EMG persisting for 2

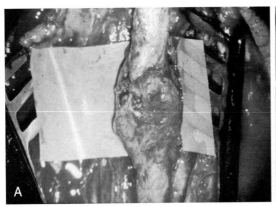
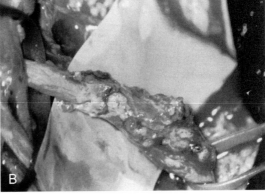

**Figure 18-6.** (A) Operating microscopic picture of an accessory neuroma in continuity. This lesion did not transmit a nerve action potential 4 months after injury and required resection and repair. (B) Another severe lesion in continuity involved the accessory nerve and also required resection.

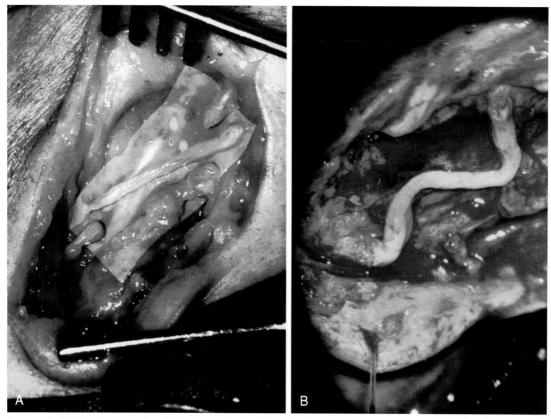

**Figure 18–7.** *(A)* This operative site in the posterior triangle shows a neuroma in continuity of cranial nerve XI. This has been resected because no nerve action potential could be recorded across it. *(B)* A sural nerve graft is laid between the proximal and distal stumps. The graft is sewn in a somewhat redundant fashion to allow for graft shrinkage and neck movement. Most trapezius function returned after several years.

months or longer. Early experience had shown that a proportion of such lesions were in continuity even if the mechanism was operative injury. As a result, exploration was delayed for several months after onset of palsy in most iatrogenic injuries as well as in the stretch injuries unassociated with prior operation. Approximately one half of such injuries were found to be in continuity. Some were regenerating and had a transmitted NAP, and thus had a neurolysis only, and the others required resection and repair. One exception was provided by an iatrogenic case in which the surgeon involved recognized that the nerve was divided, did not repair it acutely, and sent it for secondary repair. Another exception was a case in which the pathologist reported a nerve segment of approximate caliber for accessory nerve along with the lymph node submitted. In these cases, repair was done relatively early but nonetheless sec-

ondarily. Accessory nerves injured by glass or knife wounds were also repaired relatively early or soon after they were first seen.

## NONOPERATIVE CASES

Those patients not selected for operation usually improved significantly with time or were, as in two cases, referred very late. Three other patients presented with function that was partial but was thought to be acceptable. Three patients treated conservatively remained unchanged over 1 to 2 years of further follow-up. Another patient who had injury caused by irradiation had a progressive loss of not only trapezius but also SCM function, and eventually developed a complete palsy.

Table 18–2 shows the initial grades seen in a group of 34 patients, as well as their latest grade

**TABLE 18–2**
Nonoperative Case Results*
(n = 34)

| Grade | Initial Grade | Final Grade |
|-------|---------------|-------------|
| 5 | 0 | 10 |
| 4 | 6 | 11 |
| 3 | 14 | 8 |
| 2 | 8 | 2 |
| 1 | 4 | 0 |
| 0 | 2 | 3 |

*Thirty-four patients are listed beside their clinical grades at presentation and at the end of follow-up (11 months or more).

**TABLE 18–3**
Operations — Accessory Nerve (n = 44)

| Operation | No. of Cases |
|-----------|--------------|
| Neurolysis | 8 |
| Ligature removal | 1 |
| End-to-end repair | 13 |
| Local nerve graft | 11 |
| Sural nerve graft | 7 |
| Neurotization (C2, C3) | 2 |
| Burial into muscle | 2 |

on follow-up. Only patients with some sequential follow-up are included in this table. Average length of follow-up in this group was 16.1 months, with a range of 11 to 96 months.

## OPERATIVE CASES

Table 18–3 depicts the operations done in 44 patients for whom there were follow-ups available of 10 months or more.[2] The results by grade are shown in Table 18–4, which includes 40 patients with 2 or more years of follow-up. Eight patients had a neurolysis because a NAP was recorded across their lesion in continuity, and seven of these were seen in follow-up. Outcome in this group was dramatic, with improved abduction and restoration of shoulder carriage and a good shrug. Another patient who had removal of a suture from around the accessory nerve recovered well without further repair. If repair was necessary, improvement usually occurred, with most patients reaching a grade 3 or

higher level. Four of these patients reached a grade 5 level. As can be seen from Table 18–4, there were a few exceptions, and recovery with repair, even of this nerve, is not guaranteed. Average follow-up for all of the repairs was 24.2 months (range 10 to 42 months).

There were four failures of repair. Two of the failures were graft repairs. Two other patients had attempted placement of grafts directly into muscle, and this did not work. By comparison, neurotization, in which SCM branches were swung down and sewn to grafts which were attached to distal accessory branches, had some degree of recovery.

If managed correctly, the outcome with accessory palsy was usually good, and this has been the case in other smaller series.[10,15,16] On the other hand, recovery was usually not perfect. Shoulder shrug was often recovered, but some winging of the scapula and lack of full abduction was not an infrequent outcome. Even with good recovery, the shoulder on the affected side was often carried by the patient at a lower level than on the contralateral side. Most

**TABLE 18–4**
Results of Surgery* (n = 40)

| | Neurolysis | | | Repair | |
|-------|------------------------|-------------------------|-------|------------------------|-------------------------|
| Grade | Preoperative (n = 7) | Postoperative (n = 7) | Grade | Preoperative (n = 33) | Postoperative (n = 33) |
| 5 | 0 | 2 | 5 | 0 | 4 |
| 4 | 0 | 3 | 4 | 0 | 12 |
| 3 | 0 | 2 | 3 | 0 | 9 |
| 2 | 0 | 0 | 2 | 0 | 4 |
| 1 | 1 | 0 | 1 | 5 | 3 |
| 0 | 6 | 0 | 0 | 28 | 1 |

*The preoperative and postoperative clinical grades of 40 patients who underwent neurolysis (7) or repair (33) of accessory nerve. Only those available for follow-up for 2 or more years are included.

of these patients were able to return to some type of work, but there were exceptions, particularly if the work involved heavy labor, heavy lifting, or climbing ladders.

## Bibliography

1. Becker GD and Parell GJ: Technique of preserving spinal accessory nerve during radical neck dissection. Laryngoscope 89:827–831, 1979.
2. Donner T and Kline D: Extracranial spinal accessory nerve injury. Neurosurgery, 32:907–911, 1993.
3. Eisen A and Bertrand G: Isolated accessory nerve palsy of spontaneous origin. A clinical and electromyographic study. Arch Neurol 27:496–502, 1972.
4. Hanford JM: Surgical excision of tuberculosis lymph nodes of neck. Report of 131 patients with follow-up results. Surg Clin North Am 13:301–303, 1933.
5. Havelius U, Hindfelt B, Brismar J, and Cronqvist S: Carotid fibromuscular dysplasia and paresis of lower cranial nerves (Collet-Sicard Syndrome). J Neurosurg 56:850–853, 1982.
6. Hudson A, Tramner B, and Tymianski M: General principles of iatrogenic nerve injury illustrated by re-operation on the accessory nerve. Submitted for publication, 1993.
7. King R and Motta G: Iatrogenic spinal accessory nerve palsy. Ann R Coll Surg Engl 65:35–37, 1983.
8. Marini SG, Rook JL, Green RF, and Nagler W: Spinal accessory nerve palsy: An unusual complication of coronary artery bypass. Arch Phys Med Rehabil 72: 247–249, 1991.
9. Olarte M and Adams D: Accessory nerve palsy. J Neurol Neurosurg Psychiatry 40:1113–1116, 1977.
10. Osgaard O, Eskesen V, and Rosenbon J: Microsurgical repair of iatrogenic accessory nerve lesions in the posterior triangle of the neck. Acta Chir Scand 153:171–173, 1987.
11. Soo KC, Guiloff RJ, Oh A, et al.: Innervation of the trapezius muscle: A study in patients undergoing neck dissections. Head Neck 12:488–495, 1990.
12. Straus WL and Howell AB: The spinal accessory nerve and its musculature. Q Rev Biol 11:387–405, 1936.
13. Swann KW and Heros RC: Accessory nerve palsy following carotid endarterectomy: Report of two cases. J Neurosurg 63:630–632, 1985.
14. Weitz JW, Weitz SL, and McElhinney AJ: A technique of preservation of spinal accessory nerve function in radical neck dissection. Head Neck Surg 5:75–78, 1982.
15. Woodhall B: Trapezius paralysis following minor surgical procedures in the posterior cervical triangle. Ann Surg 136:375–380, 1952.
16. Wright TA: Accessory spinal nerve injury. Clin Orthop 108:15–18, 1975.

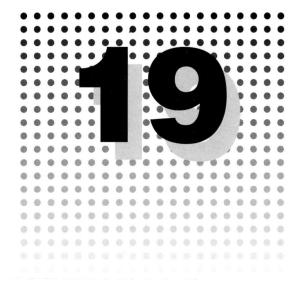

# Reconstructive
# Procedures

## SUMMARY

Neither of us is an orthopedist, plastic surgeon, or physiatrist. Nonetheless, we have seen our patients benefit from well-indicated reconstructive procedures and well-thought-out physical therapy programs. The number of substitutive procedures developed to replace a lost leg or arm, and especially hand function, is a tribute to human ingenuity. Despite this, there are times when only a direct neural repair will suffice. We are proponents of neural repair whenever possible, but realize there are limits to recovery, particularly for distal hand and foot function.

Tendon transfer for a radial palsy in which residual loss is finger or thumb extension may be the only useful treatment and, in addition, is extremely effective. Either a Brand or Riordan transfer or a Zancolli procedure to decrease clawing in the little and ring fingers and improve their extension, has been used frequently for ulnar palsies in this series. Harder to achieve is successful substitution for loss of distal thumb flexion and opposition because of median palsy, but a well-balanced transfer is capable of achieving this. Partial Achilles or posterior tibial transfer can be helpful for foot drop if done by an experienced reconstructionist. Unfortunately, an equally effective transfer for complete femoral palsy is not available, and knee fusion or use of a usually bulky knee brace is not very popular with either the patient or the physician. Effective substitution for brachial plexus palsies is very difficult, especially if a flail arm is present. On the other hand, if loss in the limb does not involve all elements and if direct repair for them is not possible, reconstructive procedures can be quite valuable. Shoulder fusion to provide an improved carrying angle for the limb is useful providing flexion of the arm is spared to begin with or is gained by neural repair. Substitution for loss of biceps/brachialis or brachioradialis can be done by transfer of the latissimus dorsi or of a portion of the pectoralis major or by sliding functional flexor musculature to a site above the elbow. Function in one of these muscle groups must be spared to begin with or must be restored to nearly normal by neural repair for these procedures to be useful in the patient with a severe stretch injury.

The limb with an injured nerve does not heal by being placed at rest for long. Early and sustained physical and occupational therapy is a must. Both the patient and the patient's family should be taught to supplement structured therapy with home exercises. In the totally paralyzed limb, range of motion activities are a necessity until recovery begins to occur.

## INTRODUCTION

There is little question that substitutive procedures such as tendon transfers and fusion are indicated for many severe peripheral nerve injuries. In fact, the practical results of such reconstructive procedures are viewed by some as more successful for restoration of function than those produced by neural repair alone.[7,12,18,22] Although this remains controversial, there are recognized limits to effective neural regeneration to distal muscles, particularly with severe proximal nerve injury. In some settings, tendon transfers may be indicated in the early weeks or months after nerve injury. On the other hand, as long as the extremity's range of motion is maintained and the limb is cared for adequately, tendon transfer or other substitutive procedures can usually be delayed until the neural regenerative process has completed itself. Obviously, use of a tendon transfer hinges on whether musculature with spared innervation has sufficient power so that a portion can be sacrificed or borrowed for transfer. Suitable muscles and attendant tendons must be available. For example, a patient with plexus palsy without function in forearm muscles doesn't have suitable muscle to transfer to substitute for loss of hand function, nor does the typical patient with a severe plexus stretch palsy usually have suitable muscles to transfer to substitute for lack of biceps.

A very important factor is whether an orthopedic, hand, or plastic surgeon is available who has had proper training and sufficient experience in these techniques. A transfer that produces an intrinsic plus or intrinsic minus hand can be more deleterious than no transfer at all. What follows is only an overview of this field, because we are neurosurgeons and not reconstructive or orthopedic surgeons. Fuller texts and explanations are available and should be consulted for further detail.[2,5,6,8,9,24,27]

## MEDIAN LOSS

If median nerve regeneration fails to provide satisfactory thumb opposition, a variety of effective procedures is available.[18,21] A tendon inserted into the distal end of the thumb's metacarpal bone can be activated by a normal ulnar forearm muscle flexor (Figure 19–1). The linkage usually is directed through a tendon pulley

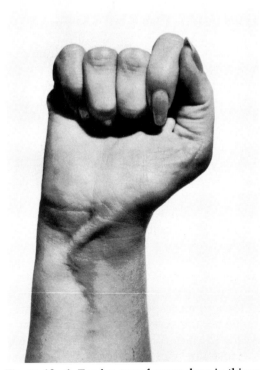

**Figure 19–1.** Tendon transfer was done in this patient to provide some abduction and opposition of the thumb for a severe median palsy. Transferred tendon can be seen running subcutaneously and obliquely across the wrist.

close to the pisiform bone. This gives a pulling movement that closely mimics opposition. With extensive motor loss that involves ulnar forearm muscles as well, it may be necessary to fuse the thumb's metacarpal in a fixed position of partial opposition. Unfortunately, it is difficult to compensate for total loss of median-innervated sensory function. This makes an attempt at direct repair of median injury, regardless of level or extent of injury, worth a try.

## ULNAR LOSS

One of the major disabilities with ulnar palsy is difficulty in extending the ring finger and especially the little finger at the proximal interphalangeal and distal interphalangeal joints. This is a result of loss of lumbrical ability to set the metacarpophalangeal joints so that the extensor communis can effectively straighten out these fingers. The result is a claw deformity of these fingers. Claw is worse with distal ulnar than proximal ulnar lesions because proximally innervated flexor profundi to little and ring fingers still work and are unopposed by an effective extensor mechanism.

Substitution for lumbrical function by the transfer of a portion of the median-innervated flexor superficialis through lumbrical canals to extensor expansions of the digits is quite successful. The flexor superficialis can be extended by fascia obtained either from the pyriformis muscle in the leg or the palmaris longus tendon in the forearm and hand.[21] In our experience, the Brand technique has provided a hand with which most patients are happy regardless of whether there is significant ulnar nerve regeneration.[3] Such a procedure is needed for many severe ulnar lesions and should be done early enough so that fixed clawing of the fingers does not develop.

Particularly difficult to treat by either reconstructive or neural operations is a combined ulnar and median palsy[21] (Figure 19–2). Sometimes a combination of tendon transfer plus arthrodesis is useful.[13]

## RADIAL LOSS

Direct neural repair is the first order of business for most serious radial injuries and is usu-

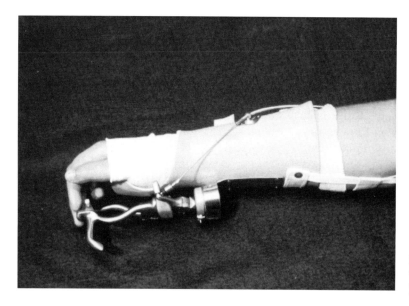

**Figure 19-2.** A type of orthosis occasionally used to provide some degree of grip.

ally effective. Paradoxically, tendon transfers are also much more effective for this type of neural loss than for that associated with median or ulnar nerve in cases in which nerve repairs are less successful.

Transfer of median- or ulnar-innervated flexor tendons to the dorsum of the wrist and to finger and thumb extensor regions can readily provide extensor function for the limb with a radial nerve injury. Some workers believe that this technique can be saved until the results of nerve repair are known, especially because the radial nerve regenerates so well. Others believe just as strongly that because such a procedure is an effective substitute for radial palsy, it should be done as soon as feasible.[10,15,17] A splint or similar device is provided in the meantime to prevent contracture and to assist finger flexion. A dynamic dorsiflexion splint with outrigger, rubber bands, and finger slings is a particularly effective device under these circumstances (Figure 19-3). We have usually waited and selected the weaker extensor functions for substitutive procedures, although the few extensor transfers done early have not been regretted. If the injury is not reparable or tendons are not available for transfer, wrist fusion in a position of partial extension is effective. Fusion places the hand in a more functional position, permitting what lumbrical function there is to extend the fingers while the median-innervated abductor pollicis brevis can pull the thumb away from the palm somewhat. Median- and ulnar-innervated

flexor superficialis and profundus muscles can flex the fingers, making a fist—a function that is not very effective with wrist drop unless the wrist is provided some degree of extension.

## BRACHIAL PLEXUS LOSS

Effective substitution for loss resulting from plexus injury is difficult to obtain. All too frequently, most of the muscles of the limb are severely paralyzed so that the possibilities for substitution or transfer are limited[16,23] (Figure 19-4).

Substitution for absent and irrecoverable biceps/brachialis function is a possibility if either sufficient latissimus dorsi or pectoralis is preserved and can be moved to the elbow region.[28] Unfortunately, most plexus injuries severe enough to result in total loss of biceps are usually too extensive in regard to neural input to latissimus dorsi or pectoralis to permit their transfer. A flexorplasty in which flexor mass is moved proximal to the elbow can be effective if the forearm muscles are innervated, but this is usually not the case.[11] An obvious exception is provided by the occasional C5-C6 stretch injury that does not reinnervate spontaneously and cannot be successfully repaired. Because forearm flexors are spared or minimally involved, a flexorplasty may work well.

Substitutive procedures for loss of shoulder abduction with proximal brachial plexus

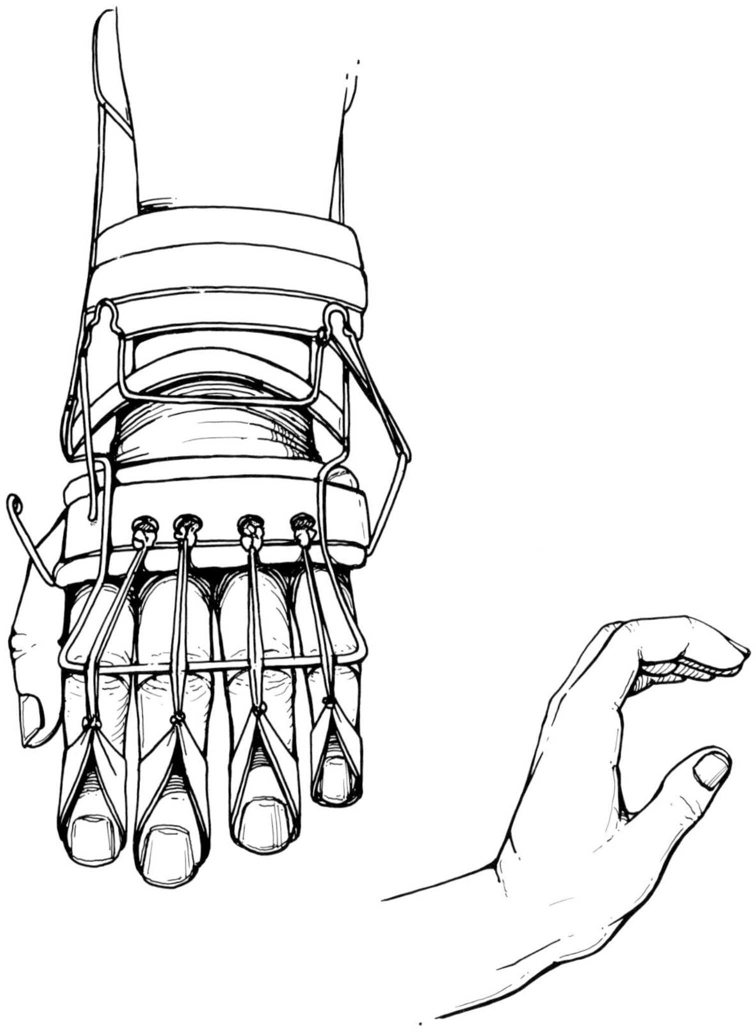

Dynamic Dorsiflexion Splint
With Outrigger Finger Pads and Rubber Bands

**Figure 19–3.** A brace used for radial palsy, especially if median- and ulnar-innervated finger flexion is present. This is called a dynamic dorsiflexion splint with outrigger, rubber bands, and finger pads. This brace places wrist and fingers in an optimal position *(smaller drawing)* and permits finger flexion against resistance.

injuries remain controversial. Fusion of the glenohumeral joint is probably the procedure of choice when the plexus injury spares hand function.[11,12,20,26] Shoulder fusion is most valuable if biceps/brachialis works or also can be substituted for, because provision of a more functional shoulder makes forearm flexion useful. Such fusions, properly done, do not totally fixate shoulder movement but rather permit the scapular muscles to provide improved abduction and shoulder rotation (Figure 19–5). Shoulder fusion remains one of the most popular and frequently used reconstructive procedures, particularly for severe brachial palsy involving the shoulder.[19] Less certain is transfer of a portion of the lateral trapezius to provide ac-

tive abduction of the shoulder. It can be difficult to achieve a balanced and therefore usable transfer with this operation.

The question of amputation arises with severe, irreparable brachial plexus injuries, particularly if there is some proximal shoulder and upper arm sparing, making the use of a prosthesis a strong possibility. The more distal the amputation site, the more useful the prosthesis is and the more likely it is that the amputee will use it (Figure 19–6). In general, even if the outlook is extremely poor, we usually wait for several years before advising amputation. By this time, it is clear to all, including the patient, that there is no hope for recovery, and the procedure is much more readily accepted. Before this is

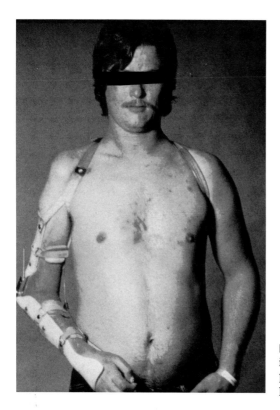

**Figure 19–4.** Some patients find an orthosis of help during the period of waiting for nerve regeneration after plexus injury; others refuse to wear either orthoses or prostheses with any consistency.

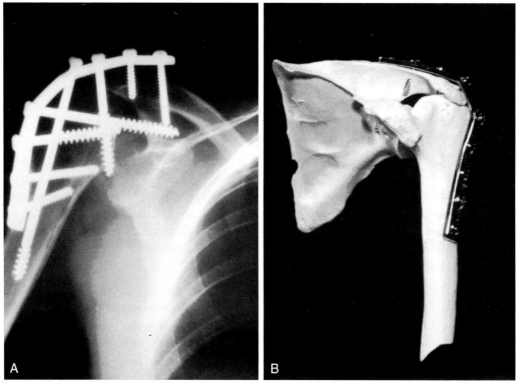

A

B

**Figure 19–5.** (*A* and *B*) Glenohumeral joint fusion can be useful in cases of poor abduction after irreparable or failed repair of outflow to axillary nerve. Patients obtain proximal control by way of trapezius, serratus anterior, and, if not part of the pattern of paralysis, latissimus dorsi and pectoralis major muscles. This procedure is especially useful if there is return of biceps or brachioradialis but not shoulder abduction, and especially if hand function is spared or recovers but proximal muscles do not.

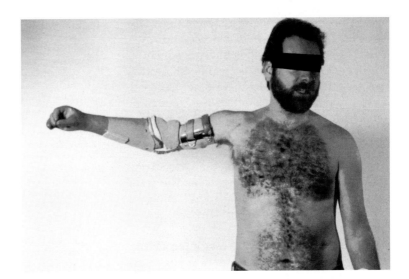

**Figure 19–6.** This patient with a flail arm had successful restoration of shoulder and biceps function by graft repair of the upper elements of the plexus. Lower elements were torn out of their foramina and could not be repaired. As a result, he had a forearm-level amputation and was then fitted with a prosthesis.

done, every attempt should be made to restore shoulder and upper arm function so that the amputation can be as distal as possible.[26] Earlier amputation may be indicated if severe nerve injury is also associated with severe vascular, soft tissue, or bony injury. In addition, some patients with flail arms opt for relatively early amputation of the limb, which they view as a useless impediment.

## LOWER EXTREMITY NEURAL LOSS

Several reconstructive procedures have been recommended to provide dorsiflexion of the foot if this is lost due to peroneal palsy. Unfortunately, dorsal transfer of tibial-innervated tendon is difficult to achieve in a balanced fashion and tends not to hold up in some patients who are large in stature and heavy in weight.[1] Nonetheless, some workers with a large experience with the lower extremity, such as Millesi, have success with such a transfer and may even do this at the time of peroneal nerve repair if outlook for neural recovery is limited.

Fusion at the ankle level also works better in small, light individuals than in the heavier-set persons, in whom it may break down and be a source of pain. A spring-loaded kick-up foot brace or even a plastic shoe insert dorsiflexion splint is far preferable to stabilization of the ankle and foot, because the brace permits an almost normal walking pattern. Many patients,

after they are taught to use the kick-up brace or shoe insert dorsiflexion splint, are quite happy with it and may not even wish anything further to be done about their peroneal nerve palsy.[25] If both peroneal- and tibial-innervated muscles are lost, triple arthrodesis of the ankle is sometimes necessary to provide as stable a foot or base for walking as possible. Substitution for tibial loss is not satisfactory because provision of powerful enough plantar flexion to step off or walk more normally cannot be provided adequately by transfer of extensor tendons. With tibial sensory loss, great attention needs to be given to protection of the insensitive foot.[4] This may require a customized shoe or shoe insert. The major effort, though, must be directed toward educating the patient regarding the insensate foot, how to avoid injury to it, and how to inspect the foot for injury and skin changes.

Reconstructive procedures available for patients with complete femoral nerve palsy are limited. Fusion of the knee in extension is not a very satisfactory substitute for a functional quadriceps. Similarly, braces to stabilize the knee and thigh are bulky, uncomfortable, and expensive and often are not worn by the patient. Some attempt at repair of the femoral nerve should be made whenever possible.

Use of direct stimulation to paralyzed muscle while awaiting recovery of peripheral nerve function has been advocated by many. To our knowledge, there is no objective or well-controlled evidence to date that the eventual result with such daily stimulation is any better than that gained from frequent passive motion of the paralyzed extremity.[14] In many cases, however, daily stimulation provides encouragement to the patient as well as his or her family, for they can see muscles contract that do not have voluntary contraction. It may also encourage an otherwise reluctant patient to attend physical therapy sessions. However, if the procedure becomes a time-consuming or painful one, it may prevent the patient from using the extremity for the functions of day-to-day living, and he or she may not even learn the substitutive and trick movements that patients learn when left to their own devices.

Further discussion on the use of reconstructive procedures for rehabilitation can be found in this book's individual chapters on various nerves as well as the brachial plexus.

## Bibliography

1. Bourrel P: Transfer of the tibialis posterior to the tibialis anterior, and of flexor hallucis longus to the extensor digitorum longus in peroneal palsy. Ann Chir 21: 1451–1456, 1967.
2. Boyes JH: Bunnell's Surgery of the Hand, 5th Ed. Philadelphia, JB Lippincott, 1970.
3. Brand P: Tendon transfers in the forearm. In Flynn J, Ed: Hand Surgery. Baltimore, Williams & Wilkins, pp. 331–342, 1966.
4. Brand P and Ebner JD: Pressure sensitive devices for denervated hands and feet. J Bone Joint Surg 51A: 109–116, 1969.
5. Chase RA: Atlas of Hand Surgery. Philadelphia: WB Saunders, 1984.
6. Gelberman R, Ed: Operative Nerve Repair and Reconstruction. Philadelphia, JB Lippincott, 1991.
7. Goldner JL: Function of the hand following peripheral nerve injuries. American Academy of Orthopedic Surgeons Instruction Course Lectures 10. Ann Arbor, Michigan, JW Edmonds, 1953, p. 268.
8. Green DP: Operative Hand Surgery. New York, Churchill Livingstone, 1988.
9. Jupiter J, Ed: Flynn's Hand Surgery. Baltimore, Williams & Wilkins, 1991.
10. Kettlekamp DB and Alexander H: Clinical review of radial nerve injury. J Trauma 7:424–432, 1967.
11. Leffert R: Brachial Plexus Injuries. London, Churchill Livingstone, 1985.
12. Leffert R: Reconstruction of the shoulder and elbow following brachial plexus injury. In Omer GE and Spinner M, Ed: Management of Peripheral Nerve Problems. Philadelphia, WB Saunders, 1980.
13. Littler JW: Tendon transfer and arthrodesis in combined median and ulnar nerve paralysis. J Bone Joint Surg 31A:225–234, 1949.
14. Liu CT and Lewey FH: The effect of surging currents of low frequency in man on atrophy of denervated muscles. J Nerve Ment Dis 105:571–581, 1947.
15. Mackinnon S and Dellon A: Surgery of the Peripheral Nerve. New York, Thieme Medical Publishers, 1988.
16. Narakas A: Thoughts on neurotization or nerve transfers in irreparable nerve lesions. Clin Plast Surg 11:153–159, 1984.
17. Omer GE: Evaluation and reconstruction of forearm and hand after acute traumatic peripheral nerve injuries. J Bone Joint Surg 50A:1454–1460, 1968.
18. Omer GE: Tendon transfers for the reconstruction of the forearm and hand following peripheral nerve injuries. In Omer GE and Spinner M, Eds: Management of Peripheral Nerve Problems. Philadelphia, WB Saunders, 1980.
19. Richards RR: Operative treatment for irreparable lesions of the brachial plexus. In Gelberman R, Ed: Operative Nerve Repair and Reconstruction. Philadelphia, JB Lippincott, 1991.
20. Richards RR, Sherman RM, Hudson AR, and Waddell JP: Shoulder arthrodesis using a pelvic reconstruction plate: A report of 11 cases. J Bone Joint Surg 70A: 416–421, 1988.
21. Riordan DC: Tendon transplantations in median nerve and ulnar nerve paralysis. J Bone Joint Surg 35A: 312–320, 1953.
22. Seddon HJ: Surgical Disorders of the Peripheral Nerves. Baltimore, Williams & Wilkins, 1972.
23. Simard J and Sypert G: Closed traction avulsion injuries of the brachial plexus. Contemp Neurosurg 50:1–6, 1983.
24. Tibiana R: The Hand, Vol. 2. Philadelphia, WB Saunders, 1985.
25. White JC: The results of traction injuries to the common peroneal nerve. J Bone Joint Surg 40B:346–351, 1968.
26. Wynn-Parry CB: The management of traction lesions of the brachial plexus and peripheral nerve injuries to the upper limb: A study in teamwork. Injury 11:265–285, 1980.
27. Zancolli E: Structural and Dynamic Basis of Hand Surgery. Philadelphia, JB Lippincott, 1979.
28. Zancolli E and Mitre H: Latissimus dorsi transfer to restore elbow flexion. J Bone Joint Surg 55A:1265–1272, 1973.

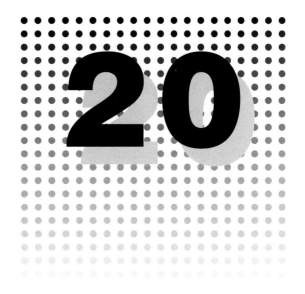

# Pain of
# Nerve Origin

# SUMMARY

Pain caused by a nerve lesion may be the major reason a patient seeks medical help. Such pain can be difficult to treat successfully, but early and accurately focused intervention, if such is afforded by both the patient and the referring physician, can make a difference. Skillful management of nerve-associated pain requires an exact characterization of the nature of the pain and associated findings. Far too many patients are mistakenly designated as having true causalgia or reflex sympathetic dystrophy, leading to incorrect and usually abortive pain syndrome management. These are both very specific diagnoses, and once they have been seen and recognized, other pain syndromes will not be mistaken for them. True causalgia and sometimes reflex sympathetic dystrophy temporarily respond to sympathetic blockade and vigorous physical therapy and may occasionally be cured without surgical sympathectomy.

Most serious pain associated with nerve lesions is not sympathetically mediated, is neuritic, and is often helped by proper surgical management of the neural injury and aggressive physical therapy. Neuritic pain may have an element of autonomic dysfunction but usually requires a different treatment regimen. Early mobilization of the limb and activities to encourage use of what can be moved are important, as are several medications thought to reduce the firing of irritable nerve fibers. Neuritic pain usually, but not always, diminishes with time. By comparison, pain caused by denervation of large muscles such as those of the shoulder or leg always dissipates with time as does that related to regeneration. Most patients with severe pain associated with stretch injury to the plexus improve with time if managed aggressively with early physical therapy and well-selected drugs, but there are exceptions, and these patients are candidates for dorsal root entry zone lesions. Finally, the terrible pain caused by disuse with secondary swelling of the limb, joint changes, and tendon shortening should not be permitted to occur. Nerves do not heal by rest. A limb with paralysis needs motion if secondary pain such as that experienced with a shoulder-hand syndrome or Achilles tendon shortening is to be prevented.

# INTRODUCTION

Not all nerve injuries result in significant pain, but those that do are challenges to manage. Unfortunately, many patients suffer from a painful limb after nerve injury because of prolonged and often unnecessary immobility or fixation of the limb. Tensile strength, even of a sutured nerve, is maximal by 3 weeks after repair.[12,29] Even if there is a question of tension and its effect on a neural repair site, the period of complete immobilization should seldom extend beyond 3 weeks.[25] Nerves do not heal by being placed at rest, nor do limbs with functional loss improve with immobility. Sometimes, the latter is necessary because of concomitant bony, tendon, or vascular injuries. After this necessary period of immobility for healing of these associated injuries, the limb with nerve injury must be moved regularly. Even with a limb in a cast, joints that are not encased need to be moved many times a day. Joint stiffness, tendon shortening, and swelling in an unused extremity are not only painful but can lead to a chronic pain syndrome and consequently a useless limb. Prevention includes a large dose of repetitive encouragement on the part of the physician, nurse, therapist, and often the patient's family.[34]

# REGENERATIVE PAIN

As nerve regenerates, there may be associated paresthesias, variously described as tingling electric shocks or even a burning feeling. The paresthesias or dysesthesias tend to be especially bothersome during the early months of the regenerative process.[22,23] The paresthesias that occur with regeneration should not be mistaken for neuritic pain or causalgia. Although patients complain of these paresthesias, after the physician describes the regenerative nature and cause of the bothersome sensation, they are more accepting of the condition and more likely to work with the involved extremity. Such a pain pattern is self-limited, as is the regenerative process itself. The patient who is frequently irritated by regenerative paresthesias may benefit from amitriptyline and carbamazepine as well as repetitive use of the limb, especially by exercises designed to desensitize it.

## DENERVATIONAL PAIN

The acute phase of denervation of muscles, especially of large ones such as infraspinatus, deltoid, biceps, triceps, quadriceps, or gastrocnemius-Achilles, can be quite painful.[21] Pain may be severe enough to require relatively strong analgesic drugs. Fortunately, after the acute phase has run its course and the muscle is atrophic, the pain either diminishes markedly or disappears entirely. This may not be the case, however, if joint stiffness or severe tendon shortening has occurred because of overzealous immobilization during the period of active denervation.

## CAUSALGIA AND REFLEX SYMPATHETIC DYSTROPHY

The term causalgia should be reserved for cases of true causalgia: a very characteristic and exquisite burning pain that begins in the distribution of an injured peripheral nerve and then spreads beyond it. This severe pain is accompanied by hyperesthesia and autonomic disturbances (Table 20–1). Usually, the patient tends to protect the extremity from contact and does not permit it to be handled or manipulated by the examiner. Even if the patient's attention is distracted, the individual with true causalgia or reflex sympathetic dystrophy (RSD) does not permit the involved hand or foot to be handled.[16] Of great importance is the fact that the pain and, to a lesser extent, autonomic disturbance do respond to sympathetic block and subsequent sympathectomy[8] (Figure 20–1). Using these criteria, there is a low incidence of true causalgia and RSD, even with severe nerve injuries. The incidence has ranged from only 2

**TABLE 20–1**
## Major Characteristics of True Causalgia

1. Severe burning pain begins in a nerve's distribution and soon spreads to involve other distributions and then the whole extremity. It can have associated paresthesias and hyperesthesia.
2. It is associated with autonomic hyperfunction with vasodilation and increased sweating, but can alternate with autonomic hypofunction and result in a limb that is cool, blanched, cyanotic, or without ability to sweat.
3. The patient with true causalgia seldom permits the limb to be manipulated, even if his or her attention is distracted by the examiner.
4. True causalgia is almost always caused by a major injury to a major mixed motor/sensory nerve such as the median, ulnar, or tibial division of sciatic.
5. Both autonomic abnormalities and the pain are helped at least temporarily by sympathetic block. Definitive and more lasting relief usually can be obtained by a thorough sympathectomy.

to 2.5 percent, at least in our civilian experience. Many patients believed to have causalgia when they were evaluated elsewhere did not meet our criteria for this diagnosis and subsequently gained substantial relief by resection and repair of their usually almost complete peripheral nerve lesions. In a few instances in which the lesion was less complete, operative manipulation of the nerve and release of a complicating entrapment were of help.

Mayfield and others have determined that a complete sympathectomy well proximal to the site of pain should be done to insure success in the properly selected patient with true causalgia.[11,25,28] Nonetheless, such a thorough sympathectomy will not relieve pain if it is not sympathetically mediated. It is in the cases of so-called minor causalgia or findings suggesting causalgia, but to a lesser extent than true causalgia, that controversy exists.[8,17] RSD is one of these syndromes. The diagnosis is harder to make than that for true causalgia, and sympathetic block or chemical blockade or sympathectomy is less certain of producing lasting relief.[3,25] The clinician must listen and look for a burning pain mixed with autonomic symptoms, and, as with true causalgia, manipulation of the extremity, even with distraction, should be difficult or not permitted by the patient at all. In some cases of minor causalgia, such as RSD, a Sudeck dystrophy occurs. This is a dystrophic condition affecting the ankle, foot, or hand with mild autonomic changes and finally osteoporo-

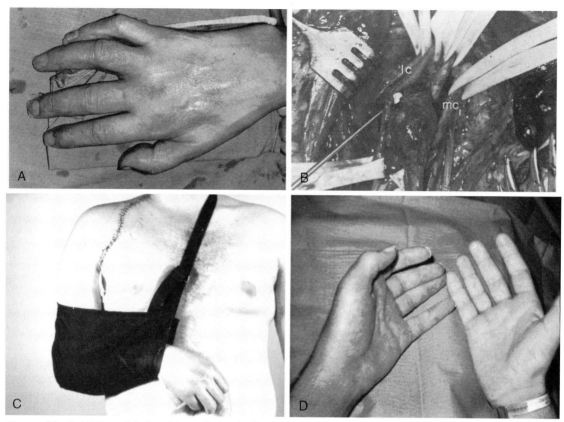

**Figure 20–1.** *(A)* Causalgic hand in patient who had sustained a gunshot wound to the plexus nearly a year before. Loss in the distribution of each plexus element was incomplete, but severe hand pain prohibited effective use of the limb. *(B)* A moderate-sized pseudoaneurysm was found, involving axillary artery and stretching and displacing cord-to-nerve segments of plexus. The aneurysm was resected and a neurolysis of the plexus was done. This gave relief of the severe hand pain for 72 hours only. lc = lateral cord; mc = medial cord. *(C)* A cervical sympathetic block was done, which temporarily relieved the pain. As a result, a cervical sympathectomy was done through a supraclavicular approach, and this reversed the pain syndrome completely. The patient eventually made a complete recovery. *(D)* In another patient, a postsympathectomy hand to the left is compared with a more normal one to the right.

sis after relatively minor injuries such as a sprain. Sympathectomy may be of some value for RSD but is usually not useful for other causalgia-like syndromes affecting the upper extremity.

RSD is often caused by a relatively minor injury or an operation involving the wrist, hand, ankle, or foot and may be compounded by a period of prolonged immobilization or, in a few cases, by too early use of the affected part. Symptoms and findings seen in a patient with suspected RSD can vary somewhat depending on the phase or time after onset of the disorder (Tables 20–2, 20–3, and 20–4).[26] The majority of these patients are depressed, and it is difficult to be certain whether affective symptoms were the cause or the result of RSD in the fully devel-

oped case. Most of the signs of RSD are the signs of disuse atrophy. Sympathectomy may help, but only if well-done blocks indicate substantial relief, and only if the individual can be convinced to use the affected extremity after sym-

**TABLE 20–2**
Reflex Sympathetic Dystrophy
Stage I—Acute Phase

1. Stage I usually occurs during the first 3 months after injury.
2. Burning pain is out of proportion with the degree of injury and usually in the distribution of a nerve, and hyperesthesia and allodynia are present.
3. There is edema and ruborous and usually warm skin; on the other hand, skin can be cool and blanched.
4. Sweating is usually increased, but at times can be decreased.

**TABLE 20-3**
Reflex Sympathetic Dystrophy
Stage II—Subacute or Dystrophic Phase

1. Stage II usually occurs 3 to 6 months after injury.
2. Constant pain usually involves all of the distal portion of the extremity. Usually, hyperesthesia and allodynia persist.
3. There is secondary joint stiffness and cool, cyanotic-appearing skin, with hair loss.
4. Osteoporosis may be present and bone scan (three-phase) may be abnormal.

pathectomy.[6,25,28] On the other hand, some clinicians believe that such a syndrome can only be reversed by repetitive stress and use of the affected extremity, and that blockade or obliteration of the sympathetically mediated portion of the syndrome has limited value. For the leg, weight-bearing on the affected foot is a must. Without this during the recuperative phase, eventual function of the leg is compromised. For the hand, there is no substitute for its repetitive use, even though sympathetic blocks or sympathectomy have given some relief. Campbell prefers to categorize patients with causalgia-like symptoms and response to sympatholytic agents as those with sympathetically mediated pain.[3] In his experience, use of intravenous phentolamine relieves most of these symptoms and, if used recurrently, may correct the disorder without surgery.

## NEURITIC PAIN RELATED TO NEURAL INJURY

This type of pain can be severe and can be associated with paresthesias and hyperesthesia mixed with hypoesthesia as well as pain with a burning quality.[2,5] Neuritic pain does not have associated autonomic dysfunction, is not

helped by sympathetic ablation, but may be helped by surgical repair or manipulation of the injured or involved nerve (Table 20-5). Experience suggests the need for local exploration and correction of the nerve lesion associated with neuritic pain if possible (Figure 20-2). The examiner may be misled into thinking a nerve injury is incomplete because of sensory overlap or branching from adjacent nerves or, even more often, because of shared or anomalous innervation syndromes, particularly in the hand.[19,32] This may lead to belief that a resection cannot be done, and so the patient's pain problem persists. The presence of fine fibers in the area of injury or even beyond it may be responsible for pain, yet the lesion should be resected because this type of regeneration does not lead to good function.[1,11] Such an approach is dependent on operative recording. If no nerve action potential is recorded in the early months, or if one with poor amplitude and conduction of less than 20 msec is recorded 9 or more months after injury, then the lesion associated with severe pain needs to be resected and repaired. Medications such as amitriptyline and carbamazepine or related drugs can sometimes control neuritic pain.[10] Unfortunately, such medications are not always effective, nor is surgical correction of the lesion. Nonetheless, one or both of these tacts are usually worth a try.

Implantation of stimulating electrodes either above or below the injury and use of chronic transcutaneous stimulation have produced relief of pain in some patients.[13,14] Here again, however, caution is advised. Sometimes, operation on the injury itself not only relieves pain but assists regeneration, which implantation of stimulating electrodes certainly does not do.[3,11] Although relief of pain is one of our prime obligations as physicians and especially as neurosurgeons, an equally important goal in manage-

**TABLE 20-4**
Reflex Sympathetic Dystrophy
Stage III—Chronic Phase

1. Stage III usually occurs 6 months or longer after injury.
2. Constant, intense pain is present in a patient with a stiff and atrophic extremity.
3. There is soft tissue atrophy; thin, cool, and grey-appearing skin; poor sweating; and hair loss.
4. Secondary joint changes can occur, and Sudek dystrophy may be a feature.

**TABLE 20-5**
Usual Characteristics of Neuritic Pain

1. Severe pain occurs in the distribution of an injured nerve.
2. Sensory and/or motor loss can be partial or complete.
3. Pain can have a burning quality along with paresthesias, but autonomic dysfunction does not predominate.
4. Local tenderness in the region of the injury site and local Tinel sign are likely but not always present.
5. Pain may be helped by amitriptyline, carbamazepine, and related drugs. Surgical repair or manipulation of the responsible neural lesion may be curative in some cases.

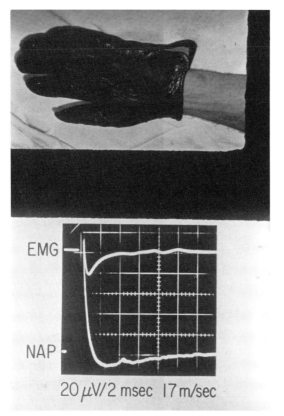

EMG

NAP

20 μV/2 msec   17 m/sec

**Figure 20 – 2.** Patient had gunshot wound to forearm 1 year earlier that involved the median nerve. Neurolysis of nerve had been done elsewhere because loss was incomplete, with sparing of thenar intrinsic function. Patient had severe neuritic pain which had some elements of causalgic pain. He wore a glove over the hand, even in very hot weather *(upper inset)*. Pain did not respond to sympathetic blocks. At exploration, a neuroma in continuity was found. This transmitted only a very small nerve action potential, and no motor function could be evoked by stimulating either above or below the lesion *(lower inset)*. The lesion was resected, and an end-to-end repair was done, with considerable improvement in pain and return of sensation to a grade of 3 to 4 over several years. Thenar function was not lost. In retrospect, this patient had one type of a Martin-Gruber anastomosis with abductor pollicis brevis and opponens pollicis fibers traveling to hand in ulnar nerve. Most of the pain was neuritic and resulted from an almost complete lesion in continuity which had regenerated poorly.

ment of peripheral nerve injuries is provision of useful function for the extremity.

Many pain syndromes become established relatively early at a central level.[18,33] The severe pain associated with some stretch and avulsive injuries to the plexus may require dorsal root entry zone (DREZ) lesions as devised by Nashold.[20,35] Because there are definite risks of paresis or paralysis and truncal sensory loss associated with these and other central procedures for severe pain, patients must be well selected.[27,30] Pain should be persistent and severe despite intensive physical therapy and closely supervised pharmacologic management. The latter usually includes trials of slowly increased dosages of Tegretol, Elavil, Pamelor, Klonopin, Mexitil, or related medications.[1,15] Both of us have had experience in the management of many patients with nerve injury, with remarkably low incidences of RSD and of patients requiring DREZ lesions in both practices. There are, nonetheless, some patients who do require DREZ lesioning for their severe phantom limb pain or sympathectomy for causalgia or RSD.

Our belief is that the best results are obtained by vigorous physical therapy with an at-home exercise program carried out by the patient with the help of the therapist. This, coupled with an appropriate explanation of the organic and psychic phenomena to both patient and family, can either prevent or ameliorate the majority of these severe pain syndromes.

## Case Summaries — Pain of Nerve Origin

### Case Number 1

This 48-year-old man received a 22-caliber gunshot wound to the lower third of the forearm. The wound was debrided elsewhere, and the median nerve was found partially transected and was sutured. A neuroma formed which led to several operations in an attempt to trim the neuroma and relieve the resulting severe neuritic pain. A more distal carpal tunnel release was done in the hope that manipulation of the median nerve at the proximal palmar and wrist levels would be of help.

On referral several years after the accident, there was a palpable and tender neuroma under one of several well-healed forearm scars. Thenar muscles such as abductor pollicis brevis and opponens pollicis worked well (grade 4 to 5) and were only mildly atrophic. Lumbricals to the forefinger and long finger worked well, but sensation in the median distribution graded only 2. Electromyographic and conductive studies were done and showed that input to the hand muscles, including those of the thenar eminence, was primarily of ulnar origin. Thus, the patient had a predominantly ulnar-innervated hand. Tapping over the forearm neuroma gave paresthesias and pain in the fingers and thumb.

At exploration, the median was not only scarred but was also quite neuromatous. Stimulation either above or below the lesion gave no distal muscle function. In addition, there was no transmission of a nerve action potential across the lesion. As a result, the neuroma was resected, and an end-to-end nerve repair was done. This was effective in relieving the patient's pain, and over a 2.5-year period, median sensation improved to grade 3 to 4. There was no change postoperatively in thenar or lumbrical function.

## Comment

Use of simple stimulation to the median nerve during one of the prior operations would not have produced thenar contraction. This would have indicated the dominant input to hand intrinsics by the ulnar nerve and might have suggested the need for earlier resection of the median neuroma. Pain due to nerve injury often requires operation on the nerve injury and its correction for relief.

## Case Number 2

A similar situation to that seen in case number 1 was found in a retired, 50-year-old Air Force sergeant who sustained a gunshot wound involving the median nerve. He had undergone several operations in which neurolysis was done, presumably because this was considered to be a partial nerve lesion. In addition, recurrent sympathetic blocks had been done to assuage causalgic-like pain. The blocks were only partially successful when in place.

He was evaluated 1.5 years after injury at LSUMC and had a Tinel sign giving severe hand pain over the original wound entry site at the distal forearm level. Electromyographic studies suggested only partial denervation of median-innervated thenar muscles. At operation, however, the lesion in continuity did not transmit a nerve action potential, nor did stimulation give distal muscle function. Resection of the neuroma and suture repair gave good pain relief, and sensory function graded 4 by 3 years, with motor function remaining at 3 to 4.

## Comment

Muscles usually innervated by median or ulnar nerves may in fact have anomalous input.

## Case Number 3

This 37-year-old man complained bitterly of right ankle and foot pain that was of a burning as well as a dysesthetic nature. He related its onset to a midshaft fracture of the right femur as a result of being thrown from a motorcycle 6 years before. To his knowledge, he had had no functional deficit either before or after his fracture management. The latter included initial balanced skeletal traction followed by rod placement. The rod had been removed several years after placement, but his foot and ankle symptoms had not changed. Some time in the first week or so after his discharge from the hospital, he noted tingling in the sole of the foot, and then over a period of a few months burning pain began in the sole of the foot and eventually involved the ankle and whole foot. Pain was worse with weight-bearing but was also present without activity; pain was also worse at night and only partially relieved by analgesics. It was not helped by several sympathetic blocks, even when the foot was made warm and hyperemic. Other types of anesthetic blocks helped only if the foot was made numb.

When seen by our service, the patient had deep tenderness in the posterior thigh and on very hard percussion over the course of the sciatic nerve. At that level, there was a mild Tinel sign radiating to the posterior calf. There was mild weakness of toe flexion, but plantar flexion, inversion, dorsiflexion of foot and toes, and eversion were normal. He tolerated manipulation of the foot and leg, although he reported a mild reduction in touch on the plantar surface of the foot and some dysesthesias there when it was stroked. Radiographs showed a well-healed midshaft femoral fracture with some but not excessive callus. Electromyographs revealed very chronic and mild denervational changes in most tibial division muscles. There was no evidence of a more recent denervational change. Imaging studies done elsewhere did not indicate any swelling or mass effect involving the sciatic nerve. Scans of the lumbar spine showed mild degenerative changes.

At surgical exploration, both extra- and intraneural scar involved the posterior tibial nerve just after it split away from the peroneal division at the junction of the middle and lower third of the thigh. The lesion conducted a good-sized NAP, although velocity across the lesion was only 40 msec. Both an external and a partial internal neurolysis were done and neither inspection nor direct recording from groups of fascicles indicated the need for resection. Fortunately, even though the patient reported increased numbness on the sole of the foot postoperatively, motor function remained good and most important, pain decreased, although it did not stop completely. Over the intervening 5.5 years of follow-up, the patient has experienced increased use of the limb but still reports some dysesthesias if it is bumped or he comes down too hard on the sole of the foot. He is able to maintain a relatively sedentary occupation in sales but does not feel capable of running or participating in most sports.

# PAINFUL NEUROMAS

Neuromas involving sensory nerves such as the dorsal cutaneous branch of the ulnar, superficial sensory radial, antebrachial cutaneous nerves, and the sural and saphenous nerves are

**Figure 20–3.** (A) Neuroma on a sensory portion of the cervical plexus caused by a laceration. The patient had pain and paresthesias whenever this portion of the neck was bumped or stroked. (B) Neuroma on dorsal cutaneous nerve at the forearm level caused by a lacerating injury. Remainder of ulnar nerve is to the right and is headed toward Guyon canal. After resection, proximal nerve was trimmed sharply and fasciculi were grasped with fine-tipped bipolar forceps and bovied in an attempt to seal them shut. The freshly trimmed stump was left deep to the flexor carpi ulnaris. See also color figure.

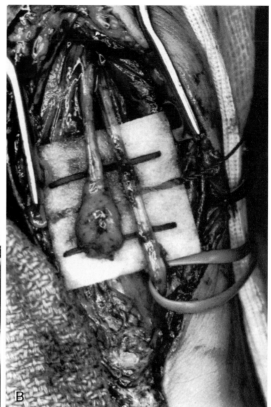

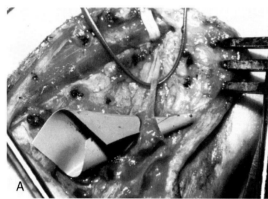

best treated by wide resection without repair.[15,31] Attempts at the latter too often lead to recurrent pain and paresthesias after regeneration occurs through the site. In addition, the sensory territories served by these nerves are of low functional importance, so that numbness in their distribution is preferable to painful paresthesias, dysesthesias, or hyperesthesia in their innervational territories (Figure 20–3).

One of us prefers sharp section of the nerve well above the neuroma and resection of the latter along with 5 to 10 cm of proximal and distal nerve. The fine bipolar tips are then used under loupe or microscopic magnification to individually seal shut the proximal tips of each fascicle. The treated end is then buried beneath muscle or other substantial soft tissue planes in the proximal limb.[4] The nerve end is not sutured to muscle or other tissue. This approach appears to reduce the incidence of recurrent neuromata, although, as with every other technique ever devised for painful neuromas, there is no guarantee of success. Wherever possible, neuroma, as well as nerve well proximal and distal to it, needs resection. Mackinnon and Dellon have

shown that neuromata in distal limb, especially of the superficial sensory radial in the forearm, can attract branches from adjacent sensory nerves, such as the lateral sensory portion of the musculocutaneous nerve or one of the antebrachial cutaneous nerves.[15] This observation favors not only excision of the neuroma but also scar and other tissue around it.

## AFFECTIVE RESPONSES ASSOCIATED WITH PAIN

Anxiety and depression are understandable symptoms in a patient who has suffered a nerve injury. The surgeon should recognize these affective responses and ensure that these do not hinder progress. A depressed patient does not exercise the limb sufficiently, and stiffness and autonomic changes supervene. It is far more difficult to treat the resulting stiff, atrophic, painful limb than to prevent its occurrence. A depressed patient must not be allowed to assume a passive attitude, expecting the therapist to do the work. There is no substitute for an active range of movement regimen performed by the patient at home.

Malingering may occasionally be diagnosed. In this situation, the patient deceives the surgeon by complaining of disability in excess of the organic disorder and usually exaggerates the pain syndrome. More common is functional exaggeration of organic disability in a situation in which the patient is hoping for secondary financial gain. Inappropriate tests and therapies fix the patient's attention more and more on the nerve injury, so that it is subsequently difficult to resolve the problem by active and passive exercise and encouragement.

There are a number of operations used for pain associated with peripheral nerve injury. Two of the most popular are lumbar and cervical sympathectomy. These procedures are, in our experience, sometimes used on poorly selected patients and thus may be overused. Nonetheless, an adequate description of the essential steps in accomplishing a sympathectomy is important, especially in a book devoted to nerve injuries.

## LUMBAR SYMPATHECTOMY

The patient is anesthetized in a supine position using an intratracheal technique.[7,24] A roll or several folded sheets are placed under the flank on the side to be done. Hip and knee are partially flexed by placing a pillow beneath the ipsilateral knee. This tends to relax the psoas muscles somewhat. A skin incision is made in the flank obliquely from the tip of the lower ribs towards the inguinal region. The incision is usually 10 to 12 cm in length. External oblique muscle fibers are split in the direction they run and are kept apart by a self-retaining retractor. The internal oblique is then split in the direction of its fibers. Usually, the assistant holds these muscle edges apart with small Richardson or Army-Navy retractors. Then, the transversalis fibers are bluntly separated by the gloved fingers in a lateral or inferior direction. This latter maneuver permits visualization of the extraperitoneal fat. Index and middle fingers are then inserted through the muscle splitting incision, and their palmar surfaces are pressed against the transversalis muscle laterally.

Fingers are then used to dissect a plane of cleavage between fat and posterior peritoneum and the posterior abdominal wall. The gloved hand then slides over the inner surface of the quadratus lumborum to the lateral psoas muscle and then up over this muscle group. In this fashion, some of the peritoneal fat lies on the palmar surface of the hand and peritoneum is above or superior to the back of the operator's hand. Either a cotton strip or a large cotton ball with an attached string can be held in place by the fingers while a Grant bladder or other curved retractor such as a Deaver is placed.[9] This is used to elevate the peritoneum and its enclosed abdominal contents. This retractor is also used to help expose the lateral portion of the lumbar vertebrae. Another curved abdominal retractor can then be inserted more cephalad at or above the attachments of the crus of the diaphragm.

The lumbar sympathetic chain is then usually found lying in the gutter formed by the rounded portion of the bodies of the vertebrae and the more medial portion of the belly of the psoas. The sympathetic chain can be elevated with a long-handled nerve hook so that rami, and then finally both ends close to the diaphragmatic crus and at the lumbosacral promontory, can be sectioned. The chain may lie beneath lumbar arterial branches on the left side or lumbar bridging veins on the right side, and these may need to be coagulated or tied off before the chain is dissected out. In addition, on the right side, some of vena cava may lie over the sympathetic chain and may need gentle elevation to expose the chain more completely. After resection of a length of this chain, muscle levels are closed in layers. Subcutaneous tissues and skin are tacked down to external oblique muscle to avoid a dead space and subsequent fluid collection in the flank.

## CERVICOTHORACIC SYMPATHECTOMY

This portion of the sympathetic chain can be most conveniently approached either by a supraclavicular or dorsal thoracic approach.[7,9,24] In recent years, some thoracic surgeons have removed the chain by a transaxillary approach or a transpleural approach. A technique for cervicothoracic sympathectomy using an endoscopic approach has also been described and is in use by some surgeons.

Because we are familiar with exposure of the supraclavicular brachial plexus, this fairly straightforward approach to this portion of the sympathetic chain is described here. Usually, the operation is done with the patient supine and anesthetized with an intratracheal technique. Several folded sheets are placed under the ipsilateral shoulder. The head is turned away from the surgical site. The incision is placed parallel with the clavicle and an inch or so superior to it. Platysma muscle is exposed and divided transversely and in the same direction as the transverse skin incision. Some of the clavicular portion of the sternocleidomastoid muscle is removed from the clavicle. A Richardson or similar retractor is placed beneath the sternocleidomastoid, and this is elevated somewhat and retracted medially to expose supraclavicular fat over the anterior scalene. Omohyoid is usually dissected out of supraclavicular fat and divided, although it can sometimes be retracted cephalad by a Penrose drain. Supraclavicular fat is mobilized, taking care especially on a left-sided approach to identify and, if possible, protect the thoracic duct. If this is entered and lymph leaks, the duct can be coagulated by the bipolar forceps or sometimes sutured shut. Thoracic duct is more likely to be preserved on the left side if fat is mobilized medially. On the right side, because the main lymph channels are not as superior, supraclavicular fat can be mobilized laterally.

Supraclavicular artery and vein or transverse cervical vessels then need to be divided. The anterior scalene is then palpable, and the phrenic nerve is seen coursing over its anterior aspect. The latter is mobilized by a combination of sharp dissection with a No. 15 scalpel blade and use of fine-nosed Metzenbaum scissors. The phrenic can have two branches, and both need to be preserved. The medial edge of the anterior scalene is freed of vessels, some of which may need to be coagulated with the bipolar forceps. The upper trunk and the distal portion of the C5 spinal nerve are freed from the anterior scalene's lateral edge. C6 is identified as it courses under the anterior scalene and is gently freed from its underside. Lower or inferior anterior scalene is freed from underlying subclavian artery, which is then protected by a sponge or

moist cotton strip. We prefer to pass heavy sutures beneath the superior and inferior aspects of the scalene muscle. These sutures are used to elevate the muscle as it is divided at either end. In this fashion, a segment of anterior scalene is removed.

C7 and middle trunk can usually be identified and protected. Medial or middle scalene is then identified. Along its medial border lies the C8 nerve root or spinal nerve, and then attached to the latter is the T1 spinal nerve. The cervical dorsal sympathetic chain is at right angles to the T1 spinal nerve, usually lying anterior to it but posterior to the vertebral artery. Some of the subclavian artery can be skeletonized and gently elevated with a vein hook. This tents up the vertebral artery. Posterior to the origin of vertebral from subclavian artery, the stellate or inferior cervical ganglion can usually be palpated. This has a somewhat rubbery feel, much like an eraser. Rami approaching this and entering and leaving the T1 spinal nerve can be seen, especially with the help of loupes or the operating microscope. The sympathetic chain is then traced down into the mediastinum. This exposes several levels or about 3 to 4 cm of the more caudal chain. These are dissected out and either coagulated or clipped at both ends and then divided. Some surgeons prefer to include the lower half of the stellate ganglion, although this increases the likelihood of an accompanying Horner syndrome.

It is easy, unfortunately, to enter apical pleura at this level. If that occurs, we close pleura, usually by use of a 4-0 silk suture on a small needle, such as is used for dural closure. The anesthetist is asked to perform a Valsalva maneuver on the patient as the suture is tied shut to evacuate any intrapleural blood or irrigation fluid as thoroughly as possible. At the end of the closure, a Valsalva is done after the wound is filled with saline to check for pleural leak. A drain may or may not be placed, and closure is in layers, primarily to subcutaneous and skin levels. A mildly compressive dressing is then applied to the neck. A chest radiograph taken in the recovery room may be of help.

### Bibliography

1. Burchiel KJ and Ochoa JL: Surgical management of posttraumatic neuropathic pain. Neurosurg Clin North Am 2:117–126, 1991.

2. Campbell JN, Raja SN, and Meyer RA: Myelinated afferents signal the hyperalgesia associated with nerve injury. Pain 32:89–94, 1988.

3. Campbell JN, Raja SN, and Meyer RA: Painful sequelae of nerve injury. In Dubner R, Ed: Pain Research and Clinical Management. Proceedings, 5th World Congress on Pain. Amsterdam, Elsevier, 1988.

4. Dellon AL and Mackinnon S: Treatment of the painful neuroma by neuroma resection and muscle implantation. Plast Reconstr Surg 77:427–436, 1986.

5. Devor M: The pathophysiology and anatomy of damaged nerve. In Wall PD and Melzack R, Eds: Textbook of Pain. New York, Churchill Livingstone, 1984.

6. Goldner JL: Function of the hand following peripheral nerve injuries. American Academy of Orthopedic Surgeons Instruction Course Lectures 10. Ann Arbor, Mich, JW Edmonds, 1953, p. 268.

7. Hardy R and Bay J: Surgery of the sympathetic nervous system. In Schmidek H and Sweet W, Eds: Operative Neurosurgical Techniques. New York, Grune & Stratton, 1988.

8. Hendler N: Reflex sympathetic dystrophy and causalgia. In Tollison CD, Ed: Handbook of Chronic Pain Management. New York, Williams & Wilkins, 1989.

9. Kempe L: Operative Neurosurgery. New York, G Thieme, 1978.

10. Killian JM and Fromm GH: Carbamazepine in the treatment of neuralgia. Arch Neurol 19:129–136, 1968.

11. Kline DG and Hudson AR: Complications of peripheral nerve repair. In Greenfield L, Ed: Complications in Surgery. Philadelphia, JB Lippincott, 1985, pp. 695–708.

12. Liu CT, Benda CF, and Lewey FH: Tensile strength of human nerves. Arch Neurol Psychiatry 59:322–336, 1948.

13. Loeser J, Black R, and Christman A: Relief of pain by transcutaneous stimulation. J Neurosurg 43:308–314, 1978.

14. Long D: Neuromodulation for the control of chronic pain. Surg Rounds 5:25–34, 1982.

15. Mackinnon S and Dellon A: Surgery of the peripheral nerve. New York, Thieme Medical Publishers, 1988.

16. Mayfield FH: Causalgia. American Lecture Series. Springfield, IL, Charles C Thomas, 1951.

17. Mayfield FH: Reflex dystrophies of the hand. In Flynn JE, Ed: Hand Surgery. Baltimore, Williams & Wilkins, 1966, p. 1095 (see also pp. 738–750).

18. Melzack R and Wall PD: Pain mechanisms: A new theory. Science 150:971–979, 1965.

19. Murphey F, Kirklin JW, and Finlaysan AI: Anomalous innervation of the intrinsic muscles of hand. Surg Gynecol Obstet 83:15–23, 1946.

20. Nashold BS and Ostahl RH: Dorsal root entry zone lesions for pain relief. J Neurosurg 51:59–69, 1979.

21. Noordenbos W: Pain. Amsterdam, Elsevier, 1959.

22. Ochoa J: Pain in local nerve lesions. In Culp WJ and Ochoa J, Eds: Abnormal Nerves and Muscles as Impulse Generators. New York, Oxford University Press, 1982.

23. Ochs G: Painful dysesthesias following peripheral nerve injury: A clinical and electrophysiological study. Brain Res 4:228–240, 1989.

24. Poppen J: Neurosurgical Techniques. Philadelphia, WB Saunders, 1960.

25. Seddon HJ, Ed: Surgical Disorders of the Peripheral Nerves. Baltimore, Williams & Wilkins, 1972.

26. Schwartzman RJ and McLellan TL: Reflex sympathetic dystrophy. A review. Arch Neurol 44:555–561, 1987.

27. Simard J and Sypert G: Closed traction avulsion injuries of the brachial plexus. Contemp Neurosurg 50:1–6, 1983.

28. Sunderland S: Nerve and Nerve Injuries. Baltimore, Williams & Wilkins, 1968.

29. Tarlov IM: How long should an extremity be immobilized after nerve suture? Ann Surg 126:336–376, 1947.

30. Thomas D and Sheely J: Dorsal root entry zone lesions (Nashold's procedure) for pain relief following brachial plexus avulsion. J Neurol Neurosurg Psychiatry 46:924–928, 1983.

31. Tindall S: Painful neuromas. In Williams R and Regachary S, Eds: Neurosurgery. New York, McGraw-Hill, 1985, pp. 1884–1886.

32. Weddell G, Guttmann L, and Guttmann E: The local extension of nerve fibers into denervated areas of skin. J Neurol Psychiatry 4:206, 1941.

33. White JC and Sweet WH: Pain and the Neurosurgeon: A Forty Year Experience. Springfield, IL, CC Thomas, 1969.

34. Wynn-Parry CB: Rehabilitation of the Hand. London, Butterworths, 1966.

35. Zorub D, Nashold BS, and Cook WA: Avulsion of the brachial plexus: I. A review with implications on the therapy of intractable pain. Surg Neurol 2:347–353, 1974.

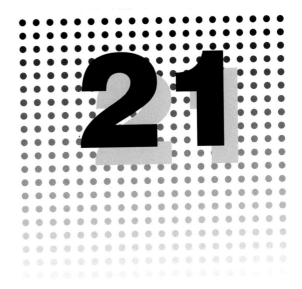

# Tumors Involving Nerve

# SUMMARY

Tumors involving nerve provide some of the most challenging and at times vexatious lesions to manage when dealing with a broad spectrum of peripheral nerve problems. Magnification, use of intraoperative recordings, and knowledge of the gross and microscopic pathology are important to the surgeon undertaking tumor resection. An understanding of the tumor's disposition concomitant with an awareness of the involved as well as spared fascicles can improve the surgeon's ability to resect benign neural sheath tumors. Summarized in this chapter are the presentations, operative techniques used, and outcomes of a series of 288 benign neural sheath tumors. The success rate for excision without significant deficit for schwannomas in this series was almost 90%. This figure was 80% for solitary neurofibromas not associated with von Recklinghausen disease (VRD), and that represents a departure from the standard in most literature, especially where only biopsy is recommended for the majority of these lesions. Successful resection of VRD-associated neurofibromas was 66%. On the other hand, it was difficult to gain any satisfactory results with plexiform tumors. Postoperative pain and likelihood of functional deficit were less of a problem if the benign neural sheath tumor had not been biopsied or operated on at a previous time.

Malignant neural sheath tumors and neurogenic sarcomas of nerve require especially discriminating management. Our operative experience and outcomes with 21 such lesions are presented. In recent years, some attempt at limb-sparing management has been studied, although amputation of the limb or forequarter amputation was done in 10 of the 21 patients. A relatively large operative experience with benign tumors or masses secondarily involving nerve is also presented. This subset included 21 ganglion cysts, 10 vascular tumors or lesions, 7 lipomas, and 6 desmoid tumors. Although usually palliative, resection of secondary or metastatic cancer involving plexus or nerve can help pain considerably and occasionally even reverse deficit in selected cases. Twenty-five such lesions, most of which involved brachial plexus, are discussed. Less efficacious appears to be surgery for irradiation plexitis, either with or without associated metastatic disease. Fourteen such cases are summarized. Finally, an unusual surgical entity involving nerve, hypertrophic neuropathy or "onion whorl disease," is discussed based on our experience to date with 13 histologically verified samples.

This is a fascinating and challenging facet of peripheral neuropathology. There are two broad categories of tumors involving nerve. The first is composed of those of neural sheath origin. Electron microscopy and microchemistry have aided in the classification of these tumors. Despite sophisticated analysis of the pathology, however, the issue of the exact cellular origins of various neural sheath tumors remains unsettled. These tumors begin within nerve, grow in it, and can project from it.[16,86] There are two subcategories: benign and malignant. Included in the benign group are schwannomas and neurofibromas. Examples of malignant tumors of neural sheath origin are neurogenic or fibrogenic sarcomas.

The second category includes tumors of non–neural sheath origin. These can also be subdivided further into benign and malignant lesions. Benign but not necessarily nicely behaved ones include ganglions, hemangiomas, lipomas, desmoids, lymphangiomas, myoblastomas, ganglioneuromas, and even a rare hemangioblastoma or an occasional meningioma.

Malignant tumors can arise from other structures and either involve nerve by direct extension or metastasize to it. Most often seen is infiltration or compression by breast cancer or by pulmonary cancer such as Pancoast tumor, extension or encasement by osteogenic sarcoma, or neural involvement by soft tissue sarcoma of non-neural sheath origin.[2] Metastatic disease can also spread to nerve or adjacent sites from a distant origin and secondarily involve it. This is rare but does occur. Examples in our clinics have been provided by primary tumors such as lymphoma and melanoma.

# CLASSIFICATION OF NERVE SHEATH TUMORS

Classification of neural sheath tumors has been widely disputed.[3,7,23,52,66,75,91] Our discussion here follows that of Lusk and colleagues.[53] Controversy concerning nomenclature hinges on whether the tumor arises from Schwann cells, which produce myelin, or from the fibroblasts that are responsible for producing the endoneurium and epineurium of nerves. Virchow described three different types of peripheral nerve tumors in 1857, using the term "neuroma fibrillare amyelinicum" for the tumor subsequently described by von Recklinghausen.[89] Verocay is credited with first describing a nerve tumor as a special entity in 1910.[87] He referred to the origin as being from the fibrous neural sheaths but did not describe the cell of origin. Verocay introduced the term "neurinoma." Because this term translated into "nerve tumor," however, most authors have recommended that it be discarded.[7,34,56,74] Mallory thought that these tumors arose from the fibroblasts and so coined the term "perineurial fibroblastoma."[55] His view was strongly supported by Penfield in 1930.[66] By 1935, Stout, who later authored the first Armed Forces Institute of Pathology fascicle on peripheral nerve tumors, introduced the term "neurilemoma," an inclusive term indicat-

ing the neuroectodermal origin of these tumors.[83] Then, in 1943, Ehrlich and Martin proposed "schwannoma" to indicate specifically a Schwann cell origin of peripheral nerve tumors[23] (Figure 21 – 1). This latter term is now preferred because, as Russell and Rubinstein pointed out in 1959, the term neurilemoma refers to membranes and not the Schwann cell whose multiplication results in tumor.[74]

In 1968, Fisher and Vusevski demonstrated by electron microscopy that Schwann cells have a distinctive basement lamella that clearly differentiates them from fibroblasts.[24] The epineurium is composed of fibroblasts and in no way differs from mesenchymal tissues elsewhere in the body. However, the cells that compose the perineurial layer investing each nerve fascicle, although they look like fibroblasts under light microscopy, possess basement membranes by electron microscopy. In addition, these "perineurial fibroblasts" also form tight junctions, accounting in part for the blood-nerve barrier diffusion properties representative of the peripheral nervous system.[37,74] Because Schwann cells have basement membranes, it may be that these perineurial fibroblasts are simply non – myelin-producing Schwann cells (Figure 21 – 2).

Differentiation of solitary neurofibroma from schwannoma should be straightforward with current histopathologic techniques, but this is not always the case.[92] Both tumors have been thought to arise from the Schwann cells, mainly because electron microscopy has shown promi-

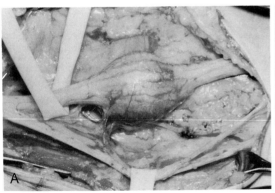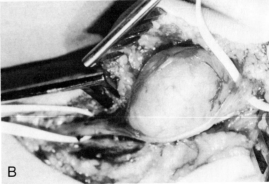

**Figure 21 – 1.** *(A)* Typical operative appearance of a neural sheath tumor, in this case a schwannoma involving tibial nerve in the popliteal fossa. Note that the surgical exposure has included nerve well proximal and distal to the lesion. *(B)* In another similar lesion, peripheral fascicles basketted around the mass have been dissected away. Entering and exiting fascicles did not transmit a nerve action potential, so they were sectioned to permit total removal of the mass.

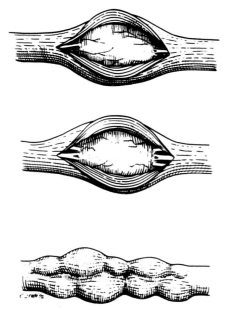

**Figure 21–2.** Drawing shows the usual appearance of a schwannoma *(top)*, a solitary neurofibroma *(middle)*, and a plexiform neurofibroma *(bottom)*. (From Donner T, Voorhies R, and Kline D: Neural sheath tumors of major nerves. J Neurosurg 81:362–373, 1994.)

nent basement membranes in both. Yet the two tumors radically differ from one another in their gross pattern of fascicular involvement, with the neurofibroma intertwining itself within at least a few fascicles of origin and the schwannoma growing extrinsically to its parent fascicles. It is our contention that the perineurial fi-

broblast, a more embryologically primitive cell, gives rise to the more "invasive" neurofibroma and that the Schwann cell, which seems to be a more highly differentiated cell, gives rise to the comparatively more benign schwannoma.

The Antoni Type A tissue of the schwannoma, with its compact array of cells, differs from the somewhat less compact and myxomatous matrix of the typical neurofibroma (Figures 21–3 and 21–4). The Antoni A tissue is very cellular and has spindle-shaped cells that may palisade to form Verocay bodies. A less compact and somewhat loose matrix, which stains poorly if at all with hematoxylin and eosin (H & E) and a mucopolysaccharide stain such as alcian blue or a reticulum stain, is characteristic of the Antoni Type B pattern seen in some schwannomas. This contrasts with the prominent mucopolysaccharide and reticulum staining and myxomatous matrix of the neurofibroma. At present, mucopolysaccharide staining is one histologic test that helps to differentiate these two benign tumors of neural origin. Unfortunately, the intensity of any stain can vary considerably according to the technique used, the technician performing the staining, and the preparation of the tissue. The numerous collagen fibrils seen in the myxocollagenous background of a neurofibroma tend also to stain more intensely with a reticulum stain than in a schwannoma. The neurofibroma has fewer Schwann cells and is mixed together with distorted axon complexes with myelinated

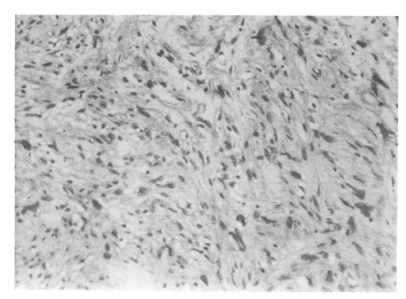

**Figure 21–3.** Usual histologic appearance of a schwannoma with Antoni Type A tissue including a compact array of Schwann cells. (H & E stain.)

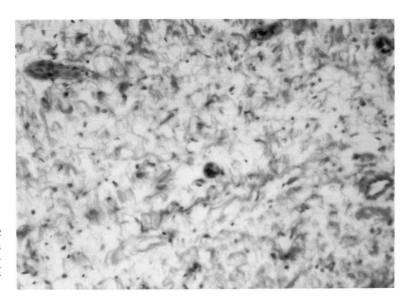

**Figure 21–4.** Usual histologic appearance of a neurofibroma with a relatively loose, somewhat myxomatous matrix. (H & E stain.)

and unmyelinated axis cylinders. Vasculature is less prominent in neurofibromas than in schwannomas and is less likely to be thickened, hyalinized, or thrombosed.

Some of the immunohistochemical and electron microscopic features currently used to differentiate Schwann cells, perineurial cells, and endoneurial fibroblasts are summarized in Table 21–1. These tests are helpful for differentiating individual cells but are more difficult to use in identifying a specific type of tumor. However, if they are used to supplement light microscopic histologic criteria, they can be quite valuable, especially in making a decision whether or not a tumor is of neural sheath origin.[92]

The terminology for malignant neural sheath tumors has been equally confusing. Some neuropathologists have categorized them as either malignant schwannomas or malignant neurofibromas. These tumors can be indistinguishable,

although the presence of mucopolysaccharide staining favors malignant neurofibroma. Harkin and Reed stated that malignant degeneration of solitary benign schwannomas rarely, if ever, occurs, except in the presence of von Recklinghausen disease (VRD).[34] On the other hand, they think that the nerve sheath fibrosarcoma is the most common type of malignancy in patients with neurofibromatosis.

Histologically, all characteristics of malignancies such as pleomorphism and mitotic figures serve to differentiate these tumors from their benign counterparts. Tumor assessment needs to be done by a pathologist who is experienced in this difficult and at times confusing field. Distinctions between a variant of a benign and perhaps ancient schwannoma with mitoses and a neurogenic sarcoma can be difficult. From a practical point of view, we agree with others that the major feature distinguishing a mesenchymal fibrosarcoma from a "neurogenic sar-

**TABLE 21–1**

Immunohistochemical and Electron Microscopic Features of Neural Cells

| | S-100 Protein | EMA | Tight Junctions | Pinocytotic Vesicles | Basement Membrane | Laminin | Type IV Collagen | Fibronectin |
|---|---|---|---|---|---|---|---|---|
| Schwann cell | (+) | (−) | (−) | (−) | (+) | (+) | (+) | (−) |
| Perineurial cell | (−) | (+) | (+) | (+) | (+) | (+) | (+) | (+) |
| Endoneurial fibroblast | (−) | (−) | (−) | (−) | (−) | (−) | (−) | (+) |

EMA = Epithelial membrane antigen; (+) = present; (−) = absent.
Data collected by R. M. Voorhies, M.D.; from Theaker et al.: Histopathology 13:171–179, 1988; Ariza et al.: Am J Surg Pathol 12:678–683, 1988; Nakajima et al.: Am J Surg Pathol 6:715–727, 1982; Jaahola et al.: J Clin Invest 84:253–261, 1989.

coma" is the latter's origin within a nerve. We prefer the nomenclature of "malignant neural sheath tumors" or "neurogenic sarcoma" in our clinic, although in the past we have used the phrase "malignant schwannoma" as well. Our cases of malignant fibrosarcoma involving brachial plexus and other nerves were differentiated by their gross appearance because they did not seem to arise in the center of a plexus element or nerve.

## BENIGN TUMORS OF NEURAL SHEATH ORIGIN

### Schwannoma

This tumor usually presents as a palpable but painless mass.[9] Tapping or percussing it may, however, give a Tinel sign in the distribution of the nerve in which the tumor arises.[11] Loss of function is rare unless a biopsy or unsuccessful attempt at removal has been done. Then, residual mass may be quite painful and loss in the nerve's distribution may be severe. On some occasions, peripheral nerve schwannomas can be present in a patient with VRD, although neurofibromas are much more common in this setting.[17] Incidence seems to be higher in females than in males, but this gender preference is not as strong as it is with neurofibromas. The tumor tends to spread apart or "basket" the fascicles and displace them to its periphery[90] (Figure 21–5). The larger lesions appear to stretch and elongate the fascicles greatly but do it so slowly,

since tumor growth usually takes years, that function is usually not lost, at least not without surgical intervention.[20,25] Frequently, one or two relatively small fascicles enter the tumor proximally, and there is a similar connection distally. If tested electrically, these connections do not on stimulation produce distal muscle function, nor do they conduct a nerve action potential (NAP) through tumor to more distal elements. There is usually a capsule of variable thickness about the tumor, and although fascicles may be adherent to the outer surface of this layer, they are seldom incorporated in it or by the tumor itself[28] (Figures 21–6 and 21–7).

The cellular makeup of a schwannoma is quite characteristic, although it may be difficult to differentiate from a neurofibroma.[33,73] Origin is from a cell with a basement lamella, and this cell of origin is probably more differentiated than a more primitive cell such as a perineurial fibroblast.[48] The most likely candidate is the Schwann cell or its related progenitors. Cells of the tumor produce a somewhat compact array of cells and what is termed Antoni Type A tissue. If tissue is stained with mucopolysaccharide or reticulum stains, these studies are less positive than those seen with a neurofibroma.

Steps in removal of schwannoma are fairly straightforward (Figures 21–8 and 21–9). Despite this, serious complications can occur if great care is not taken with the dissection.[21,72,73] The surgeon needs to dissect away and preserve other nerves or elements; dissect down to the capsule and split away the capsule while pre-

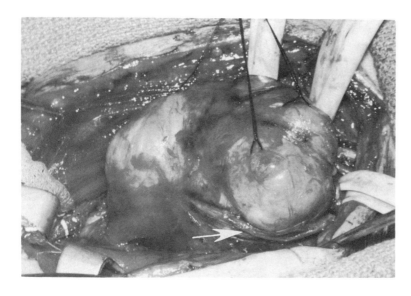

**Figure 21–5.** Large schwannoma partially worked away from surrounding fascicles (*arrow*).

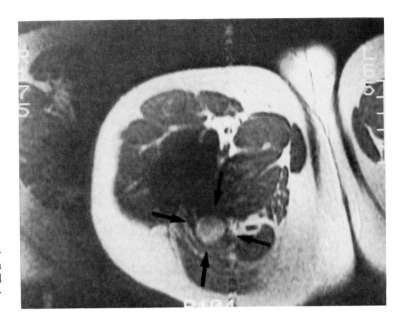

**Figure 21-6.** Magnetic resonance imaging scan of thigh showing sciatic nerve enlarged by neural sheath tumor (*arrows*).

serving fascicles basketted around the lesion; dissect fascicles off by gentle but blunt dissection; sacrifice any nonfunctional proximal or distal connections, and remove tumor as a single mass where possible. Intraoperative stimulation and recording across fascicles entering and leaving each pole of the intracapsular portion of the tumor usually show them to be nonfunctional.

An alternative approach is to open the capsule, enucleate its tumorous contents, and then tease away and resect the capsule from the spared fascicles.[10,62] This should be done thor-

oughly so as to reduce the chance of recurrence, although some surgeons believe that leaving the capsule behind does not increase the incidence of recurrence. Some schwannomas reach a great size and extend beyond the immediate region of nerve. These lesions are of course more difficult to remove, which makes the possibility of recurrence greater.[31]

## Neurofibromas

These intraneural masses are more likely to be painful than the schwannomas, and percussion over them usually produces a dramatic Tinel sign.[15] Like schwannomas, these tumors can, along with their nerve of origin, be displaced side to side, but they cannot be moved up and down or from a proximal to a distal direction. As with schwannomas, pain can become a very severe problem if there has been prior biopsy or attempted removal.[19] There are two large groups of neurofibromas. The first is a solitary tumor unassociated with other such tumors.[13] This can be fusiform or plexiform, but with solitary lesions it is much more likely to be the former.[18] The second group of neurofibromas is seen in conjunction with VRD (Figure 21-10). Although fusiform lesions are more likely to be seen with VRD than plexiform or up-and-down lesions, the latter is more common in this group than in the solitary neurofi-

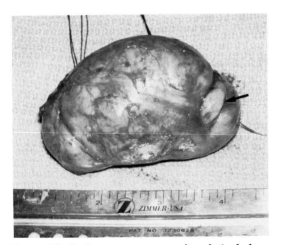

**Figure 21-7.** Gross appearance of a relatively large neural sheath tumor. Entering fascicular structure, which was nonfunctional, is indicated by an arrow.

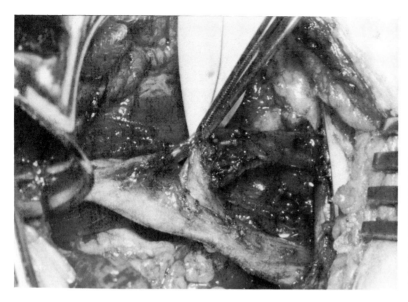

**Figure 21-8.** Plexus elements after resection of a large schwannoma at a clavicular level. Forceps are grasping entering fascicle, which was nonfunctional on stimulation and more distal recording. As a result, this fascicle and a similar exiting, distal fascicle were sectioned.

bromas. Solitary tumors are much more likely to occur in females than males, and, for reasons unclear at this time, they are more likely to be found on the right side of the body than the left side. Those associated with VRD have a more equal distribution between the sexes, and they are seen equally on both sides of the body. On the other hand, neurofibromas associated with VRD tend to present or announce themselves earlier than do solitary neurofibromas (Figure 21-11).

The cell of origin of the neurofibroma is prob-

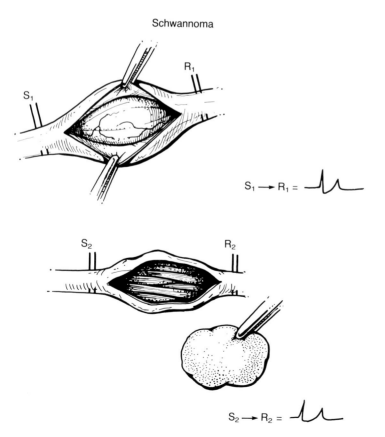

**Figure 21-9.** Usual steps in removal of a schwannoma. Fascicles are dissected from around the tumor mass after a baseline nerve action potential (NAP) has been recorded across the lesion. The entering fascicle is stimulated, and a recording is taken from the exiting fascicle, usually giving a flat trace. These fascicles are sectioned, and tumor is usually removed as a solitary mass. NAP recording after removal of the mass shows preservation of the potential. (Adapted from Lusk M, Kline D, and Garcia C: Tumors of the brachial plexus. Neurosurgery 21:439-453, 1987.)

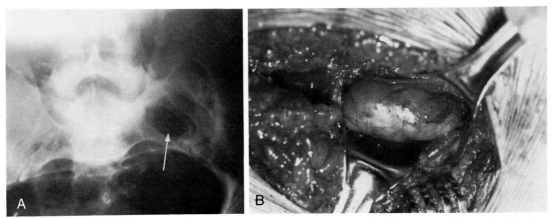

**Figure 21–10.** (A) Several sacral foramina were enlarged in this radiograph of a patient with von Recklinghausen disease (arrow). (B) Exposure of a sacral neurofibroma. Tumor was approached posterolaterally.

ably more primitive than that for schwannomas, and a stem type of cell such as a perineurial fibrocyte may be its progenitor.[75] The tumor itself is histologically less compact than a schwannoma (Antoni Type B tissue). In addition, mucopolysaccharide and reticulum stains are more positive. There is more of a tendency for neurofibromas to arise from the motor portion of the nerve and schwannomas from the sensory portion.

Neurofibromas associated with VRD are found in patients with other stigmata of that disease.[76] The manifestations of this disease are protean. Included are café au lait spots, skin tags or smaller subcutaneous tumors, salt and pepper changes in the skin, and central nervous system tumors such as acoustic neurilemoma or tumors arising from the nerve roots of the spine. Other patients have tumors and skin changes that are limited to one region of the body or neural system. This is termed regional neurofibromatosis. On occasion, larger neurofibromas,

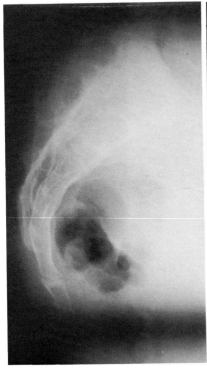

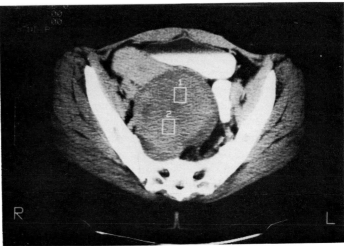

**Figure 21–11.** (A) Lateral radiograph of sacrum showing posterior displacement and deformity by a large neurofibroma. (B) Computed tomography scan showing the giant presacral neurofibroma. Removal required a pelvic exposure with mobilization of bladder, identification of ureters and great vessels, and mobilization of descending colon.

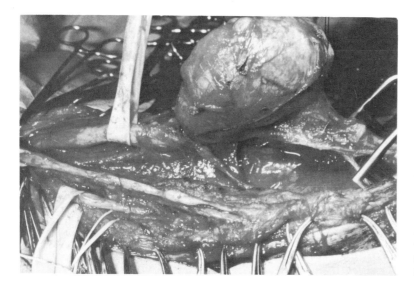

**Figure 21–12.** Large neurofibroma. Distal exiting fascicles have been sectioned, and in this case, the distal end of the tumor was gradually elevated as surrounding and primarily underlying fascicles were dissected away from it and spared.

especially those associated with VRD, can undergo malignant transformation. Whether this is really a change in the cell's potential for mitosis, or whether cells with such potential are there from the beginning, is not known.

Removal of neurofibromas is more intricate and more likely to lead to functional loss than surgery for schwannomas. For this reason, subtotal excision is sometimes indicated.[27] Under these circumstances, the chances of recurrence are increased. On the other hand, 80% of the solitary neurofibroma group operated on by us had gross total removal without further deficit.[21] This figure falls to 66% in those lesions associated with VRD because those are more likely to be of a plexiform nature.[21] Steps in the removal of neurofibromas include the following (see Figures 21–12 and 21–13): dissection away of adjacent and sometimes adherent nerves or elements; splitting away of fascicles from the surface and mobilization from around the periphery of the tumor; dissection between the fascicles and the capsule, which is left attached to tumor or, alternatively, opening and evacuation of the contents of the tumor, followed by dissection away from fascicles. It is important to dissect out fascicles at the proximal and distal poles of the tumor and to dissect them toward it (Figure 21–14). Fascicles entering and leaving the tumor are tested by stimulation of proximal ones and recording of NAPs from distal ones.[44] If traces are flat, the entering and leaving fascicles can be sacrificed. The tumor can then be removed as a solitary mass of tissue. If NAPs are positive across entering and leaving

fascicles, these fascicles need to be traced into and out of the tumor or its capsule and spared as much as possible.

Despite the above, functional fascicles some-

## Neurofibroma

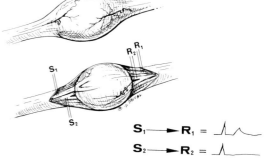

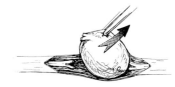

**Figure 21–13.** Steps in exposure and resection of a solitary intraneural neurofibroma. Initial exposure is well proximal and distal to the tumor *(top)*. Fascicles are dissected away from the periphery of the tumor and at both poles *(middle)*. Intraoperative nerve action potential studies usually show flat traces from one or more fascicles entering and exiting tumor, permitting their section. Tumor is elevated and dissected away from fascicular bed *(bottom)*. (Adapted from Lusk M, Kline D, Garcia C: Tumors of the brachial plexus. Neurosurgery 21:439–453, 1987.)

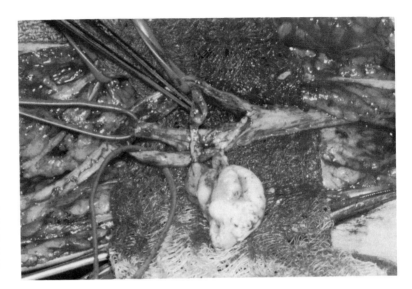

**Figure 21–14.** Relatively small neurofibroma of ulnar nerve at the elbow level, which has been worked free of most of the fascicular structure. See also color figure.

times have to be sacrificed to gain tumor resection; fascicular defects may have to be replaced by grafts.[21] Unfortunately, this may be difficult because of lengthy neural involvement in the plexiform lesions or in other large and lengthy tumors associated with VRD. Even a fusiform large lesion can be associated with multiple smaller neurofibromas or neurofibromatous change in nerve both above and below the lesion.

There is a form of VRD known as regionalized VRD in which multiple tumors affect one limb or region of anatomy without tumors elsewhere and without the usual systemic stigmata of the disease except in that area. Frequently, multiple tumors are intrinsic to one or more nerves in a given region. These intrinsic tumors involve a different quadrant or cross section of nerve at different levels. This disposition of multiple tumors makes satisfactory resection without significant deficit very difficult, especially if tumors are large and tend to be plexiform rather than globular. Regionalized VRD can also be associated with large café au lait spots, multiple small spots of skin discoloration, skin tags, and even subcutaneous neurofibromas, but all are usually confined to one limb or region of the body.

Neural sheath tumors involving the brachial or pelvic plexus pose special challenges. This topic has been covered in detail elsewhere.[15,19,21,25,28,32,40,45,50,53,59,60,65,71,82]

## Results in Benign Neural Sheath Tumors

Tables 21–2 through 21–4 show the distribution of 288 schwannomas, solitary neurofibromas, and neurofibromas associated with VRD among various peripheral nerves. These were all operated on at LSUMC and were confirmed histologically by a variety of studies. Included are 121 benign neural sheath tumors involving brachial plexus. Results for some of these plexus lesions were summarized in 1987.[53] Eighty-seven other lesions involved other upper extremity nerves, and 80 involved lower extremity nerves. A 1994 report updated

**TABLE 21–2**

Benign Neural Sheath Tumors— Brachial Plexus Region

| | Schwannoma | NF | NF-VRD | TOTALS |
|---|---|---|---|---|
| Supraclavicular brachial plexus | 24 | 37 | 14 | 75 |
| Infraclavicular brachial plexus | 6 | 14 | 8 | 28 |
| Axillary nerve | 2 | 4 | 3 | 9 |
| Musculocutaneous | 3 | 2 | 1 | 6 |
| Other | 2 | 1 | 0 | 3 |
| TOTALS | 37 | 58 | 26 | 121 |

NF = Neurofibroma; NF-VRD = neurofibroma in patient with von Recklinghausen disease.

**TABLE 21–3**
## Benign Neural Sheath Tumors — Upper Extremity

| | Schwannoma | NF | NF-VRD | TOTALS |
|---|---|---|---|---|
| Median Nerve | | | | |
|   Arm | 5 | 7 | 3 | 15 |
|   Elbow/Forearm | 3 | 3 | 2 | 8 |
|   Wrist | 6 | 3 | 3 | 12 |
| Ulnar Nerve | | | | |
|   Arm | 2 | 7 | 7 | 16 |
|   Elbow/Forearm | 1 | 6 | 3 | 10 |
|   Wrist/Hand | 1 | 3 | 4 | 8 |
| Radial Nerve | | | | |
|   Arm | 4 | 2 | 3 | 9 |
|   Elbow | 1 | 2 | 2 | 5 |
|   PIN/SSR | 1 | 1 | 2 | 4 |
| TOTALS | 24 | 34 | 29 | 87 |

NF = Neurofibroma; NF-VRD = neurofibroma in patient with von Recklinghausen disease; PIN = posterior interosseous nerve; SSR = superficial sensory radialis nerve.

the LSUMC operative results with benign neural sheath tumors involving major nerves.[21]

Tables 21–5 through 21–7 compare the preoperative grade with that found on follow-up postoperatively. Table 21–8 summarizes these findings. Eighty-nine percent of schwannomas were excised without significant residual loss, although, as can be seen from Table 21–5, 15 of these 76 lesions did have mild (grade 4 function) and 8 more serious (grade 3 or less) deficit after resection. As can be seen also from this table, 31

**TABLE 21–4**
## Benign Neural Sheath Tumors — Lower Extremity

| | Schwannoma | NF | NF-VRD | TOTALS |
|---|---|---|---|---|
| Pelvic plexus | 4 | 7 | 5 | 16 |
| Femoral nerve | 4 | 6 | 2 | 12 |
| Sciatic nerve | | | | |
|   Buttock | 2 | 3 | 2 | 7 |
|   Thigh | 5 | 7 | 5 | 17 |
| Tibial nerve | 5 | 4 | 5 | 14 |
| Peroneal nerve | 3 | 3 | 3 | 9 |
| Saphenous nerve | 1 | 0 | 0 | 1 |
| Sural nerve | 0 | 0 | 2 | 2 |
| Obturator nerve | 0 | 1 | 1 | 2 |
| TOTALS | 24 | 31 | 25 | 80 |
| GRAND TOTALS TABLES 21–2, 21–3, 21–4 | 85 | 123 | 80 | 288 |

NF = Neurofibroma; NF-VRD = neurofibroma in patient with von Recklinghausen disease

**TABLE 21–5**
## Schwannoma (n = 76)

| Postoperative Grade | Preoperative Grade | | | | | |
|---|---|---|---|---|---|---|
| | 5 | 4 | 3 | 2 | 1 | 0 |
| 5 | 41 | 9 | 3 | | | |
| 4 | 4 | 6 | 3 | 1 | 1 | |
| 3 | | 2 | 2 | | | |
| 2 | | | 2 | 1 | | |
| 1 | | | | | 1 | |
| 0 | | | | | | |

The preoperative and postoperative motor grades of involved muscle groups in patients with resected schwannomas. Overall, 17 patients improved, 8 worsened, and in 51, grades remained the same. Of the 51 with no change, 41 had normal strength at presentation.

of the schwannoma patients had some reduction in function already present before our operation (Figure 21–15). Solitary neurofibromas could be excised in 80% of cases without serious deficit. Table 21–6, however, does show 24 with mild (grade 4 function) deficit and 20 with more serious (grade 3 or less) deficit. Again, incidence of preoperative deficit was high because of prior biopsy or attempted removal, with some loss noted on presentation to us in 58 patients. Somewhat surprising were the results in the VRD-associated lesions, of which 66% could be excised without serious deficit. The following information describes details connected with each of these three types of benign neural sheath tumor.

### Schwannoma

Eighty-five patients underwent operation for removal of 85 tumors in this group (Figures 21–16, 21–17, and 21–18). There were 42 males

**TABLE 21–6**
## Solitary Neurofibroma (n = 99)

| Postoperative Grade | Preoperative Grade | | | | | |
|---|---|---|---|---|---|---|
| | 5 | 4 | 3 | 2 | 1 | 0 |
| 5 | 32 | 16 | 6 | 1 | | |
| 4 | 9 | 5 | 9 | | 1 | |
| 3 | | 2 | 5 | 2 | | 1 |
| 2 | | 1 | 2 | 1 | 2 | |
| 1 | | | | 1 | 2 | |
| 0 | | | | | | 1 |

The preoperative and postoperative motor grades of involved muscle groups in patients with resected neurofibromas. Overall, 38 patients improved, 15 worsened, and 46 had no change in grade.

**TABLE 21–7**
Von Recklinghausen Neurofibroma
(n = 48)

| Postoperative Grade | Preoperative Grade | | | | | |
|---|---|---|---|---|---|---|
| | 5 | 4 | 3 | 2 | 1 | 0 |
| 5 | 10 | 8 | 2 | | | |
| 4 | 2 | 4 | 5 | 1 | | |
| 3 | | 2 | 2 | | | |
| 2 | | 1 | | 3 | 1 | 1 |
| 1 | | | | 1 | 1 | 1 |
| 0 | | | | | 1 | 2 |

The preoperative and postoperative motor grades of involved muscle groups in von Recklinghausen disease patients with resected neurofibromas. Overall, 18 patients improved, 8 worsened, and 22 were unchanged by operation.

**TABLE 21–8**
Benign Neural Sheath Tumors*—
Resection Without Serious Deficit

| | Number of Cases | % Good Result |
|---|---|---|
| Schwannoma | 76 | 89 |
| Neurofibroma | 99 | 80 |
| Neurofibroma-VRD | 48 | 66 |
| TOTAL | 223 | |

VRD = Von Recklinghausen disease.
*Includes 9 diffuse or "plexiform" tumors, 6 associated with VRD and 3 without VRD, either subtotally resected or resected totally with repair. Prior attempted removal or biopsy decreased chances of resection without added deficit and sometimes resulted in need for repair.

and 43 females. The average age at presentation was 40.2 years. Seventy-six patients were available for follow-up 3 to 96 months postoperatively (mean time was 16.7 months). Included in this group was one patient whose median nerve tumor was of the giant cell histologic variant and another patient who had VRD and whose ulnar nerve tumor had the gross and microscopic appearance of a schwannoma. All tumors except two large pelvic schwannomas were completely excised. Graft repair of nerve was required in two patients who had damage from prior operations.

Eighty-two (96%) of the 85 patients presented with a palpable mass (Figures 21–19 and 21–20). All but one of these patients experienced referred dysesthesias (Tinel sign) on tapping or percussing over the masses.

Table 21–5 shows the pre- and postoperative motor grade for the 76 patients with excised schwannomas who had sufficient follow-up. Thirty-one patients had preoperative weakness. Of these, 17 (55%) improved postoperatively, 10 (32%) were unchanged, and 4 (13%) worsened. Among the 45 who had intact strength preoperatively, 41 (91%) maintained full strength, and 4 (9%) decreased to a grade of 4. Twenty-four patients (31%) presented with pain syndromes. Of these, 20 patients had pain that was purely radicular in nature, and four had pain which, while radicular, had a component of spontaneous pain localized to the site of the tumor. Of the 20, 15 (75%) had complete resolution of their pain syndromes at last follow-up, 2 (10%) had partial resolution, 1 (5%) had no change in the severity of pain, and 2 (10%) patients had increased pain (Table 21–

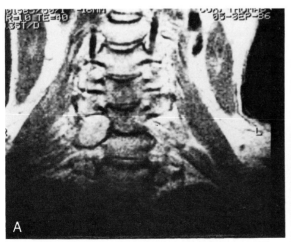
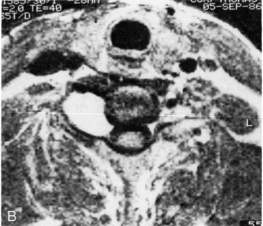

**Figure 21–15.** Magnetic resonance imaging scan of two different intraforaminal spinal nerve tumors as viewed in a frontal cut (A) and cross-sectional cut (B).

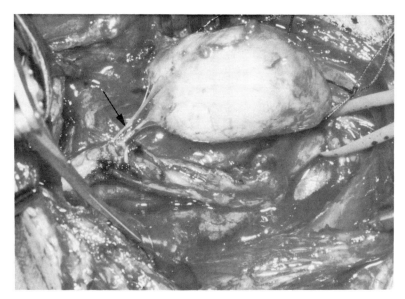

**Figure 21–16.** Schwannoma before sacrifice of several relatively small entering *(arrow)* and leaving fascicles. Most of the larger fascicles have been worked away from the tumor and spared. This tumor was located in the vagal nerve and had produced hoarseness but not paralysis of the vocal cord.

9). The four patients with pain localized to the site of the tumor had relief of this problem as well as relief of radicular pain. Four (8%) of 52 patients who had no pain syndrome preoperatively had onset of some but not severe pain postoperatively.

Thirty-seven of the 85 patients had undergone previous operations, only three of which were attempts at complete resection of tumor. These 37 included 7 of the patients who experienced decline in motor function and the 4 patients who had onset of new pain postoperatively. Also, the only patients who required graft repair of nerves had undergone "biopsy" or subtotal removal elsewhere, during which fascicles had been divided (7 patients).

One schwannoma of the plexus, which was thought to have been totally excised at the first operation, recurred. This tumor was re-excised and has not subsequently recurred after 5 years of follow-up.

## Case Summary — Schwannoma

A 26-year-old female noted pain radiating from behind the knee down to the heel of her foot while riding a ski lift. She subsequently felt a lump there and noted that if it

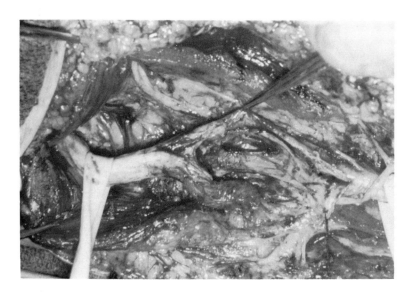

**Figure 21–17.** Bed of plexus after removal of a large schwannoma involving C7 to middle trunk. Despite what was thought to be a thorough removal, tumor recurred 2 years later and was re-resected without deficit. The patient has had no new recurrence in 4 years of further follow-up.

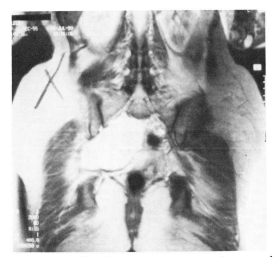

**Figure 21–18.** Magnetic resonance image of schwannoma arising from sacral plexus. Tumor was approached transabdominally after mobilizing bowel and bladder and identifying the ureter and great vessels. Fortunately, it could be shelled out and away from the fascicles of the pelvis plexus elements with preservation of function.

was bumped, a shock went into her calf. Computed tomography scan showed a popliteal fossa mass. Function on examination both clinically and by electromyography was normal in the leg.

At operation several months later, a 3 × 2.5 cm mass was found in the tibial nerve. Most of the fascicles could be dissected away along with the capsule. Two smaller fascicles entering and leaving the tumor were tested by NAPs and did not conduct. The tumor was removed as a single mass, and the capsule was then teased from fascicles. There was some decrease in toe flexion and intrinsics, but good plantar flexion, inversion, and sensation on the sole of the foot postoperatively. At follow-up 8 years later, there was full sciatic including tibial function.

Initial pathologic examination suggested the possibility of malignancy because mitotic figures were seen in what was otherwise an "epithelial-like" schwannoma. A second pathologic opinion stressed that the tumor was cellular and had mitotic activity but was well differentiated and most likely benign. A final opinion described spindle cells with Antoni A and B tissue. The tumor was thought to be somewhat cellular but nonetheless a benign schwannoma. There has been no evidence of recurrence over an 8-year period.

### Comment

The diagnosis of a malignant nerve tumor results in radical treatment. The correct interpretation using light and electron microscopy and at times histochemical studies is therefore critical. In this case, the benign nature of the tumor was eventually discerned.

### Non-VRD or Solitary Neurofibroma

In 121 patients not thought to meet the criteria for VRD, 123 solitary neurofibromas were removed. There were 66 males and 55 females. The average age at presentation was 39.1 years. Ninety-nine patients were available for follow-up at 4 to 72 months postoperatively (mean, 15.8 months) (Table 21–6). All tumors in this group were excised completely. Six patients (5%) required graft repair of nerve. Ninety-two patients had a palpable mass. All of these patients had a Tinel sign with percussion of the mass (Figure 21–21).

Fifty-eight patients presented with a motor deficit of some degree. Within this subgroup, 38 (66%) experienced improved long-term function, 14 (24%) did not change, and 6 (10%) had some further decrease in function noted at last

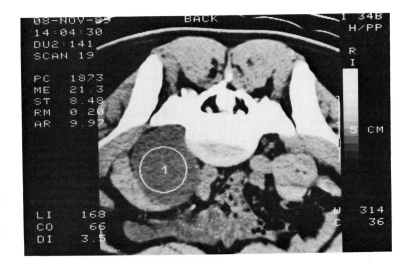

**Figure 21–19.** Large pelvic neural sheath tumor arising from lumbar root and displacing psoas laterally. Origin was lumbar roots destined for femoral nerve outflow.

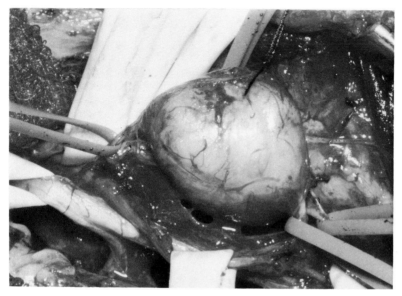

**Figure 21–20.** Fascicles have been worked down and off the periphery of this large schwannoma. Entering (plastic loop to the left) and exiting (plastic loops to far right) fascicles are shown in this photograph.

follow-up. Forty-one (41%) of the 99 patients had normal function at presentation. Thirty-two (78%) maintained normal function, and 9 (22%) had postoperative weakness of some degree.

Forty-six of these patients presented with spontaneous pain syndromes. The pain was radicular in all 46, with only 2 patients complaining of additional pain at the site of the tumor. Postoperatively, pain resolved completely in 29 (63%), partially in 11 (25%), and not at all in 3 (6%) and was made worse in 3 (6%) (Table 21–9). New pain syndromes were encountered in 7 (13%) of the remaining 53 patients, although all were mild.

Fifty-three patients had undergone prior operations, including 11 attempts at complete removal of the tumor. Of great importance, 7 of the 9 patients who experienced new postoperative paresis, 12 of 15 patients whose paresis worsened, and each of the 4 who had new pain syndromes had undergone previous operations (Figures 21–22 and 21–23).

## Von Recklinghausen's Neurofibroma

There were 57 patients who had neurofibromatosis type I in this series: 25 males and 32 females (Figures 21–24 and 21–25). In addition, there were two patients, one male and one female, who met the criteria for NF-5 or segmental neurofibromatosis. The average age at presentation was 27.7 years. From these patients, 80 tumors were removed (maximum of 7 in a single patient). Six of these were plexiform tumors. Many patients had multiple discrete tumors along the length of a single nerve. When this was encountered, smaller tumors (<1 cm) were left alone. Of the tumors that were resected, 58 were completely removed, and 16 were subtotally removed. Tumor left behind in these latter patients usually consisted of small fragments adherent or intrinsic to functional fascicles. The incompletely removed tumors included a 30-cm pelvic tumor and a 25-cm tumor arising from the proximal brachial plexus which extended deeply into the mediastinum. About

**TABLE 21–9**

Resolution of Pain After Operation on Benign Neural Sheath Tumors

| | Resolved | Improved | Unchanged | Worse Pain | New Pain |
|---|---|---|---|---|---|
| Schwannoma | 15/20 (75%) | 2/20 (10%) | 1/20 (5%) | 2/20 (10%) | 4/52 (8%) |
| Solitary neurofibroma | 29/46 (63%) | 11/46 (25%) | 3/46 (6%) | 3/46 (6%) | 7/53 (13%) |
| Von Recklinghausen neurofibroma | 10/23 (43%) | 7/23 (31%) | 4/23 (17%) | 2/23 (9%) | 4/25 (16%) |

The outcome for patients with and without radicular pain syndromes preoperatively. The first four columns represent results in patients who presented with pain syndromes. The last column represents the number of patients who had no pain preoperatively and yet developed pain after surgery.

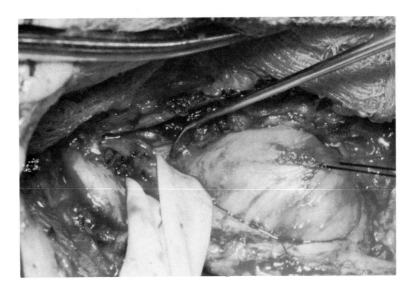

**Figure 21–21.** Large neurofibroma of the lower trunk of the plexus. Upper and middle plexus trunks are retracted laterally by the Penrose drains. Most of the fascicular structure was inferior to the mass of the tumor itself. Entering and leaving fascicles were nonfunctional, and the tumor could be excised without serious deficit, although C8-T1 distribution sensation in the hand graded 4 postoperatively.

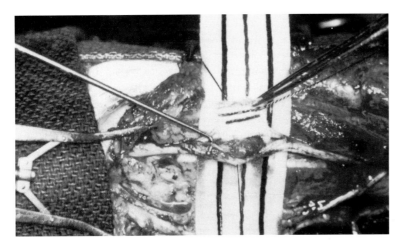

**Figure 21–22.** Small recurrent neurofibroma of ulnar nerve at the level of the wrist. Nerve hook is beneath the entering fascicles.

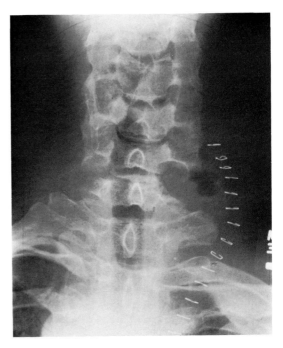

**Figure 21–23.** Postoperative anteroposterior radiograph of cervical region after posterior subscapular removal of a relatively large intraforaminal neurofibroma involving the C7 spinal nerve. Note the extent of the bone removal and placement of skin staples.

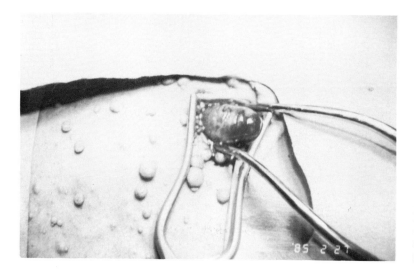

**Figure 21-24.** Cutaneous changes typical of von Recklinghausen disease, with surgical exposure of partially removed neurofibroma located in the parascapular area.

10% of each of these tumors was left behind. Six patients (10%) required graft repair of nerves after removal of tumor. Three patients required reoperation 12 to 21 months postoperatively at the site of the original tumor removal; however, each of these three had documented small tumors near the site of the initially removed tumor, so it was impossible to ascertain whether these later tumors represented recurrences or simply progression of the smaller lesions. One patient had subsequent occurrence of a malignant tumor at the site of a resected neurofibroma that was histologically benign.[53]

Forty-eight patients had sufficient follow-up (see Table 21-7). Twenty-three (48%) had presented with radicular pain syndromes. Ten patients (43%) had complete resolution of pain, 7 (31%) had partial resolution, and 4 (17%) had no change after surgery. In 2 patient (9%), pain was worse after operation (see Table 21-9). Of the 25 patients who presented without pain, 4 (16%) experienced new but, fortunately, usually mild pain syndromes.

Thirty-six patients presented with weakness. Of these, 18 (50%) had improved at last follow-up, 12 (33%) had no change in their preoperative strength, and 6 (17%) worsened (see Table 21-7). Among the 12 patients who had normal strength at presentation, 2 (17%) worsened.

Only 6 patients in this group had undergone prior operations for tumor removal or biopsy. None of these 6 had untoward effects from our surgery (Figure 21-26).

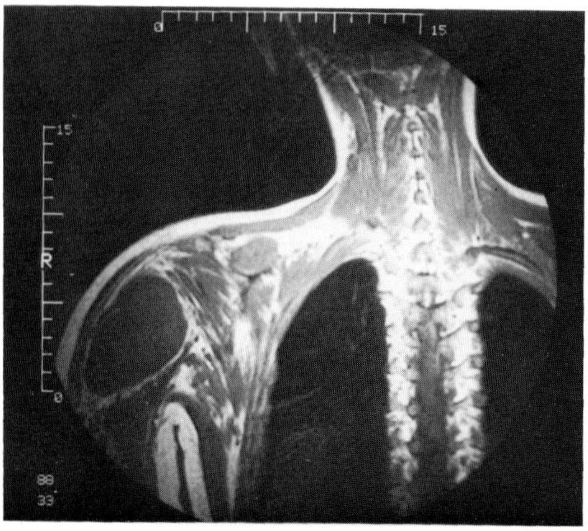

## Plexiform Neurofibroma

Nine patients with plexiform neurofibromas were encountered (Figures 21-27 and 21-28). Only two of these patients had a palpable mass. The tumors were treated by partial excision in five, internal neurolysis with gross total excision in one, internal neurolysis with subtotal excision in one, and division of the involved nerve proximal and distal to the tumor with graft repair in two. These last two patients had trace only strength in the associated muscles preoperatively, and neither of these had recovered function at last follow-up. The tumor recurred in four patients. The time to symptomatic recurrence, as judged by progressive loss of strength,

**Figure 21-25.** Magnetic resonance image of large neurofibroma of the axillary nerve in a patient with von Recklinghausen disease.

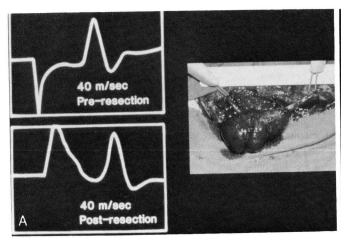

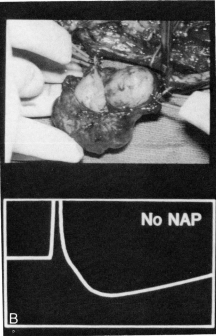

**Figure 21–26.** *(A)* Nerve action potential (NAP) testing of a large neurofibroma of tibial nerve associated with von Recklinghausen disease. Both electrical conductivity and clinical function were maintained after tumor removal. *(B)* NAP testing by stimulation of entering fascicle (to the left) and recording from exiting fascicle (to the right). There was no NAP, so these fascicles could be sacrificed.

ranged from 4 to 19 months after the initial procedure. All patients in this group had lower motor scores at last follow-up than preoperatively. Three of these patients had pain syndromes. Pain had lessened in severity with the passage of time after operation, but this was thought to be largely an effect of tumor progression rather than technical success.

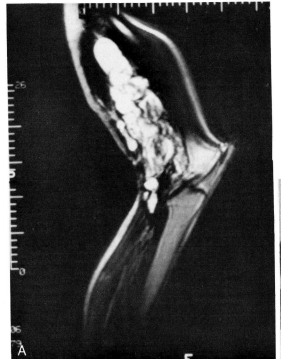

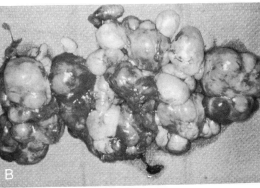

**Figure 21–27.** *(A)* Magnetic resonance image showing multiple, extensive plexiform neurofibromas involving sciatic nerve at the thigh and knee levels. Only a subtotal surgical removal was possible in this case of regionalized von Recklinghausen disease. Some of the multiple tumors removed are seen in the surgical specimen *(B)*. Painful recurrence later led to a second decompressive operation.

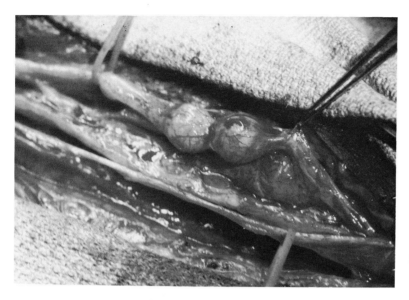

**Figure 21 – 28.** Plexiform neurofibroma involving tibial nerve in an up-and-down fashion. Partial decompression was done because of severe neuritic pain. Lesions extended from proximal thigh level of the tibial division of sciatic down to the ankle level of the posterior tibial nerve.

## Summary and Analysis of Operative Results

Table 21 – 8 summarizes the operative experience with 223 benign neural sheath tumors referable to ability to resect them without additional serious deficit in limb function.

Table 21 – 9 provides an analysis of operative outcomes on benign neural sheath tumors referable to pain. Eighty-five percent of patients with either schwannomas or neurofibromas and presenting with pain had resolution or significant improvement of their pain; this figure was 74% for VRD-associated lesions. Onset of new pain postoperatively was 8% for schwannomas, 13% for solitary neurofibromas, and 16% for VRD neurofibromas. Most of the time, new pain postoperatively could be managed pharmacologically and diminished after a few months.

## Complications

Expected complications included neural loss and new postoperative pain as detailed above (see also Figure 21 – 29). Several patients with plexus tumors approached anteriorly had transient phrenic paralysis, and two approached posteriorly had scapular winging, which was also transient. There were two patients with plexus tumors who required thoracentesis postoperatively and one who required a chest tube for 3 days. There were two wound infections.

Both were superficial, and both responded to antibiotic and local wound care.

## MALIGNANT NEURAL SHEATH TUMORS OR NEUROGENIC SARCOMAS

Neurogenic sarcomas can occur without a background of VRD.[14,79] Neural sheath malignancies were nonetheless more frequent in our patients with VRD than in those without VRD, although the number of solitary malignant tumors not associated with VRD was greater. Those neurogenic sarcomas associated with

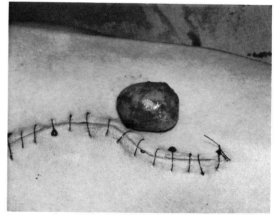

**Figure 21 – 29.** Need for an up-and-down exposure for removal of even a small neural sheath tumor is evident in this photograph. Unless this is done, nerve of origin or adjacent nerves can be damaged.

VRD tended to present at a younger age than those which were solitary. There was no gender preference in either group, and these malignant neural sheath tumors appeared to have no special laterality. Irradiation has also been implicated as an inductive factor in the occasional neurogenic sarcoma.[26]

Pain with or without progressive loss of function was the most common presenting complaint. Most frequently, painful paresthesias in the distribution of the involved nerve gradually worsened, prompting further medical and eventually surgical investigation.[88] In some cases, the patient noticed a lump or mass that was painful when it was palpated or bumped (Figure 21–30). In other cases, an initial mild loss became more severe, progressing relatively rapidly. It was rare for these patients to present initially with metastasis to lung, bone, liver, or spleen.

Other clinical findings that might suggest a malignant neural sheath tumor include a relatively rapid increase in size of a mass over a period of weeks to months and a large size on initial presentation.[38] Such malignant tumors tend to be more firm and more fixed to adjacent structures than their benign counterparts such as a schwannoma or even a neurofibroma[47] (Figure 21–31). As with the benign neural sheath tumors, though, the mass can usually be moved side to side but not up and down. Percussion or deep palpation over them gives pain radiating distally and sometimes proximally in the distribution of the nerve or element of origin. As with more benign tumors, computed tomography and especially magnetic resonance imaging with contrast can demonstrate them well. These studies do not at this time differentiate benign and malignant neural sheath tumors.

Despite some differentiating features on physical examination, the majority of these malignant neural sheath tumors are not suspected as being malignant until biopsy or attempted removal. Either procedure in relatively inexperienced hands can lead to neural loss, just as with the more benign neural sheath tumors. Loss is more likely with the malignant tumor than with the benign lesion, not only because of its more intrinsic nature in relation to the nerve or element of origin, but also because of its adherence to adjacent neural structures and other soft tissues such as vessels, muscle, and even bone (Figure 21–32).

## Operations and Results with Malignant Neural Sheath Tumors

Treatment usually includes local resection followed by amputation well proximal to the level of involvement (Table 21–10). This may be followed by irradiation or chemotherapy or both,[29] although the latter two treatment modalities have a variable and unpredictable effect

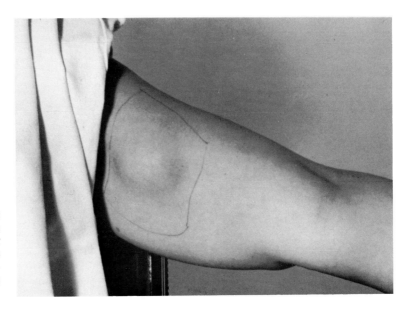

**Figure 21–30.** Painful mass in medial arm associated with progressive sensory and motor loss. At operation, this was found to be a neurogenic sarcoma arising from median nerve.

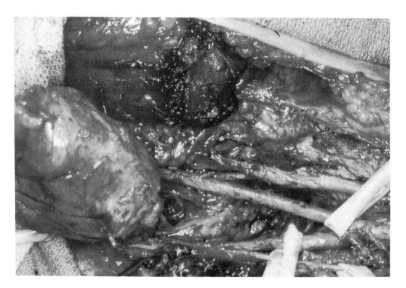

**Figure 21–31.** Neurogenic sarcoma elevated away from cords of plexus. The patient was elderly and did not wish a forequarter amputation. Recurrence at a skin level was treated successfully by irradiation several years later, and the patient survived another 8 years without other recurrence before succumbing to heart disease.

on these malignancies. After the lesion has been identified, we try to get as wide a resection of the tumor and surrounding tissues as possible (Figures 21–33 and 21–34). This approach is more workable for distal neural sheath tumors than for ones on the proximal limb, where wide resection removes vessels vital to preservation of the limb or adjacent nerves and may lead to a paralyzed extremity. Recommended is amputation of the limb well proximal to the lesion, but only after the lesion has been verified pathologically as malignant, and provided there is no evidence of metastasis by radiography and computed tomography scan of lungs (Figure 21–35), bone scan, and liver and spleen scan. For proximal thigh lesions involving sciatic or distal femoral nerves, amputation may mean hip disarticulation. For a distal brachial plexus lesion involving cords of the plexus or their proximal outflows, this translates into a forequarter amputation with removal of scapula, clavicle, and shoulder as well as transection and ligation of subclavian vessels and division of plexus elements at a spinal nerve level.

Several groups experienced with soft tissue sarcomas of various types involving the upper or lower extremities have developed programs for limb salvage.[6] This usually includes wide local resection of the tumor and adjacent tissues, leaving a good margin of soft tissue free of tumor. Then, local soft tissue irradiation can be delivered with implanted rods and supplemented if necessary by external radiation treatment. The long-term results with this limb-sparing approach in a large series of patients remain to be determined. Usually, the two

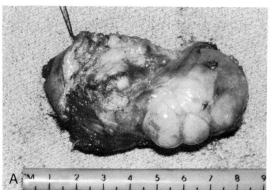
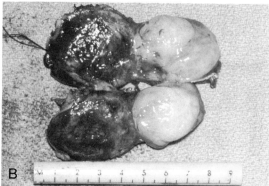

**Figure 21–32.** (A) Resected neurogenic sarcoma. (B) Section of tumor shows hemorrhagic change in one nodule of the tumor.

**TABLE 21–10**
Management of Malignant Tumors of Neural Sheath Origin (n = 21)

| | No. of Cases | VRD | LR | LRM | Irradiation | | AMP | 4 Qrt | Av.Fu. | Deaths |
|---|---|---|---|---|---|---|---|---|---|---|
| | | | | | Ports | Rods | | | | |
| Neurogenic Sarcomas | | | | | | | | | | |
| Brachial plexus | 9 | 4 | 7 | 2 | 5 | 0 | 1* | 4 | 52 mo | 4 (23 mo) |
|   Sciatic | 2 | 1 | 0 | 2 | 0 | 0 | 0 | 2 | 18 mo | 0† |
|   Peroneal | 1 | 0 | 0 | 1 | 0 | 1 | 0 | 0 | 18 mo | 0 |
|   Tibial | 1 | 1 | 1 | 0 | 1 | 0 | 1 | 0 | 30 mo | 0 |
|   Femoral | 2 | 1 | 0 | 2 | 1 | 1 | 1 | 0 | 38 mo | 0 |
|   Ulnar | 2 | 0 | 0 | 2 | 1 | 1 | 0 | 0 | 37 mo | 1 (37 mo) |
| Fibrosarcomas | | | | | | | | | | |
|   Brachial plexus | 2 | 0 | 2 | 0 | 2 | 0 | 0 | 0 | 39 mo | 0 |
|   Femoral | 1 | 0 | 0 | 1 | 1 | 0 | 0 | 1 | 18 mo | 1 (18 mo) |
| Neuroblastoma | | | | | | | | | | |
|   Sacral plexus | 1 | 0 | 1 | 0 | 1 | 0 | 0 | 0 | 38 mo | 0 |
| TOTALS | 21 | 7 | 11 | 10 | 12 | 3 | 3 | 7 | 40 mo | 6 (24.5 mo) |

4 Qrt = Forequarter amputation of shoulder and arm or hip disarticulation; AMP = amputation; Av.Fu. = average follow-up; LR = local resection; LRM = local resection with margin; VRD = von Recklinghausen disease; ( ) = average postoperative survival.
*Surviving with known residual tumor proximal to amputation site at 6 years.
†One patient had positive findings on lung scan at last follow-up.

major options are discussed with the patient and the family, and a conjoint decision is made favoring one approach or the other. In the last decade, our experience with limb sparing that included wide local resection followed by rod irradiation has been favorable, but a larger series of cases with follow-up beyond 5 years is needed.[6] To date, at a plexus level, forequarter amputation has given the longest survival in both VRD- and non–VRD-associated distal plexus malignancies. Those located more proximally and arising from the plexus have had to be treated by as thorough resection as possible and not wide local resection because that would have resulted in a flail as well as devascularized arm. Such a resection was followed by irradiation and also by chemotherapy in several cases.

Neuroblastoma has been reported involving nerve.[34] We have not had experience with this lesion involving a major upper extremity nerve or brachial plexus but did resect one involving the pelvic plexus.

## Case Summary—Neurogenic Sarcoma

This 40-year-old physician had noticed paresthesias in the right hand for a few months, followed by right

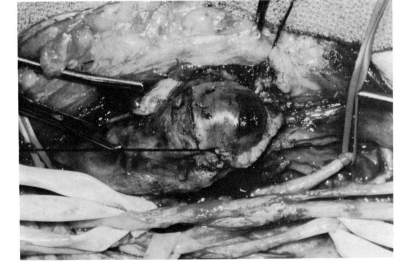

**Figure 21–33.** Malignant tumor involving brachial plexus at a cord level. Most of the cords of the plexus have been dissected away and are encircled by Penrose drains, and axillary artery is encircled by a plastic loop to the right.

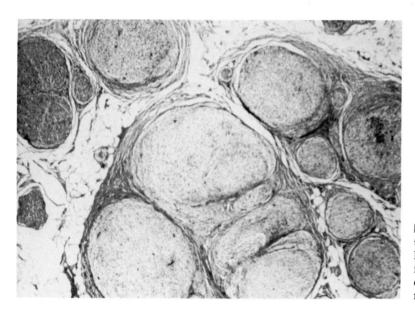

**Figure 21-34.** Neurogenic tumor in this photomicrograph has spread throughout the fascicular structure of nerve of origin, much proximal to the main mass of tumor itself.

shoulder, wrist, and hand weakness. Computed tomography and magnetic resonance imaging of the neck revealed a large supraclavicular brachial plexus mass. Needle biopsy suggested a malignant tumor, most likely a neurogenic sarcoma. Upon examination, partial dysfunction in the distribution of the C5- and C6-innervated muscles was noted. Loss was severe in the distribution of the C7, C8, and T1 elements. An operative procedure was undertaken. The lesion was approached by a poste-

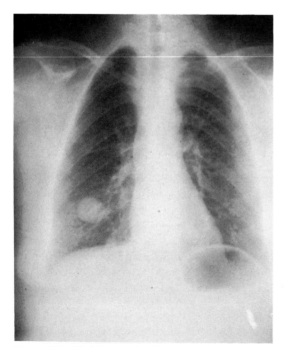

**Figure 21-35.** Metastasis of neurogenic sarcoma to lung from lesion involving sciatic nerve at a buttock level.

rior subscapular operation with resection of the first rib. After excision of the posterior scalene muscle, the posterior portion of a mass 8 cm in diameter was revealed. Tumor was then dissected circumferentially with maintenance of the capsule or outer rind of the tumor. A plane of dissection was found posteriorly, superiorly, and laterally, but inferiorly and medially, the tumor was more adherent and the capsule had to be entered to remove tumor from superior and medial pleura and deeper mediastinal structures. The tumor was relatively soft in consistency and moderately vascular. Removal of some tumor from the C5, C6, and C7 roots and upper and middle trunks was necessary, as well as removal of a good bit attached to the C8 and T1 roots and lower trunk. Tumor was also attached to the subclavian vessels, first rib, apical pleura, and anteromedial mediastinum. A section of pleura 4 cm in diameter was resected and replaced by a graft of fascia lata. Tumor entered widened foramina at the C6-C7 and C7-T1 levels. Foramina were entered for tumor removal, but a small amount within the spinal canal was not removed. After tumor dissection, NAP recordings were performed. There were good-sized NAPs from C5 and C6 to upper trunk, moderate-sized NAPs from C7 to middle trunk, but only a trace of a NAP from C8 or T1 to lower trunk. At the end of the surgical procedure, a chest tube was placed over the fifth intercostal space. Permanent histologic sections confirmed the diagnosis of malignant schwannoma or neurogenic sarcoma.

The chest tube was removed on the fifth postoperative day. The patient gained good pain relief and surprisingly recovered some C8 and T1 spinal nerve function, in that hand-intrinsic function improved. This occurred over an 8-month period despite radiation therapy and chemotherapy. The patient survived a little over 4 years postoperatively and then died from disseminated disease.

**Comment**

Local control of the tumor was obtained by an extensive but only palliative operation. This operation was not curative, and neither irradiation nor chemotherapy could halt the spread of the disease.

# BENIGN TUMORS OF NON-NEURAL SHEATH ORIGIN

By and large, this is a fortunate category. These tumors secondarily involve nerve and tend to produce symptoms because of nerve compression rather than origination in nerve[8,69,78] (Figure 21–36). There are exceptions, however, provided by desmoids, myoblastomas, lymphangiomas, or the rare extraspinal meningioma, which can be quite adherent to epineurium and difficult to remove, and in which recurrence is more likely.[92] Some ganglions remain or are extraneural and can compress nerve, and others either dissect to an intraneural level or originate there. As a result, removal of these lesions can be either incomplete or accompanied by deficit. Hemangioma or hemangiopericytoma can envelop nerve or elements of the brachial plexus, but the extremely rare hemangioblastoma can arise in nerve, as can rare tumors of congenital origin such as a triton tumor of the plexus. The various origins of these benign tumors can be inferred from Table 21–11.

## Desmoid Tumors

This lesion is of mesenchymal origin and is usually positioned in muscle. The tumor is very fibrous and also very adherent to neighboring nerves as well as other structures.[53] Although desmoids are benign, they tend to be invasive of soft tissues. If close to nerve, such a tumor can envelop and be quite adherent to it (Figure 21–37). The most frequent site of origin is abdominal musculature, but desmoids can involve neck, shoulder, upper arm, and lower extremity. Despite what would appear to be gross total excision, recurrence is common, especially if wide resection is difficult because of contiguous important neural or vascular structures. Tumors we have operated on in the area of the plexus have been difficult to completely eliminate and have tended to recur. Despite this, several have been successfully re-resected. One extensive le-

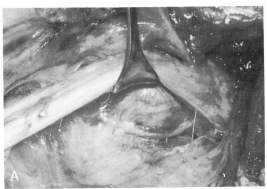

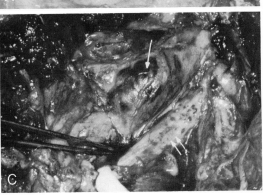

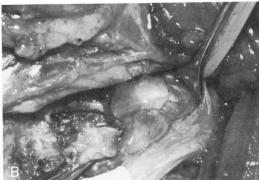

**Figure 21–36.** *(A)* Ganglion located in the sciatic notch region and compressing sciatic nerve, which is retracted superiorly with a vein retractor. *(B)* Epidermoid tumor in the region of the sciatic notch displacing sciatic nerve laterally. *(C)* Aneurysmal dilatation of vein *(single arrow)* in juxtaposition to sciatic nerve *(double arrow)* just distal to the sciatic notch.

**TABLE 21-11**

Operated Benign Tumors of Non-Neural Sheath Origin Involving Nerve (n = 61)

| Tumor Type | No. of Cases | Tumor Type | No. of Cases |
|---|---|---|---|
| Ganglion Cysts (21) | | Vascular Tumors or Lesions (10) | |
| Peroneal | 12 | Hemangioma | |
| Femoral | 1 | Ulnar | 2 |
| Tibial | 1 | Peroneal | 1 |
| Sciatic | 1 | Hemangiopericytoma | |
| Posterior interosseous nerve–Radial | 1 | Median | 1 |
| Ulnar–Guyon canal | 1 | Brachial Plexus | 1 |
| Median | 2 | Glomus Tumor | |
| Suprascapular | 2 | Peroneal branch | 1 |
| Epidermoid Cyst (1) | | Digital | 1 |
| Sciatic | 1 | Venous Angioma* | |
| Cystic Hygroma (1) | | Median | 1 |
| Accessory | 1 | Tibial | 1 |
| Desmoid (6) | | Hemangioblastoma | |
| Brachial plexus | 2 | Median | 1 |
| Median | 1 | Triton Tumor (1) | |
| Radial | 1 | Brachial plexus | 1 |
| Peroneal | 1 | Lymphangiomas (2) | |
| Sciatic Complex | 1 | Median/Ulnar | 1 |
| Meningioma (2) | | Brachial plexus | 1 |
| Brachial plexus | 2 | Myositis Ossificans (2) | |
| Lipomas (7) | | Radial | 1 |
| Median | 4 | Brachial plexus | 1 |
| Posterior interosseous nerve–Radial | 1 | Osteochondroma (4) | |
| Ulnar | 1 | Radial | 1 |
| Musculocutaneous | 1 | Peroneal | 2 |
| Ganglioneuroma (2) | | Brachial plexus | 1 |
| Brachial plexus | 2 | Hidradenitis (2) | |
| Myoblastoma or Granular Cell Tumors (2) | | Ulnar | 1 |
| Brachial plexus | 2 | Median/Ulnar | 1 |

*Two additional venous aneurysms were extrinsic to nerve and felt to be compressing in one case the femoral nerve and in another the sciatic nerve.

sion at the axillary level led to progressive neural loss, required two resections, recurred a third time, and finally, because of an almost flail arm and severe pain, required a forequarter amputation.

## Case Summary—Desmoid Tumor

A 12-year-old girl presented to her pediatrician with a large buttock mass. A desmoid tumor was removed from the buttock musculature. Within two years, there

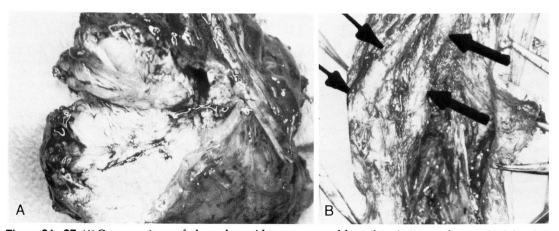

**Figure 21-37.** *(A)* Gross specimen of a large desmoid tumor resected from the sciatic complex at a thigh level. *(B)* Sciatic complex just proximal to popliteal space and relatively cleared of desmoid. These neural elements are scarred and thickened.

was a recurrence which had extended to the thigh level. This required an extensive dissection at both the buttock and thigh level to free sciatic nerve of tumor and to remove tumor from buttock and from hamstring muscles. Fortunately, most sciatic function could be preserved. However, in a few more years tumor was at the popliteal and proximal calf level with adherence to popliteal vessels as well as tibial and peroneal nerves. This required another extensive operation, which was followed over the next 2 years by several procedures at the midcalf level. The tumor seemed to move progressively down the limb. Later, the patient required a number of procedures for recurrent tumor at the level of the ankle, dorsum of the foot, and, more recently, in relation to the toes and their web spaces. Fortunately, there is no sign of recurrence at the buttock, thigh, or calf levels. Because of determination, grit, and an active exercise program, she has completed college and has a successful career as a television newscaster, and it has now been more than 25 years since the discovery of her disease.

### Comment

During dissection, it may be difficult to determine where desmoid ends and more normal tissues begin because the latter are often infiltrated by the tumor. The pattern of centrifugal growth seen in this case is most unusual.

There are other, even rarer tumors that can be quite intrinsic to nerve even though they are benign. An example is provided in Figure 21–38, which shows a congenital tumor involving brachial plexus.

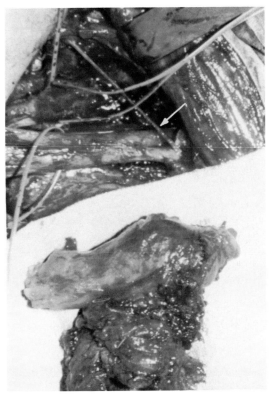

**Figure 21–38.** Triton tumor was resected from upper elements of suprascapular plexus *(top)*. Phrenic nerve is seen running obliquely across the field *(arrow)*. Resected specimen is seen at the bottom.

## Myoblastoma or Granular Cell Tumor

These tumors rarely involve nerve, but when they do, they are adherent and require careful dissection for their removal. We have seen two involving the brachial plexus.[53] Both were adherent and involved the extraforaminal portions of the spinal nerves as well as plexus trunks. One could be removed using careful dissection under magnification. The second patient had been initially operated on elsewhere, had severe lower element loss, and required operation from a posterior approach with resection of scar and recurrent tumor from upper mediastinum as well as plexus. Because deficit was severe, pain was a problem, and lower roots to trunks were involved over a length, the latter elements were resected along with recurrent tumor and scar. This tumor had some mitotic figures, and a small recurrence was treated with chemotherapy 2 years later. There has been no further recurrence with another 3 years of follow-up. Pain relief has been good despite loss of hand-intrinsic function.

These tumors are formed of a mixture of plump and somewhat angular cells with acidophilic granules.[3] Cells tend to be rather compactly arranged or aligned. Mitotic figures are few in number, but occasionally the tumor takes on an invasive behavior as in our second example above.[7] For the purposes of this discussion, we have categorized these tumors as benign, but they can take on malignant characteristics. More usual sites where major nerves are not involved by myoblastoma or granular cell tumor include the breast, peritoneum, tongue, bronchi, and the submucosal layer of the gastrointestinal tract.

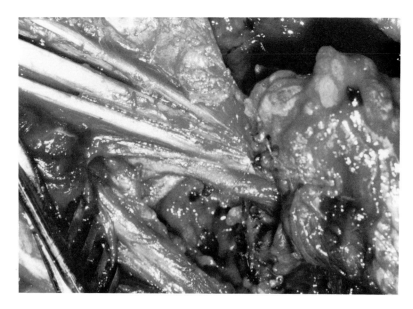

**Figure 21–39.** Lymphangioma undergoing dissection away from cords of the plexus. Mass of the tumor is pulled up and to the right.

## Lymphangiomas

If these tumors involve nerve, they have many of the same characteristics as myoblastomas.[12] They tend to spread as a sheet of tumorous tissue enveloping structures rather than forming a true mass lesion (Figure 21–39).

One lymphangioma involving the medial portion of the upper arm enveloped proximal median and ulnar nerves, and these required a neurolysis. There was some residual although mild reduction in hand-intrinsic muscle strength. Another lymphangioma was contiguous with brachial plexus elements. This was operated on successfully by a posterior subscapular approach. The first rib was resected, and tumor was successfully removed from C7, C8, and T1 spinal nerves and the middle and lower trunks.

## Meningiomas

Although they are rare, we have had experience with two meningiomas involving the peripheral nervous system. One was quite small and one was quite large. The small one involved the C7 spinal nerve. An intraspinal component had been successfully removed elsewhere, and residual intraforaminal scar and tumor were subsequently removed by a posterior subscapular approach to this spinal nerve. The second lesion was far more difficult (Figure 21–40). It involved supraclavicular plexus from spinal nerve to divisional level of the trunks, and there had been four prior attempts at removal. Using an extensive anterior approach, we performed partial graft repair of C6 to upper trunk divisions and C7 to the middle trunk of the plexus after tumor resection. Loss postoperatively was in the upper and middle trunk distributions. Some of this was recovered as a result of time and the graft repairs. Major residual deficit has persisted as poor shoulder abduction. Follow-up magnetic resonance imaging done 2 years

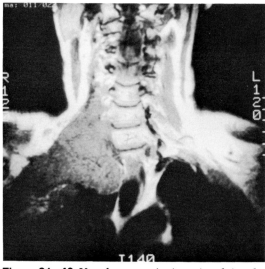

**Figure 21–40.** Very large meningioma involving the right brachial plexus. This unusual lesion was associated with severe loss and had been operated on several times with recurrence after each procedure.

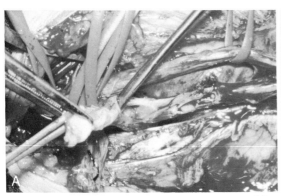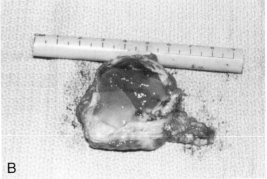

**Figure 21–41.** *(A)* Wall of a ganglion cyst is teased from fascicles of the peroneal divisions. Nerve superior to this is the tibial portion of the sciatic nerve. *(B)* Resected ganglion cyst which has been opened to show typical mucoid contents.

later indicated recurrence along the paraspinal portions of the lower roots and plexus trunks to divisions beneath the clavicle and over the pleural apex.

## Ganglion Cysts

Most of these arise from joints and are present in areas that do not involve nerves, such as the dorsum of the hand or wrist.[78] There are, however, many important exceptions (Figure 21–41). At the wrist and hand level, such cysts have been seen in our clinic compressing median nerve or its thenar sensory branch at the wrist, ulnar nerve or its superficial and deep branches in the Guyon canal, and the superficial sensory radial branches at the wrist. These lesions present with not only a mass but tenderness, pain, and paresthesias in the distribution of the nerve or branches involved. Other joint sites at which we have seen ganglions involving major nerves include the elbow and proximal forearm, where posterior interosseus or median nerve has been compressed. Quite rare is femoral or sciatic compression caused by hip-level ganglions, but they do occur at that site, and we have operated on one example of each. More difficult to explain in terms of origin is compression of the suprascapular nerve by a ganglion (Figure 21–42). These cases present somewhat like a spontaneous suprascapular neuropathy, although occasionally there is an initiating history of heavy lifting or trauma to the shoulder

**Figure 21–42.** Ganglion *(arrow)* involving suprascapular nerve near scapular notch. Exposure was gained by splitting apart and retracting supraspinatus muscle. In some cases, these lesions extend through and below the scapular notch and require dissection of infraspinatus away from scapula.

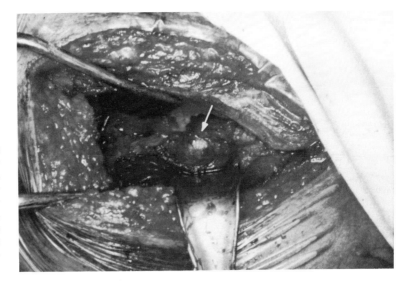

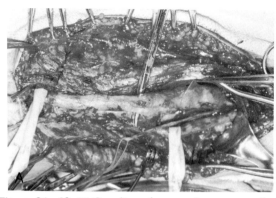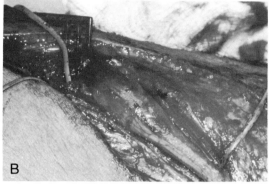

**Figure 21–43.** (A) Ganglion of peroneal nerve near the head of the fibula. This lesion had no obvious connection with the knee joint and could be dissected out by exposing the fascicles above and below and working them free of the cyst. (B) Another ganglion of the peroneal nerve, which was totally intraneural.

region. Diagnosis is usually not suspected preoperatively unless a computed tomography or magnetic resonance imaging scan of the scapular region has been done. In the cases operated on by us, the ganglions did not appear to arise from the shoulder joint. Both cysts were in the region of the scapular notch and compressed the suprascapular nerve at that level.

The second type of ganglion cyst is located in nerve (compare Figures 21–41 and 21–43 with Figures 21–42 and 21–44). It may arise from a joint and grow into the nerve or arise de novo within the nerve and not, at least when operated on, have a discernible connection to a joint. The most frequent site for such intraneural cysts is the peroneal nerve behind the head of the fibula.[76]

To date, 12 ganglion cysts have had operative removal at knee level. One has recurred and re-

quired a second removal 2.5 years after the first operation. Two were very extensive, could not be totally removed without severe deficit, and were decompressed. A third patient was a 12-year-old girl who presented with both foot drop and a cystic mass behind the knee. At operation, the intraneural ganglion extended proximally not only into thigh but also to the buttock level of the sciatic nerve. Only a decompression could be done, and, as might be expected, there has been no reversal of foot drop; on the other hand, tibial distribution loss has not developed.

An interesting patient presented with a large ganglion cyst at the level of the ankle. This cyst recurred after a prior partial decompression procedure and again after our first operation. At a second operation 5 months later, cyst was once more evacuated and capsule was removed again, but this time several fascicles were re-

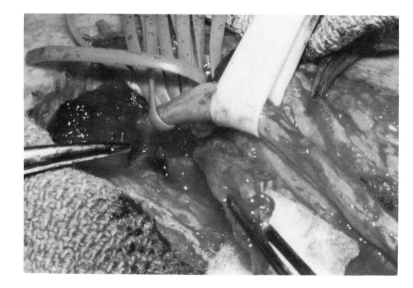

**Figure 21–44.** Extraneural ganglion is being teased away from beneath peroneal nerve at the head of the fibula. Proximal is to the right and distal is to the left in this picture. Origin of this lesion was from the knee joint.

sected and replaced by sural grafts. So far there has not been any recurrence, but follow-up has only extended to 3 years.

## Lipomas

These fatty tumors are benign, are usually globose or ovoid, are subcutaneous, and do not usually involve nerves. If they do, removal is not easy and neural damage can result (Figure 21–45). Although the usual lipoma does not envelop nerve, it can grow quite large and can lie atop or adjacent to nerve. Therefore, nerves can be easily damaged if removal of the lipoma is not carefully done. Less frequently, the fatty tumor envelops nerve. If this occurs at a plexus level, removal is difficult, especially if there has been a prior unsuccessful surgical attempt.

Unfortunately, there is also a small but significant group of patients who have a hamartomatous condition, in which there is a significant fatty-fibrous mass within nerve. If this is present, it usually involves the median nerve at the palmar and sometimes the wrist level. The usual management is section of the carpal tunnel ligament and decompression rather than an attempt to remove lipomatous tissue. We have managed three examples of this disorder in that fashion. Despite several decompressive operations in a fourth patient, there was persistent and progressive neuritic pain and severe paresthesias. This required a third operation with internal neurolysis and individual neurolysis of fascicles as well as digital branches. A mixture

of scar and lipoma was resected, but a portion of the complex was severely involved and no longer transmitted NAPs. Partial resection of the median and several digital branches led to their replacement with sural grafts and eventually to partial but incomplete recovery of sensation and thenar function.

Seddon and others have described four lipomatous conditions that can affect nerve[76,78]: neural compression by a solitary lipoma; "macrodystrophia lipomatosa," which produces an overgrowth of hand or fingers; an encapsulated lipoma located in the nerve; and lipofibromatous hamartoma of nerve. We have seen several examples of the first type treated elsewhere in which nerve was inadvertently resected and required repair. We have also seen the second type but not operated on it. We have seen only one example of the third type but have seen four examples of the final type involving median nerve at wrist and hand, which required carpal tunnel release and neurolysis at wrist and hand levels.

## TUMORS WITH MAJOR CALCIFICATION OR BONY INVOLVEMENT

### Myositis Ossificans

This strange disorder results in a firm to very hard mass of tissue which can envelop contiguous structures such as nerves, vessels, muscles,

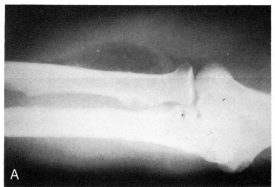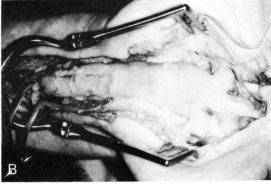

**Figure 21–45.** *(A)* Radiograph of elbow region with area of hypodensity over radius. This radiographic appearance is pathognomonic of a lipoma. At surgery, this lesion was found compressing the posterior interosseus nerve. *(B)* Lipohamartoma (lipofibromatous hamartoma) involving median nerve at the level of wrist and palm. The patient presented with symptoms like a carpal tunnel syndrome. At the time of carpal tunnel release, diffuse, fatty infiltration of the nerve was found. (From Hudson A, Gentilli F, Kline D: Peripheral nerve tumors. *In* Schmidek H and Sweet W, Eds: Operative Neurosurgical Techniques, 2nd Ed. New York, Grune & Stratton, 1988.)

and tendons. A factor that may play a role in pathogenesis of these lesions is trauma, either spontaneous or associated with prior surgery. In one obvious case, a man received a contusion of the lateral upper arm and subsequently developed a mass there. As the mass grew, the patient developed a partial radial palsy. Triceps function was spared but brachioradialis graded 2, extensor communis 2, extensor pollicis longus 3, and wrist extensors were 2 to 3. A large calcified mass arising in triceps was removed. It had compressed radial nerve as it came around the humerus in the radial groove. It was adherent to but had not invaded the nerve. With removal of this fibrotic calcified mass and neurolysis of the nerve, function in the radial distribution improved dramatically. Radial grades at 1.5 years' follow-up were excellent. Another patient, a 32-year-old male, had partial resection of a large axillary mass of fibromyositis. At reoperation for resection of residual tumor and exploration of plexus, grafts from medial and lateral cords were placed to both median and ulnar nerves. At follow-up 4 years later, there was no recurrence. Most of the median function had returned, as had flexor carpi ulnaris and profundus to little finger. There was no recovery of ulnar-innervated hand-intrinsic function.

A related disorder was seen in a 30-year-old young man who had sustained a severe left brachial plexus stretch injury as a result of a motorcycle accident. The limb was flail and the patient had a Horner sign. Attempt at operative repair elsewhere had been unsuccessful and was terminated because of severe bleeding. He presented with a large, partially calcified mass incorporating plexus but at a supra- and infra-clavicular level. In exposing what was left of the plexus elements in this large calcified mass, axillary artery was reinjured in several places. A graft repair of infraclavicular plexus elements was finally accomplished, but the grafts were 7.5 to 15 cm in length. On the second postoperative day, embolization to the radial artery occurred and the limb had to be subsequently amputated at an upper arm level. Recovery would probably not have occurred, because of the length of grafts necessary to restore some degree of continuity and the severe scarring encountered.

Although origin is different, an occasional li-

poma can become calcified after trauma or prior surgery. An example was a lipoma behind the knee of a teenage girl which not only calcified but appeared to have hemangiomatous changes after a prior partial removal. It involved peroneal nerve and required an extensive dissection for removal. Fortunately, most of the peroneal function was preserved, with grades postoperatively in anterior compartment muscles averaging 4.

## Osteochondroma

Several of these unusual bony lesions involved nerve. One tumor involved humerus in a middle-aged male. There was severe radial distribution deficit preoperatively. Loss slowly reversed over a 2-year period after removal of the bony tumor and neurolysis of the radial nerve. Another tumor arose from proximal fibula and had to be dissected free from peroneal nerve and the proximal portions of the superficial and deep branches. A similar problem arose in a young man who had bony proliferation of both fibular heads and bilateral entrapment of the peroneal nerves. A fourth patient had a large osteochondroma arising in the paraspinal region. This had arisen spontaneously and was associated with a thoracic outlet syndrome. Symptoms included pain and paresthesias in the upper arm and forearm with abduction of the arm or use of the arm above the horizontal. A posterior subscapular approach was used for resection of both the tumor and the posterior portion of the first rib, followed by neurolysis of the plexus.

## Osteogenic Sarcoma

On occasion, osteogenic sarcoma or Ewing sarcoma can also incorporate nerve. Such a tumor arising from tibia and involving posterior tibial nerve was removed as a conjoint procedure with orthopedics. This required some dissection and mobilization of the peroneal nerve as well as extensive neurolysis of the tibial nerve from knee to the midshaft area of the tibia.

# VASCULAR MASSES AND TUMORS

Clots, particularly those associated with trauma or, less frequently, with anticoagulation, can compress nerves and lead to serious loss. Tumors of vascular origin and other arterial or venous anomalies can either envelop or compress nerve or, less frequently, arise within it. Examples are provided by hemangiomas, various angiomas, pseudoaneurysms, arterial venous fistulae, hemangiosarcomas, and hemangioblastomas[11,53,54,62,64] (Table 21–12).

Our experience with hemangiomas includes two in which resection elsewhere led to neural loss. In one instance, a large hemangioma of the forearm was resected, leading to ulnar loss. On secondary exploration, a 12.7-cm gap was found in the forearm involving the ulnar nerve. Five centimeters were made up by an ulnar transposition at the elbow. The remaining gap was closed by sural nerve grafts. Only partial recovery of ulnar function occurred. Nonetheless, NAPs could be evoked through the grafts and recorded distally several years later.

Another patient had partial loss in the axillary and medial cord distributions secondary to resection of a large hemangioma involving the axilla. Fortunately, most of this loss was reversed over a 3-year period and after a neurolysis.

## Venous Aneurysms or Angioma

Two examples of this lesion intrinsic to nerve were seen. In both cases, enlargement of the lesion occurred whenever the involved limb was placed in a dependent position. The first patient worked stocking shelves in a food supermarket (Figure 21–46). If he stocked shelves above the waist, he was asymptomatic, but if he worked on the lower shelves, he developed a tender swelling at the wrist and experienced paresthesias in the median distribution of the hand. He gradually developed atrophy of the thenar eminence. A venous aneurysm or angioma was found involving median nerve at a distal forearm-to-wrist level. It was intrinsic to nerve and seemed fed by small arterioles proximally and was partially drained by veins distally. An internal neurolysis was done, and fascicles were cleared of angioma under magnification. He did well for 3 years although there was no reversal of thenar atrophy. Then, a mass recurred and numbness redeveloped in the median distribution. Resection and replacement with grafts was necessary 4.5 years after his initial presentation. There has been no recurrence. He has had partial sensory but not motor recovery. The lesion was sinusoidal, and its walls had more of a venous than an arterial structure. Indeed, enlargement with dependency could be readily demonstrated at the operating table, and the contained blood was bluish rather than red.

A similar lesion was seen in a 22-year-old woman, but it involved posterior tibial nerve behind the knee. Branches of this nerve were incorporated in a venous aneurysm-like structure just proximal to their entry into and deep to the gastrocnemius soleus muscle. Involved branches were dissected proximally and cleared of aneurysmal investment. This dissection included an internal neurolysis of the distal tibial

**TABLE 21–12**
Vascular Masses Associated With or Without Injury

| Nerve(s) Affected | Hematoma | Pseudoaneurysm | Arteriovenus Fistula | Venous Aneurysm | Hemangioma | Glomus Tumor |
|---|---|---|---|---|---|---|
| Brachial plexus | 4 | 7 | 0 | 0 | 1 | 0 |
| Femoral | 2 | 3 | 0 | 1* | 0 | 0 |
| Tibial or peroneal | 2 | 1 | 1 | 1 | 0 | 1 |
| Sciatic | 2 | 1 | 0 | 1* | 0 | 0 |
| Pelvic plexus | 4 | 0 | 0 | 0 | 0 | 0 |
| Radial | 0 | 0 | 0 | 0 | 1 | 0 |
| Median | 0 | 0 | 1 | 1 | 1 | 1 |
| Ulnar | 0 | 0 | 1 | 0 | 0 | 0 |
| TOTALS | 14 | 12 | 3 | 4 | 3 | 2 |

*These venous aneurysms were extrinsic to the nerve but felt to be compressing it.

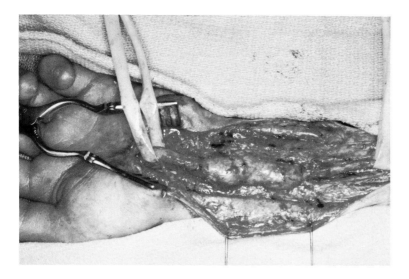

**Figure 21–46.** Venous angioma or aneurysm involving distal forearm-level median nerve. Patient worked stocking shelves in a store. While stocking lower shelves, he experienced painful paresthesias in the median distribution that dissipated when he worked on higher shelves. The lesion was resected by clearing individual fascicles of vessels and scar. Five years later, however, this venous angioma recurred and required resection and sural graft repair of the median nerve. See also color figure.

nerve itself. Resection was accomplished without loss of function, and there has been no recurrence over a 15-year period of follow-up.

Two additional patients appeared to have some degree of nerve compression with paresthesias and without deficit as a result of venous aneurysm extrinsic to nerve. One case involved sciatic nerve close to its exit from the sciatic foramen. Another patient with a history of venous insufficiency had a saphenous vein varix involving femoral sensory branches.

## Pseudoaneurysms

Pseudoaneurysms occur because of a penetrating injury to vessel which permits dissection of blood into the vessel's wall, expanding the wall and forming a sizable encapsulated mass. These vascular masses usually occur because of injury to the axillary artery. Presentation and behavior at that site are discussed in the chapter concerning the brachial plexus and gunshot wounds. We have also seen pseudoaneurysms on the femoral artery, usually caused by femoral angiography, and on the popliteal vessel, because of severe penetrating injury behind the knee. In the three femoral cases, neural involvement was severe, and these severely stretched nerves required replacement by grafts extending from pelvis to thigh. In the one pseudoaneurysm involving popliteal artery seen to date, neurolysis of tibial and peroneal nerves as well as resection of the mass sufficed. Pseudoaneurysm can cause a partial injury to nerve or plexus elements to extend, resulting in more se-

vere and complete loss. As such, this lesion is one of the few mechanisms producing progressive loss of nerve function after the original injury. Delayed onset of pain and paresthesias after a penetrating injury near a major vessel and nerve and an expanding mass with or without a palpable thrill or bruit heard on auscultation should suggest the possibility of a pseudoaneurysm. Neural loss may be progressive, and unless the lesion is resected in a timely fashion, deficit may become permanent.

## Arteriovenous Fistulas or Malformations

These vascular anomalies can occur close enough to nerve to directly involve it. Sometimes, the fistula is only in the vicinity of injured nerve and yet the patient has neural symptoms. The lesion is caused by the same, usually penetrating wound that involved the nerve. It usually does not result, in itself, in further neural loss. There is an occasional exception, however. A classic example of this was provided by a 14-year-old boy who sustained an accidental rifle wound to the left elbow and developed a pulsatile enlargement of the arm around the elbow and a progressive ulnar palsy. Ulnar arterial to venous connections had formed a fistula just proximal to the elbow. The feeding artery also had an aneurysm in it proximal to the fistula site. A similar fistula involving median nerve at the elbow was seen in another patient but was related to a knife wound; origin was from the brachial artery. In the first case, a neurolysis of the ulnar and median nerves was done after coagulating or ligating arterial feeders to the fistula. Ulnar nerve was then transposed volar to elbow and buried beneath flexor carpi ulnaris and pronator teres. In the second case, the fistula was obliterated and median nerve was unroofed from upper arm to forearm by sectioning lacertus fibrosis and a portion of overlying pronator teres. Results in both cases were gratifying.

## Hemangioblastoma

These lesions are much more common in the central than the peripheral nervous system. In fact, such tumors sited in a nerve are extremely rare.[12] A lesion that was quite characteristic presented as a mass involving median nerve at the elbow level in a middle-aged woman. Findings on angiography performed because of prior attempt at biopsy which had led to quite a bit of bleeding were quite characteristic, with a vascular stain similar to what is seen with angiography in some central nervous system hemangioblastomas (Figure 21–47). This was a difficult lesion to extract because of its vascular nature and the scar from the prior attempted biopsy. It was extirpated after splitting nerve proximal and distal to the lesion into its fascicular pattern and tracing and cleaning each fascicle as it ran into and through the tumor mass. Partial median deficit resulted. Tumor has to our knowledge not recurred to date. Histology was similar to that seen in central nervous sys-

tem lesions with an endothelial-like cell pattern with hemangiocytes and hemorrhage.

## Hemangiopericytomas

These lesions can arise in mediastinum and grow superiorly to envelop or become adherent to brachial plexus. Complete removal is difficult even if plexus is not involved, but dissections are especially trying if it is. One case was approached by thoracic surgery by splitting mediastinum and removing the mediastinal portion by dissecting it away from intrathoracic paraspinal structures, including the arch of the aorta and its superior vessels. We then proceeded to dissect remaining tumor away from the lower elements of the brachial plexus.

## Glomus Tumors

These are not uncommon, but they are usually associated with a nail bed or subungual sites and are less common elsewhere on the limb. An exception was provided by a 14-year-old girl who presented with severe pain and tenderness over the lower anterior tibia. She had fallen while skiing 2 years before. The ski boot had creased this same area but had not broken the skin or fractured the tibia. She had seen many physicians and was considered by some to have a good deal of emotional overlay or to be hysterical. She would ward off all attempts to pal-

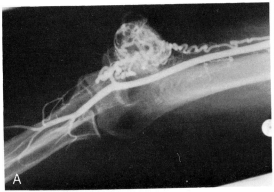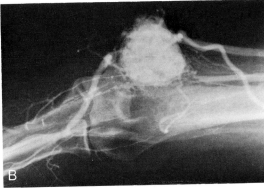

**Figure 21–47.** (A) Arterial phase of brachial angiogram of a vascular tumor involving median nerve just proximal to the elbow. Prior attempt at biopsy had led to a lot of bleeding, which suggested the need for angiography. The patient presented with partial median deficit. This deficit was slightly increased by our operation and then slowly reversed over several years. (B) Later phase in the same angiogram with relatively early venous fill. Histologically, this vascular mass proved to be a hemangioblastoma.

pate this area. After considerable persuasion, palpation showed a slight, smooth fullness there but no real palpable mass. The area was extremely tender, but light percussion did not give a Tinel sign. There was mild dysesthesia in the superficial peroneal sensory distribution. Foot function was otherwise normal, although when walking she favored this leg and was loath to bear full weight on it. She was hospitalized, and while she was asleep and with her parents' consent, the area was repalpated. She awoke with a shriek of pain. As a result, the area was surgically explored with the patient under general anesthesia. A reddish brown mass adherent to anterior periosteum of the tibia was found (Figure 21–48A). It was excised along with tibial periosteum in that area. Sensory branches of the peroneal nerve were not directly involved but lay over the mass. They were mobilized and displaced to either side of the mass. The mass proved to be a glomus tumor. Histology was characteristic (Figure 21–48B). There was a canaliculus-like arrangement of sheets of cells resembling glomus cells or pericytes. Special stains showed a characteristic stroma. Postoperatively, she was for the most part free of pain and had a normal gait for 4.5 years. Then, a painful lump recurred in that area and was re-excised when she was 19 years of age. She did relatively well in the interim but returned at age 22 with a question of recurrence. No specific mass was palpable, and tenderness

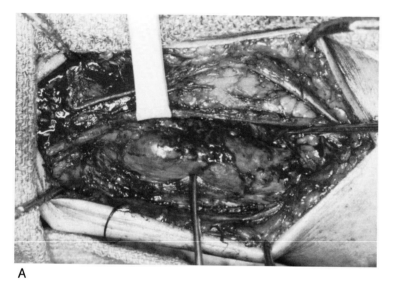

A

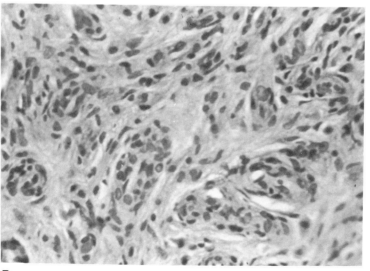

B

**Figure 21–48.** (A) Gross appearance of a fairly sizable glomus tumor located over the lower tibia. Lesion has been partially elevated from the periosteum. Nerve retracted by Penrose drain is a superficial peroneal branch. (B) Hematoxylin and eosin stain of glomus tumor resected from periosteum of lower tibia.

was not as severe as before. She declined further surgery at that time.

These unusual tumors are thought to arise from glomeruli where a small arteriole connects to an adjacent vein by way of a tiny canalicular system.[84] These microscopic structures may relate to local changes in blood flow, perfusion pressure, and regulation of heat exchange. Tumors formed from such cells can recur and, depending on the locus, can involve peripheral nerve branches, as in this case.

## MALIGNANT TUMORS OF NON–NEURAL SHEATH ORIGIN (METASTATIC TUMORS)

The largest category of metastatic tumor was related to breast carcinoma, and this usually involved the brachial plexus or one of its outflows (Figure 21–49). Each of these patients had un-

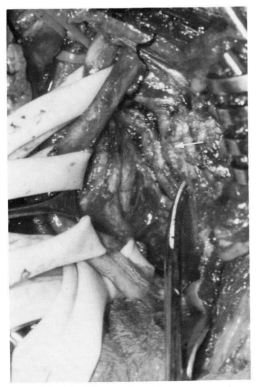

**Figure 21–49.** Metastatic pulmonary carcinoma *(arrow)* attached to proximal humerus and compressing plexus (retracted to the left) at a cord level. Plexus elements and major vessels have been dissected away from the tumor and are retracted medially by Penrose drains. See also color figure.

dergone prior mastectomy followed by irradiation. Differential diagnosis when breast carcinoma was part of the historical background included neural injury secondary to radiation fibrosis, recurrent carcinoma with invasion of the plexus, or both.[46] The specific diagnosis often cannot be resolved without operation or biopsies at multiple sites. Nonetheless, several criteria suggest carcinomatous compression or invasion, including a palpable or a definite mass on computed tomography or magnetic resonance imaging scan and involvement of specific plexus elements, especially lower trunk, medial cord, or its outflows. Less definite but also suggestive of carcinoma are severe pain, especially in the distribution of specific plexus elements, and absence of lymphedema.[85]

Other workers have cited presence of myokymia on electromyogram as favoring irradiation plexitis, but this can be present when both carcinomatous invasion and irradiation plexitis are present, which is not infrequent in these patients.[51] Other proposed criteria which have been thought to favor carcinoma have included presence of Horner syndrome, a history of radiation doses less than 6000 rads, and presentation in the first few years after mastectomy. Unfortunately, we as well as others have seen cases of irradiation plexitis without carcinoma in which one or more of these latter features have been present.[53] Certainly, the onset of irradiation plexitis is quite variable and, in our experience, can even begin up to 18 years after the course of radiation therapy. The tendency to exclude irradiation plexitis as the diagnosis because of a great delay in onset of plexus symptoms or loss should be avoided.

If metastatic tumor involves plexus or nerve, the first order of business is decompression of the neural elements involved. En bloc removal of tumor and adjacent tissues, although indicated for malignant tumors of neural sheath origin, is not indicated for non–neural sheath tumors involving plexus. Instead, as much tumor as possible should be removed to thoroughly decompress the neural elements. Further treatment with irradiation or chemotherapy is individualized for each patient and involves input from an oncologist and a radiotherapist.

In the ten cases of metastatic breast cancer that we have operated on, as much of the tumor

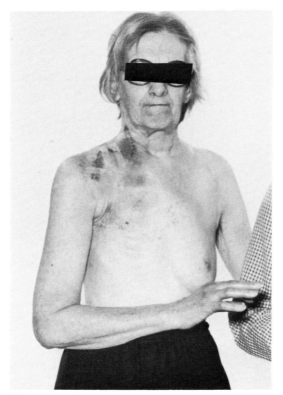

**Figure 21–50.** Breast carcinoma treated by mastectomy and irradiation with subsequent pain, paresthesias, and progressive loss in the distribution of the brachial plexus. This is a photograph taken of a patient a few days after neurolysis of the plexus for irradiation plexitis.

contiguous to plexus or nerve was removed as possible, and a thorough neurolysis of the elements or nerve involved was done (Figure 21–50). Scar secondary to irradiation made dissection difficult but not impossible. We were fortunate in these cases to find that tumor, although often adherent to epineurium, had not invaded the nerve or element itself. Operation usually reduced the pain associated with such lesions but did not reverse loss, especially if it was severe or complete to begin with. Follow-up, as expected, has usually shown death from metastatic disease within 1 to 5 years.

The seven cases of pulmonary metastatic disease involved brachial plexus and in most instances were caused by direct extension of the tumor rather than true metastasis (Figure 21–51). Operations on the plexus were palliative and included subtotal resection of tumor and decompression. Several were done from a posterior subscapular approach with first rib resection. In two patients, this approach was combined with a laminectomy to decompress tumor extending into the spinal canal. In another patient, a high open cervical and contralateral cordotomy was done to further palliate pain. Three of these patients lived beyond 3 years (3.5, 4, and 5 years, respectively) before succumbing to further metastasis or further direct extension of their disease. Occasionally, a benign neural

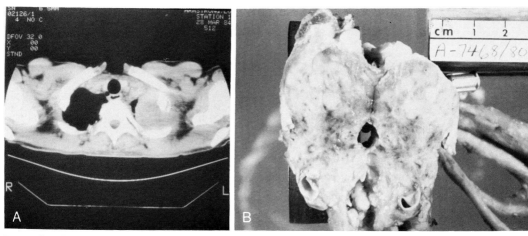

**Figure 21–51.** (A) Pancoast tumor involving left brachial plexus and seen on transverse cut of a computed tomography scan of the superior lung fields. (B) Pathologic specimen of large Pancoast tumor involving plexus elements, which are seen to the right.

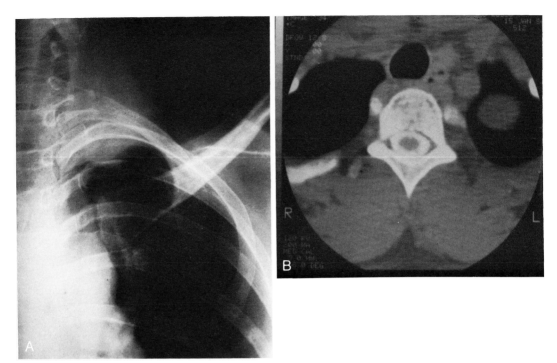

**Figure 21–52.** Chest radiograph *(A)* and computed tomography scan *(B)* of two different apical lung tumors which required plexus dissection rather than thoracotomy. Both lesions were schwannomas. These studies should be compared to the malignancy seen in Figure 21–51*A*.

sheath tumor involving a lower plexus element can indent the apex of the lung and mimic a Pancoast tumor (Figure 21–52).

It is possible, though, for malignant disease to spread or metastasize directly to nerve, presumably by the bloodstream. Examples of this were seen in three instances involving brachial plexus and one case of a lymphoma that spread

to the radial nerve. Two patients with metastatic melanoma had large lesions, one involving plexus at a divisional level and the other lateral cord to musculocutaneous outflow (Figure 21–53). Gross total excision was possible, but other metastatic lesions appeared in lung and bone 2 and 3.5 years later, even though both the original and the metastatic sites were thought to be

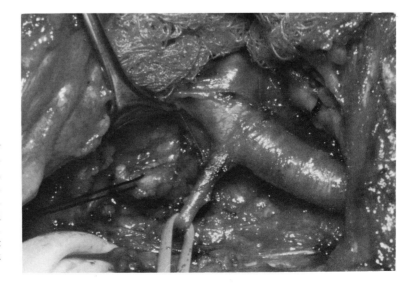

**Figure 21–53.** Nodule of metastatic melanoma (held by traction suture) nestled next to the subclavian artery and proximal to the origin of the vertebral artery, which is retracted downward by a plastic loop. Tumor was adherent to but not invading the C8 to lower trunk junction of the plexus.

adequately treated by irradiation. In the radial nerve case, a physician with central nervous system lymphoma presented 3 years after craniotomy and cranial irradiation with a complete radial palsy at the midhumeral level. At exploration, a lymphoma was found within the substance of the radial nerve (Figure 21–54). No other sign of lymphoma, either residual in the brain or elsewhere, was found for 5 years, and then the patient succumbed with extensive pulmonary lymphoma.

The Ewing sarcoma which involved tibial nerve has been discussed under "Tumors with Major Calcification or Bony Involvement," even though in the case cited it was clearly a malignancy. Occasionally, a malignancy arising from blood vessels such as an angiosarcoma can secondarily involve nerve.[57]

Operative indications for metastatic lesions included pain and paresthesias, progressive deficit, and usually a palpable and very tender mass. Local resection was done in all 25 cases, but in only 2 could an extended margin be obtained (Table 21–13). Pain was improved in 20 of 25 cases. Despite this, some further loss of function occurred in 10 cases, and in only 3 of these was some type of repair possible. None of these patients recovered more function from the repair itself. Most cases had already received radiation treatment to the area of concern, but if that was not the case (7 patients), this was done postoperatively. Average follow-up was 23 months. There were 14 deaths during follow-up in these patients. Average survival time between our operation and expiration was only 15 months.

## BRACHIAL PLEXUS TUMORS OPERATED ON BY A POSTERIOR SUBSCAPULAR APPROACH

Twenty-two patients presented with brachial plexus tumors which were then operated on by a posterior approach (Table 21–14).[22] The mean age in this group was 40 years. Twelve of the 22 patients had prior biopsy or partial tumor removal. Fourteen tumors involved the C8 or T1 nerve roots or the lower trunk, or some combination of these, and most tumors, regardless of level, had an intraforaminal component.

### Schwannomas

There were five schwannomas, one being associated with VRD. Only two patients with schwannomas presented with some degree of pain. No patients had either a severe or moderate neurologic deficit, but one had a mild sensory deficit.

The schwannoma in this series involved the lower elements. One of them mimicked an apical lung tumor and was first approached by a thoracic surgeon who performed a thoracotomy and recognized the nature of the lesion. The tumor was not biopsied or removed but was

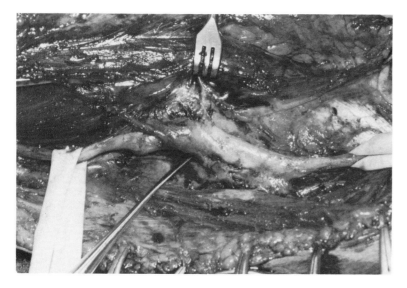

**Figure 21–54.** Lymphoma metastatic and intrinsic to radial nerve. There was total loss of function distal to the triceps branch. After a resection, a graft repair was done. Subsequent irradiation of this area probably contributed to lack of radial recovery. (From Van Bolden A, Kline D, Garcia C, et al.: Isolated radial nerve palsy from primary malignant lymphoma of brain. Neurosurgery 21:905–909, 1988.)

**TABLE 21-13**
Operated Carcinomas Involving Nerve (n = 25)

| | No. of Cases | LR | LRM | Repair/X-ray* | Improved Pain | Maintained Function | Av.Fu. | Deaths |
|---|---|---|---|---|---|---|---|---|
| Breast | | | | | | | | |
|   Brachial plexus | 9 | 9 | 0 | 0/0 | 6 | 5 | 20 mo | 5 (16 mo) |
|   Radial | 1 | 0 | 1 | 0/0 | 1 | 1 | 18 mo | 0 |
| Lung | | | | | | | | |
|   Brachial plexus | 7 | 7 | 0 | 1/0 | 5 | 5 | 18 mo | 5 (8 mo) |
| Melanoma | | | | | | | | |
|   Brachial plexus | 2 | 2 | 0 | 0/2 | 2 | 2 | 27 mo | 1 (18 mo) |
| Bladder | | | | | | | | |
|   Brachial plexus | 1 | 1 | 0 | 0/0 | 1 | 1 | 14 mo | 0 |
| Skin (Squamous) | | | | | | | | |
|   Ulnar | 1 | 1 | 0 | 1/1 | 1 | 0 | 14 mo | 1 (14 mo) |
| Ewing Sarcoma | | | | | | | | |
|   Peroneal | 1 | 1 | 0 | 0/1 | 1 | 1 | 72 mo | 0 |
| Lymphoma | | | | | | | | |
|   Radial | 1 | 0 | 1 | 1/1 | 1 | 0 | 60 mo | 1 (60 mo) |
| Head and Neck | | | | | | | | |
|   Brachial plexus | 1 | 1 | 0 | 0/1 | 1 | 0 | 4 mo | 1 (4 mo) |
| Thyroid | | | | | | | | |
|   Brachial plexus | 1 | 1 | 0 | 0/1 | 1 | 0 | 42 mo | 0 |
| TOTALS | 25 | 23 | 2 | 3/7 | 20 | 15 | 23 mo | 14 (15 mo) |

Av.Fu. = Average follow-up; LR = local resection of tumor; LMR = local resection with margins; ( ) = average postoperative survival.
*Repair was by grafts; x-ray by external beam from a cobalt source.

subsequently resected with sparing of C8, T1, and lower trunk function.[9] Each schwannoma was completely resected by use of microsurgical technique and NAP recordings, with preservation of the involved element. One other patient underwent total resection of a C7-C8 level schwannoma by the posterior subscapular approach, combined with a posterior C1-C2 laminectomy for removal of a C2 neurofibroma.

**TABLE 21-14**
Brachial Plexus Tumors Operated Posteriorly (n = 22)

| | Schwannomas | Solitary NF | NF-VRD | Malignant NST | Other |
|---|---|---|---|---|---|
| Number of cases | 5 | 5 | 5 | 3 | 1 lymphangioma 1 plasmocytoma 2 ganglioneuroma |
| Male/Female | 2/3 | 2/3 | 1/4 | 2/1 | 1/3 |
| Mean Age (yr) | 49 | 54 | 13.5 | 49 | 40 |
| Prior Treatment | | | | | |
|   Biopsy | 3 | 1 | 0 | 3 | 1 |
|   Partial removal | 0 | 0 | 2 | 0 | 2 |
|   TAR/ant. scalen. | 0 | 1 | 0 | 0 | 1 |
|   Cerv. laminect. | 0 | 0 | 1 | 0 | 0 |
|   Radiation therapy | 0 | 0 | 0 | 0 | 1 |
| Clinical Presentation | | | | | |
|   Pain | 2 | 2 | 0 | 2 | 2 |
|   No or mild deficit | 5 | 4 | 4 | 2 | 3 |
|   Moderate or severe deficit | 0 | 1 | 1 | 1 | 1 |
| Gross Total Resection | 5 | 4 | 2 | 2 | 4 |
| Postoperative Status | | | | | |
|   Intact | 5 | 3 | 4 | 2 | 3 |
|   Deficit | 0 | 2 | 1 | 1 | 1 |
|   Scapular winging | 0 | 0 | 1 | 0 | 0 |

ant.scalen. = Anterior scalenectomy; Cerv. laminect. = cervical laminectomy; NF = neurofibroma; NST = neural sheath tumor; TAR = transaxillary first rib resection; VRD = von Recklinghausen disease.

## Neurofibromas

Ten neurofibromas involving the plexus were operated on by a posterior approach (Table 21–14). Five cases were associated with VRD; these included four females and one male, with a mean age of 23.5 years. The other five cases presented with a solitary neurofibroma; these included three females and two males who were significantly older (mean age 54 years) than those with VRD. Four of the ten patients had undergone a prior operation on their tumor. In eight patients, the tumors involved lower elements. Two patients presented with pain as the only symptom, seven had a mild-to-moderate neurologic deficit, and one presented with complete middle-trunk functional loss after trans-axillary first-rib resection and scalenectomy. With the use of magnification with loupes and NAP recordings, complete resection could be achieved in six cases. Almost complete but subtotal removal was performed in four cases. Two patients with solitary neurofibromas and one with VRD had less function after surgery than preoperatively. All three patients had undergone prior operations on their tumor. The mean follow-up period for all 10 neurofibroma patients was 3 years.

## Malignant Nerve Sheath Tumors

Two cases of neurogenic sarcomas (malignant schwannomas) and one case of fibrosarcoma were treated by wide local resection through a posterior subscapular approach. The patient with fibrosarcoma underwent both a posterior and a subsequent anterior approach for further tumor removal and then received irradiation. The patient was followed for 5 years without recurrence but has since been lost to follow-up evaluation. The two patients with malignant schwannoma had extensive but subtotal tumor removal from a subscapular approach. Postoperatively, the pain was improved in both cases, but one patient had some increase in his neurologic deficit. Both patients died from widespread metastatic disease, one at 16 months and the other at 4 years postoperatively.

## Miscellaneous Tumors

There were four additional patients with brachial plexus tumors (Table 21–14). Two patients had secondary involvement of the brachial plexus by a soft-tissue tumor. One lesion was a lymphangioma involving both the C8 and T1 nerve roots. The patient had undergone partial tumor resection by an anterior approach elsewhere and presented to us with severe pain and some sensory deficit. Removal of the residual tumor was achieved by a posterior approach. His pain was improved, and neurologic status was intact postoperatively. The other patient had a plasmacytoma involving the lower three roots. She had undergone resection of the mediastinal part of the tumor as well as irradiation. The recurrent tumor, which involved the brachial plexus, was resected through a posterior subscapular approach. The tumor exhibited some malignant changes, with no demarcation from the lower roots. As a result, a wide local resection of the tumor and of the C7, C8, and T1 elements was performed. Postoperatively, the patient was free of pain and, as expected, had no distal function in the distribution of the lower nerve roots. A recurrence of the tumor 2 years postoperatively was treated by chemotherapy, and the patient has survived another 3 years without further recurrence. Two additional patients, a 5-year-old girl and a 63-year-old physician, had ganglioneuromas successfully resected from the mediastinum as well as from lower plexus elements.

## Discussion of Brachial Plexus Tumors Approached Posteriorly

In 1987, Lusk and colleagues[53] reported on a series of tumors involving the brachial plexus. Among the 56 patients with 57 tumors, 10 were operated on through a posterior approach because of involvement of proximal or lower plexus elements.

Among the 22 patients with brachial plexus tumors operated on posteriorly in our updated series, 13 had undergone partial anterior removal or a biopsy before our operation, and 14 tumors involved the C8 and T1 spinal nerves or lower trunk. These considerations made the posterior route more attractive than the anterior approach. The posterior subscapular approach was extremely useful in exposing both the intra- and extraforaminal part of dumbbell-shaped tumors, most of which were neurofibromas.

An earlier report had included seven malignant neurogenic plexus tumors and emphasized that management must be individualized. Although the posterior approach is advantageous for malignant tumors involving spinal nerves, wide local resection and postoperative radiotherapy are usually the only choices at this level. In such cases, forequarter amputation is not effective because of the medial extent of the tumor.

## POSTIRRADIATION PLEXOPATHY

Fourteen patients who previously underwent irradiation for cancer were operated on for painful brachial plexopathy[22] (Table 21–15). There were 11 women and 3 men, with a mean age of 50 years. The primary malignancy was breast cancer in 8 cases, Hodgkin disease in 3, pulmonary cancer in 2, and thyroid cancer in one. The time interval between radiotherapy and onset of disabling symptomatology and surgery ranged from 15 months to 18 years (mean, 8 years). Pain was the predominant symptom, but four patients also presented with a very severe neurologic deficit. Decompression of the irradiated plexus by first-rib resection through the posterior approach was performed, as well as neurolysis and removal of scar tissue. Associated metastatic tumor was found in three cases. Follow-up evaluation was available in 12 patients; pain was improved in 8, but function had deteriorated in 7. One of the patients who did not improve subsequently underwent amputation of a severely painful flail arm.

Among the 14 patients classified as having postirradiation brachial plexopathy, tumor metastatic to the plexus was discovered intraop-

**TABLE 21–15**
Postirradiation Brachial Plexitis Operated Posteriorly (n = 14)

| | Primary Cancer | | | |
|---|---|---|---|---|
| | **Breast** | **Hodgkin** | **Lung** | **Thyroid** |
| Number of Cases | 8 | 3 | 2 | 1 |
| Male/Female Ratio | 0/8 | 1/2 | 2/0 | 0/1 |
| Mean Age (yr) | 54 | 40 | 56.5 | 40 |
| Mean Interval Between Radiation Therapy and Plexopathy (yr) | 8.8 | 9 | 4.5 | 3 |
| Prior Operation | | | | |
|   Mastectomy | 8 | 0 | 0 | 0 |
|   Thoracotomy | 0 | 1 | 2 | 0 |
|   Neck dissection | 0 | 0 | 0 | 1 |
|   Biopsy of plexus | 1 | 1 | 0 | 0 |
|   Cervical laminectomy | 0 | 0 | 1 | 0 |
|   Carpal tunnel release | 1 | 0 | 0 | 0 |
|   Transaxillary first rib resection | 1 | 0 | 0 | 0 |
| Clinical Presentation | | | | |
|   Severe pain | 4 | 2 | 1 | 1 |
|   Mild or moderate pain | 4 | 1 | 1 | 0 |
|   No or partial deficit | 5 | 2 | 2 | 0 |
|   Moderate to severe deficit | 3 | 1 | 0 | 1 |
| Brachial Plexus Lesion | | | | |
|   All roots | 3 | 1 | 0 | 1 |
|   Upper roots | 2 | 1 | 0 | 0 |
|   Lower roots | 3 | 1 | 2 | 0 |
|   Cancer found at operation | 2 | 0 | 1 | 0 |
| Postoperative Status | | | | |
|   Pain improved | 5 | 1 | 1 | 1 |
|   Pain unchanged | 3 | 2 | 1 | 0 |
|   Added plexus deficit | 4 | 2 | 0 | 1 |
|   Scapular winging | 1 | 0 | 0 | 0 |

eratively in three cases. The original lesion was breast cancer in two and pulmonary cancer in one. In this subset, the interval between radiotherapy and onset of symptoms was 10 years, 3.5 years, and 15 months, respectively. Loss of function in these three patients was probably caused by the metastasis to the plexus as well as by changes resulting from irradiation. The presence of severe actinic changes, with large amounts of scar tissue, was the predominant operative finding. These three patients are categorized as having actinic plexitis in this section.

## Case Summary—Actinic Plexitis

This 39-year-old, right-handed woman had a simple mastectomy in 1982 for breast cancer. Postoperatively, she received 23 radiation treatments and 6 months of chemotherapy. She underwent reconstructive surgery with an attempted placement of a breast prosthesis but developed skin infection and had to have a skin graft. She had noticed progressive hand and forearm weakness and severe arm and hand pain for several years. Subsequently, she underwent a first-rib resection through a transaxillary approach but believed that her hand weakness and pain increased postoperatively.

On examination, the hand and forearm were swollen and somewhat stiff. In the supraclavicular area, there was a mild fullness, and the skin was thickened and had telangiectasia. Tapping on this area elicited a Tinel sign with electrical shocks radiating down to the fingers. Supra- and infraspinatus muscles were graded 5, deltoid, biceps, and brachioradialis muscles were 4, and triceps had only trace strength at 1. There was no wrist flexion or extension, no thumb or finger flexion or extension, and no hand-intrinsic muscle function. These findings were consistent with a complete actinic plexopathy in the outflows of the C7, C8, and T1 roots or spinal nerves.

The patient underwent a posterior subscapular approach to the plexus. The residual first rib was removed, as was an elongated C7 transverse process. The plexus demonstrated an anatomical variation, being postfixed with a contribution from the T2 nerve root. A large amount of scar tissue was removed from the lower elements. Histologic examination of tissue from this area revealed not only dense fibrocollagenous tissue but also metastatic carcinoma of breast origin. After neurolysis, NAP recordings gave no electrical response from C8, T1, or T2 to the lower trunk and none from C7 to the middle trunk. The postoperative course was uneventful. Neurologic function remained the same as preoperatively. However, good pain relief was achieved.

**Comment**

Direct operation on the plexus may give some pain relief in carefully selected cases. It is difficult to improve function, particularly of the hand. This patient succumbed to metastatic carcinoma 2 years later.

Table 21–16 includes some of the points of differentiation between secondary neoplasm involving plexus and irradiation plexitis. Unfortunately, none of these features has absolute value, and that includes findings on needle biopsy, because the neoplasm or the associated irradiation plexitis changes can be missed depending on what was sampled. An absolute diagnosis can be provided only by operating on the plexus and submitting multiple samples of tissue to the pathologist. In many cases, however, a combination of the differential findings provided in Table 21–16 will favor one diagnosis or the other.

**TABLE 21–16**

## Features Differentiating Secondary Neoplasm of Plexus and Irradiation Plexitis

**Features Favoring Irradiation Plexitis**

1. Slowly progressive onset of paralysis and/or sensory change, sometimes but often not painless; paresthesias are often the dominant symptom.
2. Onset more likely in later years after diagnosis of breast cancer, but there are exceptions to this.
3. No evidence of metastasis elsewhere.
4. Neuroimaging may show plexus thickening but not a discrete mass; needle biopsy shows no neoplasm but heavy scar instead.
5. Electromyography may show fasciculations/myokymia.

**Features Favoring Secondary Neoplasm**

1. Rapidly progressive with severe pain.
2. Onset more likely in months to early years after original diagnosis of breast cancer, but there are exceptions to this.
3. Evidence of metastasis elsewhere.
4. Neuroimaging shows localized mass or needle biopsy shows neoplasm (could have intermixed irradiation plexitis as well).

Adapted from Wilbourn AJ: Brachial plexus disorders. *In* Dyck P and Thomas PK, Eds: Peripheral Neuropathy. Philadelphia, WB Saunders, 1993.

# LOCALIZED HYPERTROPHIC NEUROPATHY ("ONION WHORL DISEASE")

This uncommon disorder results in thickening of a peripheral nerve. Because of the unusual nature of the lesion, its occurrence is usually marked by the publication of a case report or the presentation of a few cases.[5,30,36,41,63,80] Despite this, we suspect that it occurs more frequently than the sporadic case reports would suggest. Characteristic of the disease is a localized but not focal enlargement of one or sometimes two major nerves of the limb. The lesion does not spread to other nerves or to other sites in the body. Progressive deficit of function occurs, and most attempts to treat it are unsuccessful unless the lesion is resected and the nerve repaired. The latter usually requires grafts because the lesion has an up-and-down nature. The grafts are likely to be lengthy because the process involves a significant length of the nerve. Reported results with this approach have been limited both by number of cases done and by functional outcomes.[4,39,42,43,68,77]

Histologically, there is a striking proliferation of perineurial cells surrounding each individual myelinated fiber. There is a marked endoneurial fibrosis and also fibrotic replacement of the perineurium. Myelin is either lost or greatly diminished in thickness. The fibrous tissue tends to whorl around the fibers. This characteristic histologic feature of the disease has led to the term "onion whorl disease." Compartmentation, in which the axon is surrounded by fibrous tissue and also seems to be encircled by its own perineurium, is also characteristic. This produces hypertrophic fascicles (Figure 21–55). Some studies using S-100 protein as an immunocytochemical marker as well as other histologic characteristics suggest that the whorls of fibrous tissue around the fibers originate from perineurial cells.[42,58,67,81] Intraneurial tumors and other nontumorous and nontraumatic causes of nerve enlargement should be in the differential diagnosis.[49,63,70] They include amyloidosis, Hansen disease, and Charcot-Marie-Tooth disease (Figure 21–56).[1,61] It is not clear whether onion whorl lesions are of tumorous or traumatic origin. Some of the histologic observations favor the latter even though a clear history of trauma involving nerve is often absent. Interruption of the perineurial blood-nerve barrier may be the initial stimulus to these hypertrophic changes, but the cause of this interruption is still uncertain.[42]

Onion whorl disorder usually presents in children or the young. There are occasional exceptions, however, and several of our patients were young adults. To date, we have had operative experience with 13 patients with localized hypertrophic neuropathy (Table 21–17).

Distribution of the cases in our series include

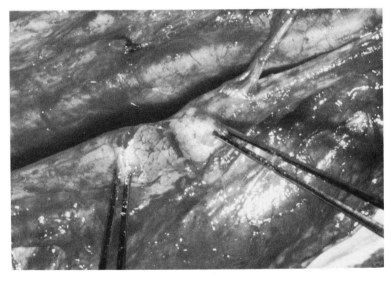

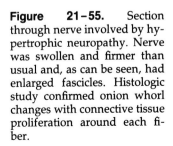

**Figure 21–55.** Section through nerve involved by hypertrophic neuropathy. Nerve was swollen and firmer than usual and, as can be seen, had enlarged fascicles. Histologic study confirmed onion whorl changes with connective tissue proliferation around each fiber.

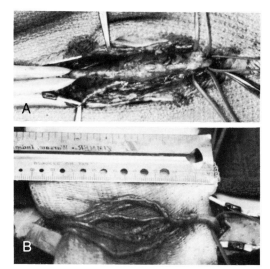

**Figure 21–56.** (A) Exposure of median nerve at the palmar level in a 4-year-old child with Déjérine-Sottas disease. Preoperative symptoms included pain, local tenderness, paresthesias, and an enlarging mass at the palmar level. (B) A carpal tunnel release and an internal neurolysis were done.

brachial plexus (2), median (3), ulnar (2), radial (1), and sciatic complex (5). Loss of function in each of the involved nerves was severe both clinically and electrically but still incomplete. As a result, early cases were treated by neurolysis, either external or internal, and of course removal of tissue for histologic studies. This approach, however, neither reversed the loss nor halted its progression, and in several cases, it increased the loss. As a result, later encounters with this unusual entity have led to resection and replacement of the lost segment with grafts. Exceptions have been lengthy lesions in nerves such as the peroneal or proximal ulnar nerve, in which resection of the lesion and lengthy graft repair seldom yield significant return. On the

**TABLE 21–17**
Localized Hypertrophic Neuropathy
(n = 13)

| Location | No. of Cases |
|---|---|
| Brachial Plexus | 2 |
| Sciatic Complex | 5 |
| Radial | 1 |
| Median | 3 |
| Ulnar | 2 |
| TOTAL | 13 |

other hand, more focal lesions have been resected and replaced with grafts and have had some recovery. The following four cases demonstrate some of the features of this unusual lesion and the difficulties in managing it.

## Case Summaries — Localized Hypertrophic Neuropathy

### Case Number 1

A 12-year-old boy presented with a painless but slowly progressive foot drop. Weakness had begun 3 years before. In addition to both clinically severe weakness and denervational change in evertors, anterior tibialis, and extensor hallucis, there was mild weakness and electromyographic change in tibial-innervated muscles. At surgical exploration, a fusiform swelling of the sciatic nerve 8 cm in length was found just proximal to its bifurcation and extending into both tibial and peroneal nerves (Figure 21–57). A NAP could be recorded from proximal sciatic to tibial nerve, but only a small response to the peroneal nerve beyond its enlargement could be recorded. An internal neurolysis of both divisions of the sciatic nerve was done. Postoperatively, peroneal loss was nearly complete and tibial function was reduced further from its preoperative status. Follow-up over a 7-year period showed full recovery of tibial function but no significant return of peroneal function. Fragments of fascicles removed were characteristic of hypertrophic neuropathy.

### Comment

Unfortunately, loss in the distribution of a nerve involved by this disease is usually progressive. Loss is neither reversed nor slowed by neurolysis alone.

### Case Number 2

A 9-year-old boy had a 1.5-year history of foot drop without a definite history of trauma. However, he had been involved in a number of organized youth sports including football and soccer. Exploration was done at the buttock level because of weakness and denervational change in the lateral (short) head of the biceps femoris. Sciatic nerve was swollen at the level of the buttocks over a 5-cm distance. The tibial division was split away from the peroneal division, and the latter was resected and replaced with sural grafts. Over a 5-year period, tibial function was maintained, but peroneal function only partially returned, and a shoe insert foot brace was still necessary for a normal gait. Resected segments of the peroneal division of the sciatic nerve were characteristic of localized hypertrophic neuropathy.

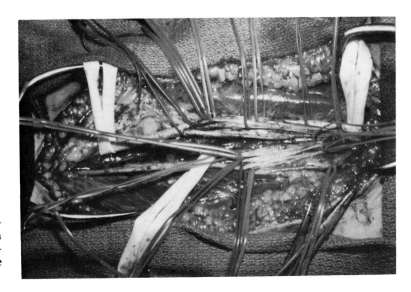

**Figure 21–57.** Internal neurolysis on sciatic complex; both divisions were involved by hypertrophic neuropathy. See also color figure.

**Comment**

Sciatic nerve was evaluated and repaired in a split fashion. It remains difficult to obtain results with proximal peroneal division repair.

**Comment**

Results in this patient were good even though junction was imperfect. Despite incomplete recovery, the patient's performance of daily activities was unimpeded.

**Case Number 3**

A 16-year-old girl had a history of progressive weakness of the left foot and ankle and trouble walking on her heels. There was a family history of diabetes mellitus, but the patient had been tested repeatedly for this and had no known diabetes. On examination, there was anterior compartment atrophy in the left leg, and peronei graded 4, anterior tibialis 1, extensor hallucis longus 0, and extensor communis 1. Electromyography showed severe denervation in the distribution of the deep branch with less change in that of the superficial branch.

At operation, a segment of the peroneal nerve over the head of the fibula was hypertrophied. This hypertrophy extended into the deep branch of the nerve. Deep branch fascicles were split away from superficial branch fascicles, and each was individually tested by NAP recording.The superficial branch fascicles and their distal branch conducted, but the deep branch did not. Testing of adjacent sural branches showed good NAP conduction. As a result, the deep branch fascicles and more distal branch were resected and replaced with three sural grafts a little over 4 cm in length.

By 4 years postoperatively, toe extension, including extensor hallucis longus, graded 3 to 4, eversion was 5, but anterior tibialis was only 1 to 2. The patient was able to walk without a brace, went swimming, and was able to do most activities. Resected tissue showed a well-established and prominent hypertrophic neuropathy (onion bulb neuropathy).

**Case Number 4**

Another 16-year-old girl had a 4-year history of a painless progressive loss of function in the C5, C6, C7 distribution of the left brachial plexus. Severe shoulder and upper arm atrophy ensued. At exploration, fusiform enlargement of the upper three plexus roots and the upper and middle trunk was found (Figure 21–58). A NAP could be evoked to the anterior and posterior divisions of the upper trunk by stimulation of C5, but not by stimulation of C6. Conduction from C7 to middle trunk was absent. C6 and its contribution to upper trunk were resected, and an attempt was made to preserve some of the C5 input by splitting it away from C6 input to upper trunk. C7 through middle trunk was resected. Resected segments were replaced by sural grafts 5 to 8 cm long. Again, the resected segments proved to be characteristic of onion whorl disease. Follow-up over 3.5 years showed recovery of deltoid to grade 3 to 4, biceps 2 to 3, and triceps 3. There was no recovery of brachioradialis or supination. Shoulder and upper arm atrophy had reversed only partially.

**Comment**

Recovery of proximal plexus outflow of C6 to biceps and C7 to triceps was partial but good. Recovery of more distal outflow to brachioradialis and supinator did not occur.

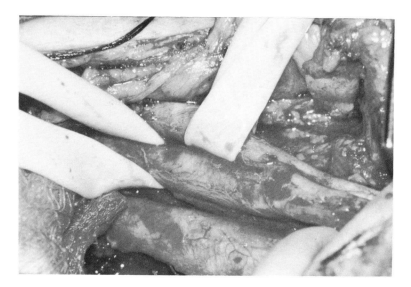

**Figure 21–58.** Hypertrophic neuropathy or onion whorl change involving C5 and C6 to upper trunk and C7 to middle trunk. Elements were quite swollen and firm. After nerve action potential recording, most of the involved plexus was resected and replaced by grafts.

## References

1. Appenzeller O and Kornfeld M: Macrodactyly and localized hypertrophic neuropathy. Neurology 24:767–771, 1974.
2. Ariel I: Current concepts in the management of peripheral nerve tumors. In Omer G and Spinner M, Eds: Management of Peripheral Nerve Lesions. Philadelphia, WB Saunders, 1986.
3. Bataskis JG: Tumors of the Head and Neck: Clinical and Pathological Considerations. Baltimore, Williams & Wilkins, 1974, pp. 231–240.
4. Bilbao JM, Khoury NJS, Hudson AR, and Briggs SJ: Perineurioma (localized hypertrophic neuropathy). Arch Pathol Lab Med 108:557–560, 1984.
5. Boker DK, Schonberg F, and Gullotta F: Localized hypertrophic neuropathy—A rare, clinically almost unknown syndrome. Clin Neuropathol 3:228–230, 1984.
6. Bolton J, Vauthey J, Farr G, et al.: Is limb-sparing surgery applicable to neurogenic sarcomas of the extremities? Arch Surg 124:118–121, 1989.
7. Burger PC and Vogel FS: Surgical Pathology of the Nervous System and Its Coverings. New York, John Wiley & Sons, 1982.
8. Byrne JJ: Nerve tumors. In Gelberman R, Ed: Operative Nerve Repair and Reconstruction. Philadelphia, JB Lippincott, 1991.
9. Byrne JJ and Cahill JM: Tumors of major peripheral nerves. Am J Surg 102:724–727, 1961.
10. Campbell R: Tumors of peripheral and sympathetic nerves. In J Youmans, Ed: Neurologic Surgery, 3rd Ed. Philadelphia, WB Saunders, 1990.
11. Cravioto H: Neoplasms of peripheral nerves. In Wilkins R and Rengachary E, Eds: Neurosurgery. Baltimore, Williams & Wilkins, 1988.
12. Curtis RM and Clark GL: Tumors of the blood and lymphatic vessels. In Gelberman R, Ed: Operative Nerve Repair and Reconstruction. Philadelphia, JB Lippincott, 1991.
13. Cutler EC and Gross RE: Neurofibroma and neurofibrosarcoma of peripheral nerves, unassociated with von Recklinghausen's disease: A report of 25 cases. Arch Surg 33:733–779, 1936.
14. D'Agostino AN, Soule EH, and Miller RH: Primary malignant neoplasm of nerves (malignant neurilemomas) in patients without manifestations of multiple neurofibromatosis (von Recklinghausen's disease). Cancer 16:1003–1014, 1963.
15. Dart L, MacCarty CS, Love JG, and Dockerty MD: Neoplasms of the brachial plexus. Minn Med 53:959–964, 1970.
16. DasGupta T: Tumors of the peripheral nerves. Clin Neurosurg 25:574–590, 1978.
17. DasGupta TK, Brasfield RD, and Strong EW: Benign solitary schwannomas (neurilemomas). Cancer 24:355–366, 1969.
18. DaSilva AL and deSouza RP: Neurofibroma solitario do plexobraquial. Hospital (Rio) 65:853–859, 1964.
19. DeSouza FM, Smith PE, and Molony TJ: Management of brachical plexus tumors. J Otolaryngol 8:537–540, 1979.
20. Dodge HW and Craig WMcK: Benign tumors of peripheral nerves and their masquerade. Minn Med 40:294–301, 1957.
21. Donner T, Voorhies R, Kline D: Neural sheath tumors of major nerves. J Neurosurg 81:362–373, 1994.
22. Dubuisson A, Kline D, and Weinshel S: Posterior subscapular approach to the brachial plexus: Report of 102 cases. J Neurosurg 79:319–330, 1993.
23. Ehrlich H and Martin H: Schwannomas (neurilemomas) in the head and neck. Surg Gynecol Obstet 76:577–583, 1943.
24. Fisher ER and Vusevski VD: Cytogenesis of schwannomas (neurilemomas), neurofibromas, dermatofibromas and dermatofibrosarcomas as revealed by electron microscopy. Am J Clin Pathol 49:141–154, 1968.
25. Fisher R and Tate H: Isolated neurilemomas of the brachial plexus. J Neurosurg 32:463–467, 1970.
26. Foley KM, Woodruff JM, Ellis FT, and Posner JB: Radiation-induced malignant and atypical peripheral nerve sheath tumors. Ann Neurol 7:311–318, 1980.
27. Gatch WD and Ritchey JO: Neurofibromyxoma treated by conservative operation. Ann Surg 75:181, 1992.
28. Godwin JT: Encapsulated neurilemoma (schwannoma) of the brachial plexus: Report of eleven cases. Cancer 5:708–720, 1952.
29. Goldman R, Jones S, and Heu Sinkueld RS: Combination chemotherapy of metastatic malignant schwannoma with vincristine, adriamycin, cyclophosphamide,

and imidazole carbaxamide. Cancer 39:1955–1957, 1977.

30. Grossiord A, Lapresle J, Lacert P, and Appeloig E: A propos d'une forme localisee de nevrite hypertrophique. Rev Neurol 119:248–252, 1968.

31. Gyhra H, Israel J, Santander C, and Acuna D: Schwannoma of the brachial plexus with intrathoracic extension. Thorax 35:703–704, 1980.

32. Handler SD, Sanalis RF, Jenkins HA, and Weiss AJ: Management of brachial plexus tumors. Arch Otolaryngol 103:653–657, 1977.

33. Harkin J: Differential diagnosis of peripheral nerve tumors. In Omer G and Spinner M, Eds: Management of Peripheral Nerve Lesions. Philadelphia, WB Saunders, 1980.

34. Harkin JC and Reed RJ: Tumors of the peripheral nervous system. In Atlas of Tumor Pathology, Fascicle 3. Washington, DC, Armed Forces Institute of Pathology, 1969.

35. Hashimoto H, Enjoiji M, Kajima T, et al.: Malignant neuroepithelioma (peripheral neuroblastoma): A clinicopathologic study of 15 cases. Am J Surg Pathol 7:309–318, 1983.

36. Hawkes CH, Jefferson JM, Jones EL, and Smith WT: Hypertrophic mononeuropathy. J Neurol Neurosurg Psychiatry 37:76–81, 1974.

37. Hudson A and Kline D: Peripheral nerve tumors. In Schmidek H and Sweet W, Eds: Operative Neurosurgical Techniques, 2nd Ed., New York, Grune & Stratton, 1993.

38. Hutchinson R, Jenkins H, Canalis R, et al.: Neurogenic sarcoma of the head and neck. Arch Otolaryngol 105:267–271, 1979.

39. Imaginario JDG, Coelho B, Tome F, and Luis MLS: Nevrite interstitielle hypertrophique monosymptomatique. J Neurol Sci 1:340–347, 1964.

40. Inoune M, Kawano T, Matsumura H, et al.: Solitary benign schwannoma of the brachial plexus. Surg Neurol 20:103–108, 1983.

41. Iyer VG, Garretson HD, Byrd RP, and Reiss SJ: Localized hypertrophic mononeuropathy involving the tibial nerve. Neurosurgery 23:218–221, 1988.

42. Johnson PC and Kline DG: Localized hypertrophic neuropathy: Possible focal perineurial barrier defect. Acta Neuropathol 77:514–518, 1989.

43. Kline DG: Comment on Reyes RADL, Chason JL, Rogers JS, and Ausman JI: Hypertrophic neurofibrosis with onion bulb formation in an isolated element of the brachial plexus. Neurosurgery 8:397–399, 1981.

44. Kline DG, Donner T, and Voorhies RM: Management of tumors of peripheral nerve. In Tindall G, Cooper P, and Barrow D, Eds: The Practice of Neurologic Surgery. Baltimore, Williams & Wilkins, 1994.

45. Kline DG, Kott J, Barnes G, and Bryant L: Exploration of selected brachial plexus lesions by the posterior subscapular approach. J Neurosurg 49:872–880, 1978.

46. Kori SH, Foley KM, and Posner JB: Brachial plexus lesions in patients with cancer: 100 cases. Neurology 31:45–50, 1981.

47. Kragh LV, Soule EH, and Masson JK: Benign and malignant neurilemmomas of the head and neck. Surg Gynecol Obstet 111:211–218, 1960.

48. Kruche W: Pathologie der Peripheren Nerven. In Olivecrona VH, Tonnis W, Kerenkel W, Eds: Handbuch der Neurochirurgie. Vol 7, Pt 3. Berlin, Springer-Verlag, 1974.

49. Lallemand RC and Weller RO: Intraneural neurofibromas involving the posterior interosseous nerve. J Neurol Neurosurg Psychiatry 36:991–996, 1973.

50. Lang K: Neurinom in Sinne von Verocay des plexus brachialis. Centralbl Chir 67:857–858, 1940.

51. Lederman RJ and Wilbourn AJ: Brachial plexopathy: Recurrent cancer or radiation? Neurology 34:1331–1335, 1984.

52. Lewis D and Hart D: Tumors of peripheral nerves. Ann Surg 92:961–983, 1930.

53. Lusk M, Kline D, and Garcia C: Tumors of the brachial plexus. Neurosurgery 21:439–453, 1987.

54. Lusli EJ: Intrinsic hemangiomas of peripheral nerves: Report of 2 cases and review of the literature. Arch Pathol 53:266–270, 1952.

55. Mallory FB: The type cell for the so-called dural endothelioma. J Med Res 41:349–364, 1920.

56. Masson P: Experimental and spontaneous schwannomas. Am J Pathol 8:384–417, 1932.

57. McCarthy WD and Pack GT: Malignant blood vessel tumors: A report of 56 cases of angiosarcoma and Kaposi's sarcoma. Surg Gynecol Obstet 91:465–470, 1950.

58. Mitsumoto H, Wilbourn AJ, and Goren H: Perineurioma as the cause of localized hypertrophic neuropathy. Muscle Nerve 3:403–412, 1980.

59. Narakas A: Brachial plexus surgery. Orthop Clin North Am 12:303–323, 1981.

60. Noterman J, D'Haens J, Nubourgh Y, and Colle H: Les tumeurs du plexus brachial. Neurochirurgie 28:139–141, 1982.

61. Ochoa J and Neary D: Localized hypertrophic neuropathy, intraneural tumour, or chronic nerve entrapment? Lancet 1:632–633, 1975.

62. Ott WO: The surgical treatment of solitary tumors of the peripheral nerves. Texas State J Med 20:171–175, 1924.

63. Peckham NH, O'Boynick PL, Meneses A, and Kepes JJ: Hypertrophic mononeuropathy: A report of two cases and review of the literature. Arch Pathol Lab Med 106:534–537, 1982.

64. Peled I, Isosipovich Z, Rousso M, and Wexler MR: Hemangioma of the median nerve. J Hand Surg 5:363–365, 1980.

65. Pellegrini G, DeFirmas JL, and Lalizout D: Neurinomas du plexus cervical et du plexus brachial. Rev Otoneuroophtalmol 41:270–274, 1969.

66. Penfield W: Tumors of the sheaths of the nervous system: Section 19. In Cytology and Cellular Pathology of the Nervous System, Vol. 3. New York, Paul B Hoeber, 1932.

67. Perentes E, Nakagawa Y, Ross GW, et al.: Expression of epithelial membrane antigen in perineurial cells and their derivatives. An immunohistochemical study with multiple markers. Acta Neuropathol 75:160–165, 1987.

68. Phillips LH, Persing JA, and Vandenberg SR: Electrophysiological findings in localized hypertrophic neuropathy. Muscle Nerve 14(4):335–341, 1991.

69. Posch JL: Soft tissue tumors of the hand. In Jupiter J, Ed: Flynn's Hand Surgery. Baltimore, Williams & Wilkins, 1991.

70. Reyes RADL, Chason JL, Rogers JS, and Ausman JI: Hypertrophic neurofibrosis with onion bulb formation in an isolated element of the brachial plexus. Neurosurgery 8:397–399, 1981.

71. Richardson R, Siqueira E, Ol S, and Nunez X: Neurogenic tumors of the brachial plexus: Report of two cases. Neurosurgery 4:66–70, 1979.

72. Rizzoli H and Horowitz N: Peripheral nerve tumors. In Horowitz N and Rizzoli H, Eds: Postoperative Complications of Extracranial Neurological Surgery. Baltimore, Williams & Wilkins, 1987.

73. Rosenberg AE, Dick HM, and Botte MJ: Benign and malignant tumors of peripheral nerve. *In* Gelberman R, Ed: Operative Nerve Repair and Reconstruction. Philadelphia, JB Lippincott, 1991.

74. Russell DS and Rubinstein LJ: Pathology of Tumors of the Nervous System, 4th Ed., Baltimore, Williams & Wilkins, 1977, pp. 293–297.

75. Saxen E: Tumours of the sheaths of the peripheral nerves (studies on their structures, histogenesis and symptomatology). Acta Pathol Microbiol Scand 26 (suppl 79):1–135, 1948.

76. Seddon H: Surgical Disorders of the Peripheral Nerves. Baltimore, Williams & Wilkins, 1972, pp. 153–170.

77. Simpson DA and Fowler M: Two cases of localized hypertrophic neurofibrosis. J Neurol Neurosurg Psychiatry 29:80–84, 1966.

78. Smith R and Lipke R: Surgical treatment of peripheral nerve tumors of the upper limb. *In* Omer G and Spinner M, Eds: Management of Peripheral Nerve Lesions. Philadelphia, WB Saunders, 1980.

79. Snyder M, Batzdorf U, and Sparks F: Unusual malignant tumors involving the brachial plexus: A report of two cases. Am Surg 45:42–48, 1979.

80. Snyder M, Cancilla PA, and Batzdorf U: Hypertrophic neuropathy simulating a neoplasm of the brachial plexus. Surg Neurol 7:131–134, 1977.

81. Stanton C, Perentes E, Phillips L, and Vandenberg SR: The immunohistochemical demonstration of early perineurial change in the development of hypertrophic localized neuropathy. Hum Pathol 19:1455–1457, 1988.

82. Stevens JC, David DH, and MacCarty CS: A 32-year experience with the surgical treatment of selected brachial plexus lesions with emphasis on its reconstruction. Surg Neurol 19:334–345, 1983.

83. Stout AP: Tumors featuring pericytes: glomus tumor and hemangiopericytoma. Lab Invest 5:217–223, 1956.

84. Stout AP: Tumors of the peripheral nervous system. *In* National Research Council Committee on Pathology, Eds: Atlas of Tumor Pathology, Section 2, Fascicle 6. Washington, DC, Armed Forces Institute of Pathology, 1949.

85. Thomas JE and Colby MY Jr: Radiation-induced or metastatic brachial plexopathy? A diagnostic dilemma. JAMA 222:1392–1395, 1972.

86. Thomas JE, Piepgras DG, and Scheithauer B: Neurogenic tumors of the sciatic nerve. A clinic and clinicopathologic study of 35 cases. Mayo Clin Proc 58:640–647, 1983.

87. Verocay J: Zur Kenntnis der Neurofibrome. Beitr Pathol Anat Allg Pathol 48:1, 1910.

88. Vieta JO and Pack GT: Malignant neurilemmomas of peripheral nerves. Am J Surg 82:416–431, 1951.

89. Virchow R: Ueber einen Fall von vielfachen Neuromen (sogenannta Faser-Kern-geschwuelsten) mit ausgezeichneter lokaler Recidivfaehigkeit. Virchows Arch A Pathol Anat Histol 12:144, 1857.

90. Whitaker WG and Droulias C: Benign encapsulated neurilemmomas: A report of 76 cases. Ann Surg 42:675–678, 1976.

91. Woodhall B: Peripheral nerve tumors. Surg Clin Am 34:1167–1172, 1954.

92. Woodruff J: The pathology and treatment of peripheral nerve tumors and tumor-like conditions. Cancer J Clin 43:290–308, 1993.

# Appendix 1

## SUMMARIZING CLINICAL DATA

There are many disadvantages to summarizing clinical data, including the fear of misleading the reader based on averaged rather than individual case results. Despite this observation, one possible advantage is an opportunity to compare results among different nerves, operations done on them, and the influence of level of injury. Examples of this type of comparison can be seen throughout the book and in Tables 1 and 2.

As expected, results with management of radial or median nerve injuries were substantially better than those for the ulnar nerve. On the other hand, the majority of patients with ulnar nerves repaired at either the elbow or wrist level recovered significant useful function, and this was a pleasant surprise. Not unexpectedly, those numbers dropped considerably when only grade 4 or better results were tabulated. Patients with median repairs also fared better than might have been predicted, and this even included lesions at either the arm or elbow

levels. Recovery of function in both grade 3 and grade 4 categories was not as good as that of the radial at an arm level, but came close to it, and elbow-level scores were quite comparable.

If neurolysis rather than repair was done on lesions in continuity because of a positive nerve action potential across the lesion, average results in 90% to 100% of cases achieved a grade 3 recovery, irrespective of nerve involved or level of injury. These values reduced for grade 4 recoveries but did not fall to less than 80%, except for median and ulnar lesions at an arm level.

If figures for repair of each of the three upper extremity nerves are averaged, there is a gradation for results. Outcomes were superior for primary repair (which were also done for the less serious and sharper transecting injuries), next best for secondary repair, and least successful for graft repair (usually the more severe lesions having an element of stretch or contusion that required resection).

As subsets of data relating type of injury to

**TABLE 1**
LSUMC Operative Results Based on 378 Serious Upper Extremity Lesions*

| Nerve Involved/Operation | Lesion Level | | |
|---|---|---|---|
| | Upper Arm | Elbow | Forearm or Wrist |
| Radial Nerve/Neurolysis† | | | |
|   Grade 3 or better | 100 | 90 | 94 |
|   Grade 4 or better | 90 | 83 | 89 |
| Radial Nerve/Repair‡ | | | |
|   Grade 3 or better | 72 | 81 | 79 |
|   Grade 4 or better | 60 | 62 | 60 |
| Median Nerve/Neurolysis | | | |
|   Grade 3 or better | 90 | 93 | 93 |
|   Grade 4 or better | 78 | 87 | 90 |
| Median Nerve/Repair | | | |
|   Grade 3 or better | 68 | 75 | 81 |
|   Grade 4 or better | 45 | 64 | 68 |
| Ulnar Nerve/Neurolysis | | | |
|   Grade 3 or better | 90 | 92 | 100 |
|   Grade 4 or better | 79 | 83 | 92 |
| Ulnar Nerve/Repair | | | |
|   Grade 3 or better | 41 | 69 | 56 |
|   Grade 4 or better | 15 | 31 | 40 |

*Percent with functional return using LSUMC grading system. Does not include brachial plexus lesions, peripheral nerve tumors, or nerve entrapment cases.
†Neurolysis was usually based on a positive nerve action potential transmitted across a lesion in continuity.
‡Repair category included end-to-end repairs, graft repairs, and split or partial repairs.

**TABLE 2**

LSUMC Operative Results Based on 378 Serious Upper Extremity Lesions
Irrespective of Level and Method of Injury*

| Type of Injury | Percentage With Grade 3 or Better Return |
|---|---|
| Transections | |
|   Primary suture | 78 |
|   Secondary suture | 70 |
|   Grafting | 63 |
| In Continuity | |
|   Neurolysis—Based on a positive nerve action potential | 92 |
|   Suture—Based on a negative nerve action potential | 75 |
|   Grafting—Based on a negative nerve action potential | 66 |

*LSUMC grading system for whole nerve used. Does not include brachical plexus lesions, peripheral nerve tumors, or nerve entrapment cases.

level and operation are reviewed, there may be reasons why outcomes for median injuries were nearly comparable to those of the radial:

1. Gunshot wounds did well in either series, but there were fewer of those involving radial at an arm level than median. Conversely, not all fracture-associated lesions in the radial series had successful recovery, but most in the median did.
2. On the other hand, median lesions of most types had a higher incidence of associated vascular injuries, especially at arm and elbow level, than did radial lesions.
3. The elbow-level median series included a number of injection injuries, usually caused by venipuncture, and loss was usually partial to begin with in these nerves. The fact that median injuries at an elbow level did slightly better than radial in the neurolysis category is somewhat misleading because more of the radial injuries having a transmitted nerve action potential at this level had a complete distal loss of function than did the median lesions in continuity. As a result, it was harder for the radial series at this level to recover as extensively after having a neurolysis, even based on a transmitted nerve action potential, than the median series.

This type of analysis emphasizes the importance of the demography for individual subsets of injury and the need to deal with detail when attempting to predict outcomes with any type of nerve operation. Other considerations, such as time interval between injury and operation, patient age, effect of other associated nerve injuries, and the individual operative experience need to be factored in as well.

# Appendix 2

# ADDITIONAL MUSCLE
# TESTING PROCEDURES

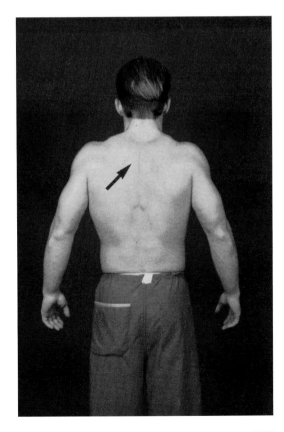

**Figure 1.** The back should not be neglected as a site for inspection and grading of muscle function. In this instance, the model is bracing the shoulders backward as if at military attention. The arrow points to contraction of the left rhomboid. This muscle receives input from C5 to dorsal scapular nerve. Grading is difficult but can be done by comparing both sides: 0 = absent, 1 = trace, 3 = contraction present but not full, 4 = reduced bulk but good contraction, and 5 = full contraction with normal bulk.

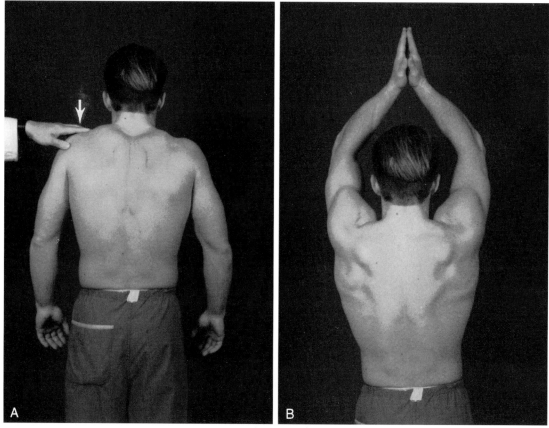

**Figure 2.** (A) Trapezius function is tested in a number of ways. In this photograph, the subject is shrugging the shoulder up against pressure from the examiner's hand (see *arrow*). Contraction of the superior portion of the muscle can be observed and palpated. (B) The lower or thoracic portion of the trapezius helps to hold the scapula against the chest wall and helps rotate it to permit full and smooth shoulder abduction. Thus, scapular function can be observed as the shoulder is abducted. The function of lower trapezius can also be checked by having the subject push forward or across the chest with the partially flexed arm and observing whether or not the scapula protrudes or "wings." Degree of elevation of shoulder against resistance, amount of scapular winging, and shoulder abduction ability can be combined to provide a grade for trapezius and thus accessory nerve function.

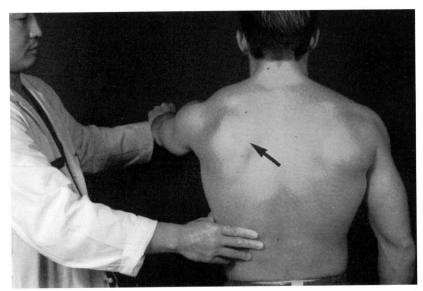

**Figure 3.** In this healthy subject, the examiner is testing the subject for winging of the scapula with the shoulder flexed or abducted forward and the subject pushing forward with the arm fully extended at the elbow. Scapular winging under these circumstances is caused by serratus anterior palsy. This muscle is the sole destination for fibers carried in the long thoracic nerve. Loss of this muscle's function also affects smooth abduction of the arm, especially above the horizontal. Degree of winging in region of arrow and secondary difficulty in shoulder abduction can be used to define a grading system.

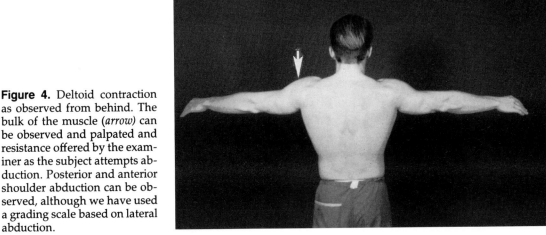

**Figure 4.** Deltoid contraction as observed from behind. The bulk of the muscle (*arrow*) can be observed and palpated and resistance offered by the examiner as the subject attempts abduction. Posterior and anterior shoulder abduction can be observed, although we have used a grading scale based on lateral abduction.

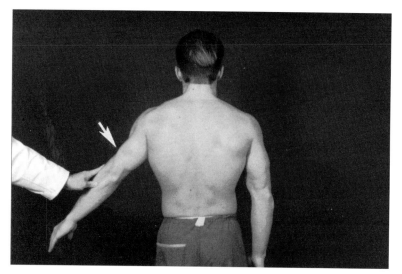

**Figure 5.** The first 30 degrees or so of shoulder abduction is provided by supraspinatus located superior to the spine of the scapula. The arrow indicates the direction for counterpressure used to test the supraspinatus. This muscle receives input from suprascapular nerve, which receives fibers primarily from C5 but also from C6. This muscle can be readily graded against gravity.

**Figure 6.** Latissimus dorsi serves as an internal rotator and partial adductor of shoulder and arm. For example, the muscle contracts and plays a major role during climbing by adducting the shoulder to help pull the individual up. The muscle is most readily tested by having the patient cough and palpating its mass in the posterolateral lower chest as the muscle contracts. Grading is by comparison to the contralateral and usually normal muscle.

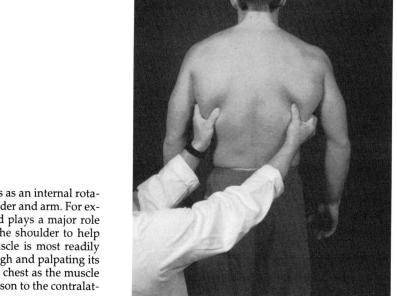

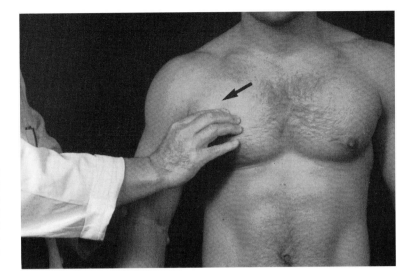

**Figure 7.** Pectoralis major serves as an adductor, but its clavicular head also provides a downward thrust to the shoulder and arm. Pectoralis can be palpated *(arrow)* and observed as the shoulder is adducted in different positions.

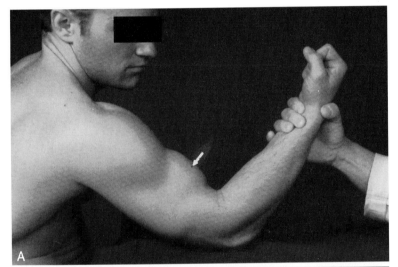

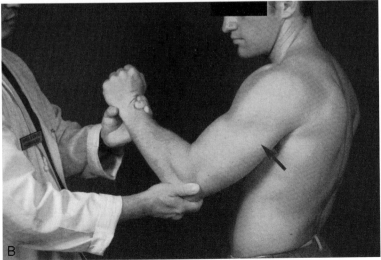

**Figure 8.** *(A)* Biceps *(arrow)* is easily tested. Elbow is placed on a flat surface, and forearm is flexed upward against resistance. Strength can be compared to contralateral biceps. *(B)* Testing triceps muscle *(arrow)*. Subject extends forearm against the examiner's resistance at a forearm level or, as in this example, at a wrist level. Muscle can be observed and palpated as it contracts, and it can be readily graded.

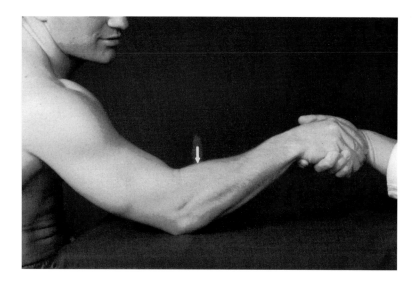

**Figure 9.** Testing pronator teres *(arrow)*. The subject has grasped the examiner's hand, and he is attempting to place the hand palm down against resistance.

**Figure 10.** Dorsiflexion of the wrist is observed in this photograph. Dorsiflexion against resistance can be tested by applying pressure at the point indicated by the arrow. The two muscles primarily responsible for this function are the extensor carpi radialis and the extensor carpi ulnaris. The functions of these muscles can be readily differentiated and graded.

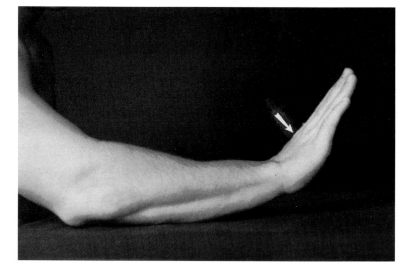

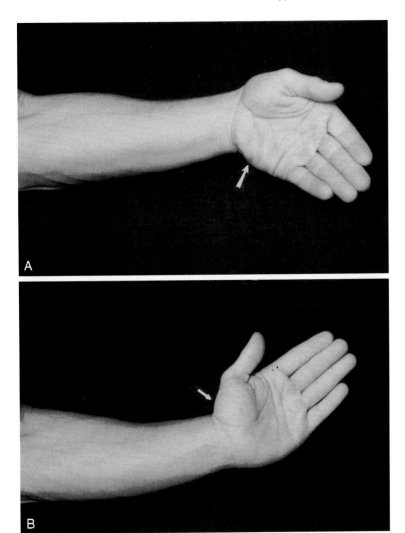

**Figure 11.** Flexor carpi ulnaris (A) and flexor carpi radialis (B) are easily examined and graded by asking the patient to flex against resistance at the points shown by the arrows.

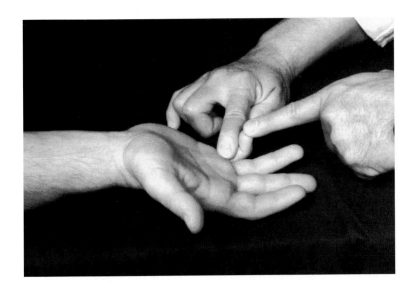

**Figure 12.** Testing flexor profundus of the little finger. The proximal phalanges are stabilized by one of the examiner's forefingers while the patient flexes the distal little finger phalanx against the examiner's other forefinger.

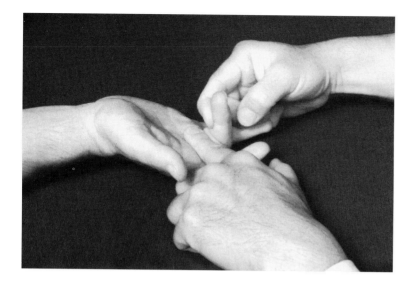

**Figure 13.** Testing flexor superficialis, in this instance of the ring finger. Metacarpal phalangeal joint is fixed by downward pressure of the examiner's left forefinger, and the opposite forefinger is used to resist and grade flexion of the first and second phalanges.

**Figure 14.** Flexor pollicis longus is tested by "suspending" and fixing the thumb's metacarpal phalangeal joint. The distal phalanx is then flexed downward in the direction of the arrow and against the examiner's forefinger and its strength is graded.

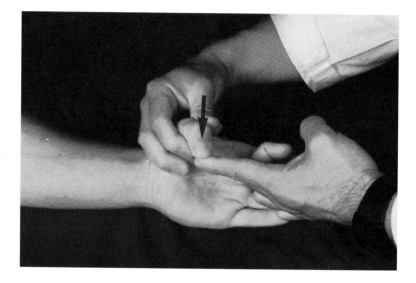

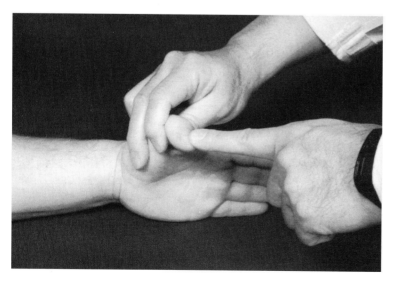

**Figure 15.** Positioning for testing the extensor pollicis longus is similar to that for flexor pollicis longus. The examiner's forefinger resists extension of the thumb's distal phalanx.

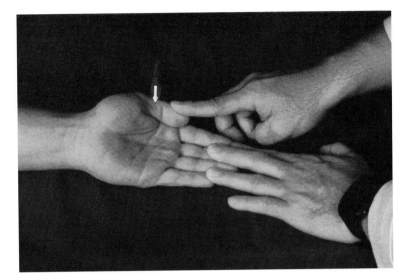

**Figure 16.** Attempt to abduct thumb away from palm at right angles and against the examiner's resistance *(arrow)*. This maneuver tests abductor pollicis brevis.

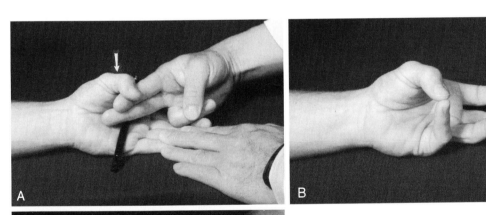

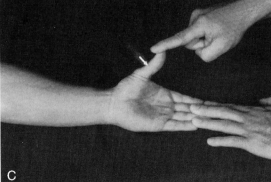

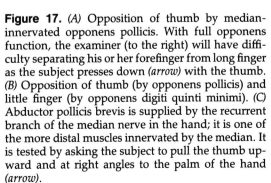

**Figure 17.** *(A)* Opposition of thumb by median-innervated opponens pollicis. With full opponens function, the examiner (to the right) will have difficulty separating his or her forefinger from long finger as the subject presses down *(arrow)* with the thumb. *(B)* Opposition of thumb (by opponens pollicis) and little finger (by opponens digiti quinti minimi). *(C)* Abductor pollicis brevis is supplied by the recurrent branch of the median nerve in the hand; it is one of the more distal muscles innervated by the median. It is tested by asking the subject to pull the thumb upward and at right angles to the palm of the hand *(arrow)*.

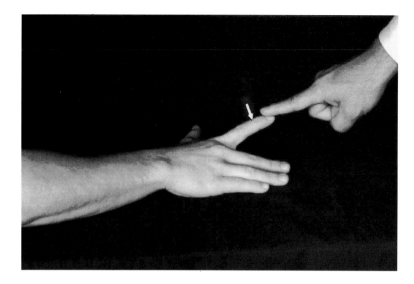

**Figure 18.** Testing extensor communis input to forefinger. The palm and fingers have been placed flat on the table. The subject is asked to lift the forefinger upward against gravity and, as in this case, some pressure. Arrow shows direction of resistance against this motion.

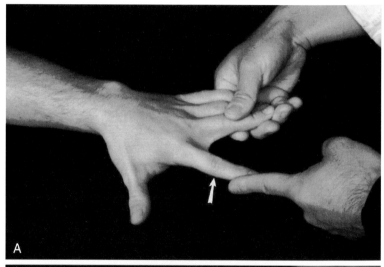

A

**Figure 19.** (A) Proper method for testing interosseous function (in this case, the first dorsal interosseous). The subject is given a target (the examiner's forefinger) which is placed volar to the palmar plane. If this spatial consideration is ignored, and the target is at the plane of the palm or more dorsal, then extensor communis will contribute to the abduction motion provided by the interosseous. (B) If target is dorsal to palmar level, as in this example using little finger, then extensor digiti quinti minimi is tested. Arrows indicate direction of resistance applied against these motions.

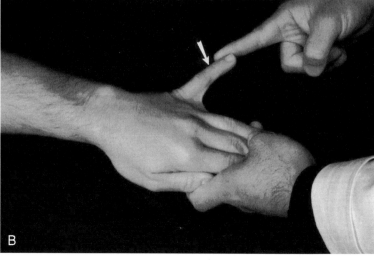

B

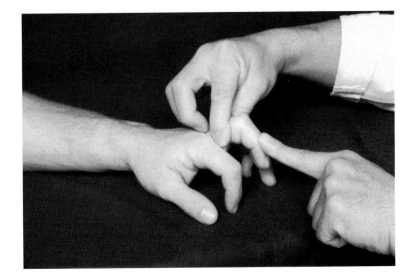

**Figure 20.** One method of testing for lumbrical function. In this example, the metacarpophalangeal joint has been extended by the examiner. The subject is attempting to extend the second phalanx against gravity and some pressure.

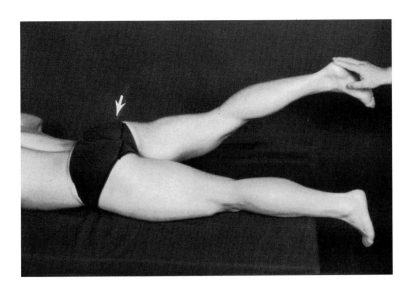

**Figure 21.** Hip extension and lateral rotation by gluteus maximus *(arrow)* can be tested with the patient placed prone. With the knee extended, the patient is asked to lift the leg posteriorly, in this case against pressure provided by the examiner's hand on the heel. Hip abduction provided by gluteus medius can also be tested in this position.

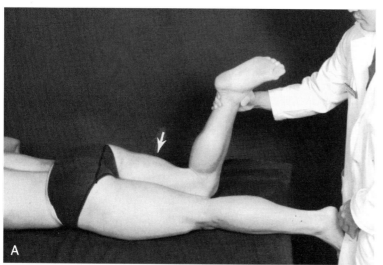

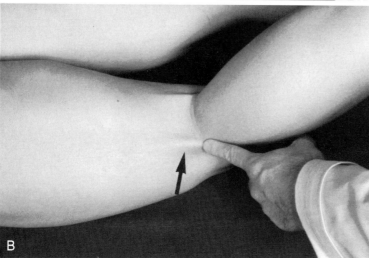

**Figure 22.** (A) Hamstring function can also be tested with the patient prone. Leg is flexed back on thigh, and hamstring muscle (arrow) is observed and palpated. (B) Short or lateral head of biceps femoris, which is innervated by peroneal division of the sciatic, can be readily palpated. Loss of this function implies a proximal peroneal division lesion. The examiner is palpating this tendon (arrow) just proximal to its insertion into the head of the fibula as the patient flexes the knee against resistance.

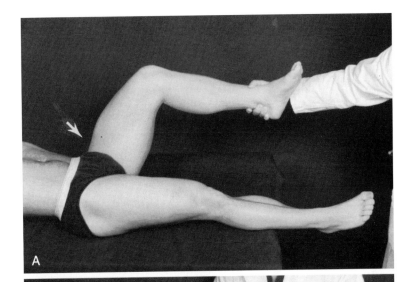

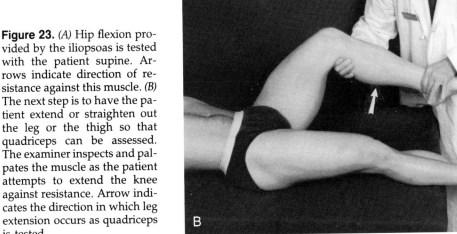

**Figure 23.** *(A)* Hip flexion provided by the iliopsoas is tested with the patient supine. Arrows indicate direction of resistance against this muscle. *(B)* The next step is to have the patient extend or straighten out the leg or the thigh so that quadriceps can be assessed. The examiner inspects and palpates the muscle as the patient attempts to extend the knee against resistance. Arrow indicates the direction in which leg extension occurs as quadriceps is tested.

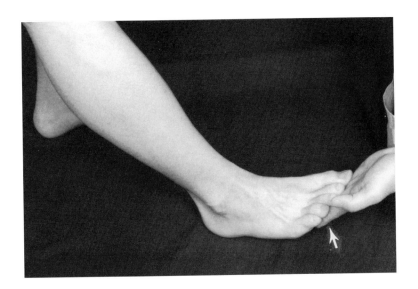

**Figure 24.** Plantar flexion provided by gastrocnemius-soleus can be tested by having the patient place his or her heel flat on the floor and push down with the sole of the foot on the examiner's hand *(arrow)*. To eliminate the effect of gravity, the patient can be placed supine with leg extended. Patient is then asked to push the foot down or to plantar flex. The calf muscle can be readily palpated by the examiner.

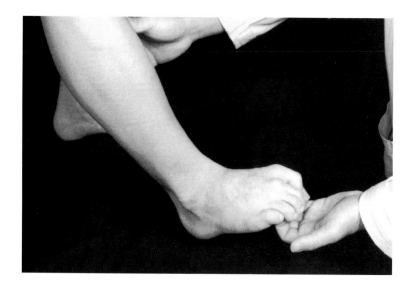

**Figure 25.** Toe flexion can be assessed by asking the patient to grasp the examiner's fingers with his or her toes. This function is best tested by matching it against the contralateral toe flexors.

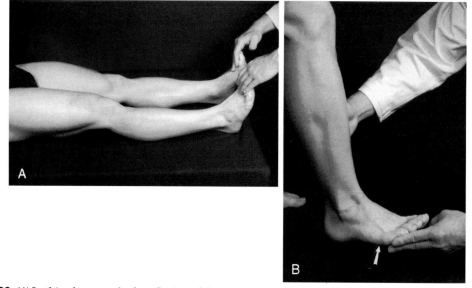

**Figure 26.** *(A)* In this photograph, dorsiflexion of the toes and feet with patient supine is assessed by the examiner, who is providing resistance with one hand on each foot for comparison. *(B)* Eversion provided by peronei is readily tested by having the patient dorsiflex and flare the foot laterally. This proximal anterolateral compartment muscle can also be readily observed and palpated. Arrow indicates direction of resistance on foot to test eversion.

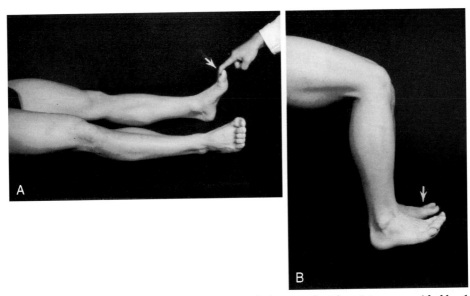

**Figure 27.** *(A)* The patient's left extensor hallucis longus is being tested with resistance provided by the examiner's forefinger *(arrow)*. *(B)* Poor toe extension against gravity is noted in patient's left foot *(arrow)* compared with excellent contraction against gravity in the right foot.

# Appendix 3

. . . . . . . . . . . . . . . . . . . . . . . . . . . . . . . . . . . . . . . . . . . . . . . . . .

## "THIRTEEN YEARS DOWN THE TRACK" BY SIR SYDNEY SUNDERLAND

(Read posthumously before The Sunderland Society, Seattle, September 1993, by Edward Almquist, M.D., and George Omer, M.D.)*

It is a little more than 13 years since this group first met at the Harrison Conference Centre of Glen Cove, Long Island, New York, on July 17 and 18, 1980. If we use the creation of this society as a useful point of reference, we are now 13 years down the track, which brings to mind the words of that enlightened British philosopher-surgeon, Wilfred Trotter, when he wrote that "even the most assiduous workman will from time to time stand back to get a more general view of his work and to contemplate its wider relations. Indeed, such intermissions are necessary if he is to escape the tyranny of detail."

As I reflect back over past events, I find that I am asking questions to which, in my autumn years and in my present circumstances, I am no longer capable of providing answers. It is perhaps not surprising that I should use the occasion of this Seattle meeting in an attempt to satisfy my curiosity. This presentation, then, has been designed solely to stimulate discussion and debate.

My first two questions relate to axon regeneration.

## QUESTION 1:

What is the greatest distance that a neuron, originally supporting a short axon, can be expected to regenerate a new and functionally effective axon?

This is relevant to the planning and undertaking of some cross-innervations. Are we demanding too much of the provider neuron in these cases?

And here a note of caution. Beware of experi-

ments on small animals, where the distances involved are too short to provide an acceptable experimental model.

## QUESTION 2:

My second difficulty concerns the vexing question of neurotropism as a factor assisting useful functional regeneration after nerve repair. If neurotropism, which now appears to be back in business, is doing what it is supposed to do, how are we to explain the following facts?

1. Great importance is assigned to correct axial alignment of the nerve ends during repair. Experience tells us that neurotropism does not compensate for malalignment.
2. Neuromas form at suture lines because regenerating axons grow just as readily into the interfascicular connective tissue as into fasciculi.
3. It has been demonstrated experimentally that motor regenerating axons will enter and grow down sensory endoneurial tubes, and this obviously occurs in autografting.

It seems to me that neurotropism as an aid to functional regeneration remains seriously flawed, although others may think differently.

## QUESTION 3:

Despite the wealth of information that has accumulated in recent years, are the results of nerve repair today consistently better and more predictable than in the past? I suspect that the answer must be only marginally so, largely because of our inability to exploit the mass of information that is now available to the surgeon. We now appear to be in an unfortunate position in which much detailed information is available

---

*Permission to publish this address was given by Lady Gwen Sunderland, George Omer, M.D., and Edward Almquist, M.D., in the spring of 1994.

on the factors adversely affecting functional regeneration but little can be done in the way of corrective measures to offset their pernicious influences.

Let us take a closer look at only three of these unfriendly factors.

1. If a length of nerve has been destroyed and the fascicular patterns at the nerve ends in no way correspond, correct alignment of the nerve ends still remains largely a matter of guesswork. Malalignment during the repair remains a potential source of error until we have a foolproof method for ensuring correct coaptation of the nerve ends. Are we any closer to a solution to this problem?

2. As yet nothing can be done to prevent the loss of those regenerating axons that enter functionally unrelated endoneurial tubes and the interfascicular epineurium. This leaves reinnervation both imperfect and incomplete.

3. Scarring at the site of coaptation of the nerve ends remains a variable and unpredictable quantity in regard to both its density and the manner in which it obstructs and misdirects the passage of regenerating axons across the nerve end interface. Will it ever be possible to control and standardize the behavior of fibroblasts and healing at that site in order to provide a framework that will facilitate the orderly passage of regenerating axons? The dilemma here, of course, is to achieve this without threatening the integrity and strength of the union.

After a searching audit of all known possible sources of error, one can only conclude that unexpected shortfalls in recovery will be inevitable and should be expected. It seems that the outcome after any nerve repair continues to carry an element of doubt and uncertainty.

## QUESTION 4:

We come now to the question of the plasticity of neural mechanisms within the central nervous system and the role that it plays in bringing about that further improvement that continues long after it can be attributed to any peripheral phenomena. Clearly this late improvement in response to remedial training must involve readjustments to, and the reorganisation of, flexible central mechanisms, enabling the motivated patient to compensate for incomplete and imperfect patterns of peripheral reinnervation.

There is much supporting clinical evidence to favor the existence of such central mechanisms and their far greater potential in the very young than in the adult. This evidence throws no light on their nature or modus operandi.

The question then becomes, "Would knowing more about these central mechanisms inevitably lead to further and substantially improved recoveries?" Here one suspects that it will be well into the future before speculation has been replaced by reality.

## QUESTION 5:

My fifth and last question goes to the core of evaluating and recording motor and sensory recovery after nerve repair. Historically, the method currently in use for doing this is a continuum of that adopted and later published in 1954 in the postwar British Medical Council Report on peripheral nerve injuries. Faced with a rapid influx of war injuries in large numbers in the early 1940s, a standard method of evaluating and grading recovery was established to meet the clinicians' needs for one that was simple, clear, precise, and easily and quickly obtained; one that could be readily converted to a simple coding system; and one that could be used to quantify recovery so that, ultimately, the data collected could be used for comparing the recovery of one nerve with that of another, and the recovery of one nerve under different circumstances. All this was planned in the interest of determining management policy for the treatment of large number of patients with the least possible delay.

To cut through the detail, there finally emerged from the deliberations an M0 to M5 grading for motor recovery and one of S0 to S5 for sensory recovery, each representing recognizable steps in recovery and with defined criteria for each of the five grades. With minor modifications over the years, this method has become entrenched in clinical practice and in the literature.

My question is, should we be satisfied with this method of recording recovery?

In response to this question, it seems to me that there are good grounds for subjecting it to a searching audit. In the first place, it lacks a useful functional basis and is, at the same time, flawed and inadequate in other respects.

When the method was introduced, it was emphasized that it was to be limited to testing and grading the power of individual muscles and that the sensory grading was to be confined exclusively to the primary sensory elements of pain (using graded pin prick and spring algesiometers), tactile sensibility (using a standardized series of Von Frey hairs), thermal sensibility (using recording techniques ranging from the simple to the complex), two-point sensory discrimination (using the points of a compass), position sense, and localization. Moving two-point discrimination and vibration sense were added at a later date. Despite the fact that the restoration of function is the central objective of nerve repair, it was specifically stated at that time that usefulness as a criterion of recovery was to be rejected, and that testing useful functional recovery was to be avoided because of the complexities involved and, presumably, because this would add to the delay in finalizing management policy.

These were serious omissions, and in their absence it is difficult to accept the claim that the results gave a clear picture of the ultimate outcome. On the contrary, because restoration of function is the name of the game, published results leave the reader with a totally inadequate picture of the ultimate outcome, limited as it is to individual movements and the primary elements of sensibility. To the patient, this information is meaningless. What is important to the patient is what can be done with, for example, the affected hand and digits when they are called upon to perform the wide range of both simple and complex tasks that are required in the course of conducing daily activities.

Again, not only does the method fall short of what is required, but it may easily lead to misleading reporting. In my own experience, repeated testing at short intervals often gave conflicting results.

Turning now to the motor grading of M0 to M5, this relates to individual reinnervated muscles acting solely as prime movers. This, however, is an oversimplistic approach to the evaluation of useful motor function. Concentrating solely on its action as a prime mover in this way neglects the muscle's important role as an antagonist, synergist, and fixator in the execution of a wide range of movements to give them refinement and precision. A residual paresis, therefore, not only impairs a muscle's function as a prime mover but also, and importantly, destabilises the actions of other normally innervated muscles. The latter is not covered by the test for motor recovery.

Furthermore, this method of grading and recording recovery disregards the importance of sensory mechanisms in motor performance and of motor functions in sensory discrimination and stereognosis. The latter is not possible in the absence of movement. Though a variety of tests is now available for testing and evaluating tactile discrimination, the recording of sensory recovery is still based on the primary elements of sensory function.

Despite these deficiencies, the method remains entrenched in clinical practice. Persisting confidence in it is also evidenced by the reporting of new devices and techniques to facilitate testing and by the efforts taken, in the belief that measurement brings respectability, to provide, in exact numerical terms, values for each of the primary sensory components. No great accuracy can be claimed for these measurements because they relate to functions with fluctuating fortunes, and as one who has spent hours engaged in this practice, it soon became clear that it was a fruitless attempt to quantify the unquantifiable. As Trotter reminded us 52 years ago, "The affectation of scientific exactitude in circumstances where it has no meaning is perhaps the fallacy of method to which medicine is not most exposed."

Finally, we return to the original claim that the method of coding recovery, as originally introduced, gave a "good picture" of the ultimate outcome. It is difficult to decide whether this is a statement of fact or just an expression of expectation because, to the best of my knowledge, the claim has never been subjected to a searching examination in an attempt to ascertain if the code did in fact equate with the restoration of useful function. Too much has to be inferred in order to make the method as decisive as some writers over the years have claimed.

In other words, when you read of a recovery grading, for example, of M4S4, what does it really tell you about the ability of the patient to use the affected digits and hand in a purposeful way to provide for a wide range of selected manual tasks and skills of a type required for the performance of his or her daily activities? End results as currently recorded are capable of grave misrepresentation.

There is, I believe, good reason for concluding that the coding system of M0 to M5 and S0 to S5 fails to cover modern requirements as these relate to complex motor and sensory functions. Despite the fact that it represents an attempt to bring objectivity into what are essentially subjective events, and no matter how useful it may be for monitoring the progress of recovery, the system is totally inadequate for recording a meaningful end result assessment. For the latter it needs to be amended and extended.

Moberg was absolutely correct in directing attention to the flaws inherent in the use of oversimplistic procedures, but even his criticism did not go far enough. Nevertheless, his "pick up" testing method represented a distinct improvement.

In recent times, the pick up test has admittedly undergone considerable modification, elaboration, and improvement, and a variety of tests is now available for evaluating tactile discrimination. However, if the literature is any guide, much of what is currently written on the subject indicates that the main thrust of their use is to follow the progress of recovery as this occurs during a regime of motor and sensory re-education directed to restoring function to the hand. In this respect, it is important to distinguish between recording an end result assessment and monitoring the progress of recovery during re-educational therapy.

If medical records and published papers on this subject are to be kept within reasonable limits, then it becomes necessary to convert end result information on assessment. Needed is a coding scale that can convey to the reader, elsewhere and at a later date, a clear picture of the residual function of the hand and digits as this is reflected in the performance of the patient's daily activities. Furthermore, each grade in the scale would need to be based on clearly defined criteria, so that each grade represents clearly defined differences in the ultimate outcome of the repair, and each grade conveys to both recorder and reader the same clear and precise picture of the status of the recovery for that grade. Only in this way could the scale be used with confidence for comparing one set of results with another, one technique with another, and one management policy with another.

Briefly, this would, of course, call for the selection of suitable tasks that would need to be standardized and approved by some international body for universal acceptance and use. Clearly, there are problems in such an undertaking, but it should not be beyond the wit of man to reduce the type of tests required to achieve this to manageable proportions and to convert them to some reliable and practical coding system.

Clearly, this list of questions could be extended, but I believe I have said sufficient to indicate that the saga of nerve injury, nerve regeneration, and nerve repair is still far from complete, and it is imperative not only that research should be continued but, even more importantly, that it should be specifically directed to meeting the needs of those faced with the management of nerve injuries.

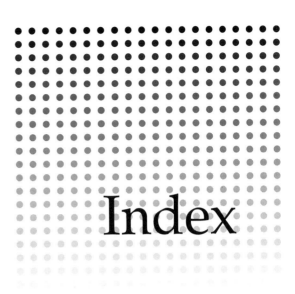

# Index

Note: Page numbers in *italics* refer to illustrations; page numbers followed by t indicate tables.